Malaria: Diagnosis and Treatment

Malaria: Diagnosis and Treatment

Editor: Beckham Hill

MURPHY & MOORE
www.murphy-moorepublishing.com

www.murphy-moorepublishing.com

MURPHY & MOORE

Cataloging-in-Publication Data

Malaria : diagnosis and treatment / edited by Beckham Hill.
p. cm.
Includes bibliographical references and index.
ISBN 978-1-63987-348-7
1. Malaria. 2. Malaria--Diagnosis. 3. Malaria--Treatment. 4. Malaria--Prevention. 5. Fever.
6. Protozoan diseases. I. Hill, Beckham.
RC156 .M35 2022
616.936 2--dc23

Murphy & Moore Publishing,
1 Rockefeller Plaza,
New York City, NY 10020, USA

ISBN 978-1-63987-348-7 (Hardback)

Contents

Preface

Malariology is the scientific study of malaria and issues related to this disease. It also focuses on the biology of malarial parasites and the factors that affect their transmission to humans by anopheline vectors. Malaria is an infectious disease that spreads by Anopheles mosquitoes, and affects humans and other animals. It is caused by Plasmodium parasites that spread through the bites of infected female mosquitoes also called malaria vectors. Symptoms of malaria occur 10-15 days after the bite of an infected mosquito. Primary symptoms include headache, fever and chills. Children with severe malaria may develop cerebral malaria, severe anemia and respiratory distress in relation to metabolic acidosis. This book explores all the important aspects of malariology in the present day scenario. Such selected concepts that redefine this field have been presented in it. This book includes contributions of experts and scientists which will provide innovative insights into this field.

This book is a comprehensive compilation of works of different researchers from varied parts of the world. It includes valuable experiences of the researchers with the sole objective of providing the readers (learners) with a proper knowledge of the concerned field. This book will be beneficial in evoking inspiration and enhancing the knowledge of the interested readers.

In the end, I would like to extend my heartiest thanks to the authors who worked with great determination on their chapters. I also appreciate the publisher's support in the course of the book. I would also like to deeply acknowledge my family who stood by me as a source of inspiration during the project.

Editor

1

Neutrophils and Malaria

Elizabeth H. Aitken, Agersew Alemu and Stephen J. Rogerson*

Department of Medicine at Royal Melbourne Hospital, Peter Doherty Institute, University of Melbourne, Melbourne, VIC, Australia

Edited by:
Ashraful Haque,
QIMR Berghofer Medical Research Institute, Australia

Reviewed by:
Tobias Bald,
QIMR Berghofer Medical Research Institute, Australia
Ashley Vaughan,
Seattle Children's Research Institute, United States
Mattias Svensson,
Karolinska Institutet (KI), Sweden

***Correspondence:**
Elizabeth H. Aitken
elizabeth.aitken@unimelb.edu.au

Neutrophils are abundant in the circulation and are one of the immune system's first lines of defense against infection. There has been substantial work carried out investigating the role of neutrophils in malaria and it is clear that during infection neutrophils are activated and are capable of clearing malaria parasites by a number of mechanisms. This review focuses on neutrophil responses to human malarias, summarizing evidence which helps us understand where neutrophils are, what they are doing, how they interact with parasites as well as their potential role in vaccine mediated immunity. We also outline future research priorities for these, the most abundant of leukocytes.

Keywords: neutrophil, malaria, *Plasmodium*, immunity, antibody mediated immunity, polymorphonuclear (PMN)

INTRODUCTION

Neutrophils (also known as polymorphonuclear cells) are the most common white blood cell in the body (1). They can clear pathogens by phagocytosis; by producing reactive oxygen species (ROS) and other antimicrobial products; or by formation of neutrophil extracellular traps (NETs) (2). Additionally, they also play a role in the activation and regulation of the immune response, by cytokine and chemokine secretion (3), and possibly antigen presentation (4). Their importance in controlling infection can be highlighted by the increased susceptibility to fungal and bacterial infections seen in individuals suffering from neutrophil deficiencies (5). Malaria is a disease caused by infection with *Plasmodium spp.* parasites. It causes severe morbidity and mortality, and young children and pregnant women are especially susceptible to disease. Malaria is a large public health burden with an estimated 216 million cases of malaria being reported in 2016, resulting in an estimated 445,000 deaths (6). Globally most disease caused by infection with *Plasmodium spp.* is caused by *P. falciparum* (6). Pathology is thought to be due to a combination of the sequestration of infected red blood cells (iRBC) in the microvasculature, endothelial activation, as well as pro-coagulant and importantly pro-inflammatory responses (7). In this review, we assess the literature examining how neutrophils and *Plasmodium spp.* parasites interact, and the mechanisms by which neutrophils can play an active role in parasite clearance.

NEUTROPHIL DYNAMICS AND RECRUITMENT TO SITES OF PARASITE SEQUESTRATION

Changes in peripheral blood neutrophil levels have been described during *Plasmodium spp.* infections. In controlled human malaria infections (CHMI) in non-immune individuals, neutrophil numbers are stable during the asymptomatic liver stage (8). In naturally-infected individuals, patterns of change in peripheral blood neutrophil numbers vary with the cohort studied. Using hematological data from over 3,000 children, Olliaro et al. estimated that peripheral blood neutrophil counts increase about 43% (95% CI 26–35%) during acute uncomplicated malaria, and that the level of increase is positively associated with parasitaemia (9). In semi-immune travelers neutrophil counts were higher in those with severe malaria compared to those with uncomplicated malaria, while in non-immune travelers, though neutrophil counts increased with the presence of infection, neutrophil counts did not vary with disease severity (10). A study in HIV-infected individuals showed no difference in neutrophil numbers when comparing those with and without asymptomatic *P. falciparum* infection (11), whereas pregnant women with *P. falciparum* infection had lower numbers of peripheral blood neutrophils than uninfected women (12). Differences between cohorts are likely due to disease status classification (clinical malaria or asymptomatic parasitemia), immune status and/or age.

Neutrophils are a heterogenous population and this is important because different neutrophil subsets can have varying functional properties, for example CD177+ neutrophils are also positive for Proteinase 3, and IL17+ neutrophils have increased ROS production [reviewed in (13)]. We know that neutrophils from individuals infected with *Plasmodium spp.* behave differently compared to those from non-infected individuals (14–18), and a subset of neutrophils with impaired oxidative burst have been observed in individuals infected with *P. falciparum* (18), suggesting that neutrophil subsets change during the course of infection. In individuals challenged with LPS, inflammation results in the release of a neutrophil subset that suppresses T cell activation (19), whether this occurs during *P. falciparum* infection is unclear but it is one example of why work to identify neutrophil subsets in *Plasmodium spp.* infections would likely yield valuable information into the role of neutrophils in malaria.

Neutrophils are generally the first circulating cells to respond to an invading pathogen. However, how and whether neutrophils are recruited to the sites of iRBC sequestration is still unclear. We know very little regarding neutrophil expression of receptors involved in migration and adhesion. There is no evidence that neutrophil adhesion molecule CD11a changes with infection (18), and expression by neutrophils of other adhesion molecules such as CD18, CD11b, and CD62L is still unstudied. There is more information on the expression of neutrophil receptors on endothelial cells. Expression of receptors on endothelial cells involved in neutrophil adhesion and migration are likely increased with infection. Intercellular adhesion molecule-1 (ICAM-1), vascular cell adhesion molecule-1 (VCAM-1) and the endothelial leukocyte adhesion molecule E-selectin are increased on endothelial cells after exposure to iRBC *in vitro* [reviewed in (20)] and this is supported by observations showing increased levels of soluble E-selectin and soluble ICAM-1 in the blood of *P. falciparum* infected individuals (21). Regarding chemokines involved in neutrophil recruitment, neutrophil chemoattractant protein CXCL8 is increased in peripheral blood of patients with severe malaria [reviewed in (22)] (23) as well as in the cerebral spinal fluid (CSF) of children with cerebral malaria and in the placentas of women with malaria in pregnancy [reviewed in (22)]. In addition, *P. falciparum* antigen can induce the production of neutrophil recruitment chemokines CXCL1 and Interleukin 8 (IL8) production by endothelial cells and the production of Interleukin 8 (IL8) by placental syncytiotrophoblast [reviewed in (22)]. Interestingly, although increased expression of neutrophil chemoattractants occurs, studies of malaria pathology rarely show significant neutrophil infiltration at sites of sequestration.

Low numbers of neutrophils were reported in the brain microvasculature in autopsy samples from children in Malawi (14), and neutrophil numbers were not significantly higher in placentas infected with *P. falciparum* or *P. vivax* compared to non-infected placentas (24, 25). An exception is chronic *P. falciparum* placental malaria, which can be accompanied by massive intervillous inflammation, with increased numbers of CD15+ granulocytes (predominantly neutrophils) (26). When the lungs were studied, one study from Thailand showed no difference in neutrophil levels (measured by the presence of elastase positive cells) between fatal *P. falciparum* malaria with or without pulmonary oedema and controls who died from trauma (27). By contrast, in fatal *P. vivax* infection, interstitial lung infiltrates consisting of CD15+ cells were reported from Brazil. Caveats are that some individuals suffered co-pathologies and there was no non-infected control group for comparison (28).

The "snap shots" of pathogenesis provided by tissue samples, together with neutrophils' short half-life (29), mean that it is hard to exclude neutrophil recruitment to sites of infection, however the data to date suggest recruitment is not always happening; why is this? One possible answer is that *Plasmodium spp.* infection inhibits neutrophil chemotaxis. Neutrophils from individuals with symptomatic *P. falciparum* malaria have reduced chemotaxis compared to non-infected healthy controls (15) and this is restored 7 days after treatment, suggesting the involvement of parasite antigens. Neutrophils from individuals with cerebral malaria have reduced chemotaxis to Interleukin 8 (IL8) and N-formyl-L-methionyl-L-leucyl-phenylalanine (fMLP) (14), and this reduction in chemotaxis may be partly due to increased free heme (14, 18) and/or decreased neutrophil expression of IL8 receptor CXCR2 (as reported in *P. vivax* malaria) (14, 30). Additionally, blood-stage parasite antigens inhibit proinflammatory protein S100-calcium binding protein (S100P) stimulated chemotaxis of the neutrophil cell line HL-60 *in vitro* (31, 32). Whether the reduced chemotaxis observed *ex vivo* explains the lack of neutrophil recruitment to the sites of parasite sequestration is still uncertain and warrants further investigation (20, 21, 33).

NEUTROPHILS AND PARASITE CLEARANCE: PHAGOCYTOSIS, ROS AND NETS

Neutrophil Phagocytosis of *Plasmodium spp.*

Phagocytosis is one way that neutrophils play a role in the clearance of malaria parasites. Neutrophils express immunoglobulin (Ig) binding receptors Fcγ receptor I (FcγRI) (after activation), FcγRII and FcγRIII as well as complement receptors complement receptor 1 (CR1) and CR3. Together these can facilitate phagocytic uptake of antigen opsonised with components such as IgG or C3b [reviewed in (34)] (**Figure 1A**). Neutrophils are known to phagocytose iRBC *in vivo* as observed in blood films from children (35) and in bone marrow aspirates which show phagocytosis of merozoites and occasionally

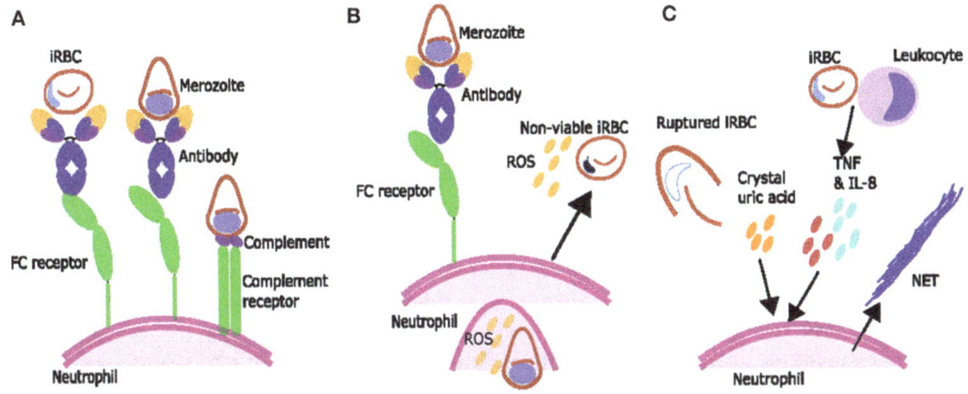

FIGURE 1 | Proposed mechanisms of parasite clearance by neutrophils during *Plasmodium spp.* infection. **(A)** Neutrophils can phagocytose blood stage parasites after opsonization with antibodies and possibly opsonization with complement. **(B)** Neutrophils exposed to merozoite antigen opsonized with antibody produce reactive oxygen species (ROS) which can inhibit intraerythrocytic parasite growth. **(C)** Components associated with *Plasmodium spp.* infection including inflammatory cytokines TNF and IL-8 produced by leukocytes and crystal uric acid released upon infected red blood cell (iRBC) rupture may induce neutrophils to produce neutrophil extracellular traps (NETs).

trophozoites by neutrophils and neutrophil metamyelocytes (neutrophil precursors undergoing granulopoiesis) (36).

Neutrophil phagocytosis of merozoites is influenced by several factors. Phagocytosis of merozoites opsonised with non-immune serum has been observed *in vitro* (37) and has possibly been observed *ex vivo* in the blood of ex-service men who had returned from Vietnam infected with *P. falciparum* (38). Neutrophil phagocytosis of merozoites opsonised with non-immune serum is possibly dependent on complement, as heat inactivation decreases phagocytosis, and can be increased if the neutrophils are pre-treated with factors such as tumor necrosis factor (TNF), interferon γ (IFNγ), IL1β or granulocyte-macrophage colony-stimulating factor (GM-CSF) (37). Antibody toward merozoite antigens also promotes phagocytosis, which is much higher if merozoites are opsonised with immune serum compared to non-immune serum (37).

Unlike phagocytosis of merozoites, which may involve complement, phagocytosis of iRBC is largely dependent on the presence of Ig. Neutrophils isolated from malaria infected children can phagocytose schizonts *in vitro* (16), but neutrophils from American service men infected with *P. falciparum* (38) (with limited previous exposure to *P. falciparum* and therefore little Ig toward the iRBC) did not. In addition, sera from individuals living in endemic areas promote phagocytosis of iRBC and this activity is dependent on IgG in the serum (39) and independent of complement (40, 41). It is not known if Ig mediated phagocytosis of parasites by neutrophils is associated with protection from disease.

Intra-erythrocytic gametocytes are not very susceptible to neutrophil phagocytosis (40). However, it is possible that neutrophil phagocytosis of extracellular gametes while in the mosquito gut could play a role in transmission-blocking immunity. Neutrophils phagocytose gametes *in vitro* in conditions similar to those of the mosquito gut when immune sera is present and this phagocytosis is dependent on gametocyte antibodies, especially IgG (40). *In vivo* it has been shown that neutrophils also phagocytose gametes inside mosquito midguts, and that this phagocytosis is enhanced by the presence of immune serum in the blood meal (40). However, although the presence of neutrophils and individual sera in the blood meal decreases infectivity (42), there is no evidence of an association between levels of neutrophil phagocytosis, promoted by serum *in vitro*, and the ability of that serum to affect mosquito infectivity in experimental settings (40).

In rat models, neutrophils phagocytose exoerythrocytic parasites (43), however *ex-vivo* evidence of a role of neutrophil phagocytosis and immunity toward this parasite stage in humans (both *in vitro* and *ex vivo*) is lacking.

Key unanswered questions include the importance of neutrophil phagocytosis in protection from infection or disease and in blocking of transmission. Studies examining associations between antibody induction of neutrophil phagocytosis of different parasite life cycle stages and patient outcomes could help determine the importance of neutrophil phagocytosis in protection from disease.

Reactive Oxygen Species and *Plasmodium spp.* Infection

Neutrophils can clear pathogens by respiratory burst, the conversion of oxygen to superoxide by nicotinamide adenine dinucleotide phosphate oxidase (NAPDH) oxidase (NOX). This superoxide is converted into hydrogen peroxide and hydroxyl radicals, together referred to as ROS. NOX is located on both the neutrophils plasma and phagosomal membranes and the ROS it produces can diffuse across membranes. This means that ROS are present in the phagosome, intracellular and also extracellular spaces [reviewed in (44)] and can therefore play a role in killing both phagocytosed intracellular as well as extracellular parasites.

ROS from activated neutrophils are capable of inhibiting parasite growth *in vitro*, and studies using various ROS inhibitors or scavengers suggest singlet oxygen, rather than hydrogen peroxide or superoxide, is responsible for this inhibition (45, 46). Growth inhibition by ROS occurs during the intra-erythrocytic development stage of the parasite (45, 46) (**Figure 1B**), rather than during merozoite invasion of erythrocytes, which is not inhibited by ROS production from stimulated neutrophils *in vitro* (47). *Ex vivo* data suggests that during malaria infection neutrophils are activated to produce ROS and that ROS may have a role in parasite clearance. Neutrophils from children with malaria inhibit parasite growth *in vitro* better than neutrophils from uninfected children or adults (16) and oxygen consumption is higher [indicating activation and production of ROS (48)] in neutrophils from people with symptomatic acute malaria compared to controls (17). In addition, children with faster parasite clearance times have neutrophils which produce more ROS (49).

ROS production by neutrophils is influenced by a number of factors, including the host's genetic background (50). In the presence of antigen neutrophils produce higher amounts of ROS with immune serum compared to non-immune serum (51) or compared to IgG depleted serum (52), supporting a role for IgG-Fc interactions in ROS production (52) (**Figure 1B**). Regarding complement, one study suggests serum heat inactivation reduces ROS production (51) and another showed that heat inactivation changes the dynamics of ROS production (53). However, the activation of neutrophils to produce ROS by heat-inactivated serum (52) and by purified IgG (52, 53) suggests that the full complement cascade is not necessary.

The ability of Ig to induce ROS has been called antibody dependent respiratory burst (ADRB), and assays measure different components of this process. In solid-phase assays (where the antigen is bound on a plate), ROS are secreted from the neutrophil and this process is largely dependent on FcγRIIa. By contrast, when neutrophils phagocytose whole merozoites the resulting ADRB and associated ROS production occur within the neutrophil are only partially dependent on FcγRIIa (53). Antibodies capable of inducing respiratory burst are acquired with exposure to *Plasmodium spp.* In a small cohort study, sera taken after an immune episode and incubated with merozoites induced more neutrophil ROS production than sera taken during the malaria episode, and sera from adults induced more neutrophil ROS production than sera from young children (54). ADRB toward merozoite antigens was higher in a holo-endemic area compared to a meso-endemic area (52) and increased with age (55), and antibodies capable of inducing respiratory burst have been associated with protection from malaria. Individuals whose serum induced a high ADRB toward merozoites were less likely to experience clinical malaria when compared to those whose serum induced a low ADRB (52, 55), and a combined measure of ability of an individual's serum sample to induce both ADRB and growth inhibition has been associated with protection from severe malaria (56). Supporting a role for ADRB in protection from disease, polymorphisms of FcγRIIIb [a neutrophil receptor that is involved in IgG dependent ROS production (57)] that improve neutrophil Fc-Ig binding are associated with protection from febrile malaria (58, 59).

Antibodies opsonising merozoites or merozoite antigens can induce ROS production by neutrophils, whereas there is no evidence that antibodies opsonising iRBCs result in a major ROS response (17, 51, 52, 54, 60). The reasons for this difference are unclear as IgG are known to recognize the surface of iRBC (61). The merozoite antigens which are targets for ADRB include *Plasmodium falciparum* merozoite surface protein-5 (PfMSP5), MSP1-19 and MSP1, as indicated by correlations between IgG antibodies to these antigens and ADRB (55, 62, 63), and by antigen/antibody depletion assays with MSP1 or its C terminal domain MSP1-19 (62, 63). See **Figure 1B** for diagram for ROS production.

Antibodies which induce ROS may be similar to those which promote merozoite phagocytosis, as the functions are correlated in neutrophils responding to opsonised merozoites (54). Antibody subclass may be important: mouse-human chimeric IgG toward MSP1-19 is sufficient to induce NADPH-mediated oxidative burst (and degranulation) from neutrophils, but mouse-human chimeric IgG3 toward the same antigen is not (64). Multiple antibody isotypes may be involved ROS production. Recombinant human IgA toward merozoite antigen is a potent inducer of ROS (65), but IgA's importance in ROS production in malaria is unclear as IgG depletion from serum appears to be sufficient to eliminate most ADRB toward merozoite antigen (52). Further research is needed to identify the characteristics of antibody responses to malaria antigens that effectively elicit neutrophil ADRB.

Evidence for NETS in Malaria

Neutrophil extracellular trap (NET) formation has evolved as an important innate strategy for killing extracellular pathogens, and occurs when activated neutrophils degranulate and release neutrophil antimicrobial factors into the extracellular environment. NETs are mesh-like extracellular structures made up of decondensed chromatin and histones decorated with different antimicrobial granular proteins that can capture, neutralize and kill a diversity of microbes (66). There are several factors which might induce NET formation during *Plasmodium* infections (**Figure 1C**). Crystal uric acid [a potent inducer of NETosis (67)] and its precursor hypoxanthine are released upon iRBC rupture [reviewed in (68)]. In addition, cytokines such as TNF and IL8 which are increased during *Plasmodium* infections [reviewed in (69)], and H_2O_2 secreted by immune cells stimulated by *Plasmodium spp.* antigen [reviewed in (70)] have been shown to induce NETosis *in vitro* [reviewed in (67)] (**Figure 1C**). NET-like structures which stain positive for DNA with 4′,6-Diamidino-2-Phenylindole, Dihydrochloride (DAPI) have been found in peripheral blood of children with uncomplicated *P. falciparum* infections (71), however it is unclear if these structures were produced in response to *Plasmodium* antigen (as opposed to another stimulus) and/or if they are derived from neutrophils (as opposed to monocytes) (72). There is some qualitative evidence that neutrophils can produce NETs in response to *P. falciparum* antigen *in vitro* (73) however, quantitative evidence that neutrophils produce

NETs in response to *P. falciparum* and evidence that NETs are present in tissues and contribute to pathology of *Plasmodium* infection in humans is still lacking. When brain tissue sections from 4 children with fatal cerebral malaria (CM) and associated retinopathy and 5 with CM without retinopathy (indicating an alternative diagnosis) were stained with antibodies toward NET markers neutrophil elastase and citrillinated histones, no NETs were seen (14). There are no published studies looking for NETS in other human tissues. Possible explanations for the lack of evidence of NETs in *ex-vivo* brain tissue include neutrophils making NETs that the parasites break down. *P. falciparum* asexual blood stage parasites expresses a DNase virulence factor which may be able to break down NETs, as they are made of DNA (74) (**Figure 1C**). Alternatively, it may be that NETs are simply not being formed. If neutrophils phagocytose bulky antigens via opsonisation and/or phosphatidylserine (PS) exposure sometimes they cannot make NETs [reviewed in (75)] (**Figure 1C**) and we know during malaria infection neutrophils do phagocytose bulky antigens (such as merozoites and iRBC) by these mechanisms (**Figure 2**) (37, 39, 76). Further, research is needed to clarify whether NETs do play an active role in *Plasmodium spp.* infections.

Neutrophils, Severe Malaria and Parasite Adhesion

As well as playing a role in parasite clearance, neutrophils may contribute to the pathology of severe malaria syndromes, but there is limited supporting data from human studies on this topic. In CM, neutrophil proteins in plasma [including neutrophil primary granule proteins, neutrophil elastase, myeloperoxidase and proteinase 3 (PRTN3)] are associated with disease (14) and it has been hypothesized that neutrophil products contribute to CM pathology, with elastase damaging the endothelium (77, 78), and inflammatory factors such as TNF [reviewed in (79)] and ROS [reviewed in (80)] increasing expression of the iRBC adhesion receptor, ICAM-1 (81) on endothelial cells to promote parasite adhesion. Also, PRTN3 can cleave endothelial protein C receptor (EPCR) from endothelial cells and contribute to the procoagulant state observed in severe malaria [reviewed in (14)]. On the other hand neutrophil products may also reduce parasite adhesion, for example by PRTN cleavage of EPCR (82) as it is a receptor for parasites associated with severe malaria (83). Also, neutrophil elastase, released by activated neutrophils, can cleave iRBC antigens involved in *P. falciparum* iRBC cytoadherence to C32 melanoma cells (84).

It has also been suggested that neutrophils play a role in the pathology of the liver during *Plasmodium spp.* infections (85). Neutrophil activation by type I Interferon is associated with increased serum levels of transaminases in *P. vivax* malaria and together with murine data showing type I IFN modulates neutrophil migration to the liver in mice, suggests type I IFN are responsible for neutrophil mediated liver pathology in malaria (85). Human evidence showing that neutrophils are present in the liver during infection and could cause damage is lacking. Further studies using human samples to identify the role of neutrophils in severe malaria are needed.

Factors Inhibiting Neutrophil Responses

Although neutrophils can clear parasites in a variety of ways, several mosquito and parasite antigens can modify neutrophil responses to the parasite's advantage (**Figure 2**). For example, mosquito salivary proteins can alter neutrophil function. Secretion of the protein agaphelin in the mosquito's salivary glands is increased upon infection with *P. falciparum*, and agaphelin can inhibit neutrophil elastase activity, neutrophil chemotaxis and NET formation in response to phorbol myristate acetate (PMA) (31) (**Figure 2**). Other salivary proteins that may also alter neutrophil function include the antigen-5 salivary proteins, which scavenge superoxide and inhibit neutrophil ROS (86) (**Figure 2A**).

Parasite antigens which can inhibit neutrophil function include histamine-releasing factor (an ortholog of mammalian histamine-releasing factor), which was shown to inhibit neutrophil IL6 production in the liver in a murine malaria model, and subsequently promoted liver stage parasite development (87). Also, *P. falciparum* protein MSP1-19 can block neutrophil responses to proinflammatory protein S100P, inhibiting neutrophil chemotaxis *in vitro* (32) (**Figure 2B**). There is clearly an interesting dynamic between neutrophils and *Plasmodium*, with each trying to take advantage and control the other. Identification and understanding of neutrophil parasite interactions may result in the identification of novel therapeutic targets and warrants further investigation.

Parasite-neutrophil interactions may also result in susceptibility to other diseases. Malaria infection (especially with severe anemia) has been associated with susceptibility to non-typhoidal salmonella (NTS) bacteraemia (88, 89) and this is thought to occur due to impaired neutrophil function. *In vitro* observations suggest that neutrophil phagocytosis of parasite products results in them being less capable of phagocytosing bacteria (47). *Ex vivo* observations show reduced ability for neutrophils to generate ROS during malaria (18), and this reduced function was associated with increased haemolysis and heme oxygenase-1 (HO-1) expression in infected individuals (18) (**Figure 2A**); similar findings have been reported in asymptomatic infection (90). Mouse data suggests that haemolysis during infection induces HO-1 and results in impaired maturation of neutrophils (91). In addition mouse data shows that IL10 [which is also associated with infection in children (90)] inhibits neutrophil migration resulting in altered clinical presentation of NTS (92).

Pigmented Neutrophils as a Marker of Disease Severity

Neutrophils with malaria pigment can be seen in the peripheral blood during *Plasmodium* infection. In children, the percentage of neutrophils with pigment in the peripheral blood increases with disease severity (93, 94) and is positively correlated with parasitaemia (93, 95). The percentage of neutrophils with pigment has also been positively associated with mortality due to severe malaria in adults and children (94, 96), and in parasitaemic pregnant women high numbers of pigmented neutrophils in the peripheral blood during gestation were associated with

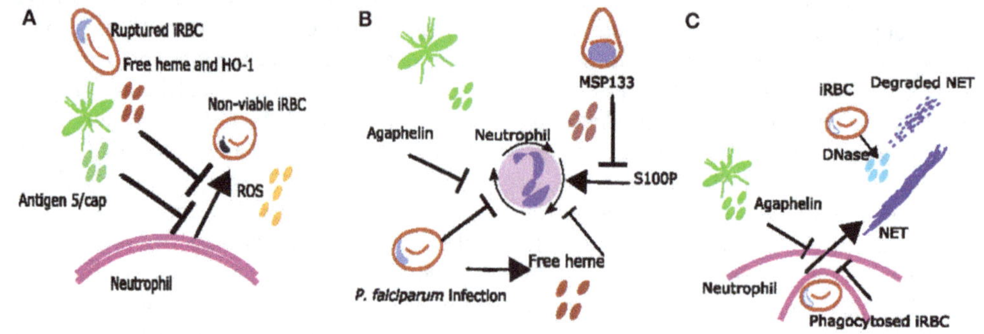

FIGURE 2 | Proposed mechanisms neutrophil inhibition during *Plasmodium spp.* infection. **(A)** Neutrophil ROS may be inhibited due to excess free heme and HO-1 or due to mosquito salivary protein antigen 5/cap. **(B)** reduced neutrophil chemotaxis may be due to exposure to free heme, merozoite protein MSP133 or mosquito salivary protein agaphelin. **(C)** It is possible that phagocytosis of bulky parasite antigens inhibits neutrophils from producing NETs during *Plasmodium spp.* infections and that any NETs produced are degraded by parasite DNase.

lower birth weights at delivery (97). The predictive value of pigmented neutrophils (94, 96, 97) suggest that they could indicate sequestered biomass, and because pigment-containing neutrophils are cleared from the circulation after about 72 h (29) it is likely they are a marker of recent pigment phagocytosis. Pigment containing neutrophils have also been associated with disease severity in *P. knowlesi* malaria (98).

Neutrophils and Antimalarials

A number of *in vitro* studies have investigated whether neutrophil activity may be affected by antimalarial drugs. At non-physiological levels chloroquine, quinine, proguanil, and mefloquine all inhibit neutrophil oxidative burst (99) however at lower physiological plasma levels they, as well as sulphadoxine, cycloguanil, pyrimethamine and tetracycline, have no depressive effects on oxidative burst nor markers of oxidative metabolism (99). Likewise at high concentrations, chloroquine decreases the phagocytic activity of neutrophils and quinine, chloroquine and quinacrine inhibit neutrophil chemotaxis but at physiological concentrations they do not (100, 101). There is however some evidence that neutrophil chemotaxis and neutrophil iodination (a measure associated with phagocytosis and oxidative burst) are inhibited at physiologically relevant concentrations by pyrimethamine and by mefloquine or pyrimethamine respectively, (101). Mefloquine inhibits oxidative burst by interacting with cellular phospholipid-dependent protein kinase C (102). Amodiaquine and pyronaridine have been shown to cause neutrophil glutathione depletion in *in vitro* systems where pyronaridine is oxidized to a quinonimine metabolite, raising concerns they could be cytotoxic to neutrophils at physiological concentrations (103). However, *in vivo* studies in rats did not find any quinoneimine metabolites after receipt of pyronaridine nor is there is clinical evidence of significant toxicity associated with pyronaridine use in humans [reviewed in (104)].

As well as effects on neutrophil function, studies have raised the possibility that neutrophil numbers may be affected by antimalarials (105–107). In an analysis of data from 7 randomized trials across 13 sites in 9 countries comparing artesunate-amodiaquine to single and combination treatments (including amodiaquine mono-therapy, artesunate mono-therapy, artemether-lumefantrine, artesunate and sulphadoxine-pyrimethamine, and dihydroartemisinin) the treatment-emergent adverse event incidence of neutropenia was 11% (107). However, when neutrophil counts were compared between treatment groups there was no apparent differences (107). Interestingly, in the case of artesunate, an effect on neutrophil numbers may be dose dependent. In a clinical study conducted among Cambodian patients with uncomplicated malaria, those who received 6 mg/kg/day had lower neutrophil counts than those who received 2 or 4 mg/kg/day, also 5 of 26 patients who received 6 mg/kg artesunate developed neutropenia $<1000/mm^3$, while only 1 of 38 patients receiving 2 or 4 mg/kg/day did (105).

A Brief Overview of Neutrophils in Animal Models of Malaria

Murine models have been used to study the role of neutrophils in malaria complications including lung injury, CM and liver injury. Accumulation of neutrophils in the lungs has been associated with lung injury in multiple murine malaria models (73, 108–114) and lung injury is associated with increased TNF (108, 109), parasite sequestration in the pulmonary vasculature (113), the presence of NETs (73), neutrophil adhesion to endothelial walls, and with increased vascular permeability (110, 111) but not ICAM-1 expression (114).

In murine models of CM, neutrophils have been shown to express cytokines IL2, IL12p40, IL18, IFNγ, and TNF as well as chemoattractive-chemokines monokine-induced by gamma (MIG), macrophage inflammatory protein-1α (MIP1α) and IFNγ induced- protein 10 (IP10) (115) suggesting a role for neutrophils in cytokine and chemokine secretion. In murine CM neutrophils are detected in the microvasculature (116), and neutrophil depletion results in decreased monocyte sequestration and microhaemorrhages in the brain and prevents development of CM (117). Other neutrophil factors associated with CM include neutrophil secretion of CXCL10 which may contribute to high parasitemia and disease (118), and neutrophil expression of FcεRI (a high affinity IgE receptor) which may result in the production of proinflammatory cytokines (119).

Studies have identified a possible role for neutrophils in liver damage in murine models with neutrophil dependent liver damage being associated with free heme, NFkB activation and neutrophil infiltration (120). Neutrophil infiltration and subsequent liver damage may also be dependent on type I IFN signaling (85).

Murine models can play a valuable role in dissecting the role of neutrophils in disease, but whether the roles of neutrophils in humans and murine malaria are similar is still unclear and more work needs to be done to validate findings in humans.

A Role for Neutrophils in Vaccine Mediated Immunity

Neutrophil-antibody interactions can play an active role in parasite clearance and should be considered when evaluating vaccine mediated immunity. ADRB toward merozoite antigens is associated with protection (52, 56), but whether other antigens such as those on the asexual iRBC, gametocytes or sporozoites can trigger ADRB, or whether such responses could be associated with protection, is unknown. Likewise, although it is clear that neutrophil phagocytosis of parasite antigen, merozoites, iRBC and possibly gametocytes occurs *in vivo* (35 36, 40, 121), it is unknown whether antibodies promoting neutrophil phagocytosis are protective. Studies examining antibody mediated neutrophil functions to a variety of antigens and their associations with protection will help elucidate th role neutrophils have in antibody mediated immunity and their potential in vaccine mediated immunity.

A few studies have used animal models to investigate the role of antibody-dependent neutrophil responses in the contex of protection from disease and also vaccination. In one study murine IgG1 toward MSP1-19 was effective at inducing human neutrophil ADRB and degranulation, but these same antibodies did not protect against *P. berghei* expressing MSP1 *in vivo* (122 In another study, serum from previously challenged mice and both murine IgG1 and IgG2 could elicit ADRB from murine neutrophils in response to murine antigens *in vitro*, however vaccination of mice with MSP1-42 resulted in antibodies whic did not elicit neutrophil ADRB toward merozoites and ADRB did not contribute to vaccine mediated protection (123). On the other hand, when non-human primates were immunized with MSP-1, antibodies were produced which opsonised merozoites and elicited ADRB by neutrophils (63), suggesting that vaccination can result in generation of antibodies which activate neutrophils.

As well as their role in parasite clearance by antibody dependent mechanisms, neutrophils may also play a role in immune responses to vaccines. There is growing evidence that neutrophils have the capacity to present antigen to T-cells. Whilst they may not be as effective at antigen presentation as typical antigen presenting cells their overall impact may be significant due to their sheer numbers [reviewed in (4)]. At least in the case of irradiated sporozoites, data from murine models suggests that neutrophils are available to take up the vaccine as intradermal injection of both irradiated and wild type sporozoites result in recruitment of neutrophils (and inflammatory monocytes) to the injection site, however there was no evidence that neutrophil depletion in this model affected the establishment of a protective immune response (124). The occurrence and significance of antigen presentation by neutrophils during both natural malaria infections and vaccination is yet to be investigated.

FUTURE DIRECTIONS

Neutrophils in malaria remains understudied, undertaking the future research priorities listed below will go a long way in helping us to understand the role of neutrophils during *Plasmodium spp.* infections.

1. Identify the presence (or absence) of neutrophils at sites of parasite sequestration using *ex vivo* samples from humans.
2. Identify neutrophil subsets during infection in humans using *ex vivo* samples from humans.
3. Identify and quantify neutrophils products (including NETs) at sites of parasite sequestration and in the periphery using *ex vivo* samples from humans.
4. Investigate possible roles of neutrophils in asymptomatic *Plasmodium spp.* infection, clinical malaria and severe malaria by comparing neutrophil counts and indicators of neutrophil activation and/or inhibition between different clinical groups.
5. Using *in vitro* models investigate the role of parasite products (such as DNAse) on neutrophil function.
6. Measure antibody mediated functions of neutrophils (such as ADRB & phagocytosis) and investigate their associations with protection from disease.
7. Using *in vitro* models clarify the role of complement in neutrophil parasite interactions.
8. Identify whether neutrophils should they be considered in evaluation of antibody mediated immunity provided by vaccines.
9. Investigate the role of neutrophils in antigen presentation in the context of both natural infection and vaccination.

CONCLUSION

The role of neutrophils in protection and disease during *Plasmodium spp.* infections has been little studied, and important questions remain. Further research with a focus on neutrophil responses toward the parasite and how neutrophils play a role in parasite clearance will likely aid in the development and evaluation of vaccines for malaria.

AUTHOR CONTRIBUTIONS

All authors listed have made a substantial, direct and intellectual contribution to the work, and approved it for publication.

REFERENCES

1. Hsieh MM, Everhart JE, Byrd-Holt DD, Tisdale JF, Rodgers GP. Prevalence of neutropenia in the U.S. population: age, sex, smoking status, and ethnic differences. *Ann Intern Med.* (2007) 146:486–92. doi: 10.7326/0003-4819-146-7-200704030-00004
2. Kolaczkowska E, Kubes P. Neutrophil recruitment and function in health and inflammation. *Nat Rev Immunol.* (2013) 13:159–75. doi: 10.1038/nri3399
3. Tecchio C, Cassatella MA. Neutrophil-derived chemokines on the road to immunity. *Semin Immunol.* (2016) 28:119–28. doi: 10.1016/j.smim.2016.04.003
4. Lin A, Lore K. Granulocytes: new members of the antigen-presenting cell family. *Front Immunol.* (2017) 8:1781. doi: 10.3389/fimmu.2017.01781
5. Leiding JW. Neutrophil evolution and their diseases in humans. *Front Immunol.* (2017) 8:1009. doi: 10.3389/fimmu.2017.01009
6. World Health Organization. *World Malaria Report World Malaria Report 2017.* Geneva: World Health Organization (2017).
7. Wassmer SC, Grau GE. Severe malaria: what's new on the pathogenesis front? *Int J Parasitol.* (2017) 47:145–52. doi: 10.1016/j.ijpara.2016.08.002
8. van Wolfswinkel ME, Langenberg MC C, Wammes LJ, Sauerwein RW, Koelewijn R, Hermsen CC, et al. Changes in total and differential leukocyte counts during the clinically silent liver phase in a controlled human malaria infection in malaria-naive Dutch volunteers. *Malar J.* (2017) 16:457. doi: 10.1186/s12936-017-2108-1
9. Olliaro P, Djimde A, Dorsey G, Karema C, Martensson A, Ndiaye JL, et al. Hematologic parameters in pediatric uncomplicated *Plasmodium falciparum* malaria in sub-Saharan Africa. *Am J Trop Med Hyg.* (2011) 85:619–25. doi: 10.4269/ajtmh.2011.11-0154
10. Berens-Riha N, Kroidl I, Schunk M, Alberer M, Beissner M, Pritsch M, et al. Evidence for significant influence of host immunity on changes in differential blood count during malaria. *Malar J.* (2014) 13:155. doi: 10.1186/1475-2875-13-155
11. Jegede FE, Oyeyi TI, Abdulrahman SA, Mbah HA, Badru T, Agbakwuru C, et al. Effect of HIV and malaria parasites co-infection on immune-hematological profiles among patients attending anti-retroviral treatment (ART) clinic in Infectious Disease Hospital Kano, Nigeria. *PLoS ONE* (2017) 12:e0174233. doi: 10.1371/journal.pone.0174233
12. Bostrom S, Schmiegelow C, Abu Abed U, Minja DT R, Lusingu J, Brinkmann V, et al. Neutrophil alterations in pregnancy-associated malaria and induction of neutrophil chemotaxis by *Plasmodium falciparum. Parasite Immunol.* (2017) 39:e12433. doi: 10.1111/pim.12433
13. Silvestre-Roig C, Hidalgo A, Soehnlein O. Neutrophil heterogeneity: implications for homeostasis and pathogenesis. *Blood* (2016) 127:2173–81. doi: 10.1182/blood-2016-01-688887
14. Feintuch CM, Saidi A, Seydel K, Chen G, Goldman-Yassen A, Mita-Mendoza NK, et al. Activated neutrophils are associated with pediatric cerebral malaria vasculopathy in malawian children. *MBio* (2016) 7:e01300–15. doi: 10.1128/mBio.01300-15
15. Nielsen H, Kharazmi A, Theander TG. Suppression of blood monocyte and neutrophil chemotaxis in acute human malaria. *Parasite Immunol.* (1986) 8:541–50.
16. Brown J, Smalley ME. Inhibition of the *in vitro* growth of *Plasmodium falciparum* by human polymorphonuclear neutrophil leucocytes. *Clin Exp Immunol.* (1981) 46:106–9.
17. Salmon D, Vilde JL, Andrieu B, Simonovic R, Lebras J. Role of immune serum and complement in stimulation of the metabolic burst of human neutrophils by *Plasmodium falciparum. Infect Immun.* (1986) 51:801–6.
18. Cunnington AJ, Njie M, Correa S, Takem EN, Riley EM, Walther M. Prolonged neutrophil dysfunction after *Plasmodium falciparum* malaria is related to hemolysis and heme oxygenase-1 induction. *J Immunol.* (2012) 189:5336–46. doi: 10.4049/jimmunol.1201028
19. Pillay J, Kamp VM, van Hoffen E, Visser T, Tak T, Lammers JW, et al. A subset of neutrophils in human systemic inflammation inhibits T cell responses through Mac-1. *J Clin Invest.* (2012) 122:327–36. doi: 10.1172/JCI57990
20. Chakravorty SJ, Carret C, Nash GB, Ivens A, Szestak T, Craig AG. Altered phenotype and gene transcription in endothelial cells, induced by *Plasmodium falciparum*-infected red blood cells: pathogenic or protective? *Int J Parasitol.* (2007) 37, 975–87. doi: 10.1016/j.ijpara.2007.02.006
21. Moxon CA, Chisala NV, Wassmer SC, Taylor TE, Seydel KB, Molyneux ME, et al. Persistent endothelial activation and inflammation after *Plasmodium falciparum* Infection in Malawian children. *J Infect Dis.* (2014) 209:610–5. doi: 10.1093/infdis/jit419
22. Ioannidis LJ, Nie CQ, Hansen DS. The role of chemokines in severe malaria: more than meets the eye. *Parasitology* (2014) 141:602–13. doi: 10.1017/S0031182013001984
23. Chandrasiri UP, Randall LM, Saad AA, Bashir AM, Rogerson SJ, Adam I. Low antibody levels to pregnancy-specific malaria antigens and heightened cytokine responses associated with severe malaria in pregnancy. *J Infect Dis.* (2014) 209:1408–17. doi: 10.1093/infdis/jit646
24. Souza RM, Ataide R, Dombrowski JG, Ippolito V, Aitken EH, Valle SN, et al. Placental histopathological changes associated with Plasmodium vivax infection during pregnancy. *PLoS Negl Trop Dis.* (2013) 7:e2071. doi: 10.1371/journal.pntd.0002071
25. Carmona-Fonseca J, Arango E, Maestre A. Placental malaria in Colombia: histopathologic findings in Plasmodium vivax and P. falciparum infections. *Am J Trop Med Hyg.* (2013) 88:1093–101. doi: 10.4269/ajtmh.12-0363
26. Ordi J, Menendez C, Ismail MR, Ventura PJ, Palacin A, Kahigwa E, et al. Placental malaria is associated with cell-mediated inflammatory responses with selective absence of natural killer cells. *J Infect Dis.* (2001) 183:1100–7. doi: 10.1086/319295
27. Ampawong S, Chaisri U, Viriyavejakul P, Prapansilp P, Grau GE, Turner GD, et al. A potential role for interleukin-33 and gamma-epithelium sodium channel in the pathogenesis of human malaria associated lung injury. *Malar J.* (2015) 14:389. doi: 10.1186/s12936-015-0922-x
28. Lacerda MV, Fragoso SC, Alecrim MG, Alexandre MA, Magalhaes BM, Siqueira AM, et al. Postmortem characterization of patients with clinical diagnosis of Plasmodium vivax malaria: to what extent does this parasite kill? *Clin Infect Dis.* (2012) 55:e67–74. doi: 10.1093/cid/cis615
29. Day NP, Pham TD, Phan TL, Dinh XS, Pham PL, Ly VC, et al. Clearance kinetics of parasites and pigment-containing leukocytes in severe malaria. *Blood* (1996) 88:4694–700.
30. Leoratti FM, Trevelin SC, Cunha FQ, Rocha BC, Costa PA, Gravina HD, et al. Neutrophil paralysis in Plasmodium vivax malaria. *PLoS Negl Trop Dis.* (2012) 6:e1710. doi: 10.1371/journal.pntd.0001710
31. Waisberg M, Molina-Cruz A, Mizurini DM, Gera N, Sousa BC, Ma D, et al. *Plasmodium falciparum* infection induces expression of a mosquito salivary protein (Agaphelin) that targets neutrophil function and inhibits thrombosis without impairing hemostasis. *PLoS Pathog.* (2014) 10:e1004338. doi: 10.1371/journal.ppat.1004338
32. Waisberg M, Cerqueira GC, Yager SB, Francischetti IM, Lu J, Gera N, et al. *Plasmodium falciparum* merozoite surface protein 1 blocks the proinflammatory protein S100P. *Proc Natl Acad Sci USA.* (2012) 109:5429–34. doi: 10.1073/pnas.1202689109
33. Ding ZM, Babensee JE, Simon SI, Lu H, Perrard JL, Bullard DC, et al. Relative contribution of LFA-1 and Mac-1 to neutrophil adhesion and migration. *J Immunol.* (1999) 163:5029–38.
34. Dale DC, Boxer L, Liles WC. The phagocytes: neutrophils and monocytes. *Blood.* (2008) 112:935–45. doi: 10.1182/blood-2007-12-077917
35. Sun T, Chakrabarti C. Schizonts, merozoites, and phagocytosis in falciparum malaria. *Ann Clin Lab Sci.* (1985) 15:465–9.
36. Wickramasinghe SN, Phillips RE, Looareesuwan S, Warrell DA, Hughes M. The bone marrow in human cerebral malaria: parasite sequestration within sinusoids. *Br J Haematol.* (1987) 66:295–306.
37. Kumaratilake LM, Ferrante A. Opsonization and phagocytosis of *Plasmodium falciparum* merozoites measured by flow cytometry. *Clin Diagn Lab Immunol.* (2000) 7:9–13.
38. Trubowitz S, Masek B. *Plasmodium falciparum*: phagocytosis by polymorphonuclear leukocytes. *Science* (1968) 162:273–4.
39. Celada A, Cruchaud A, Perrin LH. Phagocytosis of *Plasmodium falciparum*-parasitized erythrocytes by human polymorphonuclear leukocytes. *J Parasitol.* (1983) 69:49–53.
40. Healer J, Graszynski A, Riley E. Phagocytosis does not play a major role in naturally acquired transmission-blocking immunity to *Plasmodium falciparum* malaria. *Infect Immun.* (1999) 67:2334–9.
41. Celada A, Cruchaud A, Perrin LH. Independence of complement on *in vitro* immune phagocytosis of *plasmodium falciparum* parasitised erythrocytes by

human monocytes and polymorphonuclear leukocytes. *Int Arch Allergy Appl Immunol.* (1984) 73:363–6.

42. Lensen AH, M. Bolmer-Van de Vegte, van Gemert GJ, Eling WM, Sauerwein RW. Leukocytes in a *Plasmodium falciparum*-infected blood meal reduce transmission of malaria to Anopheles mosquitoes. *Infect Immun.* (1997) 65:3834–7.
43. Meis JF, Jap PH, Hollingdale MR, Verhave JP. Cellular response against exoerythrocytic forms of *Plasmodium berghei* in rats. *Am J Trop Med Hyg.* (1987) 37:506–10.
44. Dupre-Crochet S, Erard M, Nubetae O. ROS production in phagocytes: why, when, and where? *J Leukoc Biol.* (2013) 94:657–70. doi: 10.1189/jlb.1012544
45. Kharazmi A, Jepsen S. Enhanced inhibition of *in vitro* multiplication of *Plasmodium falciparum* by stimulated human polymorphonuclear leucocytes. *Clin Exp Immunol.* (1984) 57:287–92.
46. Nnalue NA, Friedman MJ. Evidence for a neutrophil-mediated protective response in malaria. *Parasite Immunol.* (1988) 10:47–58.
47. Dasari P, Reiss K, Lingelbach K, Baumeister S, Lucius R, Udomsangpetch R, et al. Digestive vacuoles of *Plasmodium falciparum* are selectively phagocytosed by and impair killing function of polymorphonuclear leukocytes. *Blood* (2011) 118:4946–56. doi: 10.1182/blood-2011-05-353920
48. Robinson JM. Reactive oxygen species in phagocytic leukocytes. *Histochem Cell Biol.* (2008) 130:281–97. doi: 10.1007/s00418-008-0461-4
49. Greve B, Lehman LG, Lell B, Luckner D, Schmidt-Ott R, Kremsner PG. High oxygen radical production is associated with fast parasite clearance in children with *Plasmodium falciparum* malaria. *J Infect Dis.* (1999) 179:1584–6. doi: 10.1086/314780
50. Greve B, Hoffmann P, Vonthein R, Kun J, Lell B, Mycko MP, et al. NCF1 gene and pseudogene pattern: association with parasitic infection and autoimmunity. *Malar J.* (2008) 7:251. doi: 10.1186/1475-2875-7-251
51. Kharazmi A, Jepsen S, Andersen BJ. Generation of reactive oxygen radicals by human phagocytic cells activated by *Plasmodium falciparum. Scand J Immunol.* (1987) 25:335–41.
52. Joos C, Marrama L, Polson HE, Corre S, Diatta AM, Diouf B, et al. Clinical protection from falciparum malaria correlates with neutrophil respiratory bursts induced by merozoites opsonized with human serum antibodies. *PLoS ONE* (2010) 5:e9871. doi: 10.1371/journal.pone.0009871
53. Kapelski S, Klockenbring T, Fischer R, Barth S, Fendel R. Assessment of the neutrophilic antibody-dependent respiratory burst (ADRB) response to *Plasmodium falciparum. J Leukoc Biol.* (2014) 96:1131–42. doi: 10.1189/jlb.4A0614-283RR
54. Lunel F, Descamps-Latscha B, Druilhe P. Activation of phagocyte oxidative metabolism by opsonized *Plasmodium falciparum* merozoites. *Acta Trop.* (1990) 47:61–8.
55. Perraut R, Joos C, Sokhna C, Polson HE, Trape JF, Tall A, et al. Association of antibody responses to the conserved *Plasmodium falciparum* merozoite surface protein 5 with protection against clinical malaria. *PLoS ONE.* (2014) 9:e101737. doi: 10.1371/journal.pone.0101737
56. Murungi LM, Sonden K, Llewellyn D, Rono J, Guleid F, Williams AR, et al. Targets and mechanisms associated with protection from severe *Plasmodium falciparum* malaria in kenyan children. *Infect Immun.* (2016) 84:950–63. doi: 10.1128/IAI.01120-15
57. Crockett-Torabi E, Fantone JC. Soluble and insoluble immune complexes activate human neutrophil NADPH oxidase by distinct Fc gamma receptor-specific mechanisms. *J Immunol.* (1990) 145:3026–32.
58. Adu B, Jepsen MP, Gerds TA, Kyei-Baafour E, Christiansen M, Dodoo D, Theisen M. Fc gamma receptor 3B (FCGR3B-c.233C>A-rs5030738) polymorphism modifies the protective effect of malaria specific antibodies in Ghanaian children. *J Infect Dis.* (2014) 209:285–9. doi: 10.1093/infdis/jit422
59. Adu B, Dodoo D, Adukpo S, Hedley PL, Arthur FK, Gerds TA, et al. Fc gamma receptor IIIB (FcgammaRIIIB) polymorphisms are associated with clinical malaria in Ghanaian children. *PLoS ONE* (2012) 7:e46197. doi: 10.1371/journal.pone.0046197
60. Malhotra K, Salmon D, Le Bras J, Savel J, Vilde JL. [Stimulation of the chemiluminescence of human polymorphonuclear leukocytes in various stages of the intraerythrocyte development of *Plasmodium falciparum*]. *C R Seances Soc Biol Fil.* (1988) 182:270–8.
61. Aitken EH, Mbewe B, Luntamo M, Maleta K, Kulmala T, Friso MJ, et al. Antibodies to chondroitin sulfate A-binding infected erythrocytes: dynamics and protection during pregnancy in women receiving intermittent preventive treatment. *J Infect Dis.* (2010) 201:1316–25. doi: 10.1086/651578
62. Joos C, Varela ML, Mbengue B, Mansourou A, Marrama L, Sokhna C, et al. Antibodies to *Plasmodium falciparum* merozoite surface protein-1p19 malaria vaccine candidate induce antibody-dependent respiratory burst in human neutrophils. *Malar J.* (2015) 14:409. doi: 10.1186/s12936-015-0935-5
63. Jaschke A, Coulibaly B, Remarque EJ, Bujard H, Epp C. Merozoite Surface Protein 1 from *Plasmodium falciparum* is a major target of opsonizing antibodies in individuals with acquired immunity against malaria. *Clin Vaccine Immunol.* (2017) 24:e00155–17.
64. Lazarou M, Guevara Patino JA, Jennings RM, McIntosh RS, Shi J, Howell S, et al. Inhibition of erythrocyte invasion and *Plasmodium falciparum* merozoite surface protein 1 processing by human immunoglobulin G1 (IgG1) and IgG3 antibodies. *Infect Immun.* (2009) 77:5659–67. doi: 10.1128/IAI.00167-09
65. Shi J, McIntosh RS, Adame-Gallegos J, Dehal PK, van Egmond M, J. van de Winkel, et al. The generation and evaluation of recombinant human IgA specific for *Plasmodium falciparum* merozoite surface protein 1–19 (PfMSP1 19). *BMC Biotechnol.* (2011) 11:77. doi: 10.1186/1472-6750-11-77
66. Brinkmann V, Reichard U, Goosmann C, Fauler B, Uhlemann Y, Weiss DS, et al. Neutrophil extracellular traps kill bacteria. *Science* (2004) 303:1532–5. doi: 10.1126/science.1092385
67. Hoppenbrouwers T, Autar ASA, Sultan AR, Abraham TE, van Cappellen WA, Houtsmuller AB, et al. *In vitro* induction of NETosis: comprehensive live imaging comparison and systematic review. *PLoS ONE* (2017) 12:e0176472. doi: 10.1371/journal.pone.0176472
68. Gallego-Delgado J, Ty M, Orengo JM, van de Hoef D, Rodriguez A. A surprising role for uric acid: the inflammatory malaria response. *Curr Rheumatol Rep.* (2014) 16:401. doi: 10.1007/s11926-013-0401-8
69. Dunst J, Kamena F, Matuschewski K. Cytokines and chemokines in cerebral malaria pathogenesis. *Front Cell Infect Microbiol.* (2017) 7:324. doi: 10.3389/fcimb.2017.00324
70. Percario S, Moreira DR, Gomes BA, Ferreira ME, Goncalves AC, Laurindo PS, et al. Oxidative stress in malaria. *Int J Mol Sci.* (2012) 13:16346–72. doi: 10.3390/ijms131216346
71. Baker VS, Imade GE, Molta NB, Tawde P, Pam SD, Obadofin MO, et al. Cytokine-associated neutrophil extracellular traps and antinuclear antibodies in *Plasmodium falciparum* infected children under six years of age. *Malar J.* (2008) 7:41. doi: 10.1186/1475-2875-7-41
72. Granger V, Faille D, Marani V, Noel B, Gallais Y, Szely N, et al. Human blood monocytes are able to form extracellular traps. *J Leukoc Biol.* (2017) 102:775–781. doi: 10.1189/jlb.3MA0916-411R
73. Sercundes MK, Ortolan LS, Debone D, Soeiro-Pereira PV, Gomes E, Aitken EH, et al. Targeting neutrophils to prevent malaria-associated acute lung injury/acute respiratory distress syndrome in mice. *PLoS Pathog.* (2016) 12:e1006054. doi: 10.1371/journal.ppat.1006054
74. Chang Z, Jiang N, Zhang Y, Lu H, Yin J, Wahlgren M, et al. The TatD-like DNase of plasmodium is a virulence factor and a potential malaria vaccine candidate. *Nat Commun.* (2016) 7:11537. doi: 10.1038/ncomms11537
75. Manfredi AA, Ramirez GA, Rovere-Querini P, Maugeri N. The Neutrophil's choice: phagocytose vs make neutrophil extracellular traps. *Front Immunol.* (2018) 9:288. doi: 10.3389/fimmu.2018.00288
76. Turrini F, Ginsburg H, Bussolino F, Pescarmona GP, Serra MV, Arese P. Phagocytosis of *Plasmodium falciparum*-infected human red blood cells by human monocytes: involvement of immune and nonimmune determinants and dependence on parasite developmental stage. *Blood* (1992) 80:801–8.
77. Yang JJ, Kettritz R, Falk RJ, Jennette JC, Gaido ML. Apoptosis of endothelial cells induced by the neutrophil serine proteases proteinase 3 and elastase. *Am J Pathol.* (1996) 149:1617–26.
78. Smedly LA, Tonnesen MG, Sandhaus RA, Haslett C, Guthrie LA, Johnston RB, Jr, et al. Neutrophil-mediated injury to endothelial cells. Enhancement by endotoxin and essential role of neutrophil elastase. *J Clin Invest.* (1986) 77:1233–43. doi: 10.1172/JCI112426
79. Meager A. Cytokine regulation of cellular adhesion molecule expression in inflammation. *Cytokine Growth Factor Rev.* (1999) 10:27–39.
80. Mittal M, Siddiqui MR, Tran K, Reddy SP, Malik AB. Reactive oxygen species in inflammation and tissue injury. *Antioxid Redox Signal.* (2014) 20:1126–67. doi: 10.1089/ars.2012.5149

81. Berendt AR, Simmons DL, Tansey J, Newbold CI, Marsh K. Intercellular adhesion molecule-1 is an endothelial cell adhesion receptor for *Plasmodium falciparum*. *Nature* (1989) 341:57–9. doi: 10.1038/341057a0
82. Villegas-Mendez A, Montes R, Ambrose LR, Warrens AN, Laffan M, Lane DA. Proteolysis of the endothelial cell protein C receptor by neutrophil proteinase 3. *J Thromb Haemost.* (2007) 5:980–8. doi: 10.1111/j.1538-7836.2007.02480.x
83. Turner L, Lavstsen T, Berger SS, Wang CW, Petersen JE, Avril M, et al. Severe malaria is associated with parasite binding to endothelial protein C receptor. *Nature* (2013) 498:502–5. doi: 10.1038/nature12216
84. Janoff A, Roth WJ, Sinha S, Barnwell JW. Degradation of plasmodial antigens by human neutrophil elastase. *J Immunol.* (1988) 141:1332–40.
85. Rocha BC, Marques PE, Leoratti FM S, Junqueira C, Pereira DB, Antonelli L, et al. Type I interferon transcriptional signature in neutrophils and low-density granulocytes are associated with tissue damage in malaria. *Cell Rep.* (2015) 13:2829–41. doi: 10.1016/j.celrep.2015.11.055
86. Assumpcao TC, Ma D, Schwarz A, Reiter K, Santana JM, Andersen JF, et al. Salivary antigen-5/CAP family members are Cu2+-dependent antioxidant enzymes that scavenge O(2)(-). and inhibit collagen-induced platelet aggregation and neutrophil oxidative burst. *J Biol Chem.* (2013) 288:14341–61. doi: 10.1074/jbc.M113.466995
87. Mathieu C, Demarta-Gatsi C, Porcherie A, Brega S, Thiberge S, Ronce K, et al. *Plasmodium berghei* histamine-releasing factor favours liver-stage development via inhibition of IL-6 production and associates with a severe outcome of disease. *Cell Microbiol.* (2015) 17:542–58. doi: 10.1111/cmi.12382
88. Mabey DC, Brown A, Greenwood BM. *Plasmodium falciparum* malaria and *Salmonella* infections in Gambian children. *J Infect Dis.* (1987) 155:1319–21.
89. Bronzan RN, Taylor TE, Mwenechanya J, Tembo M, Kayira K, Bwanaisa L, et al. Bacteremia in Malawian children with severe malaria: prevalence, etiology, HIV coinfection, and outcome. *J Infect Dis.* (2007) 195:895–904. doi: 10.1086/511437
90. Mooney JP, Barry A, Goncalves BP, Tiono AB, Awandu SS, Grignard L, et al. Haemolysis and haem oxygenase-1 induction during persistent "asymptomatic" malaria infection in Burkinabe children. *Malar J.* (2018) 17:253. doi: 10.1186/s12936-018-2402-6
91. Cunnington AJ, de Souza JB, Walther M, Riley EM. Malaria impairs resistance to *Salmonella* through heme- and heme oxygenase-dependent dysfunctional granulocyte mobilization. *Nat Med.* (2011) 18:120–7. doi: 10.1038/nm.2601
92. Mooney JP, Butler BP, Lokken KL, Xavier MN, Chau JY, Schaltenberg N, et al. The mucosal inflammatory response to non-typhoidal Salmonella in the intestine is blunted by IL-10 during concurrent malaria parasite infection. *Mucosal Immunol.* (2014) 7:1302–11. doi: 10.1038/mi.2014.18
93. Amodu OK, Adeyemo AA, Olumese PE, Gbadegesin RA. Intraleucocytic malaria pigment and clinical severity of malaria in children. *Trans R Soc Trop Med Hyg.* (1998) 92:54–6.
94. Lyke KE, Diallo DA, Dicko A, Kone A, Coulibaly D, Guindo A, et al. Association of intraleukocytic *Plasmodium falciparum* malaria pigment with disease severity, clinical manifestations, and prognosis in severe malaria. *Am J Trop Med Hyg.* (2003) 69:253–9. doi: 10.4269/ajtmh.2003.69.253
95. Metzger WG, Mordmuller BG, Kremsner PG. Malaria pigment in leucocytes. *Trans R Soc Trop Med Hyg.* (1995) 89:637–8.
96. Nguyen PH, Day N, Pram TD, Ferguson DJ, White NJ. Intraleucocytic malaria pigment and prognosis in severe malaria. *Trans R Soc Trop Med Hyg.* (1995) 89:200–4.
97. Chua CL, Robinson LJ, Baiwog F, Stanisic DI, Hamilton JA, Brown GV, et al. High numbers of circulating pigmented polymorphonuclear neutrophils as a prognostic marker for decreased birth weight during malaria in pregnancy. *Int J Parasitol.* (2015) 45:107–11. doi: 10.1016/j.ijpara.2014.12.002
98. Willmann M, Ahmed A, Siner A, Wong IT, Woon LC, Singh B, et al. Laboratory markers of disease severity in *Plasmodium knowlesi* infection: a case control study. *Malar J.* (2012) 11:363. doi: 10.1186/1475-2875-11-363
99. Kharazmi A. Antimalarial drugs and human neutrophil oxidative metabolism. *Trans R Soc Trop Med Hyg.* (1986) 80:94–7.
100. Jones CJ, Jayson MI. Chloroquine: its effect on leucocyte auto- and heterophagocytosis. *Ann Rheum Dis.* (1984) 43:205–12.
101. Ferrante A, Rowan-Kelly B, Seow WK, Thong YH. Depression of human polymorphonuclear leucocyte function by anti-malarial drugs. *Immunology* (1986) 58:125–30.
102. el Benna J, Hakim J, Labro MT. Inhibition of human neutrophil protein kinase C activity by the antimalarial drug mefloquine. *Biochem Pharmacol.* (1992) 43:527–32.
103. Naisbitt DJ, Williams DP, O'Neill PM, Maggs JL, Willock DJ, Pirmohamed M, et al. Metabolism-dependent neutrophil cytotoxicity of amodiaquine: a comparison with pyronaridine and related antimalarial drugs. *Chem Res Toxicol.* (1998) 11:1586–95. doi: 10.1021/tx980148k
104. Croft SL, Duparc S, Arbe-Barnes SJ, Craft JC, Shin CS, Fleckenstein L, et al. Review of pyronaridine anti-malarial properties and product characteristics. *Malar J.* (2012) 11:270. doi: 10.1186/1475-2875-11-270
105. Bethell D, Se Y, Lon C, Socheat D, Saunders D, Teja-Isavadharm P, et al. Dose-dependent risk of neutropenia after 7-day courses of artesunate monotherapy in Cambodian patients with acute *Plasmodium falciparum* malaria. *Clin Infect Dis.* (2010) 51:e105–14. doi: 10.1086/657402
106. Gasasira AF, Kamya MR, Achan J, Mebrahtu T, Kalyango JN, Ruel T, et al. High risk of neutropenia in HIV-infected children following treatment with artesunate plus amodiaquine for uncomplicated malaria in Uganda. *Clin Infect Dis.* (2008) 46:985–91. doi: 10.1086/529192
107. Zwang J, Ndiaye JL, Djimde A, Dorsey G, Martensson A, Karema C, et al. Comparing changes in haematologic parameters occurring in patients included in randomized controlled trials of artesunate-amodiaquine vs single and combination treatments of uncomplicated falciparum in sub-Saharan Africa. *Malar J.* (2012) 11:25. doi: 10.1186/1475-2875-11-25
108. Clark IA, Cowden WB, Butcher GA, Hunt NH. Possible roles of tumor necrosis factor in the pathology of malaria. *Am J Pathol.* (1987) 129:192–9.
109. Clark IA, Ilschner S, MacMicking JD, Cowden WB. TNF and *Plasmodium berghei* ANKA-induced cerebral malaria. *Immunol Lett.* (1990) 25:195–8.
110. Senaldi G, Vesin C, Chang R, Grau GE, Piguet PF. Role of polymorphonuclear neutrophil leukocytes and their integrin CD11a (LFA-1) in the pathogenesis of severe murine malaria. *Infect Immun.* (1994) 62:1144–9.
111. Carvalho LJ, Lenzi HL, Pelajo-Machado M, Oliveira DN, Daniel-Ribeiro CT, Ferreira-da-Cruz MF. *Plasmodium berghei*: cerebral malaria in CBA mice is not clearly related to plasma TNF levels or intensity of histopathological changes. *Exp Parasitol.* (2000) 95:1–7. doi: 10.1006/expr.2000.4508
112. Lovegrove FE, Gharib SA, Pena-Castillo L, Patel SN, Ruzinski JT, Hughes TR, et al. Parasite burden and CD36-mediated sequestration are determinants of acute lung injury in an experimental malaria model. *PLoS Pathog.* (2008) 4:e1000068. doi: 10.1371/journal.ppat.1000068
113. Lin JW, Sodenkamp J, Cunningham D, Deroost K, Tshitenge TC, McLaughlin S, et al. Signatures of malaria-associated pathology revealed by high-resolution whole-blood transcriptomics in a rodent model of malaria. *Sci Rep.* (2017) 7:41722. doi: 10.1038/srep41722
114. Favre N, Da Laperousaz C, Ryffel B, Weiss NA, Imhof BA, Rudin W, et al. Role of ICAM-1 (CD54) in the development of murine cerebral malaria. *Microbes Infect.* (1999) 1:961–8.
115. Chen L, Sendo F. Cytokine and chemokine mRNA expression in neutrophils from CBA/NSlc mice infected with *Plasmodium berghei* ANKA that induces experimental cerebral malaria. *Parasitol Int.* (2001) 50:139–43. doi: 10.1016/S1383-5769(01)00063-0
116. Nacer A, Movila A, Sohet F, Girgis NM, Gundra UM, Loke P, et al. Experimental cerebral malaria pathogenesis–hemodynamics at the blood brain barrier. *PLoS Pathog.* (2014) 10:e1004528. doi: 10.1371/journal.ppat.1004528
117. Chen L, Zhang Z, Sendo F. Neutrophils play a critical role in the pathogenesis of experimental cerebral malaria. *Clin Exp Immunol.* (2000) 120:125–33. doi: 10.1046/j.1365-2249.2000.01196.x
118. Ioannidis LJ, Nie CQ, Ly A, Ryg-Cornejo V, Chiu CY, Hansen DS. Monocyte- and Neutrophil-Derived CXCL10 Impairs Efficient Control of Blood-Stage Malaria Infection and Promotes Severe Disease. *J Immunol.* (2016) 196:1227–38. doi: 10.4049/jimmunol.1501562

119. Porcherie A, Mathieu C, Peronet R, Schneider E, Claver J, Commere PH, et al. Critical role of the neutrophil-associated high-affinity receptor for IgE in the pathogenesis of experimental cerebral malaria. *J Exp Med.* (2011) 208:2225–36. doi: 10.1084/jem.20110845

120. Dey S, Bindu S, Goyal M, Pal C, Alam A, Iqbal MS, Kumar R, Sarkar S, Bandyopadhyay U. Impact of intravascular hemolysis in malaria on liver dysfunction: involvement of hepatic free heme overload, NF-kappaB activation, and neutrophil infiltration. *J Biol Chem.* (2012) 287:26630–46. doi: 10.1074/jbc.M112.341255

121. Laing AB, Wilson M. Remarkable polymorphonuclear phagocytosis of *P. falciparum*. *Trans R Soc Trop Med Hyg.* (1972) 66:523.

122. Adame-Gallegos JR, Shi J, McIntosh RS, Pleass RJ. The generation and evaluation of two panels of epitope-matched mouse IgG1, IgG2a, IgG2b and IgG3 antibodies specific for *Plasmodium falciparum* and *Plasmodium yoelii* merozoite surface protein 1–19 [MSP1(19)]. *Exp Parasitol.* (2012) 130:384–93. doi: 10.1016/j.exppara.2012.02.003

123. Llewellyn D, de Cassan SC, Williams AR, Douglas AD, Forbes EK, Adame-Gallegos JR, et al. Assessment of antibody-dependent respiratory burst activity from mouse neutrophils on *Plasmodium yoelii* malaria challenge outcome. *J Leukoc Biol.* (2014) 95:369–82. doi: 10.1189/jlb.0513274

124. Mac-Daniel L, Buckwalter MR, Berthet M, Virk Y, Yui K, Albert ML, et al. Local immune response to injection of Plasmodium sporozoites into the skin. *J Immunol.* (2014) 193:1246–57. doi: 10.4049/jimmunol.1302669

2

Development of B Cell Memory in Malaria

Ann Ly[1,2] *and Diana S. Hansen*[1,2*]

[1] *The Walter and Eliza Hall Institute of Medical Research, Parkville, VIC, Australia,* [2] *Department of Medical Biology, The University of Melbourne, Parkville, VIC, Australia*

Edited by:
*Ian Marriott,
University of North Carolina at Charlotte, United States*

Reviewed by:
*Julius Clemence Hafalla,
London School of Hygiene and Tropical Medicine (LSHTM), United Kingdom
Robin Stephens,
The University of Texas Medical Branch at Galveston, United States*

***Correspondence:**
*Diana S. Hansen
hansen@wehi.edu.au*

A single exposure to many viral and bacterial pathogens typically induces life-long immunity, however, the development of the protective immunity to *Plasmodium* parasites is strikingly less efficient and achieves only partial protection, with adults residing in endemic areas often experiencing asymptomatic infections. Although naturally acquired immunity to malaria requires both cell-mediated and humoral immune responses, antibodies govern the control of malarial disease caused by the blood-stage form of the parasites. A large body of epidemiological evidence described that antibodies to *Plasmodium* antigens are inefficiently generated and rapidly lost without continued parasite exposure, suggesting that malaria is accompanied by defects in the development of immunological B cell memory. This topic has been of focus of recent studies of malaria infection in humans and mice. This review examines the main findings to date on the processes that modulate the acquisition of memory B cell responses to malaria, and highlights the importance of closing outstanding gaps of knowledge in the field for the rational design of next generation therapeutics against malaria.

Keywords: malaria, immunity, antibodies, memory B cells, inflammation

B CELL IMMUNOLOGICAL MEMORY

Immunological memory refers to the ability of the vertebrate immune system to remember previously encountered antigens or pathogens and evoke an enhanced immune response to control infection. The capacity of the host to generate T and B cell memory underlies the basis of protective immunity induced by vaccination or after exposure to specific pathogens. The generation of T cell-dependent humoral immune memory in secondary lymphoid organs (**Figure 1**) typically begins following B cell engagement with its cognate antigen, which triggers their migration to the B cell follicle border to receive T cell help (1). Activated B cells then differentiate along one of three possible routes, leading to the rapid production of short-lived plasmablasts, generating germinal center (GC)-independent memory B cells (MBCs), or formation of GCs in B cell follicles (2, 3). GCs establish within a few days of initial antigen encounter and mature into two distinct micro-anatomical compartments: the dark zone, where B cell clones undergo proliferative expansion and somatic hypermutation of their immunoglobulin (Ig) genes, and the light zone, where B cells expressing high-affinity antibodies are selected and undergo class switch recombination (4–6). The GC reaction leads to the generation of affinity-matured MBCs and long-lived plasma cells that contribute to host protection against re-infection. Plasma cells migrate to the bone marrow and provide a continuous source of circulating high-affinity antibody (7), while MBCs recirculate in the blood and secondary lymphoid tissue (8) to induce a rapid effector response upon antigen re-encounter (9, 10).

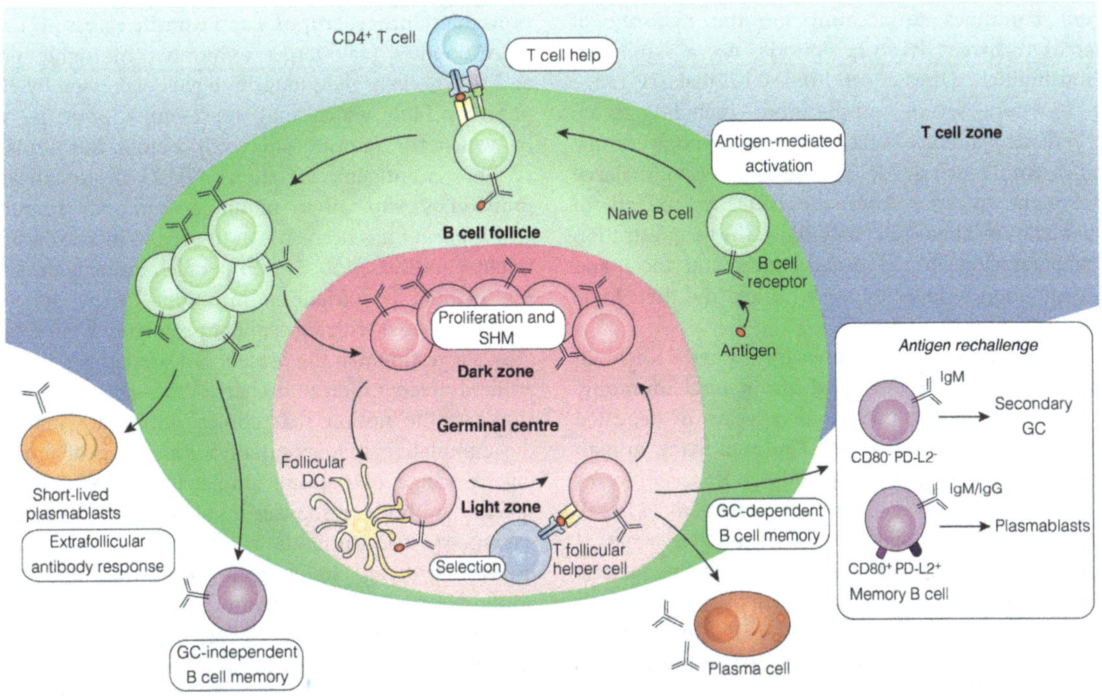

FIGURE 1 | Pathways leading to the development of B cell memory. Upon encounter with antigen, activated B cells in secondary lymphoid tissue receive helper signals from cognate CD4+ T cells at the border of the B cell follicle and T cell zones. Some of the proliferating B cells differentiate into short-lived plasmablasts that initiate an extrafollicular antibody response, some develop into early memory B cells independently of GC formation, while others aggregate into the follicle to establish a GC. Within the GC, B cells undergo proliferation and somatic hypermutation in the dark zone, followed by affinity-based selection in the light zone with the help of T follicular helper cells and follicular dendritic cells. Long-lived plasma cells and memory B cells emerge from the GC reaction. Upon antigen rechallenge, memory B cells lacking expression of the surface molecules CD80 and PD-L2, mainly of the IgM isotype, can seed secondary GCs, whereas those expressing both molecules, comprising of IgM and IgG isotypes, predominantly generate plasmablasts. GC, germinal center; DC, dendritic cell; SHM, somatic hypermutation.

Comprehensive studies of MBC biology have led to the appreciation of substantial heterogeneity among the MBC compartment, consisting of distinct subpopulations with different effector capacity upon secondary challenge (11). In humans, the expression of unique memory-specific surface markers has been extensively used to identify and characterize MBCs. Surface expression of CD27 defines a subset of antigen-experienced MBCs in humans that are class-switched and bear Ig variable region mutations (12, 13). However, CD27 expression does not universally define all MBCs, as subsequent work identified an $CD27^-$ $CD21^-$ MBC population (14). These cells, coined as atypical MBCs in malaria, express several Fc receptor-like (FcRL) inhibitory receptors, including FcRL3 and 5 (15–17).

The development of novel labeling techniques to track antigen-specific B cells in murine models has enabled the functional characterization of MBCs expressing different antibody isotypes. Whereas, IgG MBCs have been found to preferentially differentiate into plasmablasts upon antigen rechallenge, IgM MBCs appear to have the capacity to re-enter secondary GC reactions but were not enhanced in plasmablast generation (18, 19). Recent studies have uncovered additional heterogeneity within the IgM and IgG MBC pools, proposing that MBCs lacking the memory markers CD80 and PD-L2, which primarily express IgM, are dedicated to reseeding GCs, while those expressing both markers, comprising of IgM and IgG isotypes, contribute mainly to immediate antibody-secreting function (**Figure 1**) (20). Consistently, IgM-expressing MBCs have recently been shown to exhibit considerable plasticity in their differentiation capacity following rechallenge (21). This division of labor in the MBC response has been proposed to support a rapid and effective response upon antigen rechallenge while concurrently permit the generation of new MBCs (11). How these findings in murine models relate to human settings is unclear, as there is still little information about the homology between mouse and humans MBC subsets with regards to their surface marker expression usage.

A ROLE FOR MEMORY B CELS IN NATURALLY ACQUIRED IMMUNITY TO MALARIA

The global burden of malaria has more than halved since the turn of the century due to renewed eradication efforts, but progress has recently stalled as current intervention strategies are confronted with several major challenges, including the emergence of anti-malarial drug and insecticide resistance

(22). Of the six *Plasmodium* species known to infect humans, *P. falciparum* continues to account for the majority of deaths, whereas recurrent *P. vivax* episodes are a significant source of morbidities. Disease syndromes of malaria range from fever to more severe complications including acute pulmonary oedema, jaundice, severe anemia, hypoglycaemia, acidosis, and cerebral malaria (23). The pathogenesis of malarial disease is thought to arise from the concerted effects of host and parasite mechanisms, including the sequestration of blood-stage parasites in microvasculature, and local and systemic inflammation induced by the parasites and their toxic products (24, 25).

Early epidemiological observations by Robert Koch in malaria-endemic populations described that natural immunity to malaria can be achieved, but requires years of repeated exposure to *Plasmodium* parasites (26). Children living in high transmission regions become immune to the most severe forms of malaria after relatively few symptomatic infections (27–29), but remain at risk of uncomplicated malaria. After years of repeated infections with age, protection from successive malaria episodes or "clinical immunity," is acquired by the ability to substantially reduce parasite burdens (30–35). This form of protection is not paralleled by sterile immunity that prevents re-infection (36), and adults continue to be experience low-density, asymptomatic infections throughout life (37). Naturally acquired clinical immunity to malaria targets blood-stage parasites and requires antibodies, as demonstrated by studies in which the transfer of purified IgG from malaria-immune adults to children with symptomatic malaria rapidly reduced parasitemia and fever (38). Together, these observations have led to the hypothesis that the slow and imperfect acquisition of immunity to malaria reflects in the development of MBCs, and this topic has been the subject of several studies including mouse infection models as well as human settings. Here we review our current understanding on the salient features of the development of humoral immunity to malaria infection, and highlight some of the outstanding questions regarding the cellular mechanisms that underlie the slow acquisition of clinical immunity.

ANTIBODY RESPONSES TO BLOOD-STAGE MALARIA

The paramount importance of antibodies in controlling blood-stage malaria infection was proven by seminal passive-transfer experiments, in which IgG from *P. falciparum* clinically immune adults protected non-immune children from high parasitemia and clinical symptoms (38, 39). Numerous immuno-epidemiological studies subsequently demonstrated that high antibody levels against specific blood-stage parasite antigens correlate with protection from disease (40–46). Antibodies may control the development of clinical symptoms by targeting the invasion and growth of the merozoite form of the blood-stage parasite and redirect their clearance by phagocytic cells via Fc and complement receptors (47). Additionally, antibodies directed against parasite antigens expressed on infected erythrocytes can promote opsonic phagocytosis, block microvasculature adherence, disrupt rosette formation with uninfected cells, and prevent erythrocyte rupture and parasite egress (47).

Antibodies may target a number of highly polymorphic and functionally redundant antigens expressed by *Plasmodium* parasites (48), which may represent a potential mechanism by which the parasite effectively evades the human immune system via antigenic variation (49). Asymptomatically-infected individuals who fail to mount an antibody response against *P. falciparum* has been shown to predict increased susceptibility to clinical disease (50, 51). In parallel, individuals detected with multi-clonal *P. falciparum* infections in the dry season have been associated with subsequent protection from febrile malaria (52), suggesting that the presence of persisting parasites enhance antibody recognition and enable cross-reactive responses. This supports the notion that clinical immunity may depend on the cumulative acquisition of a repertoire of antibodies to a diverse range of parasite antigens or development of cross-species antibody responses (53–55). Indeed, the breadth of parasite-specific antibody responses have been identified to increase with age in endemic populations (56–58), and the antibody repertoire diversifies rapidly during infancy but plateaus in toddlers (59). Moreover, antibodies with broad reactivity against *P. falciparum* that carry a gene insertion derived from the collagen-binding protein LAIR1, have been shown to undergo somatic hypermutation that increase binding to infected erythrocytes (60). LAIR1 insertions have been further revealed to represent a relatively common mechanism of antibody diversification in African individuals, and that broadly-neutralizing antibodies against *Plasmodium* arise from these low-affinity precursors over time (61). While antigenic variation has been proposed to explain the slow acquisition immunity to malaria, there is also an increasing body of evidence suggesting that antibody responses to malaria are poorly generated. In malaria-endemic areas, substantial declines have been reported in *Plasmodium*-specific antibody responses to low or undetectable levels within months, and even weeks of a clinical episode after reduced parasite exposure, despite an initial robust response (56, 57, 62–69). Studies modeling the longevity of *P. falciparum* merozoite-specific IgG antibodies have estimated average half-lives of <10 days in children recovering from clinical malaria (67). Similarly, short antibody half-lives ranging from only 2–7 weeks has been reported in asymptomatic children during the dry season in The Gambia (68), which contrasts dramatically with those of antibody responses to viral and bacterial antigens such as vaccinia, measles and tetanus that reportedly persist for decades following a single exposure (70–72). It is possible that antibody responses measured following a clinical malaria episode may reflect the output of short-lived antibody-secreting cells, which typically produce an immediate but transient wave of antibodies to control infection. In line with this idea, antibody-secreting cells have been detected transiently in Ugandan children immediately following acute malaria, and were found to proportionally increase again upon a second clinical episode (73). Modeling studies extended these observations, estimating the longevity of both short- and long-lived antibody-secreting cells in African children to range from 2–10 days, and 3–9 years, respectively (74). Thus, together these findings suggest that a long-lived humoral response to malaria infection can potentially be sustained after decay of transient antibody-secreting cells. More detailed mechanistic investigations are much needed to determine how parasite-specific antibody responses are sustained over time and the factors that modulate the generation and maintenance of antibody-secreting cells to infection.

THE ACQUISITION OF MEMORY B CELLS TO NATURAL MALARIA INFECTION

Several studies have now shown the induction of *Plasmodium*-specific MBCs in response to malaria infection; although individuals exposed to high seasonal transmission have been reported to induce only low frequencies of MBCs or to lack detectable MBCs, even after exposure to parasitic loads sufficient and capable of inducing antibody responses (57, 75, 76). Consistent with the slow acquisition of antibody responses in endemic settings, the prevalence and breadth of *Plasmodium*-specific MBCs appear to develop incrementally with age and exposure (57, 59, 77). Longitudinal studies of children and young adults in an area of high seasonal transmission in Mali demonstrated a delayed, age-associated development of MBCs specific for *P. falciparum* merozoite antigens despite repeated infections annually (57). Moreover, the prevalence of MBCs acquired by children following acute malaria appeared to diminish substantially within the 6-month dry season, contrasting with the stable frequency of MBCs to tetanus toxoid vaccination in the same subjects (57). While seasonal transmission prevented the longevity of these cells to be determined beyond the dry season, this finding implies an impaired maintenance or generation of MBCs in children exposed to high transmission as they acquire clinical protection.

In contrast, individuals residing in areas of low transmission or subjected to fewer clinical episodes have been shown to generate stable *Plasmodium*-specific MBCs without frequent boosting (77–85). The frequencies of *P. falciparum*-specific MBCs detected in Thai adults that had experienced limited episodes reportedly remained stable over time, with an estimated half-life of approximately 7.5 years (81). Similarly, malaria-specific MBCs have been described to be well-maintained in individuals with a history of acute malaria but have since lived in the absence of persistent infection (83, 84). In parallel, low levels of exposure can effectively sustain parasite-specific antibody responses (79, 82, 84, 86, 87), with antibody half-lives estimated to be substantially longer than that of highly-exposed individuals, ranging from months to years (32, 81, 88), suggesting sustained antibody production from long-lived plasma cells. Collectively, these findings reveal that MBCs can be generated and sustained following a limited number of clinical episodes, while repeated infections in endemic areas could have a detrimental effect on the generation of B cell memory.

The characterization of malaria-specific MBCs to date has relied predominantly on *in vitro* stimulation and differentiation of circulating MBCs into antibody-secreting cells followed by detection of antigen-specific clones by ELISPOT assays. This approach precludes phenotypic analysis of the malaria-specific MBC compartment. More detailed investigations are needed to determine the ontogeny of detected MBCs and whether they contribute to effective clinical immunity in malaria-exposed individuals. Whereas, the induction of IgG-expressing MBCs has been the primary focus over the past several years, a few studies have identified IgM MBCs in malaria-exposed individuals and in malaria mouse infection models (59, 89, 90), with those induced by murine malaria found to rapidly differentiate into plasmablasts upon antigenic restimulation (89). Interestingly, MBCs isolated from malaria-exposed individuals have been described to have undergone Ig somatic hypermutations (76), and accumulate further mutations upon acute malaria, with IgM being the dominant isotype expressed prior to re-infection (59).

The use of murine infection models has also provided insight into the development of B cell memory to malaria. Although murine infection does not mirror all the features of human malaria, there are genetic and phenotypic parallels between the human parasite and rodent counterparts (91, 92). A few studies have detected the development of IgG memory B cells following non-lethal *P. chabaudi* infection (89, 90, 93, 94), associated with efficient generation of secondary GCs and enhanced control of re-infection (90, 95). In contrast, *P. yoelii* blood-stage infection has been suggested to ablate vaccination-induced MBCs (96), and further reduces the development of mature, isotype-switched MBCs against pre-erythrocytic parasite antigen, which was associated with the induction of pro-inflammatory cytokines and chemokines that may hinder effective T and B cell interactions (97).

IMMUNOLOGICAL PROCESSES MODULATING THE INDUCTION OF MEMORY B CELLS IN MALARIA

T follicular helper (Tfh) cells are a crucial subset of $CD4^+$ T cells that orchestrate B cell memory development by providing crucial survival and differentiation signals to B cells during the GC response (98), and have been shown to be important for the control of *Plasmodium* infection (99–105). The development of Tfh cells has not been extensively investigated in human malaria infection, however, a recent study identified the induction of T helper 1 (Th1) cell-like $CXCR3^+PD\text{-}1^+$ Tfh cells in the circulation of Malian children following acute *P. falciparum* malaria (106). Circulating Tfh cells have been proposed to be a surrogate measure of GC-derived Tfh cell responses to human infection (107, 108) and thus constitutes a valuable proxy to investigate Tfh cell biology in human settings. Circulating Tfh cells in malaria-exposed children were shown to express the Th1 lineage-defining transcription factor T-bet, and had limited functional capacity to support MBC responses *in vitro* (106). $CXCR3^+PD\text{-}1^+$ Tfh cells have also been identified in Brazilian adults during acute *P. vivax* malaria (109). Interestingly, their proportions positively correlated with repeated malaria episodes (109), implying that circulating Tfh cells accumulate with sustained parasite exposure. However, whether or not the detected Tfh cells facilitate the induction of MBCs that confer protection to disease over time remains to be investigated in larger cohorts and different transmission settings. In addition, circulating follicular regulatory T (Tfr) cells have been postulated to interfere with Tfh cell responses to infection (110). Tfr cells expressing the inhibitory molecule CTLA-4, have been detected at increased frequencies after acute malaria in Malian children (110). Future studies will be important in determining if the transition between susceptibility to clinical disease and asymptomatic infection is associated with the development of functional Tfh cell responses that support the induction of B cell memory populations.

Similar to human malaria, $CD4^+$ T cells induced by murine infection have been described to express a dual Th1- and Tfh-associated phenotype, including chemokine receptor CXCR5, and cytokines IL-21 and IFN-γ (99, 111, 112). Precursor Tfh cells induced in response to *P. berghei* severe malaria infection also display a Th1 cell-like phenotype, characterized by the upregulation the chemokine receptor CXCR3 and transcription factor T-bet (113). Moreover, the expression of T-bet impaired the differentiation of Tfh cell precursors into mature Tfh cells, which significantly suppressed the development of GC B cells, plasma cells and MBCs (113). Notably, genetic ablation of T-bet or neutralization of the pro-inflammatory cytokines interferon (IFN)-γ and tumor necrosis factor (TNF) promoted Tfh cell differentiation, and restored previously impaired GC responses, demonstrating that inflammatory responses associated with the induction of symptomatic malaria reduce the magnitude of MBC responses by modulating effective Tfh cell development (114). In support of this concept, exogenous IFN-γ has been shown to reduce Tfh and GC B cell responses to *Plasmodium yoelii* (102), and the blockade of CXCR3-mediated signals was found to enhance precursor Tfh cell accumulation in the spleen of malaria-infected mice, thereby favoring parasitic clearance (115). Other inflammatory pathways such as type I IFN signals have also been recognized to indirectly limit Tfh and GC B cell responses to infection (116, 117), although the precise mechanisms by which this occurs is not yet clear. Recent studies suggest that the damage-signal sensor P2X7 (118), IFN regulatory factor 3 (119), and changes in metabolism and proliferation, as well as altered gene expression of chemokine receptors (120) influence the bifurcation of Tfh and Th1 cell differentiation during murine infection. Whereas, inflammatory responses to malaria appear to dampen the magnitude of the MBC response to infection (114), effective control of blood-stage malaria and its associated pro-inflammatory responses appears to permits normal progression of Tfh cell development (113, 121), giving rise to T cell memory that responds to secondary infection (112).

Whereas, it is reasonable to assume that the aforementioned modulation of Tfh cell function by inflammatory pathways elicited in response to infection is responsible for the reduced B cell responses observed during acute infection, a direct effect of IFN-γ-mediated signaling or intrinsic expression of T-bet in B cells cannot be ruled out. *P. yoelii* infection has recently been shown to induce a subset of B cells to express the transcription factor T-bet, and deletion of B cell-specific IFN-γ receptor or T-bet deletion elevated antibody responses to infection (122, 123). Further work to establish if inflammation directly modulates the differentiation and functional capacity of B cells is needed to address this question.

ATYPICAL MEMORY B CELLS: FRIENDS OR FOES?

There is evidence that *Plasmodium* parasites can directly modulate B cell function. *In vitro* studies have shown that the parasite can directly activate human naive B cells via a cysteine rich inter-domain region of *P. falciparum* erythrocyte membrane protein 1 (124, 125) and downstream toll-like receptor signaling (126), which may lead to non-specific polyclonal activation of B cell responses. CD27-expressing B cells were observed to be the major responding population (124, 125), suggesting a potential impact on the MBC compartment. In line with this idea, acute *P. falciparum* infection has been reported to modulate systemic mediators of B cell activation and survival (127, 128), which has been associated with an early proliferation of MBC subsets, prior to the induction of GC responses following experimental human infection (128), supporting a potential role of bystander activation of non-specific MBC subsets that enables parasite evasion.

Insight into the notion that B cell memory induction in malaria may be dysregulated surfaced upon the characterization of an expansion of MBCs exhibiting an atypical phenotype following persistent malaria exposure (17, 84, 129, 130). Originally described as an exhausted subset of MBCs implicated in humoral deficiencies in HIV infection (131), a phenotypically similar $CD27^-CD21^-$ circulating MBC subset notable for their expression of inhibitory receptors, was detected in *Plasmodium*-infected individuals following acute malaria in Brazil (109), Gabon (132), Ghana (85), Gambia (77), India (133), Kenya (84, 130), Mali (15, 17, 129, 134, 135), Papua New Guinea (136, 137), Thailand (78), and Uganda (16, 73, 138), and further exacerbated by HIV co-infection (139, 140). Studies to date corroborate that the accumulation of this subset is influenced by the level of parasite exposure. Higher frequencies of atypical MBCs were found in adults compared to children with shorter exposure histories (17). Similarly, Malian adults from high transmission settings were found to have higher frequencies of these cells than Peruvian individuals residing in a low transmission area (129). A decline in the atypical MBC pool was observed during 12 months without malaria transmission (84), further substantiating a role of persistent parasite exposure in the maintenance of this population.

Recent work has investigated the function of these atypical MBCs and their relationship to classical MBCs. Evaluation of the variable gene repertoires of atypical MBCs proposed that they share a common developmental precursor to classical MBCs (15, 132, 141), however, emerging work support that atypical MBCs are phenotypically and functionally different to classical MBCs. There is still conflicting evidence on the effector capacity of atypical MBCs from malaria-infected individuals. Whereas, some support the notion that atypical MBCs are capable of secreting neutralizing antibodies (132), subsequent work contend their lack of active antibody secretion (15, 16). Atypical MBCs have been reported to express lower levels of surface IgG (136), possess reduced B cell receptor signaling, as well as impaired interleukin (IL)-6, IL-8 and antibody production *in vitro* (15, 16). Atypical MBC frequencies in malaria-exposed individuals have been shown to be positively correlated with pro-inflammatory cytokine levels such as IL-8 (136), and their expression of the inhibitory molecule FcRL5 has been proposed to be a marker of dysfunction associated with increased malaria exposure (16). FcRL5-expressing atypical-like MBCs in healthy individuals have been distinguished by their higher expression of inhibitory receptors such as PD-1 and transcription factors *Tbx21, Bcl-6*, and *Sox5* and blunted proliferation capacity compared to $FcRL5^{-}$ B cells (142). In line with these findings, recent studies revealed that atypical MBCs in Malian children express *Tbx21* (134), which encodes the Th1 transcription factor T-bet (143). Emerging evidence that T-bet becomes up-regulated in various disease contexts in subsets of B cells that share many features in common with atypical MBCs found in malaria-infected individuals. T-bet-expressing B cells have been associated with both protective and pathogenic roles depending on specific settings, which include bacterial (21), parasitic (144–146) and viral infection (147–153), cancer (154–156), autoimmune conditions (157–164), and aging (165). In malaria, atypical MBCs expressing high levels of T-bet have also been found to express decreased levels of the co-stimulatory molecule CD40 and reduced phosphorylation of B cell receptor signaling molecules (134), suggesting that T-bet expression might reduce B cell effector function. In line with this concept, the frequency of malaria episodes was found to be associated with increased $T\text{-}bet^{hi}$ MBC in a small group of children (134). On the other hand, longitudinal cohort studies have reported that low parasite density malaria is associated with persistence (78) or accumulation of atypical MBCs over time, which raises the possibility that atypical MBCs contribute to developing immunity (73, 138), although T-bet expression was not examined in these cells. Furthermore, similar atypical MBCs that express FcRL5 have been recently detected in *P. chabaudi*-infected mice (166, 167), but appear to display normal features of proliferation and Ig expression, representing a short-lived population of activated MBCs (167). Collectively, a causal relationship between atypical MBCs and immune protection or disease progression remains unclear, and more studies are urgently needed to determine the functional significance of atypical MBC expansion in the acquisition of humoral immunity to malaria and the precise contribution of the transcription factor T-bet in shaping atypical MBC function.

CONCLUDING REMARKS AND FUTURE PERSPECTIVES

Emerging evidence both in human field studies and murine infection models are beginning to address how the induction of humoral immune responses is compromised during acute malaria, and the consequences of these processes for the establishment of long-term immunological B cell memory. There is now considerable evidence that exposure to *Plasmodium* parasites is associated with altered proportions of circulating memory B cells, including an expansion of atypical memory B cells. Further studies to unravel the complexity of this diverse memory B cell compartment, in terms of origin, function and protective capacity of different subpopulations are urgently needed. Information about the level of homology between human and mouse memory B cell subsets is lacking, particularly in relation to their surface marker expression patterns, which makes it difficult to infer how findings in malaria infection models translate into human settings. Gene expression analysis studies, including how transcription factors and the cytokine environment influence these processes might be required to overcome these issues and establish functional correlations between human studies and much needed mechanistic work in mice.

Given the critical importance of antibodies and long-lived humoral memory in immunity to malaria, an in-depth understanding of the factors that delay their development is undoubtedly required to inform the design of targeted therapeutic strategies to enhance immune responses to the parasite and protect against disease susceptibility. Detailed characterization of the immune processes by which B cell memory to malaria is generated and the specific effector populations required to confer protection, will undoubtedly benefit vaccine development and optimisation efforts, especially in light of the modest efficacy levels achieved to date with current vaccination regimes at a population level (168, 169).

AUTHOR CONTRIBUTIONS

All authors listed have made a substantial, direct and intellectual contribution to the work, and approved it for publication.

REFERENCES

1. De Silva NS, Klein U. Dynamics of B cells in germinal centres. *Nat Rev Immunol.* (2015) 15:137–48. doi: 10.1038/nri3804
2. Weisel FJ, Zuccarino-Catania GV, Chikina M, Shlomchik MJ. A temporal switch in the germinal center determines differential output of memory B and plasma cells. *Immunity.* (2016) 44:116–30. doi: 10.1016/j.immuni.2015.12.004
3. Jacob J, Kelsoe G. *In situ* studies of the primary immune response to (4-hydroxy-3-nitrophenyl)acetyl. II. A common clonal origin for periarteriolar lymphoid sheath-associated foci and germinal centers. *J Exp Med.* (1992) 176:679–87.
4. Allen CDC, Okada T, Tang HL, Cyster JG. Imaging of germinal center selection events during affinity maturation. *Science.* (2007) 315:528–31. doi: 10.1126/science.1136736

5. Victora GD, Schwickert TA, Fooksman DR, Kamphorst AO, Meyer-Hermann M, Dustin ML, et al. Germinal center dynamics revealed by multiphoton microscopy with a photoactivatable fluorescent reporter. *Cell.* (2010) 143:592–605. doi: 10.1016/j.cell.2010.10.032
6. Gitlin AD, Shulman Z, Nussenzweig MC. Clonal selection in the germinal centre by regulated proliferation and hypermutation. *Nature.* (2014) 509:637–40. doi: 10.1038/nature13300
7. Slifka MK, Antia R, Whitmire JK, Ahmed R. Humoral immunity due to long-lived plasma cells. *Immunity.* (1998) 8:363–72.
8. Anderson SM, Tomayko MM, Ahuja A, Haberman AM, Shlomchik MJ. New markers for murine memory B cells that define mutated and unmutated subsets. *J Exp Med.* (2007) 204:2103–14. doi: 10.1084/jem.20062571
9. Good KL, Avery DT, Tangye SG. Resting human memory B cells are intrinsically programmed for enhanced survival and responsiveness to diverse stimuli compared to naive B cells. *J Immunol.* (2009) 182:890–901. doi: 10.4049/jimmunol.182.2.890
10. Tangye SG, Avery DT, Deenick EK, Hodgkin PD. Intrinsic differences in the proliferation of naive and memory human B cells as a mechanism for enhanced secondary immune responses. *J Immunol.* (2003) 170:686–94. doi: 10.4049/jimmunol.170.2.686
11. Weisel F, Shlomchik M. Memory B cells of mice and humans. *Ann Rev Immunol.* (2017) 35:255–84. doi: 10.1146/annurev-immunol-041015-055531
12. Klein U, Kuppers R, Rajewsky K. Evidence for a large compartment of IgM-expressing memory B cells in humans. *Blood.* (1997) 89:1288–98.
13. Tangye SG, Liu YJ, Aversa G, Phillips JH, de Vries JE. Identification of functional human splenic memory B cells by expression of CD148 and CD27. *J Exp Med.* (1998) 188:1691–703.
14. Ehrhardt GRA, Hsu JT, Gartland L, Leu C-M, Zhang S, Davis RS, et al. Expression of the immunoregulatory molecule FcRH4 defines a distinctive tissue-based population of memory B cells. *J Exp Med.* (2005) 202:783–91. doi: 10.1084/jem.20050879
15. Portugal S, Tipton CM, Sohn H, Kone Y, Wang J, Li S, et al. Malaria-associated atypical memory B cells exhibit markedly reduced B cell receptor signaling and effector function. *Elife.* (2015) 4:1748. doi: 10.7554/eLife.07218
16. Sullivan RT, Kim CC, Fontana MF, Feeney ME, Jagannathan P, Boyle MJ, et al. FCRL5 delineates functionally impaired memory B cells associated with *Plasmodium falciparum* exposure. *PLoS Pathog.* (2015) 11:e1004894. doi: 10.1371/journal.ppat.1004894
17. Weiss GE, Crompton PD, Li S, Walsh LA, Moir S, Traore B, et al. Atypical memory B cells are greatly expanded in individuals living in a malaria-endemic area. *J Immunol.* (2009) 183:2176–82. doi: 10.4049/jimmunol.0901297
18. Dogan I, Bertocci B, Vilmont V, Delbos F, Mégret J, Storck S, et al. Multiple layers of B cell memory with different effector functions. *Nat Immunol.* (2009) 10:1292–9. doi: 10.1038/ni.1814
19. Pape KA, Taylor JJ, Maul RW, Gearhart PJ, Jenkins MK. Different B cell populations mediate early and late memory during an endogenous immune response. *Science.* (2011) 331:1203–7. doi: 10.1126/science.1201730
20. Zuccarino-Catania GV, Sadanand S, Weisel FJ, Tomayko MM, Meng H, Kleinstein SH, et al. CD80 and PD-L2 define functionally distinct memory B cell subsets that are independent of antibody isotype. *Nat Immunol.* (2014) 15:631–7. doi: 10.1038/ni.2914
21. Kenderes KJ, Levack RC, Papillion AM, Cabrera-Martinez B, Dishaw LM, Winslow GM. T-Bet$^+$ IgM memory cells generate multi-lineage effector B cells. *Cell Rep.* (2018) 24:824–37.e3. doi: 10.1016/j.celrep.2018.06.074
22. World Health Organization. *World Malaria Report 2016* (2016).
23. White NJ, Pukrittayakamee S, Hien TT, Faiz MA, Mokuolu OA, Dondorp AM. Malaria. *Lancet.* (2014) 383:723–35. doi: 10.1016/S0140-6736(13)60024-0
24. Schofield L, Grau GE. Immunological processes in malaria pathogenesis. *Nat Rev Immunol.* (2005) 5:722–35. doi: 10.1038/nri1686
25. Miller LH, Ackerman HC, Su X-Z, Wellems TE. Malaria biology and disease pathogenesis: insights for new treatments. *Nat Med.* (2013) 19:156–67. doi: 10.1038/nm.3073
26. Koch R. Professor Koch's investigations on malaria: fourth report to the colonial department of the german colonial office. *Br Med J.* (1900) 1:1597–8.
27. Gupta S, Snow RW, Donnelly CA, Marsh K, Newbold C. Immunity to non cerebral severe malaria is acquired after one or two infections. *Nat Med.* (1999) 5:340–3. doi: 10.1038/6560
28. Reyburn H, Mbatia R, Drakeley C, Bruce J, Carneiro I, Olomi R, et al. Association of transmission intensity and age with clinical manifestations and case fatality of severe *Plasmodium falciparum* malaria. *JAMA.* (2005) 293:1461–70. doi: 10.1001/jama.293.12.1461
29. Griffin JT, Hollingsworth TD, Reyburn H, Drakeley CJ, Riley EM, Ghani AC. Gradual acquisition of immunity to severe malaria with increasing exposure. *Proc R Soc B.* (2015) 282:20142657. doi: 10.1098/rspb.2014.2657
30. Bejon P, Warimwe G, Mackintosh CL, Mackinnon MJ, Kinyanjui SM, Musyoki JN, et al. Analysis of immunity to febrile malaria in children that distinguishes immunity from lack of exposure. *Infect Immun.* (2009) 77:1917–23. doi: 10.1128/IAI.01358-08
31. McGregor IA, Smith DA. A health, nutrition and parasitological survey in a rural village (Keneba) in west Kiang, Gambia. *Trans R Soc Trop Med Hyg.* (1952) 46:403–27.
32. Drakeley CJ, Carneiro I, Reyburn H, Malima R, Lusingu JPA, Cox J, et al. Altitude-dependent and -independent variations in *Plasmodium falciparum* prevalence in northeastern Tanzania. *J Infect Dis.* (2005) 191:1589–98. doi: 10.1086/429669
33. Michon P, Cole-Tobian JL, Dabod E, Schoepflin S, Igu J, Susapu M, et al. The risk of malarial infections and disease in Papua New Guinean children. *Am J Trop Med Hyg.* (2007) 76:997–1008. doi: 10.4269/ajtmh.2007.76.997
34. Ndungu FM, Marsh K, Fegan G, Wambua J, Nyangweso G, Ogada E, et al. Identifying children with excess malaria episodes after adjusting for variation in exposure: identification from a longitudinal study using statistical count models. *BMC Med.* (2015) 13:183. doi: 10.1186/s12916-015-0422-4
35. Bouchaud O, Cot M, Kony S, Durand R, Schiemann R, Ralaimazava P, et al. Do African immigrants living in France have long-term malarial immunity? *Am J Trop Med Hyg.* (2005) 72:21–5. doi: 10.4269/ajtmh.2005.72.21
36. Tran TM, Li S, Doumbo S, Doumtabe D, Huang C-Y, Dia S, et al. An intensive longitudinal cohort study of malian children and adults reveals no evidence of acquired immunity to *Plasmodium falciparum* infection. *Clin Infect Dis.* (2013) 57:40–7. doi: 10.1093/cid/cit174
37. Okell LC, Bousema T, Griffin JT, Ouedraogo AL, Ghani AC, Drakeley CJ. Factors determining the occurrence of submicroscopic malaria infections and their relevance for control. *Nat Commun.* (2012) 3:1237. doi: 10.1038/ncomms2241
38. Cohen S, Carrington S, McGregor IA. Gamma-globulin and acquired immunity to human malaria. *Nature.* (1961) 192:733–7.
39. McGregor IA, Carrington SP, Cohen S. Treatment of East African *P. falciparum* malaria with West African human γ-globulin. *Trans R Soc Trop Med Hyg.* (1963) 57:170–5. doi: 10.1016/0035-9203(63)90058-0
40. Chiu CYH, Hodder AN, Lin CS, Hill DL, Li Wai Suen CSN, Schofield L, et al. Antibodies to the *Plasmodium falciparum* proteins MSPDBL1 and MSPDBL2 opsonize merozoites, inhibit parasite growth, and predict protection from clinical malaria. *J Infect Dis.* (2015) 212:406–15. doi: 10.1093/infdis/jiv057
41. Chiu CYH, Healer J, Thompson JK, Chen L, Kaul A, Savergave L, et a Association of antibodies to *Plasmodium falciparum* reticulocyte binding protein homolog 5 with protection from clinical malaria. *Front Microbiol.* (2014) 5:314. doi: 10.3389/fmicb.2014.00314
42. Richards JS, Stanisic DI, Fowkes FJI, Tavul L, Dabod E, Thompson JK, et al. Association between naturally acquired antibodies to erythrocyte-binding antigens of *Plasmodium falciparum* and protection from malaria and high-density parasitemia. *Clin Infect Dis.* (2010) 51:e50–60. doi: 10.1086/656413
43. Fowkes FJI, Richards JS, Simpson JA, Beeson JG. The relationship between anti-merozoite antibodies and incidence of *Plasmodium falciparum* malaria: a systematic review and meta-analysis. *PLoS Med.* (2010) 7:e1000218–94. doi: 10.1371/journal.pmed.1000218
44. Stanisic DI, Richards JS, McCallum FJ, Michon P, King CL, Schoepflin S, et al. Immunoglobulin G subclass-specific responses against *Plasmodium falciparum* merozoite antigens are associated with control of parasitemia and protection from symptomatic illness. *Infect Immun.* (2009) 77:1165–74. doi: 10.1128/IAI.01129-08

45. John CC, O'Donnell RA, Sumba PO, Moormann AM, de Koning-Ward TF, King CL, et al. Evidence that invasion-inhibitory antibodies specific for the 19-kDa fragment of merozoite surface protein-1 (MSP-1 19) can play a protective role against blood-stage *Plasmodium falciparum* infection in individuals in a malaria endemic area of Africa. *J Immunol.* (2004) 173:666–72. doi: 10.4049/jimmunol.173.1.666
46. Dodoo D, Staalsoe T, Giha H, Kurtzhals JA, Akanmori BD, Koram K, et al. Antibodies to variant antigens on the surfaces of infected erythrocytes are associated with protection from malaria in Ghanaian children. *Infect Immun.* (2001) 69:3713–8. doi: 10.1128/IAI.69.6.3713-3718.2001
47. Teo A, Feng G, Brown GV, Beeson JG, Rogerson SJ. Functional antibodies and protection against blood-stage malaria. *Trends Parasitol.* (2016) 32:887–98. doi: 10.1016/j.pt.2016.07.003
48. Chan J-A, Howell KB, Reiling L, Ataide R, Mackintosh CL, Fowkes FJI, et al. Targets of antibodies against *Plasmodium falciparum*-infected erythrocytes in malaria immunity. *J Clin Invest.* (2012) 122:3227–38. doi: 10.1172/JCI62182
49. Scherf A, Lopez-Rubio JJ, Riviere L. Antigenic variation in *Plasmodium falciparum. Annu Rev Microbiol.* (2008) 62:445–70. doi: 10.1146/annurev.micro.61.080706.093134
50. Mackintosh CL, Mwangi T, Kinyanjui SM, Mosobo M, Pinches R, Williams TN, et al. Failure to respond to the surface of *Plasmodium falciparum* infected erythrocytes predicts susceptibility to clinical malaria amongst African children. *Int J Parasitol.* (2008) 38:1445–54. doi: 10.1016/j.ijpara.2008.03.009
51. Kinyanjui SM, Mwangi T, Bull PC, Newbold CI, Marsh K. Protection against clinical malaria by heterologous immunoglobulin G antibodies against malaria-infected erythrocyte variant surface antigens requires interaction with asymptomatic infections. *J Infect Dis.* (2004) 190:1527–33. doi: 10.1086/424675
52. Sondén K, Doumbo S, Hammar U, Homann MV, Ongoiba A, Traore B, et al. Asymptomatic multiclonal *Plasmodium falciparum* infections carried through the dry season predict protection against subsequent clinical malaria. *J Infect Dis.* (2015) 212:jiv088–616. doi: 10.1093/infdis/jiv088
53. King CL, Davies DH, Felgner P, Baum E, Jain A, Randall A, et al. Biosignatures of exposure/transmission and immunity. *Am J Trop Med Hyg.* (2015) 93:16–27. doi: 10.4269/ajtmh.15-0037
54. Murungi LM, Kamuyu G, Lowe B, Bejon P, Theisen M, Kinyanjui SM, et al. A threshold concentration of anti-merozoite antibodies is required for protection from clinical episodes of malaria. *Vaccine.* (2013) 31:3936–42. doi: 10.1016/j.vaccine.2013.06.042
55. Arama C, Skinner J, Doumtabe D, Portugal S, Tran TM, Jain A, et al. Genetic resistance to malaria is associated with greater enhancement of immunoglobulin (Ig)M than IgG responses to a broad array of *Plasmodium falciparum* antigens. *Open Forum Infect Dis.* (2015) 2:ofv118. doi: 10.1093/ofid/ofv118
56. Crompton PD, Kayala MA, Traore B, Kayentao K, Ongoiba A, Weiss GE, et al. A prospective analysis of the Ab response to *Plasmodium falciparum* before and after a malaria season by protein microarray. *Proc Natl Acad Sci USA.* (2010) 107:6958–63. doi: 10.1073/pnas.1001323107
57. Weiss GE, Traore B, Kayentao K, Ongoiba A, Doumbo S, Doumtabe D, et al. The *Plasmodium falciparum*-specific human memory B cell compartment expands gradually with repeated malaria infections. *PLoS Pathog.* (2010) 6:e1000912. doi: 10.1371/journal.ppat.1000912
58. Finney OC, Danziger SA, Molina DM, Vignali M, Takagi A, Ji M, et al. Predicting antidisease immunity using proteome arrays and sera from children naturally exposed to malaria. *Mol Cell Proteomics.* (2014) 13:2646–60. doi: 10.1074/mcp.M113.036632
59. Wendel, He C, Qu M, Di Wu, Hernandez SM, Ma K-Y, et al. Accurate immune repertoire sequencing reveals malaria infection driven antibody lineage diversification in young children. *Nat Commun.* (2017) 8:1–14. doi: 10.1038/s41467-017-00645-x
60. Tan J, Pieper K, Piccoli L, Abdi A, Perez MF, Geiger R, et al. A LAIR1 insertion generates broadly reactive antibodies against malaria variant antigens. *Nature.* (2016) 529:105–9. doi: 10.1038/nature16450
61. Pieper K, Tan J, Piccoli L, Foglierini M, Barbieri S, Chen Y, et al. Public antibodies to malaria antigens generated by two LAIR1 insertion modalities. *Nature.* (2017) 548:597–601. doi: 10.1038/nature23670
62. Ceravolo IP, Sanchez BAM, Sousa TN, Guerra BM, Soares IS, Braga EM, et al. Naturally acquired inhibitory antibodies to *Plasmodium vivax* Duffy binding protein are short-lived and allele-specific following a single malaria infection. *Clin Exp Immunol.* (2009) 156:502–10. doi: 10.1111/j.1365-2249.2009.03931.x
63. Fruh K, Doumbo O, Muller HM, Koita O, McBride J, Crisanti A, et al. Human antibody response to the major merozoite surface antigen of *Plasmodium falciparum* is strain specific and short-lived. *Infect Immun.* (1991) 59:1319–24.
64. Cavanagh DR, Dodoo D, Hviid L, Kurtzhals JA, Theander TG, Akanmori BD, et al. Antibodies to the N-terminal block 2 of *Plasmodium falciparum* merozoite surface protein 1 are associated with protection against clinical malaria. *Infect Immun.* (2004) 72:6492–502. doi: 10.1128/iai.72.11.6492-6502.2004
65. Cavanagh DR, Elhassan IM, Roper C, Robinson VJ, Giha H, Holder AA, et al. A longitudinal study of type-specific antibody responses to *Plasmodium falciparum* merozoite surface protein-1 in an area of unstable malaria in Sudan. *J Immunol.* (1998) 161:347–59.
66. Soares IS, Oliveira SG, Souza JM, Rodrigues MM. Antibody response to the N and C-terminal regions of the *Plasmodium vivax* Merozoite Surface Protein 1 in individuals living in an area of exclusive transmission of P-vivax malaria in the north of Brazil. *Acta Trop.* (1999) 72:13–24.
67. Kinyanjui SM, Conway DJ, Lanar DE, Marsh K. IgG antibody responses to *Plasmodium falciparum* merozoite antigens in Kenyan children have a short half-life. *Malar J.* (2007) 6:82. doi: 10.1186/1475-2875-6-82
68. Akpogheneta OJ, Duah NO, Tetteh KKA, Dunyo S, Lanar DE, Pinder M, et al. Duration of naturally acquired antibody responses to blood-stage *Plasmodium falciparum* is age dependent and antigen specific. *Infect Immun.* (2008) 76:1748–55. doi: 10.1128/IAI.01333-07
69. Fonjungo PN, Elhassan IM, Cavanagh DR, Theander TG, Hviid L, Roper C, et al. A longitudinal study of human antibody responses to *Plasmodium falciparum* rhoptry-associated protein 1 in a region of seasonal and unstable malaria transmission. *Infect Immunol.* (1999) 67:2975–85.
70. Maple PA, Jones CS, Wall EC, Vyseb A, Edmunds WJ, Andrews NJ, et al. Immunity to diphtheria and tetanus in England and Wales. *Vaccine.* (2000) 19:167–73. doi: 10.1016/s0264-410x(00)00184-5
71. Hammarlund E, Lewis MW, Hansen SG, Strelow LI, Nelson JA, Sexton GJ, et al. Duration of antiviral immunity after smallpox vaccination. *Nat Med.* (2003) 9:1131–7. doi: 10.1038/nm917
72. Amanna IJ, Carlson NE, Slifka MK. Duration of humoral immunity to common viral and vaccine antigens. *N Engl J Med.* (2007) 357:1903–15. doi: 10.1056/NEJMoa066092
73. Sullivan RT, Ssewanyana I, Wamala S, Nankya F, Jagannathan P, Tappero JW, et al. B cell sub-types following acute malaria and associations with clinical immunity. *Malar J.* (2016) 15:139. doi: 10.1186/s12936-016-1190-0
74. White MT, Griffin JT, Akpogheneta O, Conway DJ, Koram KA, Riley EM, et al. Dynamics of the antibody response to *Plasmodium falciparum* infection in African children. *J Infect Dis.* (2014) 210:1115–22. doi: 10.1093/infdis/jiu219
75. Dorfman JR, Bejon P, Ndungu FM, Langhorne J, Kortok MM, Lowe BS, et al. B cell memory to 3 *Plasmodium falciparum* blood-stage antigens in a malaria-endemic area. *J Infect Dis.* (2005) 191:1623–30. doi: 10.1086/429671
76. Triller G, Scally SW, Costa G, Pissarev M, Kreschel C, Bosch A, et al. Natural parasite exposure induces protective human anti-malarial antibodies. *Immunity.* (2017) 47:1197–209.e10. doi: 10.1016/j.immuni.2017.11.007
77. Nogaro SI, Hafalla JC, Walther B, Remarque EJ, Tetteh KK, Conway DJ, et al. The breadth, but not the magnitude, of circulating memory B cell responses to *P. falciparum* increases with age/exposure in an area of low transmission. *PLoS ONE.* (2011) 6:e25582. doi: 10.1371/journal.pone.0025582
78. Changrob S, McHenry AM, Nyunt MH, Sattabongkot J, Han E-T, Adams JH, et al. Persistence of long-lived memory B cells specific to duffy binding protein in individuals exposed to *Plasmodium vivax. Sci Rep.* (2018) 8:8347. doi: 10.1038/s41598-018-26677-x
79. Min HMK, Changrob S, Soe PT, Han JH, Muh F, Lee S-K, et al. Immunogenicity of the *Plasmodium vivax* merozoite surface protein 1 paralog in the induction of naturally acquired antibody and memory B cell responses. *Malar J.* (2017) 16:354. doi: 10.1186/s12936-017-2000-z

80. Migot F, Chougnet C, Henzel D, Dubois B, Jambou R, Fievet N, et al. Anti-malaria antibody-producing B cell frequencies in adults after a *Plasmodium falciparum* outbreak in Madagascar. *Clin Exp Immunol.* (1995) 102:529–34.
81. Wipasa J, Suphavilai C, Okell LC, Cook J, Corran PH, Thaikla K, et al. Long-lived antibody and B Cell memory responses to the human malaria parasites, *Plasmodium falciparum* and *Plasmodium vivax. PLoS Pathog.* (2010) 6:e1000770. doi: 10.1371/journal.ppat.1000770
82. Clark EH, Silva CJ, Weiss GE, Li S, Padilla C, Crompton PD, et al. *Plasmodium falciparum* malaria in the Peruvian Amazon, a region of low transmission, is associated with immunologic memory. *Infect Immun.* (2012) 80:1583–92. doi: 10.1128/IAI.05961-11
83. Ndungu FM, Olotu A, Mwacharo J, Nyonda M, Apfeld J, Mramba LK, et al. Memory B cells are a more reliable archive for historical antimalarial responses than plasma antibodies in no-longer exposed children. *Proc Natl Acad Sci USA.* (2012) 109:8247–52. doi: 10.1073/pnas.1200472109
84. Ayieko C, Maue AC, Jura WGZO, Noland GS, Ayodo G, Rochford R, et al. Changes in B cell populations and merozoite surface protein-1-specific memory B cell responses after prolonged absence of detectable *P. falciparum* infection. *PLoS ONE.* (2013) 8:e67230. doi: 10.1371/journal.pone.0067230
85. Ampomah P, Stevenson L, Ofori MF, Barfod L, Hviid L. B-cell responses to pregnancy-restricted and -unrestricted *Plasmodium falciparum* erythrocyte membrane protein 1 antigens in Ghanaian women naturally exposed to malaria parasites. *Infect Immunol.* (2014) 82:1860–71. doi: 10.1128/IAI.01514-13
86. Moncunill G, Mayor A, Jiménez A, Nhabomba A, Casas-Vila N, Puyol L, et al. High antibody responses against *Plasmodium falciparum* in immigrants after extended periods of interrupted exposure to malaria. *PLoS ONE.* (2013) 8:e73624. doi: 10.1371/journal.pone.0073624
87. Torres KJ, Clark EH, Hernandez JN, Soto-Cornejo KE, Gamboa D, Branch OH. Antibody response dynamics to the *Plasmodium falciparum* conserved vaccine candidate antigen, merozoite surface protein-1 C-terminal 19kD (MSP1-19kD), in Peruvians exposed to hypoendemic malaria transmission. *Malar J.* (2008) 7:173. doi: 10.1186/1475-2875-7-173
88. Bousema T, Roeffen W, Meijerink H, Mwerinde H, Mwakalinga S, van Gemert G-J, et al. The dynamics of naturally acquired immune responses to *Plasmodium falciparum* sexual stage antigens Pfs230 & Pfs48/45 in a low endemic area in tanzania. *PLoS ONE.* (2010) 5:e14114. doi: 10.1371/journal.pone.0014114
89. Krishnamurty AT, Thouvenel CD, Portugal S, Keitany GJ, Kim KS, Holder A, et al. Somatically hypermutated *Plasmodium*-specific IgM^+ memory B cells are rapid, plastic, early responders upon malaria rechallenge. *Immunity.* (2016) 45:402–14. doi: 10.1016/j.immuni.2016.06.014
90. Stephens R, Ndungu FM, Langhorne J. Germinal centre and marginal zone B cells expand quickly in a second *Plasmodium chabaudi* malaria infection producing mature plasma cells. *Parasite Immunol.* (2009) 31:20–31. doi: 10.1111/j.1365-3024.2008.01066.x
91. Craig AG, Grau GE, Janse C, Kazura JW, Milner D, Barnwell JW, et al. The role of animal models for research on severe malaria. *PLoS Pathog.* (2012) 8:e1002401. doi: 10.1371/journal.ppat.1002401
92. Stephens R, Culleton RL, Lamb TJ. The contribution of *Plasmodium chabaudi* to our understanding of malaria. *Trends Parasitol.* (2012) 28:73–82. doi: 10.1016/j.pt.2011.10.006
93. Castillo-Méndez SI, Castillo-Méndez SI, Zago CA, Zago CA, Sardinha LR, Sardinha LR, et al. Characterization of the spleen B-cell compartment at the early and late blood-stage *Plasmodium chabaudi* malaria. *Scand J Immunol.* (2007) 66:309–19. doi: 10.1111/j.1365-3083.2007.01972.x
94. Ndungu FM, Cadman ET, Coulcher J, Nduati E, Couper E, Macdonald DW, et al. Functional memory B cells and long-lived plasma cells are generated after a single *Plasmodium chabaudi* infection in mice. *PLoS Pathog.* (2009) 5:e1000690. doi: 10.1371/journal.ppat.1000690
95. Achtman AH, Stephens R, Cadman ET, Harrison V, Langhorne J. Malaria-specific antibody responses and parasite persistence after infection of mice with *Plasmodium chabaudi chabaudi. Parasite Immunol.* (2007) 29:435–44. doi: 10.1111/j.1365-3024.2007.00960.x
96. Wykes MN, Zhou Y-H, Liu XQ, Good MF. *Plasmodium yoelii* can ablate vaccine-induced long-term protection in mice. *J Immunol.* (2005) 175:2510–6. doi: 10.4049/jimmunol.175.4.2510
97. Keitany GJ, Kim KS, Krishnamurty AT, Hondowicz BD, Hahn WO, Dambrauskas N, et al. Blood stage malaria disrupts humoral immunity to the pre-erythrocytic stage circumsporozoite protein. *Cell Rep.* (2016) 17:3193–205. doi: 10.1016/j.celrep.2016.11.060
98. Vinuesa CG, Linterman MA, Yu D, MacLennan ICM. Follicular helper T cells. *Ann Rev Immun.* (2016) 34:335–68. doi: 10.1146/annurev-immunol-041015-055605
99. Pérez-Mazliah D, Ng DHL, Freitas do Rosário AP, McLaughlin S, Mastelic-Gavillet B, Sodenkamp J, et al. Disruption of IL-21 signaling affects T cell-B cell interactions and abrogates protective humoral immunity to malaria. *PLoS Pathog.* (2015) 11:e1004715. doi: 10.1371/journal.ppat.1004715
100. Opata MM, Carpio VH, Ibitokou SA, Dillon BE, Obiero JM, Stephens R. Early Effector cells survive the contraction phase in malaria infection and generate both central and effector memory T cells. *J Immunol.* (2015) 194:5346–54. doi: 10.4049/jimmunol.1403216
101. Butler NS, Pewe LL, Traore B, Doumbo OK, Tygrett LT, Waldschmidt TJ, et al. Therapeutic blockade of PD-L1 and LAG-3 rapidly clears established blood-stage *Plasmodium* infection. *Nat Immunol.* (2011) 13:188–95. doi: 10.1038/ni.2180
102. Zander RA, Obeng-Adjei N, Guthmiller JJ, Kulu DI, Li J, Ongoiba A, et al. PD-1 co-inhibitory and OX40 co-stimulatory crosstalk regulates helper T cell differentiation and anti-*Plasmodium* humoral immunity. *Cell Host Microbe.* (2015) 17:628–41. doi: 10.1016/j.chom.2015.03.007
103. Hansen DS, Obeng-Adjei N, Ly A, Ioannidis LJ, Crompton PD. Emerging concepts in T follicular helper cell responses to malaria. *Int J Parasitol.* (2017) 47:105–10. doi: 10.1016/j.ijpara.2016.09.004
104. Wikenheiser DJ, Ghosh D, Kennedy B, Stumhofer JS. The costimulatory molecule ICOS regulates host Th1 and follicular Th cell differentiation in response to *Plasmodium chabaudi chabaudi* AS infection. *J Immunol.* (2015) 196:778–91. doi: 10.4049/jimmunol.1403206
105. Pérez-Mazliah D, Nguyen MP, Hosking C, McLaughlin S, Lewis MD, Tumwine I, et al. Follicular helper T cells are essential for the elimination of *Plasmodium* infection. *EBioMedicine.* (2017) 24:216–30. doi: 10.1016/j.ebiom.2017.08.030
106. Obeng-Adjei N, Portugal S, Tran TM, Yazew TB, Skinner J, Li S, et al. Circulating Th1-cell-type Tfh cells that exhibit impaired B cell help are preferentially activated during acute malaria in children. *Cell Rep.* (2015) 13:425–39. doi: 10.1016/j.celrep.2015.09.004
107. Locci M, Havenar-Daughton C, Landais E, Wu J, Kroenke MA, Arlehamn CL, et al. Human circulating $PD\text{-}1^+CXCR3^-CXCR5^+$ memory Tfh cells are highly functional and correlate with broadly neutralizing HIV antibody responses. *Immunity.* (2013) 39:758–69. doi: 10.1016/j.immuni.2013.08.031
108. He J, Tsai LM, Leong YA, Hu X, Ma CS, Chevalier N, et al. Circulating precursor $CCR7^{lo}PD\text{-}1^{hi}$ $CXCR^{5+}$ CD^{4+} T cells indicate Tfh cell activity and promote antibody responses upon antigen reexposure. *Immunity.* (2013) 39:770–81. doi: 10.1016/j.immuni.2013.09.007
109. Figueiredo MM, Costa PAC, Diniz SQ, Henriques PM, Kano FS, Tada MS, et al. T follicular helper cells regulate the activation of B lymphocytes and antibody production during *Plasmodium vivax* infection. *PLoS Pathog.* (2017) 13:e1006484–23. doi: 10.1371/journal.ppat.1006484
110. Kurup SP, Obeng-Adjei N, Anthony SM, Traore B, Doumbo OK, Butler NS, et al. Regulatory T cells impede acute and long-term immunity to blood-stage malaria through CTLA-4. *Nat Med.* (2017) 23:1220–5. doi: 10.1038/nm.4395
111. Carpio VH, Opata MM, Montañez ME, Banerjee PP, Dent AL, Stephens R. IFN-γ and IL-21 double producing T cells are Bcl6-independent and survive into the memory phase in *Plasmodium chabaudi* infection. *PLoS ONE.* (2015) 10:e0144654. doi: 10.1371/journal.pone.0144654
112. Zander RA, Vijay R, Pack AD, Guthmiller JJ, Graham AC, Lindner SE, et al. Th1-like *Plasmodium*-specific memory $CD4^+$ T cells support humoral immunity. *Cell Rep.* (2017) 21:1839–52. doi: 10.1016/j.celrep.2017.10.077
113. Ryg-Cornejo V, Ioannidis LJ, Ly A, Chiu CY, Tellier J, Hill DL, et al. Severe malaria infections impair germinal center responses by inhibiting T follicular helper cell differentiation. *Cell Rep.* (2016) 14:68–81. doi: 10.1016/j.celrep.2015.12.006
114. Ryg-Cornejo V, Ly A, Hansen DS. Immunological processes underlying the slow acquisition of humoral immunity to malaria. *Parasitology.* (2016) 143:199–207. doi: 10.1017/S0031182015001705

115. Ioannidis LJ, Nie CQ, Ly A, Ryg-Cornejo V, Chiu CY, Hansen DS. Monocyte- and neutrophil-derived CXCL10 impairs efficient control of blood-stage malaria infection and promotes severe disease. *J Immunol.* (2016) 196:1227–38. doi: 10.4049/jimmunol.1501562
116. Sebina I, James KR, Soon MSF, Fogg LG, Best SE, Labastida Rivera F de, et al. IFNAR1-signalling obstructs ICOS-mediated humoral immunity during non-lethal blood-stage *Plasmodium* infection. *PLoS Pathog.* (2016) 12:e1005999. doi: 10.1371/journal.ppat.1005999
117. Zander RA, Guthmiller JJ, Graham AC, Pope RL, Burke BE, Carr DJJ, et al. Type I interferons induce T regulatory 1 responses and restrict humoral immunity during experimental malaria. *PLoS Pathog.* (2016) 12:e1005945. doi: 10.1371/journal.ppat.1005945
118. Salles ÉM de, Menezes MN de, Siqueira R, Borges da Silva H, Amaral EP, Castillo-Méndez SI, et al. P2X7 receptor drives Th1 cell differentiation and controls the follicular helper T cell population to protect against *Plasmodium chabaudi* malaria. *PLoS Pathog.* (2017) 13:e1006595. doi: 10.1371/journal.ppat.1006595
119. James KR, Soon MSF, Sebina I, Fernandez-Ruiz D, Davey G, Liligeto UN, et al. IFN regulatory factor 3 balances Th1 and T follicular helper immunity during nonlethal blood-stage *Plasmodium* infection. *J Immunol.* (2018) 200:1443–56. doi: 10.4049/jimmunol.1700782
120. Lönnberg T, Svensson V, James KR, Fernandez-Ruiz D, Sebina I, Montandon R, et al. Single-cell RNA-seq and computational analysis using temporal mixture modelling resolves Th1/Tfh fate bifurcation in malaria. *Sci Immunol.* (2017) 2:eaal2192. doi: 10.1126/sciimmunol.aal2192
121. Hahn WO, Butler NS, Lindner SE, Akilesh HM, Sather DN, Kappe SHI, et al. cGAS-mediated control of blood-stage malaria promotes *Plasmodium*-specific germinal center responses. *JCI Insight.* (2018) 3:1–18. doi: 10.1172/jci.insight.94142
122. Rivera-Correa J, Guthmiller JJ, Vijay R, Fernandez-Arias C, Pardo-Ruge MA, Gonzalez S, et al. *Plasmodium* DNA-mediated TLR9 activation of T-bet$^+$ B cells contributes to autoimmune anaemia during malaria. *Nat Commun.* (2017) 8:584. doi: 10.1038/s41467-017-01476-6
123. Guthmiller JJ, Graham AC, Zander RA, Pope RL, Butler NS. Cutting edge: IL-10 is essential for the generation of germinal center B cell responses and anti-*Plasmodium* humoral immunity. *J Immunol.* (2017) 198:617–22. doi: 10.4049/jimmunol.1601762
124. Donati D, Zhang LP, Chêne A, Chen Q, Flick K, Nyström M, et al. Identification of a polyclonal B-cell activator in *Plasmodium falciparum*. *Infect Immun.* (2004) 72:5412–8. doi: 10.1128/IAI.72.9.5412-5418.2004
125. Donati D, Mok B, Chêne A, Xu H, Thangarajh M, Glas R, et al. Increased B cell survival and preferential activation of the memory compartment by a malaria polyclonal B cell activator. *J Immunol.* (2006) 177:3035–44. doi: 10.4049/jimmunol.177.5.3035
126. Simone O, Bejarano MT, Pierce SK, Antonaci S, Wahlgren M, Troye-Blomberg M, et al. TLRs innate immunereceptors and *Plasmodium falciparum* erythrocyte membrane protein 1 (PfEMP1) CIDR1 alpha-driven human polyclonal B-cell activation. *Acta Trop.* (2011) 119:144–50. doi: 10.1016/j.actatropica.2011.05.005
127. Nduati E, Gwela A, Karanja H, Mugyenyi C, Langhorne J, Marsh K, et al. The plasma concentration of the B cell activating factor is increased in children with acute malaria. *J Infect Dis.* (2011) 204:962–70. doi: 10.1093/infdis/jir438
128. Scholzen A, Teirlinck AC, Bijker EM, Roestenberg M, Hermsen CC, Hoffman SL, et al. BAFF and BAFF receptor levels correlate with B cell subset activation and redistribution in controlled human malaria infection. *J Immunol.* (2014) 192:3719–29. doi: 10.4049/jimmunol.1302960
129. Weiss GE, Clark EH, Li S, Traore B, Kayentao K, Ongoiba A, et al. A positive correlation between atypical memory B cells and *Plasmodium falciparum* transmission intensity in cross-sectional studies in Peru and Mali. *PLoS ONE.* (2011) 6:e15983. doi: 10.1371/journal.pone.0015983
130. Illingworth J, Butler NS, Roetynck S, Mwacharo J, Pierce SK, Bejon P, et al. Chronic exposure to *Plasmodium falciparum* is associated with phenotypic evidence of B and T cell exhaustion. *J Immunol.* (2013) 190:1038–47. doi: 10.4049/jimmunol.1202438
131. Moir S, Ho J, Malaspina A, Wang W, DiPoto AC, O'Shea MA, et al. Evidence for HIV-associated B cell exhaustion in a dysfunctional memory B cell compartment in HIV-infected viremic individuals. *J Exp Med.* (2008) 205:1797–805. doi: 10.1084/jem.20072683
132. Muellenbeck MF, Ueberheide B, Amulic B, Epp A, Fenyo D, Busse CE, et al. Atypical and classical memory B cells produce *Plasmodium falciparum* neutralizing antibodies. *J Exp Med.* (2013) 210:389–99. doi: 10.1084/jem.20121970
133. Patgaonkar M, Herbert F, Powale K, Gandhe P, Gogtay N, Thatte U, et al. Vivax infection alters peripheral B-cell profile and induces persistent serum IgM. *Parasite Immunol.* (2018) 40:e12580. doi: 10.1111/pim.12580
134. Obeng-Adjei N, Portugal S, Holla P, Li S, Sohn H, Ambegaonkar A, et al. Malaria-induced interferon-γ drives the expansion of Tbethi atypical memory B cells. *PLoS Pathog.* (2017) 13:e1006576. doi: 10.1371/journal.ppat.1006576
135. Portugal S, Doumtabe D, Traore B, Miller LH, Troye-Blomberg M, Doumbo OK, et al. B cell analysis of ethnic groups in Mali with differential susceptibility to malaria. *Malar J.* (2012) 11:162. doi: 10.1186/1475-2875-11-162
136. Requena P, Campo JJ, Umbers AJ, Ome M, Wangnapi R, Barrios D, et al. Pregnancy and malaria exposure are associated with changes in the B cell pool and in plasma eotaxin levels. *J Immunol.* (2014) 193:2971–83. doi: 10.4049/jimmunol.1401037
137. Ubillos I, Campo JJ, Requena P, Ome-Kaius M, Hanieh S, Rose H, et al. Chronic exposure to malaria is associated with inhibitory and activation markers on atypical memory B cells and marginal zone-like B cells. *Front Immunol.* (2017) 8:966. doi: 10.3389/fimmu.2017.00966
138. Lugaajju A, Reddy SB, Wahlgren M, Kironde F, Persson KEM. Development of *Plasmodium falciparum* specific naïve, atypical, memory and plasma B cells during infancy and in adults in an endemic area. *Malar J.* (2017) 16:37. doi: 10.1186/s12936-017-1697-z
139. Subramaniam KS, Skinner J, Ivan E, Mutimura E, Kim RS, Feintuch CM, et al. HIV malaria co-infection is associated with atypical memory B cell expansion and a reduced antibody response to a broad array of *Plasmodium falciparum* antigens in rwandan adults. *PLoS ONE.* (2015) 10:e0124412. doi: 10.1371/journal.pone.0124412
140. Frosch AE, Odumade OA, Taylor JJ, Ireland K, Ayodo G, Ondigo B, et al. Decrease in numbers of naive and resting B cells in HIV-infected kenyan adults leads to a proportional increase in total and *Plasmodium falciparum*-specific atypical memory B cells. *J Immunol.* (2017) 198:4629–38. doi: 10.4049/jimmunol.1600773
141. Zinöcker S, Schindler CE, Skinner J, Rogosch T, Waisberg M, Schickel J-N, et al. The V gene repertoires of classical and atypical memory B cells in malaria-susceptible West African children. *J Immunol.* (2015) 194:929–39. doi: 10.4049/jimmunol.1402168
142. Li H, Borrego F, Nagata S, Tolnay M. Fc receptor-like 5 expression distinguishes two distinct subsets of human circulating tissue-like memory B cells. *J Immunol.* (2016) 196:4064–74. doi: 10.4049/jimmunol.1501027
143. Szabo SJ, Kim ST, Costa GL, Zhang XK, Fathman CG, Glimcher LH. A novel transcription factor, T-bet, directs Th1 lineage commitment. *Cell.* (2000) 100:655–69. doi: 10.1016/S0092-8674(00)80702-3
144. Jöhrens K, Shimizu Y, Anagnostopoulos I, Schiffmann S, Tiacci E, Falini B, et al. T-bet-positive and IRTA1-positive monocytoid B cells differ from marginal zone B cells and epithelial-associated B cells in their antigen profile and topographical distribution. *Haematologica.* (2005) 90:1070–7.
145. Johrens K, Anagnostopoulos I, Durkop H, Stein H. Different T-bet expression patterns characterize particular reactive lymphoid tissue lesions. *Histopathology.* (2006) 48:343–52. doi: 10.1111/j.1365-2559.2005.02305.x
146. Jöhrens K, Moos V, Schneider T, Stein H, Anagnostopoulos I. Interferon-gamma and T-bet expression in a patient with toxoplasmic lymphadenopathy. *Hum Immunol.* (2010) 71:366–71. doi: 10.1016/j.humimm.2010.01.005
147. Knox JJ, Buggert M, Kardava L, Seaton KE, Eller MA, Canaday DH, et al. T-bet$^+$ B cells are induced by human viral infections and dominate the HIV gp140 response. *JCI Insight.* (2017) 2:92943. doi: 10.1172/jci.insight.92943
148. Rubtsova K, Rubtsov AV, van Dyk LF, Kappler JW, Marrack P. T-box transcription factor T-bet, a key player in a unique type of B-cell activation essential for effective viral clearance. *Proc Natl Acad Sci USA.* (2013) 110:E3216–24. doi: 10.1073/pnas.1312348110
149. Barnett BE, Staupe RP, Odorizzi PM, Palko O, Tomov VT, Mahan AE, et al. Cutting edge: B cell-intrinsic T-bet expression is required

to control chronic viral infection. *J Immunol.* (2016) 197:1017–22. doi: 10.4049/jimmunol.1500368
150. Rubtsova K, Rubtsov AV, Halemano K, Li SX, Kappler JW, Santiago ML, et al. T cell production of IFNγ in response to TLR7/IL-12 stimulates optimal B cell responses to viruses. *PLoS ONE.* (2016) 11:e0166322. doi: 10.1371/journal.pone.0166322
151. Chang L-Y, Li Y, Kaplan DE. Hepatitis C viraemia reversibly maintains subset of antigen-specific T-bet$^+$ tissue-like memory B cells. *J Viral Hepat.* (2017) 24:389–96. doi: 10.1111/jvh.12659
152. Papillion AM, Kenderes KJ, Yates JL, Winslow GM. Early derivation of IgM memory cells and bone marrow plasmablasts. *PLoS ONE.* (2017) 12:e0178853. doi: 10.1371/journal.pone.0178853
153. Naradikian MS, Myles A, Beiting DP, Roberts KJ, Dawson L, Herati RS, et al. Cutting edge: IL-4, IL-21, and IFN-γ interact to govern T-bet and CD11c expression in TLR-activated B cells. *J Immunol.* (2016) 197:1023–8. doi: 10.4049/jimmunol.1600522
154. Bürgler S, Gimeno A, Parente-Ribes A, Wang D, Os A, Devereux S, et al. Chronic lymphocytic leukemia cells express CD38 in response to Th1 cell-derived IFN-γ by a T-bet-dependent mechanism. *J Immunol.* (2015) 194:827–35. doi: 10.4049/jimmunol.1401350
155. Jöhrens K, Dietel M, Anagnostopoulos I. Three different expression patterns of T-bet in angioimmunoblastic T-cell lymphoma. *Leuk Lymphoma.* (2012) 53:152–5. doi: 10.3109/10428194.2011.606941
156. Jöhrens K, Moos V, Schneider T, Anagnostopoulos I. T-box-expressed-in-T-cells (T-bet) expression by the tumor cells of hairy-cell leukemia correlates with interferon-gamma production. *Leuk Lymphoma.* (2009) 50:1687–92. doi: 10.1080/10428190903161042
157. Rubtsova K, Rubtsov AV, Thurman JM, Mennona JM, Kappler JW, Marrack P. B cells expressing the transcription factor T-bet drive lupus-like autoimmunity. *J Clin Invest.* (2017) 127:1392–404. doi: 10.1172/JCI91250
158. Wang Z, Wang Z, Wang J, Diao Y, Qian X, Zhu N. T-bet-expressing B cells are positively associated with Crohn's disease activity and support Th1 inflammation. *DNA Cell Biol.* (2016) 35:628–35. doi: 10.1089/dna.2016.3304
159. Becker AM, Dao KH, Han BK, Kornu R, Lakhanpal S, Mobley AB, et al. SLE peripheral blood B cell, T cell and myeloid cell transcriptomes display unique profiles and each subset contributes to the interferon signature. *PLoS ONE.* (2013) 8:e67003. doi: 10.1371/journal.pone.0067003
160. Isnardi I, Ng Y-S, Menard L, Meyers G, Saadoun D, Srdanovic I, et al. Complement receptor 2/CD21- human naive B cells contain mostly autoreactive unresponsive clones. *Blood.* (2010) 115:5026–36. doi: 10.1182/blood-2009-09-243071
161. Domeier PP, Chodisetti SB, Soni C, Schell SL, Elias MJ, Wong EB, et al. IFN-γ receptor and STAT1 signaling in B cells are central to spontaneous germinal center formation and autoimmunity. *J Exp Med.* (2016) 213:715–32. doi: 10.1084/jem.20151722
162. Frisullo G, Nociti V, Iorio R, Patanella AK, Marti A, Cammarota G, et al. Increased expression of T-bet in circulating B cells from a patient with multiple sclerosis and celiac disease. *Hum Immunol.* (2008) 69:837–9. doi: 10.1016/j.humimm.2008.09.008
163. Jackson SW, Jacobs HM, Arkatkar T, Dam EM, Scharping NE, Kolhatkar NS, et al. B cell IFN-γ receptor signaling promotes autoimmune germinal centers via cell-intrinsic induction of BCL-6. *J Exp Med.* (2016) 213:733–50. doi: 10.1084/jem.20151724
164. Rubtsov AV, Rubtsova K, Fischer A, Meehan RT, Gillis JZ, Kappler JW, et al. Toll-like receptor 7 (TLR7)-driven accumulation of a novel CD11c$^+$ B-cell population is important for the development of autoimmunity. *Blood.* (2011) 118:1305–15. doi: 10.1182/blood-2011-01-331462
165. Rubtsov AV, Rubtsova K, Kappler JW, Marrack P. TLR7 drives accumulation of ABCs and autoantibody production in autoimmune-prone mice. *Immunol Res.* (2013) 55:210–6. doi: 10.1007/s12026-012-8365-8
166. Fontana MF, Baccarella A, Craft JF, Boyle MJ, McIntyre TI, Wood MD, et al. A novel model of asymptomatic *Plasmodium* parasitemia that recapitulates elements of the human immune response to chronic infection. *PLoS ONE.* (2016) 11:e0162132. doi: 10.1371/journal.pone.0162132
167. Pérez-Mazliah D, Gardner PJ, Schweighoffer E, McLaughlin S, Hosking C, Tumwine I, et al. *Plasmodium*-specific atypical memory B cells are short-lived activated B cells. *Elife.* (2018) 7:e39800. doi: 10.7554/eLife.39800
168. RTS,S Clinical Trials Partnership. Efficacy and safety of RTS,S/AS01 malaria vaccine with or without a booster dose in infants and children in Africa: final results of a phase 3, individually randomised, controlled trial. *Lancet.* (2015) 386:31–45. doi: 10.1016/S0140-6736(15)60721-8
169. Olotu A, Fegan G, Wambua J, Nyangweso G, Leach A, Lievens M, et al. Seven-year efficacy of RTS,S/AS01 malaria vaccine among young African children. *N Engl J Med.* (2016) 374:2519–29. doi: 10.1056/NEJMoa1515257

3

Evidencing the Role of Erythrocytic Apoptosis in Malarial Anemia

*Paulo R. R. Totino *, Cláudio T. Daniel-Ribeiro and Maria de Fátima Ferreira-da-Cruz*

Laboratory of Malaria Research, Instituto Oswaldo Cruz, Fundação Oswaldo Cruz, Rio de Janeiro, Brazil

Edited by:
Joao Santana Silva, University of São Paulo, Brazil

Reviewed by:
Glen C. Ulett, Griffith University, Australia
Susu M. Zughaier, Emory University, USA

****Correspondence:***
Paulo R. R. Totino
prtotino@ioc.fiocruz.br

In the last decade it has become clear that, similarly to nucleated cells, enucleated red blood cells (RBCs) are susceptible to programmed apoptotic cell death. Erythrocytic apoptosis seems to play a role in physiological clearance of aged RBCs, but it may also be implicated in anemia of different etiological sources including drug therapy and infectious diseases. In malaria, severe anemia is a common complication leading to death of children and pregnant women living in malaria-endemic regions of Africa. The pathogenesis of malarial anemia is multifactorial and involves both ineffective production of RBCs by the bone marrow and premature elimination of non-parasitized RBCs, phenomena potentially associated with apoptosis. In the present overview, we discuss evidences associating erythrocytic apoptosis with the pathogenesis of severe malarial anemia, as well as with regulation of parasite clearance in malaria. Efforts to understand the role of erythrocytic apoptosis in malarial anemia can help to identify potential targets for therapeutic intervention based on apoptotic pathways and consequently, mitigate the harmful impact of malaria in global public health.

Keywords: malaria, anemia, apoptosis, red blood cells, phagocytosis

INTRODUCTION

Kerr and colleagues introduced the term *apoptosis* in 1972 to designate a physiologic process of programmed cell death implicated in normal maintenance of tissue cell population as well as in development of pathologies such as cancer. Since then, an enormous number of studies focusing on apoptosis have been published. These studies have focused on apoptosis of nucleated cells, whose dramatic changes occurring in the nucleus, i.e., chromatin condensation and DNA fragmentation (Kerr et al., 1972; Wyllie, 1980; Totino et al., 2006), labeled apoptosis as a nucleus-dependent stereotyped process. However, pioneer studies with experimentally enucleated cells demonstrated that typical cytoplasmic and cell membrane features of apoptosis, such as membrane blebbing, cell shrinkage, loss of mitochondrial transmembrane potential, and exposure of phosphatidylserine can be induced in the absence of a nucleus (Jacobson et al., 1994; Schulze-Osthoff et al., 1994; Castedo et al., 1996), raising the possibility that apoptosis could also determine the life span of physiologically enucleated cells, i.e., the red blood cells (RBC).

Indeed, even the lack of organelles in RBCs, including those directly implicated in apoptosis induction (i.e., mitochondria and endoplasmic reticulum), does not impair activation of the cytoplasmic machinery present in the cell that coordinates the apoptotic process (Bratosin et al., 2001; Lang et al., 2012). Although the pathways leading to apoptosis in RBC are not well known, they have been shown to be initiated by an increase in cytosolic Ca^{2+} due to activation of Ca^{2+} permeable non-selective cation channels in the cell membrane, which can be triggered by a variety of xenobiotics and endogenous substances (Lang et al., 2012). In turn, influx of Ca^{2+} leads to (1) activation of caspases and calpains, which participate in cell disassembly and formation of cell membrane blebbing; (2) cell shrinkage through exit of K^+ via Ca^{2+}-sensitive K^+ channel; and (3) stimulation of cell membrane scrambling, resulting in phosphatidylserine (PS) exposure at the cell surface (Gao et al., 2012; Lang et al., 2012). This last event is critical for elimination of apoptotic cells, before cell disintegration, and subsequent release of cytoplasmic proinflammatory mediators, because PS works as an "eat me" signal for phagocytic cells that operate in an anti-inflammatory manner (Wu et al., 2006).

Similarly to apoptosis of nucleated cells, apoptosis of erythrocytes participates in the body homeostasis through physiological clearance of aged cells. It is estimated that 360 billion of senescent erythrocytes undergo apoptotic processes and are removed every day by the spleen, avoiding systemic complications related to intravascular hemolysis (Bratosin et al., 1998, 2009). On the other hand, apoptosis is also believed to contribute to anemia and vascular disorders associated with clinical conditions in which excessive rates of apoptotic RBCs are documented, including diabetes, renal insufficiency, sickle-cell anemia, chronic lead exposure (Lang et al., 2002; Myssina et al., 2003; Calderón-Salinas et al., 2011; Aguilar-Dorado et al., 2014) as well as infectious diseases such as sepsis and mycoplasmosis (Kempe et al., 2007; Felder et al., 2011).

In view of the pathophysiological significance of erythrocytic apoptosis, our group has attempted to study this erythrocytic process in malaria, a vector-borne infection caused by protozoa of the genus *Plasmodium* that infect RBCs and induce strong hematologic and vascular disturbances (Anstey et al., 2009; Grau and Craig, 2012; Carvalho et al., 2014). Our studies have shown that induction of apoptosis is not limited to parasitized RBCs (pRBCs) but also occurs in non-parasitized RBCs (nRBCs), pointing to an involvement of both pRBC and nRBC in the pathogenesis of malaria through deflagration of suicide processes (Totino et al., 2009, 2011, 2013, 2014). Thus, the present review covers evidence implicating erythrocytic apoptosis in the pathogenesis of severe anemia, a common complication of malaria that represents an important public health concern strongly related to mortality in children and pregnant women living in malaria-hyperendemic regions of sub-Saharan Africa (Schantz-Dunn and Nour, 2009; Muoneke et al., 2012).

MALARIAL ANEMIA AND RBC REMOVAL

It should not be a surprise that anemia is one of the most common disorders associated with malaria, because *Plasmodium* parasites develop an intraerythrocytic schizogony process culminating in lysis of RBCs. In non-immune children and adults infected with *P. falciparum,* the degree of anemia may correlate with parasitemia (Phillips and Pasvol, 1992; Biemba et al., 2000; Menendez et al., 2000) and in most experimental rodent malaria, acute anemia is a consequence of the rupture of high percentages of pRBCs (Lamikanra et al., 2007). Nevertheless, it is known that destruction of pRBCs alone cannot account for anemia severity in malaria patients (Ekvall, 2003; Akinosoglou et al., 2012). Acute anemia can be observed in both experimental and human infections presenting low parasitemia and even after antimalarial treatment and clearance of parasites, anemia can persist or worsen (Phillips et al., 1986; Camacho et al., 1998; Carvalho et al., 2003; Helleberg et al., 2005; Evans et al., 2006). In view of these facts, both ineffective production of RBCs by the bone marrow and premature elimination of nRBC have been postulated as important determinants of malaria anemia pathogenesis (Jakeman et al., 1999; Casals-Pascual et al., 2006; Evans et al., 2006; Thawani et al., 2014).

The extent of RBC elimination in malaria was reported in studies estimating that, for every pRBC, up to 32 nRBC are removed from circulation (Jakeman et al., 1999; Collins et al., 2003; Evans et al., 2006). In addition, there is evidence supporting that nRBC removal is mediated by phagocytic activity rather than intravascular hemolysis (Phillips et al., 1986; Abdalla, 1988; Goka et al., 2001; La Raja, 2002; Satpathy et al., 2004; Evans et al., 2006), highlighting the mononuclear phagocytic reticuloendothelial system as an important mechanism of malarial anemia pathogenesis. Indeed, besides directly participate in malarial anemia by uptake of both pRBCs and nRBCs, macrophages may also interfere with the erythropoietic process by limiting systemic bioavailability of recycled iron, the main source of which is erythrophagocytosis occurring in spleen and bone marrow (Beaumont and Delaby, 2009; Spottiswoode et al., 2014). However, the pathways underlying clearance of RBCs in malarial anemia remain elusive and therefore, apoptosis as a well-known mechanism of cell depletion participating in cytopenia of several pathologies could mediate elimination of nRBCs.

MALARIA AND ERYTHROCYTIC APOPTOSIS INDUCERS

Studies conducted by Dondorp et al. (1999) with *P. falciparum*-infected patients demonstrated that similarly to pRBCs, in which parasites induces drastic changes on the host cell membrane, nRBCs also present reduced deformability correlating with anemia severity. This phenomenon, also recorded in nRBC from *P. falciparum in vitro* culture and *P. yoelii*-infected mice (Paul et al., 2013; Huang et al., 2014), has been related to adsorption of malaria parasite antigens on the cell surface (Layez et al., 2005; Omodeo-Salè et al., 2005) and interestingly, more recently identified as a hallmark of erythrocytic apoptosis (Mindukshev et al., 2013), raising the possibility that antigens of malaria parasites have proapoptotic proprieties on RBCs.

Microbes in general could affect proapoptotic pathways in host cells. Gram-positive and gram-negative bacteria, as well as protozoan parasites, have been shown to manipulate apoptotic processes of both infected and non-infected host nucleated cells via pathogen antigens that act as apoptosis regulatory molecules through multifarious pathways, impacting on the outcome of disease (Ulett and Adderson, 2006; Rodrigues et al., 2012). A diversity of antigens produced by pathogenic bacteria such as enterotoxins, hemolysins, lethal toxins, lipotechoic acid, and lipopolysaccharide, have the ability to promote apoptosis in several types of host cells including T and B lymphocytes, dendritic cells, monocytes, macrophages, neutrophils, endothelial cells, epithelial cells (Ulett and Adderson, 2006; Carrero and Unanue, 2012). Similarly, malaria toxins glycosylphosphatidylinositol and hemozoin purified from *P. falciparum* showed proapoptotic activity in cardiomyocytes and erythroblasts, respectively (Wennicke et al., 2008; Lamikanra et al., 2009). Moreover, such apoptogenic effect of parasite factors was recorded by incubating brain vascular endothelial and neuroglia cells with *P. falciparum*-pRBC conditioned medium (Wilson et al., 2008), and induction of apoptosis in lung endothelial cells can additionally take place by physical contact due to pRBC adhesion phenomenon (Pino et al., 2003).

There are no studies further exploring the proapoptotic potential of plasmodial antigens in erythrocytic apoptosis. However, it was already reported that in *P. falciparum in vitro* cultures nRBCs are marked by PS externalization (Koka et al., 2007; Pattanapanyasat et al., 2010), and in our previous study with BALB/c mice infected by the lethal *P. yoelii* 17XL parasites, increased levels of nRBC apoptosis correlated with hiperparasitemia (Totino et al., 2013), indirectly suggesting that as do bacterial toxins (listeriolysin from *Listeria monocytogenes* and hemolysin from *Vibrio parahaemolyticus*), peptidoglycan, and *Schistosoma mansoni* egg antigens (Lang et al., 2004b; Föller et al., 2007; Kasinathan and Greenberg, 2010; Jilani et al., 2012; Abed et al., 2013), plasmodial antigens can play a role in induction of erythrocytic apoptosis.

Additionally, several host factors have the potential to modulate erythrocytic apoptosis during malaria (Lang and Lang, 2015). They may comprise: (1) proapoptotic factors whose increased levels are associated with malarial severity, such as soluble Fas ligand (sFasL), anti-erythrocyte antibodies, hematin, granzyme B, and oxidative stress (Das et al., 1993; Waitumbi et al., 2000; Hermsen et al., 2003; Issifou et al., 2003; Dalko et al., 2015) and; (2) antiapoptotic factors, i.e., erythropoietin, vitamin E, and nitric oxide, that show either reduced levels or low bioavability in malaria, and consequently, could contribute to amplify erythrocytic apoptosis induction (Burgmann et al., 1996; Kulkarni et al., 2003; Sobolewski et al., 2005).

It is also noteworthy that several routine therapeutic drugs present proapoptotic properties on erythrocytes, which has been linked to drug-associated anemia (Lang and Lang, 2015). *In vitro* studies performed by Alzoubi et al. (2014a,b) showed that the antimalarial drugs artesunate and lumefantrine have proapoptotic effect on erythrocytes, possibly through generation of oxidative stress, a feature already reported for both drugs (Xie et al., 2005; Abolaji et al., 2013). Thus, the proapoptotic effect of artesunate and lumefantrine could explain the reduction of erythrocytic blood parameters reported in healthy rats and humans (Xie et al., 2005; Kongpatanakul et al., 2009) as well as in occurrence of acute anemia in malarial patients following antimalarial drug treatment (De Nardo et al., 2013; Raffray et al., 2014; Sowunmi et al., 2015).

REMOVING nRBCs IN MALARIA BY APOPTOSIS

Although it is known that sensitization of nRBCs by antibodies and complement system contributes to malarial anemia pathogenesis ((Daniel-Ribeiro et al., 1986); (Daniel-Ribeiro and Zanini, 2000; Waitumbi et al., 2000), there is evidence indicating that the elimination of nRBCs could also occur in an opsonin-independent manner. For instance, a lack of correlation between RBC sensitization and anemia degree has been reported in some studies with malarial patients (Abdalla, 1986; Merry et al., 1986) and a shortened lifespan of nRBCs was observed during *P. yoelii* induced-anemia in a B cell-deficient environment provided by severe combined immunodeficient mice (Salmon et al., 1997). In addition, in a recently described novel model of severe malarial anemia presenting low parasitemia, $C3^{-/-}$ mice still developed acute anemia following *P. berghei* infection (Harris et al., 2012).

The participation of a nonopsonic phagocytosis in nRBC elimination and its relation to apoptosis can be sustained by data concerning the scavenger receptor CD36 and PS. CD36 is a well-known phagocytic receptor for apoptotic cells that acts via recognition of PS on the apoptotic cell surface (Greenberg et al., 2006). Experiments with both monoclonal anti-CD36 antibodies and CD36-deficient rodent macrophages have shown that CD36 plays also a role in phagocytic uptake of RBC in malaria (McGilvray et al., 2000; Patel et al., 2004; Ayi et al., 2005). In these experiments, the contribution of parasite antigens with affinity to CD36 (e.g., *P. falciparum* erythrocyte membrane protein 1—PfEMP-1) on the pRBC surface cannot be ruled out, since they were performed with pRBC. Nevertheless, intraerythrocytic plasmodia development progressively induces PS exteriorization on pRBC as a result of non-selective cation channel activation in the host RBC membrane (Eda and Sherman, 2002; Lang et al., 2004a), indicating that pRBC could be removed via PS.

Importantly, PS has been recognized as a key molecule mediating erythrophagocytosis, as *in vitro* treatment with annexin V or PS-containing liposomes is able to inhibit phagocytosis of senescent or oxidatively stressed RBC, an effect also achieved with the use of anti-CD36 antibodies (Bratosin et al., 1997; Tait and Smith, 1999; Mandal et al., 2002). In a similar way, phagocytosis of RBC from uremic patients, with increased levels of PS-exposing RBC with great propensity for phagocytosis, was also inhibited after preincubation of macrophages with glycerophosphorylserine, a structural derivate of PS (Bonomini et al., 2001), indicating that PS can mediate shortened life span of RBC in pathological conditions in which anemia is a common feature. In this context, anemia has been associated with the rates of PS-exposing RBC in peritoneal dialysis and sepsis patients (Bi et al., 2006; Shi et al., 2013) as well as with erythrophagocytosis mediated by PS in rats treated with lead or naphthoquinone—two inducers of erythrocytic apoptosis (Noh et al., 2010; Jang et al., 2011).

Hence, PS exposure on nRBCs induced to apoptosis during malaria could also be involved in anemia development, as suggested initially by our studies on lethal *P. yoelii* experimental infection, in which the levels of PS-exposing nRBCs were increased during the stage of infection marked by an acute anemia (Totino et al., 2010). Both erythrophagocytosis and PS-exposing RBCs are increased in *P. falciparum* infected-children presenting severe anemia as compared to those with uncomplicated malaria (Fendel et al., 2010). Apoptosis can also be induced by incubating RBCs from healthy individuals with plasma from *P. falciparum* patients, an effect that is not observed with plasma from *P. vivax* infections, which, comparatively to *P. falciparum*, are less prone to lead to severe disease (Totino et al., 2014). Furthermore, since CD36 is a key molecule in the RBC clearance process, resistance to severe malarial anemia reported in children with a non-sense CD36 mutation can be explained, in part, by a deficiency in phagocytosis of apoptotic nRBCs mediated by CD36-PS interaction (Pain et al., 2001; Chilongola et al., 2009).

Recently, additional evidence for the contribution of PS to malarial anemia was reported in a study of mice infected with the nonlethal (17XNL) *P. yoelii* (Fernandez-Arias et al., 2016). In this model, as observed by our group with the lethal (17XL) strain *P. yoelii* (Totino et al., 2010), there was a significant increase in the levels of PS-exposing nRBCs. In addition, it was shown that *P. yoelii* infection induces autoantibodies against PS exposed on nRBCs and that these antibodies enhance anemia when transferred to infected mice, an effect related to *in vitro* nRBC phagocytosis. Importantly, anti-PS antibodies were also detected in sera from *P. falciparum*-infected patients and the highest levels were associated with late postmalarial anemia in nonimmune travelers. Therefore, besides participating in the pathogenesis of malarial anemia by directly promoting RBC elimination via the innate immune receptor CD36, PS may also contributes antigenically as a target of acquired immune response, a novel described autoimmune phenomenon in malaria whose source needs further investigation.

Another cell event that links erythrocytic apoptosis and anemia is a change in CD47 expression. CD47 is a ubiquitous glycoprotein expressed on the cell surface that was identified as a "marker of self" by suppressing phagocytosis of normal viable cells through interaction with signal-regulatory protein alpha (SIRPα), which operates as a inhibitory receptor on phagocytes (Sosale et al., 2015). Initially identified in studies demonstrating a rapid *in vivo* clearance of CD47-deficient RBCs and an increased *in vitro* phagocytosis of normal RBCs by macrophages treated with SIRPα-blocking antibodies, the CD47/SIRPα system of cell clearance was suggested to play role in anemia of Rh_{null} individuals, given that expression of CD47 on normal RBCs is coupled to Rh antigen complex (Oldenborg et al., 2000). Indeed, the involvement of CD47 in anemia was also observed in mild autoimmune hemolytic anemia typical of experimental nonobese diabetes, which was worsened and became lethal in CD47-deficient mice (Oldenborg et al., 2002) and in patients with myelodysplastic syndrome, the degree of anemia was correlated to the levels of CD47 expressed on erythroblasts (Jiang et al., 2013). Furthermore, down-regulation of surface CD47 occurring specifically on platelets was connected to thrombocytopenia of *Escherichia coli* infected-mice (Guo et al., 2009), supporting data suggesting that CD47 participates in cytopenia of different etiological sources through cell depletion processes.

Comprehensibly CD47/SIRPα self-recognition system has been implicated in clearance of apoptotic cells. It was demonstrated that apoptosis of neutrophils and Jurkat cells is followed by decreased expression of surface CD47 (Lawrence et al., 2009; Azuma et al., 2011), while in apoptosis of several other nucleated cell types CD47, initially clustered in lipid rafts, is diffused on the cell surface, reducing its avidity for SIRPα (Lv et al., 2015). In both cases, it is believed that the inhibitory signaling triggered by CD47 via phosphorylation of the SIRPA cytoplasmic tail is discontinued and consequently, apoptotic cells are phagocytized. Therefore, elimination of RBCs contributing to the pathogenesis of malarial anemia could also be a reflex of CD47 changes during the apoptosis process.

Reduction of surface CD47 expression has been observed on RBCs maintained under conditions that induce erythrocytic apoptosis, such as blood storage and hypoxia, as detected by externalization of PS (Stewart et al., 2005; Mao et al., 2011), and there is a consensus that *in vivo* elimination of senescent RBCs, which are marked by deflagration of apoptotic processes (Bosman et al., 2005), is regulated by CD47 (Khandelwal et al., 2007; Burger et al., 2012). Nevertheless, with the exception of studies with CD47-deficient mice and Rh_{null} individuals, those addressing a relationship between RBC CD47 and anemia are limited. Two studies on warm autoimmune hemolytic anemia showed no difference in CD47 expression when comparing RBCs from patients with those from healthy individuals, suggesting that CD47 does not play a role in the development of this pathology, in which autoantibodies are well known to be involved (Ahrens et al., 2006; Barros et al., 2009). However, it has been demonstrated that CD47, as a regulator of RBC clearance, is able to overwhelm phagocytosis mediated by antibody and complement (Oldenborg et al., 2001; Olsson and Oldenborg, 2008). Therefore, the contribution of CD47 to autoimmune anemia, possibly by means of its reorganization on cell surface (not assayed in the above mentioned studies), rather than by its downexpression, cannot be excluded.

In malaria, the role of CD47 has been recently addressed (Banerjee et al., 2015; Ayi et al., 2016). Parasites of the nonlethal strain of *P. yoelii* 17XNL were mostly detected infecting young RBCs expressing high levels of CD47, suggesting that malaria parasites could take advantage of negative signaling of CD47 to avoid early elimination by phagocytosis (Banerjee et al., 2015). The authors of this study also demonstrated that absence of this molecule in deficient mice attenuated the course of parasitemia and notably, converted the lethal infection of *P. yoelii* YM into a nonlethal, self-resolving infection characterized by a very low parasite load (peak of 0.06%). Similar results in a more recent study (Ayi et al., 2016) showed that CD47-deficiency attenuated parasitemia and abolished the development of cerebral malaria in *P. berghei* ANKA-infected mice, as well as *P. falciparum*-pRBC had decreased levels of CD47, a phenomenon that was associated with both *in vitro* and *in vivo* clearance of *P. falciparum*—and *P. berghei*-pRBCs via SIRPα, respectively.

These data raise the possibility that alteration of CD47 expression on apoptotic pRBCs operates as a regulator of malaria parasite clearance. Although elimination of pRBCs has a role in pathogenesis of malarial anemia, contrary to RBC lysis that allows the propagation of merozoites at the end of schizogony, RBC apoptosis could play a beneficial role leading intraerythrocytic-developing parasites to degradation by phagocytosis and consequently reducing parasite burden that directly promotes anemia through RBC lysis. This protective role of erythrocytic apoptosis was previously demonstrated by treating *P. berghei*-infected mice with the drug aurothiomalate, which triggers apoptosis selectively in pRBCs with no effect on intraerythrocytic parasite development (Alesutan et al., 2010). This *in vivo* stimulation of pRBC apoptosis delayed the course of parasitemia and mortality of mice, suggesting that the use of drugs to selectively trigger apoptosis pathways in pRBCs could be a strategy to treat malaria in a manner not propitious to generation of parasite resistance, since drugs would target the host cell and not the parasite.

While CD47 changes on pRBCs could play a protector effect, the same is not expected for nRBCs. As mentioned above, CD47 deficiency is associated with development of anemia as a result of increased susceptibility of $CD47^{-/-}$ RBC to phagocytosis under pathological circumstances. Thus, if on one hand RBC clearance promoted by the absence of CD47 attenuates malaria parasitemia (pRBC), on the other hand it leads to anemia (nRBC), as observed in CD47-deficient mice with *P. berghei* malaria (Ayi et al., 2016). This connection between CD47, nRBC and anemia was also confirmed in a study with wild type mice infected by *P. yoelii* 17XNL that found a decline in the number of nRBCs expressing high levels CD47 when RBC counts were falling. An increase in newly formed RBCs (reticulocytes) that express high levels of CD47 was detected later at the recovery stage (Fernandez-Arias et al., 2016), implicating CD47 in the pathogenesis of malarial anemia through elimination of nRBCs.

Paradoxically, deflagration of apoptosis in nRBCs could play a protective role in malaria infection. It is well-known that apoptotic processes represent an innate mechanism against intracellular parasitism that altruistically drives parasites to degradation by phagocytosis along with host parasitized cells, thereby preventing infection of adjacent cells and pathogen propagation (Williams, 1994). Alternatively, apoptosis could act in the control of parasitemia limiting the availability of non-parasitized targeted cells susceptible to infection, as shown in *P. falciparum in vitro* culture where apoptotic nRBCs were refractory to parasite invasion (Totino et al., 2011). However, this phenomenon offering as a host protective mechanism for parasite burden control in malaria while adversely induces anemia, needs to be better examined.

APOPTOSIS AND DEFECTIVE ERYTHROPOIESIS

Besides participating in the pathogenesis of malarial anemia by mediating precocious elimination of nRBC, apoptosis could interfere with the production of new RBCs, as previously reported in severe anemia associated to *Leishmania donovani* infection in golden hamsters (Lafuse et al., 2013) as well as in anemia of chronic disease in patients with rheumatoid arthritis (Papadaki et al., 2002), in which cytokine-mediated apoptosis of erythroid cells seems to operate.

Anemia in both malaria experimental models and human infection is followed by an unexpected frequency of peripheral reticulocytes considering the loss of RBCs, indicating that impaired erythropoietic activity is an important mechanism in the pathogenesis of malarial anemia (Chang et al., 2004; Leowattana et al., 2008; Fendel et al., 2010; Anyona et al., 2012; Thawani et al., 2014). Infection by *P. chabaudi*, *P. yoelii*, and *P. berghei* was shown to inhibit development of erythroid precursors induced by erythropoietin in mice (Thawani et al., 2014), an effect also achieved by *in vitro* incubation of human erythroid cells with hemozoin or proinflamatory cytokines such as TNF and IFN-γ, whose levels are augmented during malaria (Means and Krantz, 1991; Casals-Pascual et al., 2006; Awandare et al., 2011). In addition, in a study with children presenting several degrees of malarial anemia, ineffective erythropoiesis was associated with the amount of circulating hemozoin and TNF, and deposition of hemozoin in bone marrow was related to abnormal erythroid development in postmortem analysis of children with severe anemia (Casals-Pascual et al., 2006).

In this context, proapoptotic effects of hemozoin, TNF and interferon-γ on erythroid precursors have been described *in vitro* (Dai and Krantz, 1999; Lamikanra et al., 2009; Vittori et al., 2010) and high levels of apoptotic erythroid cells were observed in bone marrow aspirates of severe malaria patients presenting erythroid hypoplasia and low percentage of peripheral reticulocytes (Anantrakulsil et al., 2005). Nevertheless, the capacity of both TNF and hemozoin to depress erythropoiesis by inducing apoptosis has not been consensually demonstrated *in vitro* (Skorokhod et al., 2010; Awandare et al., 2011) and apoptosis was not implicated in impaired maturation of erythroblasts during anemia of experimental *P. chabaudi* infection (Chang et al., 2004).

These apparently contradictory results could be related to the differences between cell lines, since *in vitro* studies with hemozoin and TFN were performed with cells from different sources, i.e., erythroid cell lines or fresh isolated $CD34^{+}$ stem cells from PBMC, which have been shown to exhibit different susceptibility to apoptosis induced by TNF or hemozoin (Lamikanra et al., 2009; Skorokhod et al., 2010; Vittori et al., 2010; Awandare et al., 2011). For instance, erythroid cells derived from human erythroleukaemia K562 cell line were susceptible to apoptosis induced by TNF, but not hemozoin, while those cells derived from normal peripheral blood $CD34^{+}$ cells were only susceptible to hemozoin-induced apoptosis, suggesting that these compounds interfere in the development of erythroid cells through distinct pathways, with hemozoin inducing apoptosis and TNF triggering non-apoptotic mechanisms in healthy (non-leukemia) cells. Indeed, a gene expression profile study of purified primary erythroid cultures incubated with either TNF or hemozoin showed recently that both stimuli were able to inhibit erythroid development, with activation of largely distinct transcriptional programs: hemozoin up-regulated genes related to regulation of transcription, cellular stress response and apoptosis, and the majority of genes up-regulated by TNF was involved in innate and adaptive immune responses to infection (Lamikanra et al., 2015).

These data explain, at least in part, the lack of a relationship between apoptosis and depressed erythropoiesis in severe anemia of *P. chabaudi* infection in A/J mice (Chang et al., 2004), with TNF probably overwhelming the proapoptotic property of hemozoin. Although there are no studies concerning the effect of TNF on hemozoin-induced apoptosis, it has been shown that *P. chabaudi* infection in A/J mice is marked by increased levels of TNF at the time of decreased reticulocyte response (Jacobs et al., 1996). Additionally, these data illustrate the well-known concept of the complex multifactorial pathogenesis of malarial anemia, in which the molecular mechanisms regulating eythropoiesis in malaria are still poorly understood; a scenario that reflects a research gap that remains challenging due to practical and ethical difficulties in obtaining bone marrow samples from patients with severe malarial anemia, whose population majority comprises children of African endemic regions.

CONCLUDING REMARKS

It has become evident that deflagration of cell death processes by apoptosis is not restrict to nucleated cells, occurring also in enucleated RBCs, and consequently, contributing to the development of anemia through precocious elimination of RBCs. In malaria infection, erythrocytic apoptosis occurs and seems to play both detrimental and protective roles by inducing anemia and controlling parasitemia, respectively (**Figure 1**). Although the magnitude and dynamics of erythrocytic apoptosis in malaria are still to be better established, the above reported connections between apoptosis and anemia open new options for development of therapy for severe malarial anemia by exploring the apoptotic machinery, as considered in other pathologies related to increased induction of apoptosis such as Alzheimer's disease, Parkinson's disease, and sepsis (Jana and Paliwal, 2007; Hattori et al., 2010). Advances that allow therapy improvement for severe malaria anemia are, indeed, urgently needed. The use of adjunctive therapy for severe malarial anemia has not been well explored, possibly due to the common requirement for blood transfusion. However, the prevalence of blood-borne infections such as HIV in malaria endemic areas limits the availability and safety of blood transfusion (Osaro and Charles, 2011). Furthermore, blood transfusion shows a trend toward presentation of severe adverse events and does not significantly decrease mortality rates, underscoring the need for new strategies for treating severe malarial anemia (Meremikwu and Smith, 2000; Obonyo et al., 2007). Thus, inhibition of cell signaling pathways leading to erythrocytic apoptosis could be explored as an alternative strategy to

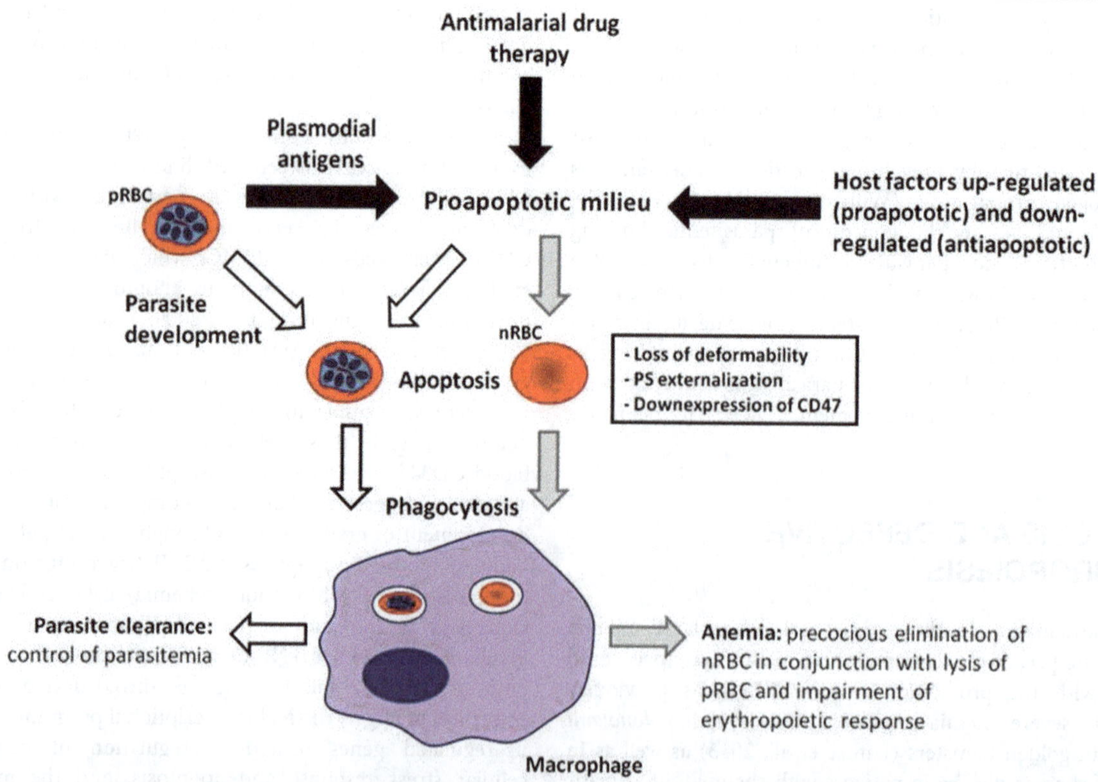

FIGURE 1 | Model of erythrocytic apoptosis involvement in the pathogenesis of malarial anemia. Both parasitic antigens and host factors modulated by malaria infection generate a favorable environment for precocious induction of erythrocytic apoptosis (black arrows), which can be enhanced by antimalarial drug treatment, and in the case of parasitized red blood cells (pRBCs), by intraerythrocytic parasite development. Erythrocytic apoptosis provokes cellular changes, i.e., cell rigidity increase, exposure of phosphatidylserine and downexpression of CD47, that drive pRBC (white arrows) and non-parasitized RBC (nRBC; gray arrows) to phagocytosis. Elimination of apoptotic nRBCs along with pRBC lysis and erythropoiesis impairment contribute to the development of malarial anemia. Uptake of apoptotic pRBCs can help control parasite load. In this manner, the pathogenic or protective role of erythrocytic apoptosis in malaria could be a result of increased apoptosis induction differentially in nRBC and pRBC, respectively.

mitigate the impact of severe anemia in mortality caused by malaria.

AUTHOR CONTRIBUTIONS

PT wrote the manuscript; CD-R and MF critically revised it for intellectual content. All authors read and approved the final manuscript.

ACKNOWLEDGMENTS

This work was supported by Instituto Oswaldo Cruz-Fiocruz; Fundação de Amparo à Pesquisa do Estado do Rio de Janeiro (Faperj) and; Conselho Nacional de Desenvolvimento Científico e Tecnológico (CNPq). CD-R and MF are recipients of a Research Productivity Fellowship from CNPq and Full Scientists of the Faperj.

REFERENCES

Abdalla, S. H. (1986). Red cell associated IgG in patients suffering from *Plasmodium falciparum* malaria. *Br. J. Haematol.* 62, 13–19. doi: 10.1111/j.1365-2141.1986.tb02895.x

Abdalla, S. H. (1988). Peripheral blood and bone marrow leucocytes in Gambian children with malaria: numerical changes and evaluation of phagocytosis. *Ann. Trop. Paediatr.* 8, 250–258. doi: 10.1080/02724936.1988.11748582

Abed, M., Towhid, S. T., Pakladok, T., Alesutan, I., Götz, F., Gulbins, E., et al. (2013). Effect of bacterial peptidoglycan on erythrocyte death and adhesion to endothelial cells. *Int. J. Med. Microbiol.* 303, 182–189. doi: 10.1016/j.ijmm.2013.01.004

Abolaji, A. O., Eteng, M. U., Omonua, O., and Adenrele, Y. (2013). Influence of coadministration of artemether and lumefantrine on selected plasma biochemical and erythrocyte oxidative stress indices in female Wistar rats. *Hum. Exp. Toxicol.* 32, 206–215. doi: 10.1177/0960327112464666

Aguilar-Dorado, I. C., Hernández, G., Quintanar-Escorza, M. A., Maldonado-Vega, M., Rosas-Flores, M., and Calderón-Salinas, J. V. (2014). Eryptosis in lead-exposed workers. *Toxicol. Appl. Pharmacol.* 281, 195–202. doi: 10.1016/j.taap.2014.10.003

Ahrens, N., Pagenkopf, C., Kiesewetter, H., and Salama, A. (2006). CD47 is expressed at normal levels in patients with autoimmune haemolytic anaemia and/or immune thrombocytopenia. *Transfus. Med.* 16, 397–402. doi: 10.1111/j.1365-3148.2006.00688.x

Akinosoglou, K. S., Solomou, E. E., and Gogos, C. A. (2012). Malaria: a haematological disease. *Hematology* 17, 106–114. doi: 10.1179/102453312X13221316477336

Alesutan, I., Bobbala, D., Qadri, S. M., Estremera, A., Föller, M., and Lang, F. (2010). Beneficial effect of aurothiomalate on murine malaria. *Malar. J.* 9:118. doi: 10.1186/1475-2875-9-118

Alzoubi, K., Alktifan, B., Oswald, G., Fezai, M., Abed, M., and Lang, F. (2014a). Breakdown of phosphatidylserine asymmetry following treatment of erythrocytes with lumefantrine. *Toxins* 6, 650–664. doi: 10.3390/toxins6020650

Alzoubi, K., Calabrò, S., Bissinger, R., Abed, M., Faggio, C., and Lang, F. (2014b). Stimulation of suicidal erythrocyte death by artesunate. *Cell. Physiol. Biochem.* 34, 2232–2244. doi: 10.1159/000369666

Anantrakulsil, S., Maneerat, Y., Wilairatana, P., Krudsood, S., Arunsuriyasak, C., Atichartakarn, V., et al. (2005). Hematopoietic feature and apoptosis in the bone marrow of severe *Plasmodium falciparum*-infected patients: preliminary study. *Southeast Asian J. Trop. Med. Public Health* 36, 543–551.

Anstey, N. M., Russell, B., Yeo, T. W., and Price, R. N. (2009). The pathophysiology of vivax malaria. *Trends Parasitol.* 25, 220–227. doi: 10.1016/j.pt.2009.02.003

Anyona, S. B., Kempaiah, P., Raballah, E., Davenport, G. C., Were, T., Konah, S. N., et al. (2012). Reduced systemic bicyclo-prostaglandin-E_2 and cyclooxygenase-2 gene expression are associated with inefficient erythropoiesis and enhanced uptake of monocytic hemozoin in children with severe malarial anemia. *Am. J. Hematol.* 87, 782–789. doi: 10.1002/ajh.23253

Awandare, G. A., Kempaiah, P., Ochiel, D. O., Piazza, P., Keller, C. C., and Perkins, D. J. (2011). Mechanisms of erythropoiesis inhibition by malarial pigment and malaria-induced proinflammatory mediators in an *in vitro* model. *Am. J. Hematol.* 86, 155–162. doi: 10.1002/ajh.21933

Ayi, K., Lu, Z., Serghides, L., Ho, J. M., Finney, C., Wang, J. C., et al. (2016). CD47-SIRPα interactions regulate macrophage uptake of *Plasmodium falciparum*-infected erythrocytes and clearance of malaria *in vivo*. *Infect. Immun.* 84, 2002–2011. doi: 10.1128/IAI.01426-15

Ayi, K., Patel, S. N., Serghides, L., Smith, T. G., and Kain, K. C. (2005). Nonopsonic phagocytosis of erythrocytes infected with ring-stage *Plasmodium falciparum*. *Infect. Immun.* 73, 2559–2563. doi: 10.1128/IAI.73.4.2559-2563.2005

Azuma, Y., Nakagawa, H., Dote, K., Higai, K., and Matsumoto, K. (2011). Decreases in CD31 and CD47 levels on the cell surface during etoposide-induced Jurkat cell apoptosis. *Biol. Pharm. Bull.* 34, 1828–1834. doi: 10.1248/bpb.34.1828

Banerjee, R., Khandelwal, S., Kozakai, Y., Sahu, B., and Kumar, S. (2015). CD47 regulates the phagocytic clearance and replication of the Plasmodium yoelii malaria parasite. *Proc. Natl. Acad. Sci. U.S.A.* 112, 3062–3067. doi: 10.1073/pnas.1418144112

Barros, M. M. O., Yamamoto, M., Figueiredo, M. S., Cançado, R., Kimura, E. Y., Langhi, D. M. Jr., et al. (2009). Expression levels of CD47, CD35, CD55, and CD59 on red blood cells and signal-regulatory protein-alpha, beta on monocytes from patients with warm autoimmune hemolytic anemia. *Transfusion* 49, 154–160. doi: 10.1111/j.1537-2995.2008.01936.x

Beaumont, C., and Delaby, C. (2009). Recycling iron in normal and pathological states. *Semin. Hematol.* 46, 328–338. doi: 10.1053/j.seminhematol.2009.06.004

Bi, S. H., Cheng, L. T., and Wang, T. (2006). The role of erythrocytes phosphatidylserine exposure in anemia in peritoneal dialysis patients. *Ren. Fail.* 28, 573–576. doi: 10.1080/08860220600839647

Biemba, G., Dolmans, D., Thuma, P. E., Weiss, G., and Gordeuk, V. R. (2000). Severe anaemia in Zambian children with *Plasmodium falciparum* malaria. *Trop. Med. Int. Health* 5, 9–16. doi: 10.1046/j.1365-3156.2000.00506.x

Bonomini, M., Sirolli, V., Reale, M., and Arduini, A. (2001). Involvement of phosphatidylserine exposure in the recognition and phagocytosis of uremic erythrocytes. *Am. J. Kidney Dis.* 37, 807–814. doi: 10.1016/S0272-6386(01)80130-X

Bosman, G. J., Willekens, F. L., and Werre, J. M. (2005). Erythrocyte aging: a more than superficial resemblance to apoptosis? *Cell. Physiol. Biochem.* 16, 1–8. doi: 10.1159/000087725

Bratosin, D., Estaquier, J., Petit, F., Arnoult, D., Quatannens, B., Tissier, J. P., et al. (2001). Programmed cell death in mature erythrocytes: a model for investigating death effector pathways operating in the absence of mitochondria. *Cell Death Differ.* 8, 1143–1156. doi: 10.1038/sj.cdd.4400946

Bratosin, D., Mazurier, J., Tissier, J. P., Estaquier, J., Huart, J. J., Ameisen, J. C., et al. (1998). Cellular and molecular mechanisms of senescent erythrocyte phagocytosis by macrophages. A review. *Biochimie* 80, 173–195. doi: 10.1016/S0300-9084(98)80024-2

Bratosin, D., Mazurier, J., Tissier, J. P., Slomianny, C., Estaquier, J., Russo-Marie, F., et al. (1997). Molecular mechanisms of erythrophagocytosis. Characterization of the senescent erythrocytes that are phagocytized by macrophages. *C. R. Acad. Sci. III* 320, 811–818. doi: 10.1016/S0764-4469(97)85017-2

Bratosin, D., Tcacenco, L., Sidoroff, M., Cotoraci, C., Slomianny, C., Estaquier, J., et al. (2009). Active caspases-8 and -3 in circulating human erythrocytes purified on immobilized annexin-V: a cytometric demonstration. *Cytometry A* 75, 236–244. doi: 10.1002/cyto.a.20693

Burger, P., de Korte, D., van den Berg, T. K., and van Bruggen, R. (2012). CD47 in erythrocyte ageing and clearance - the Dutch point of view. *Transfus. Med. Hemother.* 39, 348–352. doi: 10.1159/000342231

Burgmann, H., Looareesuwan, S., Kapiotis, S., Viravan, C., Vanijanonta, S., Hollenstein, U., et al. (1996). Serum levels of erythropoietin in acute *Plasmodium falciparum* malaria. *Am. J.Trop. Med. Hyg.* 54, 280–283.

Calderón-Salinas, J. V., Muñoz-Reyes, E. G., Guerrero-Romero, J. F., Rodríguez-Morán, M., Bracho-Riquelme, R. L., Carrera-Gracia, M. A., et al. (2011). Eryptosis and oxidative damage in type 2 diabetic mellitus patients with chronic kidney disease. *Mol. Cell. Biochem.* 357, 171–179. doi: 10.1007/s11010-011-0887-1

Camacho, L. H., Gordeuk, V. R., Wilairatana, P., Pootrakul, P., Brittenham, G. M., and Looareesuwan, S. (1998). The course of anaemia after the treatment of acute, falciparum malaria. *Ann. Trop. Med. Parasitol.* 92, 525–537. doi: 10.1080/00034983.1998.11813310

Carrero, J. A., and Unanue, E. R. (2012). Mechanisms and immunological effects of apoptosis caused by *Listeria monocytogenes*. *Adv. Immunol.* 113, 157–174. doi: 10.1016/B978-0-12-394590-7.00001-4

Carvalho, L. J., Alves, F. A., de Oliveira, S. G., do Valle Rdel, R., Fernandes, A. A., Muniz, J. A., et al. (2003). Severe anemia affects both splenectomized and non-splenectomized *Plasmodium falciparum*-infected Aotus infulatus monkeys. *Mem. Inst. Oswaldo Cruz* 98, 679–686. doi: 10.1590/S0074-02762003000500016

Carvalho, L. J., Moreira Ada, S., Daniel-Ribeiro, C. T., and Martins, Y. C. (2014). Vascular dysfunction as a target for adjuvant therapy in cerebral malaria. *Mem. Inst. Oswaldo Cruz* 109, 577–588. doi: 10.1590/0074-0276140061

Casals-Pascual, C., Kai, O., Cheung, J. O. P., Williams, S., Lowe, B., Nyanoti, M., et al. (2006). Suppression of erythropoiesis in malarial anemia is associated with hemozoin *in vitro* and *in vivo*. *Blood* 108, 2569–2577. doi: 10.1182/blood-2006-05-018697

Castedo, M., Hirsch, T., Susin, S. A., Zamzami, N., Marchetti, P., Macho, A., et al. (1996). Sequential acquisition of mitochondrial and plasma membrane alterations during early lymphocyte apoptosis. *J. Immunol.* 157, 512–521.

Chang, K. H., Tam, M., and Stevenson, M. M. (2004). Inappropriately low reticulocytosis in severe malarial anemia correlates with suppression in the development of late erythroid precursors. *Blood* 103, 3727–3735. doi: 10.1182/blood-2003-08-2887

Chilongola, J., Balthazary, S., Mpina, M., Mhando, M., and Mbugi, E. (2009). CD36 deficiency protects against malarial anaemia in children by reducing *Plasmodium falciparum*-infected red blood cell adherence to vascular endothelium. *Trop. Med. Int. Health* 14, 810–816. doi: 10.1111/j.1365-3156.2009.02298.x

Collins, W. E., Jeffery, G. M., and Roberts, J. M. (2003). A retrospective examination of anemia during infection of humans with *Plasmodium vivax*. *Am. J. Trop. Med. Hyg.* 68, 410–412.

Dai, C., and Krantz, S. B. (1999). Interferon gamma induces upregulation and activation of caspases 1, 3, and 8 to produce apoptosis in human erythroid progenitor cells. *Blood* 93, 3309–3316.

Dalko, E., Das, B., Herbert, F., Fesel, C., Pathak, S., Tripathy, R., et al. (2015). Multifaceted role of heme during severe *Plasmodium falciparum* infections in India. *Infect. Immun.* 83, 3793–3799. doi: 10.1128/IAI.00531-15

Daniel-Ribeiro, C. T., Banic, D. M., Issa-Ahmed, I., and Galvão-Castro, B. (1986). Polyclonal B-lymphocyte activation and sensitization of erythrocytes by IgG in human malaria: relevance to the development of anaemia in a holoendemic area in northwestern Brazil (Ariquemes - Rondônia). *Mem. Inst. Oswaldo Cruz* 81, 169–176. doi: 10.1590/S0074-02761986000600028

Daniel-Ribeiro, C. T., and Zanini, G. (2000). Autoimmunity and malaria: what are they doing together? *Acta Trop.* 76, 205–221. doi: 10.1016/S0001-706X(00)00099-1

Das, B. S., Patnaik, J. K., Mohanty, S., Mishra, S. K., Mohanty, D., Satpathy, S. K., et al. (1993). Plasma antioxidants and lipid peroxidation products in falciparum malaria. *Am. J. Trop. Med. Hyg.* 49, 720–725.

De Nardo, P., Oliva, A., Giancola, M. L., Ghirga, P., Mencarini, P., Bibas, M., et al. (2013). Haemolytic anaemia after oral artemether-lumefantrine treatment in a patient affected by severe imported falciparum malaria. *Infection* 41, 863–865. doi: 10.1007/s15010-013-0451-x

Dondorp, A. M., Angus, B. J., Chotivanich, K., Silamut, K., Ruangveerayuth, R., Hardeman, M. R., et al. (1999). Red blood cell deformability as a predictor of anemia in severe falciparum malaria. *Am. J. Trop. Med. Hyg.* 60, 733–737.

Eda, S., and Sherman, I. W. (2002). Cytoadherence of malaria-infected red blood cells involves exposure of phosphatidylserine. *Cell. Physiol. Biochem.* 12, 373–384. doi: 10.1159/000067908

Ekvall, H. (2003). Malaria and anemia. *Curr. Opin. Hematol.* 10, 108–114. doi: 10.1097/00062752-200303000-00002

Evans, K. J., Hansen, D. S., van Rooijen, N., Buckingham, L. A., and Schofield, L. (2006). Severe malarial anemia of low parasite burden in rodent models results from accelerated clearance of uninfected erythrocytes. *Blood* 107, 1192–1199. doi: 10.1182/blood-2005-08-3460

Felder, K. M., Hoelzle, K., Ritzmann, M., Kilchling, T., Schiele, D., Heinritzi, K., et al. (2011). Hemotrophic mycoplasmas induce programmed cell death in red blood cells. *Cell. Physiol. Biochem.* 27, 557–564. doi: 10.1159/000329957

Fendel, R., Brandts, C., Rudat, A., Kreidenweiss, A., Steur, C., Appelmann, I., et al. (2010). Hemolysis is associated with low reticulocyte production index and predicts blood transfusion in severe malarial anemia. *PLoS ONE* 5:e10038. doi: 10.1371/journal.pone.0010038

Fernandez-Arias, C., Rivera-Correa, J., Gallego-Delgado, J., Rudlaff, R., Fernandez, C., Roussel, C., et al. (2016). Anti-self phosphatidylserine antibodies recognize uninfected erythrocytes promoting malarial anemia. *Cell Host Microbe* 19, 194–203. doi: 10.1016/j.chom.2016.01.009

Föller, M., Shumilina, E., Lam, R., Mohamed, W., Kasinathan, R., Huber, S., et al. (2007). Induction of suicidal erythrocyte death by listeriolysin from *Listeria monocytogenes*. *Cell. Physiol. Biochem.* 20, 1051–1060. doi: 10.1159/000110715

Gao, M., Cheung, K. L., Lau, I. P., Yu, W. S., Fung, K. P., Yu, B., et al. (2012). Polyphyllin D induces apoptosis in human erythrocytes through Ca^{2+} rise and membrane permeabilization. *Arch. Toxicol.* 86, 741–752. doi: 10.1007/s00204-012-0808-4

Goka, B. Q., Kwarko, H., Kurtzhals, J. A., Gyan, B., Ofori-Adjei, E., Ohene, S. A., et al. (2001). Complement binding to erythrocytes is associated with macrophage activation and reduced haemoglobin in *Plasmodium falciparum* malaria. *Trans. R. Soc. Trop. Med. Hyg.* 95, 545–549. doi: 10.1016/S0035-9203(01)90036-7

Grau, G. E., and Craig, A. G. (2012). Cerebral malaria pathogenesis: revisiting parasite and host contributions. *Future Microbiol.* 7, 291–302. doi: 10.2217/fmb.11.155

Greenberg, M. E., Sun, M., Zhang, R., Febbraio, M., Silverstein, R., and Hazen, S. L. (2006). Oxidized phosphatidylserine-CD36 interactions play an essential role in macrophage-dependent phagocytosis of apoptotic cells. *J. Exp. Med.* 203, 2613–2625. doi: 10.1084/jem.20060370

Guo, Y. L., Liu, D. Q., Bian, Z., Zhang, C. Y., and Zen, K. (2009). Down-regulation of platelet surface CD47 expression in *Escherichia coli* O157:H7 infection-induced thrombocytopenia. *PLoS ONE* 4:e7131. doi: 10.1371/journal.pone.0007131

Harris, J. V., Bohr, T. M., Stracener, C., Landmesser, M. E., Torres, V., Mbugua, A., et al. (2012). *Sequential Plasmodium* chabaudi and *Plasmodium berghei* infections provide a novel model of severe malarial anemia. *Infect. Immun.* 80, 2997–3007. doi: 10.1128/IAI.06185-11

Hattori, Y., Takano, K., Teramae, H., Yamamoto, S., Yokoo, H., and Matsuda, N. (2010). Insights into sepsis therapeutic design based on the apoptotic death pathway. *J. Pharmacol. Sci.* 114, 354–365. doi: 10.1254/jphs.10R04CR

Helleberg, M., Goka, B. Q., Akanmori, B. D., Obeng-Adjei, G., Rodriques, O., and Kurtzhals, J. A. (2005). Bone marrow suppression and severe anaemia associated with persistent *Plasmodium falciparum* infection in African children with microscopically undetectable parasitaemia. *Malar. J.* 4:56. doi: 10.1186/1475-2875-4-56

Hermsen, C. C., Konijnenberg, Y., Mulder, L., Loé, C., van Deuren, M., van der Meer, J. W., et al. (2003). Circulating concentrations of soluble granzyme A and B increase during natural and experimental *Plasmodium falciparum* infections. *Clin. Exp. Immunol.* 132, 467–472. doi: 10.1046/j.1365-2249.2003.02160.x

Huang, S., Amaladoss, A., Liu, M., Chen, H., Zhang, R., Preiser, P. R., et al. (2014). *In vivo* splenic clearance correlates with *in vitro* deformability of red blood cells from *Plasmodium yoelii*-infected mice. *Infect. Immun.* 82, 2532–2541. doi: 10.1128/IAI.01525-13

Issifou, S., Mavoungou, E., Borrmann, S., Bouyou-Akotet, M. K., Matsiegui, P. B., and Kremsner, P. G. (2003). Severe malarial anemia associated with increased soluble Fas ligand (sFasL) concentrations in Gabonese children. *Eur. Cytokine Netw.* 14, 238–241.

Jacobs, P., Radzioch, D., and Stevenson, M. M. (1996). A Th1-associated increase in tumor necrosis factor alpha expression in the spleen correlates with resistance to blood-stage malaria in mice. *Infect. Immun.* 64, 535–541.

Jacobson, M. D., Burne, J. F., and Raff, M. C. (1994). Programmed cell death and Bcl-2 protection in the absence of a nucleus. *EMBO J.* 13, 1899–1910.

Jakeman, G. N., Saul, A., Hogarth, W. L., and Collins, W. E. (1999). Anaemia of acute malaria infections in non-immune patients primarily results from destruction of uninfected erythrocytes. *Parasitology* 119, 127–133. doi: 10.1017/S0031182099004564

Jana, S., and Paliwal, J. (2007). Apoptosis: potential therapeutic targets for new drug discovery. *Curr. Med. Chem.* 14, 2369–2379. doi: 10.2174/092986707781745569

Jang, W. H., Lim, K. M., Kim, K., Noh, J. Y., Kang, S., Chang, Y. K., et al. (2011). Low level of lead can induce phosphatidylserine exposure and erythrophagocytosis: a new mechanism underlying lead-associated anemia. *Toxicol. Sci.* 122, 177–184. doi: 10.1093/toxsci/kfr079

Jiang, H., Fu, R., Wang, H., Li, L., Liu, H., and Shao, Z. (2013). CD47 is expressed abnormally on hematopoietic cells in myelodysplastic syndrome. *Leuk. Res.* 37, 907–910. doi: 10.1016/j.leukres.2013.04.008

Jilani, K., Lupescu, A., Zbidah, M., Abed, M., Shaik, N., and Lang, F. (2012). Enhanced apoptotic death of erythrocytes induced by the mycotoxin ochratoxin A. *Kidney Blood Press. Res.* 36, 107–118. doi: 10.1159/000341488

Kasinathan, R. S., and Greenberg, R. M. (2010). *Schistosoma mansoni* soluble egg antigens trigger erythrocyte cell death. *Cell. Physiol. Biochem.* 26, 767–774. doi: 10.1159/000322344

Kempe, D. S., Akel, A., Lang, P. A., Hermle, T., Biswas, R., Muresanu, J., et al. (2007). Suicidal erythrocyte death in sepsis. *J. Mol. Med.* 85, 273–281. doi: 10.1007/s00109-006-0123-8

Kerr, J. F., Wyllie, A. H., and Currie, A. R. (1972). Apoptosis: a basic biological phenomenon with wide-ranging implications in tissue kinetics. *Br. J. Cancer* 26, 239–257. doi: 10.1038/bjc.1972.33

Khandelwal, S., van Rooijen, N., and Saxena, R. K. (2007). Reduced expression of CD47 during murine red blood cell (RBC) senescence and its role in RBC clearance from the circulation. *Transfusion* 47, 1725–1732. doi: 10.1111/j.1537-2995.2007.01348.x

Koka, S., Huber, S. M., Boini, K. M., Lang, C., Föller, M., and Lang, F. (2007). Lead decreases parasitemia and enhances survival of *Plasmodium berghei*-infected mice. *Biochem. Biophys. Res. Commun.* 363, 484–489. doi: 10.1016/j.bbrc.2007.08.173

Kongpatanakul, S., Chatsiricharoenkul, S., Khuhapinant, A., Atipas, S., and Kaewkungwal, J. (2009). Comparative study of dihydroartemisinin and artesunate safety in healthy Thai volunteers. *Int. J. Clin. Pharmacol. Ther.* 47, 579–586. doi: 10.5414/CPP47579

Kulkarni, A. G., Suryakar, A. N., Sardeshmukh, A. S., and Rathi, D. B. (2003). Studies on biochemical changes with special reference to oxidant and antioxidants in malaria patients. *Indian J. Clin. Biochem.* 18, 136–149. doi: 10.1007/BF02867380

Lafuse, W. P., Story, R., Mahylis, J., Gupta, G., Varikuti, S., Steinkamp, H., et al. (2013). *Leishmania donovani* infection induces anemia in hamsters by differentially altering erythropoiesis in bone marrow and spleen. *PLoS ONE* 8:e59509. doi: 10.1371/journal.pone.0059509

Lamikanra, A. A., Brown, D., Potocnik, A., Casals-Pascual, C., Langhorne, J., and Roberts, D. J. (2007). Malarial anemia: of mice and men. *Blood* 110, 18–28. doi: 10.1182/blood-2006-09-018069

Lamikanra, A. A., Merryweather-Clarke, A. T., Tipping, A. J., and Roberts, D. J. (2015). Distinct mechanisms of inadequate erythropoiesis induced by tumor necrosis factor alpha or malarial pigment. *PLoS ONE* 10:e0119836. doi: 10.1371/journal.pone.0119836

Lamikanra, A. A., Theron, M., Kooij, T. W. A., and Roberts, D. J. (2009). Hemozoin (malaria pigment) directly promotes apoptosis of erythroid precursors. *PLoS ONE* 4:e8446. doi: 10.1371/journal.pone.0008446

Lang, E., and Lang, F. (2015). Triggers, inhibitors, mechanisms, and significance of eryptosis: the suicidal erythrocyte death. *BioMed. Res. Int.* 2015:513518. doi: 10.1155/2015/513518

Lang, E., Qadri, S. M., and Lang, F. (2012). Killing me softly – suicidal erythrocyte death. *Int. J. Biochem. Cell Biol.* 44, 1236–1243. doi: 10.1016/j.biocel.2012.04.019

Lang, F., Lang, P. A., Lang, K. S., Brand, V., Tanneur, V., Duranton, C., et al. (2004a). Channel-induced apoptosis of infected host cells-the case of malaria. *Pflugers Arch.* 448, 319–324. doi: 10.1007/s00424-004-1254-9

Lang, K. S., Roll, B., Myssina, S., Schittenhelm, M., Scheel-Walter, H. G., Kanz, L., et al. (2002). Enhanced erythrocyte apoptosis in sickle cell anemia, thalassemia and glucose-6-phosphate dehydrogenase deficiency. *Cell. Physiol. Biochem.* 12, 365–372. doi: 10.1159/000067907

Lang, P. A., Kaiser, S., Myssina, S., Birka, C., Weinstock, C., Northoff, H., et al. (2004b). Effect of *Vibrio parahaemolyticus* haemolysin on human erythrocytes. *Cell. Microbiol.* 6, 391–400. doi: 10.1111/j.1462-5822.2004.00369.x

La Raja, M. (2002). Erythrophagocytosis by peripheral monocytes in *Plasmodium falciparum* malaria. *Haematologica* 87:EIM14.

Lawrence, D. W., King, S. B., Frazier, W. A., and Koenig, J. M. (2009). Decreased CD47 expression during spontaneous apoptosis targets neutrophils for phagocytosis by monocyte-derived macrophages. *Early Hum. Dev.* 85, 659–663. doi: 10.1016/j.earlhumdev.2009.09.005

Layez, C., Nogueira, P., Combes, V., Costa, F. T., Juhan-Vague, I., da Silva, L. H., et al. (2005). *Plasmodium falciparum* rhoptry protein RSP2 triggers destruction of the erythroid lineage. *Blood* 106, 3632–3638. doi: 10.1182/blood-2005-04-1574

Leowattana, W., Krudsood, S., Tangpukdee, N., Brittenham, G., and Looareesuwan, S. (2008). Defective erythropoietin production and reticulocyte response in acute *Plasmodium falciparum* malaria-associated anemia. *Southeast Asian J. Trop. Med. Public Health* 39, 581–588.

Lv, Z., Bian, Z., Shi, L., Niu, S., Ha, B., Tremblay, A., et al. (2015). Loss of cell surface CD47 clustering formation and binding avidity to SIRPα facilitate apoptotic cell clearance by macrophages. *J. Immunol.* 195, 661–671. doi: 10.4049/jimmunol.1401719

Mandal, D., Moitra, P. K., Saha, S., and Basu, J. (2002). Caspase 3 regulates phosphatidylserine externalization and phagocytosis of oxidatively stressed erythrocytes. *FEBS Lett.* 513, 184–188. doi: 10.1016/S0014-5793(02)02294-9

Mao, T. Y., Fu, L. L., and Wang, J. S. (2011). Hypoxic exercise training causes erythrocyte senescence and rheological dysfunction by depressed Gardos channel activity. *J. Appl. Physiol.* 111, 382–391. doi: 10.1152/japplphysiol.00096.2011

McGilvray, I. D., Serghides, L., Kapus, A., Rotstein, O. D., and Kain, K. C. (2000). Nonopsonic monocyte/macrophage phagocytosis of *Plasmodium falciparum*-parasitized erythrocytes: a role for CD36 in malarial clearance. *Blood* 96, 3231–3240.

Means, R. T. Jr., and Krantz, S. B. (1991). Inhibition of human erythroid colony-forming units by gamma interferon can be corrected by recombinant human erythropoietin. *Blood* 78, 2564–2567.

Menendez, C., Fleming, A. F., and Alonso, P. L. (2000). Malaria-related anaemia. *Parasitol. Today* 16, 469–476. doi: 10.1016/S0169-4758(00)01774-9

Meremikwu, M. M., and Smith, H. J. (2000). Blood transfusion for treating malarial anaemia. *Cochrane Database Syst. Rev.* 2:CD001475. doi: 10.1002/14651858.CD001475

Merry, A. H., Looareesuwan, S., Phillips, R. E., Chanthavanich, P., Supanaranond, W., Warrell, D. A., et al. (1986). Evidence against immune haemolysis in falciparum malaria in Thailand. *Br. J. Haematol.* 64, 187–194. doi: 10.1111/j.1365-2141.1986.tb07586.x

Mindukshev, I. V., Rukoiatkina, N. I., Dobrylko, I. A., Skverchinskaia, E. A., Nikitina, E. R., Krivoshlyk, V. V., et al. (2013). Characterisation of enucleated cells apoptosis: human platelets and erythrocytes. *Ross. Fiziol. Zh. Im. I. M. Sechenova* 99, 92–110.

Muoneke, V.U., Ibekwe, R.C., Nebe-Agumadu, H.U., and Ibe, B.C. (2012). Factors associated with mortality in under-five children with severe anemia in Ebonyi, Nigeria. *Idian. Pediatr.* 49, 119–123. doi: 10.1007/s13312-012-0026-4

Myssina, S., Huber, S. M., Birka, C., Lang, P. A., Lang, K. S., Friedrich, B., et al. (2003). Inhibition of erythrocyte cation channels by erythropoietin. *J. Am. Soc. Nephrol.* 14, 2750–2757. doi: 10.1097/01.ASN.0000093253.42641.C1

Noh, J. Y., Park, J. S., Lim, K. M., Kim, K., Bae, O. N., Chung, S. M., et al. (2010). A naphthoquinone derivative can induce anemia through phosphatidylserine exposure-mediated erythrophagocytosis. *J. Pharmacol. Exp. Ther.* 333, 414–420. doi: 10.1124/jpet.109.164608

Obonyo, C. O., Vulule, J., Akhwale, W. S., and Grobbee, D. E. (2007). In-hospital morbidity and mortality due to severe malarial anemia in western Kenya. *Am. J. Trop. Med. Hyg.* 77, 23–28.

Oldenborg, P. A., Gresham, H. D., Chen, Y., Izui, S., and Lindberg, F. P. (2002). Lethal autoimmune hemolytic anemia in CD47-deficient nonobese diabetic (NOD) mice. *Blood* 99, 3500–3504. doi: 10.1182/blood.V99.10.3500

Oldenborg, P. A., Gresham, H. D., and Lindberg, F. P. (2001). CD47-signal regulatory protein α (SIRPα) regulates Fcγ and complement receptor-mediated phagocytosis. *J. Exp. Med.* 193, 855–862. doi: 10.1084/jem.193.7.855

Oldenborg, P. A., Zheleznyak, A., Fang, Y. F., Lagenaur, C. F., Gresham, H. D., and Lindberg, F. P. (2000). Role of CD47 as a marker of self on red blood cells. *Science* 288, 2051–2054. doi: 10.1126/science.288.5473.2051

Olsson, M., and Oldenborg, P. A. (2008). CD47 on experimentally senescent murine RBCs inhibits phagocytosis following Fcγ receptor-mediated but not scavenger receptor-mediated recognition by macrophages. *Blood* 112, 4259–4267. doi: 10.1182/blood-2008-03-143008

Omodeo-Salè, F., Motti, A., Dondorp, A., White, N. J., and Taramelli, D. (2005). Destabilisation and subsequent lysis of human erythrocytes induced by *Plasmodium falciparum* haem products. *Eur. J. Haematol.* 74, 324–332. doi: 10.1111/j.1600-0609.2004.00352.x

Osaro, E., and Charles, A. T. (2011). The challenges of meeting the blood transfusion requirements in Sub-Saharan Africa: the need for the development of alternatives to allogenic blood. *J. Blood. Med.* 2, 7–21. doi: 10.2147/JBM.S17194

Pain, A., Urban, B. C., Kai, O., Casals-Pascual, C., Shafi, J., Marsh, K., et al. (2001). A non-sense mutation in Cd36 gene is associated with protection from severe malaria. *Lancet* 357, 1502–1503. doi: 10.1016/S0140-6736(00)04 662-6

Papadaki, H. A., Kritikos, H. D., Valatas, V., Boumpas, D. T., and Eliopoulos, G. D. (2002). Anemia of chronic disease in rheumatoid arthritis is associated with increased apoptosis of bone marrow erythroid cells: improvement following anti-tumor necrosis factor-alpha antibody therapy. *Blood* 100, 474–482. doi: 10.1182/blood-2002-01-0136

Patel, S. N., Serghides, L., Smith, T. G., Febbraio, M., Silverstein, R. L., Kurtz, T. W., et al. (2004). CD36 mediates the phagocytosis of *Plasmodium falciparum*-infected erythrocytes by rodent macrophages. *J. Infect. Dis.* 189, 204–213. doi: 10.1086/380764

Pattanapanyasat, K., Sratongno, P., Chimma, P., Chitjamnongchai, S., Polsrila, K., and Chotivanich, K. (2010). Febrile temperature but not proinflammatory cytokines promotes phosphatidylserine expression on *Plasmodium falciparum* malaria-infected red blood cells during parasite maturation. *Cytometry A* 77, 515–523. doi: 10.1002/cyto.a.20879

Paul, A., Pallavi, R., Tatu, U. S., and Natarajan, V. (2013). The bystander effect in optically trapped red blood cells due *Plasmodium falciparum* infection. *Trans. R. Soc. Trop. Med. Hyg.* 107, 220–223. doi: 10.1093/trstmh/trt010

Phillips, R. E., Looareesuwan, S., Warrell, D. A., Lee, S. H., Karbwang, J., Warrell, M. J., et al. (1986). The importance of anaemia in cerebral and uncomplicated falciparum malaria: role of complications, dyserythropoiesis and iron sequestration. *Q. J. Med.* 58, 305–323.

Phillips, R. E., and Pasvol, G. (1992). Anaemia of *Plasmodium falciparum* malaria. *Baillières Clin. Haematol.* 5, 315–330. doi: 10.1016/S0950-3536(11)80022-3

Pino, P., Vouldoukis, I., Kolb, J. P., Mahmoudi, N., Desportes-Livage, I., Bricaire, F., et al. (2003). *Plasmodium falciparum*-infected erythrocyte adhesion induces caspase activation and apoptosis in human endothelial cells. *J. Infect. Dis.* 187, 1283–1290. doi: 10.1086/373992

Raffray, L., Receveur, M. C., Beguet, M., Lauroua, P., Pistone, T., and Malvy, D. (2014). Severe delayed autoimmune haemolytic anaemia following artesunate administration in severe malaria: a case report. *Malar. J.* 13:398. doi: 10.1186/1475-2875-13-398

Rodrigues, V., Cordeiro-da-Silva, A., Laforge, M., Ouaissi, A., Silvestre, R., and Estaquier, J. (2012). Modulation of mammalian apoptotic pathways by intracellular protozoan parasites. *Cell. Microbiol.* 14, 325–333. doi: 10.1111/j.1462-5822.2011.01737.x

Salmon, M. G., De Souza, J. B., Butcher, G. A., and Playfair, J. H. (1997). Premature removal of uninfected erythrocytes during malarial infection of normal and immunodeficient mice. *Clin. Exp. Immunol.* 108, 471–476. doi: 10.1046/j.1365-2249.1997.3991297.x

Satpathy, S. K., Mohanty, N., Nanda, P., and Samal, G. (2004). Severe falciparum malaria. *Indian J. Pediatr.* 71, 133–135. doi: 10.1007/BF02723094

Schantz-Dunn, J., and Nour, N. M. (2009). Malaria and pregnancy: a global health perspective. *Rev. Obstet. Gynecol.* 2, 186–192.

Schulze-Osthoff, K., Walczak, H., Drodge, W., and Krammer, P. H. (1994). Cell nucleus and DNA fragmentation are not required for apoptosis. *J. Cell. Biol.* 127, 15–20. doi: 10.1083/jcb.127.1.15

Shi, B., Ma, G. G., Liu, H. X., Liu, J. Q., Yang, W. H., Zhang, H. Z., et al. (2013). Significance of erythrocytes phosphatidylserine exposure on occurrence of anemia in sepsis. *Chin. Crit. Care. Med.* 25, 614–617. doi: 10.3760/cma.j.issn.2095-4352.2013.10.009

Skorokhod, O. A., Caione, L., Marrocco, T., Migliardi, G., Barrera, V., Arese, P., et al. (2010). Inhibition of erythropoiesis in malaria anemia: role of hemozoin and hemozoin-generated 4-hydroxynonenal. *Blood* 116, 4328–4337. doi: 10.1182/blood-2010-03-272781

Sobolewski, P., Gramaglia, I., Frangos, J., Intaglietta, M., and van der Heyde, H. C. (2005). Nitric oxide bioavailability in malaria. *Trends Parasitol.* 21, 415–422. doi: 10.1016/j.pt.2005.07.002

Sosale, N. G., Spinler, K. R., Alvey, C., and Discher, D. E. (2015). Macrophage engulfment of a cell or nanoparticle is regulated by unavoidable opsonization, a species-specific 'marker of self' CD47, and target physical properties. *Curr. Opin. Immunol.* 35, 107–112. doi: 10.1016/j.coi.2015.06.013

Sowunmi, A., Akano, K., Ayede, A. I., Ntadom, G., Fatunmbi, B., Aderoyeje, T., et al. (2015). Temporal changes in haematocrit following artemisinin-based combination treatments of uncomplicated falciparum malaria in children. *BMC Infect. Dis.* 15:454. doi: 10.1186/s12879-015-1219-y

Spottiswoode, N., Duffy, P. E., and Drakesmith, H. (2014). Iron, anemia and hepcidin in malaria. *Front. Pharmacol.* 5:125. doi: 10.3389/fphar.2014.00125

Stewart, A., Urbaniak, S., Turner, M., and Bessos, H. (2005). The application of a new quantitative assay for the monitoring of integrin-associated protein CD47 on red blood cells during storage and comparison with the expression of CD47 and phosphatidylserine with flow cytometry. *Transfusion* 45, 1496–1503. doi: 10.1111/j.1537-2995.2005.00564.x

Tait, J. F., and Smith, C. (1999). Phosphatidylserine receptors: role of CD36 in binding of anionic phospholipid vesicles to monocytic cells. *J. Biol. Chem.* 274, 3048–3054. doi: 10.1074/jbc.274.5.3048

Thawani, N., Tam, M., Bellemare, M. J., Bohle, D. S., Olivier, M., de Souza, J. B., et al. (2014). Plasmodium products contribute to severe malarial anemia by inhibiting erythropoietin-induced proliferation of erythroid precursors. *J. Infect. Dis.* 209, 140–149. doi: 10.1093/infdis/jit417

Totino, P. R., Daniel-Ribeiro, C. T., and Ferreira-da-Cruz, M. F. (2009). Pro-apoptotic effects of antimalarial drugs do not affect mature human erythrocytes. *Acta Trop.* 112, 236–238. doi: 10.1016/j.actatropica.2009.08.002

Totino, P. R., Daniel-Ribeiro, C. T., and Ferreira-da-Cruz M., F. (2011). Refractoriness of eryptotic red blood cells to *Plasmodium falciparum* infection: a putative host defense mechanism limiting parasitaemia. *PLoS ONE* 6:e26575. doi: 10.1371/journal.pone.0026575

Totino, P. R., Magalhães, A. D., Alves, E. B., Costa, M. R. F., Lacerda, M. V. G., Daniel-Ribeiro, C. T., et al. (2014). *Plasmodium falciparum*, but not P. vivax, can induce erythrocytic apoptosis. *Parasit. Vectors* 7:484. doi: 10.1186/s13071-014-0484-8

Totino, P. R., Magalhães, A. D., Silva, L. A., Banic, D. M., Daniel-Ribeiro, C. T., and Ferreira-da-Cruz M., F. (2010). Apoptosis of non-parasitized red blood cells in malaria: a putative mechanism involved in the pathogenesis of anaemia. *Malar. J.* 9:350. doi: 10.1186/1475-2875-9-350

Totino, P. R., Pinna, R. A., Oliveira, A. C., Banic, D. M., Daniel-Ribeiro, C. T., and Ferreira-da-Cruz M., F. (2013). Apoptosis of non-parasitised red blood cells in *Plasmodium yoelii* malaria. *Mem. Inst. Oswaldo Cruz* 108, 686–690. doi: 10.1590/0074-0276108062013003

Totino, P. R., Riccio, E. K., Corte-Real, S., Daniel-Ribeiro, C. T., and de Fátima Ferreira-da-Cruz, M. (2006). Dexamethasone has pro-apoptotic effects on non-activated fresh peripheral blood mononuclear cells. *Cell. Biol. Int.* 30, 133–137. doi: 10.1016/j.cellbi.2005.09.002

Ulett, G. C., and Adderson, E. E. (2006). Regulation of apoptosis by gram-positive bacteria: mechanistic diversity and consequences for immunity. *Curr. Immunol. Rev.* 2, 119–141. doi: 10.2174/157339506776843033

Vittori, D., Vota, D., Callero, M., Chamorro, M. E., and Nesse, A. (2010). c-FLIP is involved in erythropoietin-mediated protection of erythroid-differentiated cells from TNF-α-induced apoptosis. *Cell Biol. Int.* 34, 621–630. doi: 10.1042/CBI20090085

Waitumbi, J. N., Opollo, M. O., Muga, R. O., Misore, A. O., and Stoute, J. A. (2000). Red cell surface changes and erythrophagocytosis in children with severe *Plasmodium falciparum* anemia. *Blood* 95, 1481–1486.

Wennicke, K., Debierre-Grockiego, F., Wichmann, D., Brattig, N. W., Pankuweit, S., Maisch, B., et al. (2008). Glycosylphosphatidylinositol-induced cardiac myocyte death might contribute to the fatal outcome of *Plasmodium falciparum* malaria. *Apoptosis* 13, 857–866. doi: 10.1007/s10495-008-0217-6

Williams, G. T. (1994). Programmed cell death: a fundamental protective response to pathogens. *Trends Microbiol.* 2, 463–464. doi: 10.1016/0966-842X(94)90648-3

Wilson, N. O., Huang, M. B., Anderson, W., Bond, V., Powell, M., Thompson, W. E., et al. (2008). Soluble factors from *Plasmodium falciparum*-infected erythrocytes induce apoptosis in human brain vascular endothelial and neuroglia cells. *Mol. Biochem. Parasitol.* 162, 172–176. doi: 10.1016/j.molbiopara.2008.09.003

Wu, Y., Tibrewal, N., and Birge, R. B. (2006). Phosphatidylserine recognition by phagocytes: a view to a kill. *Trends Cell Biol.* 16, 189–197. doi: 10.1016/j.tcb.2006.02.003

Wyllie, A. H. (1980). Glucocorticoid-induced thymocyte apoptosis is associated with endogenous endonuclease activation. *Nature* 284, 555–556. doi: 10.1038/284555a0

Xie, L. H., Johnson, T. O., Weina, P. J., Si, Y., Haeberle, A., Upadhyay, R., et al. (2005). Risk assessment and therapeutic indices of artesunate and artelinate in Plasmodium berghei-infected and uninfected rats. *Int. J. Toxicol.* 24, 251–264. doi: 10.1080/10915810591007229

4

Mining the Human Host Metabolome Toward an Improved Understanding of Malaria Transmission

Regina Joice Cordy[1,2*]

[1] *Department of Biology, Wake Forest University, Winston-Salem, NC, United States,* [2] *Department of Microbiology and Immunology, Wake Forest School of Medicine, Winston-Salem, NC, United States*

Edited by:
Brandon Keith Wilder,
Oregon Health & Science University,
United States

Reviewed by:
Jeremy Keith Herren,
International Centre of Insect
Physiology and Ecology, Kenya
Gabriella Fiorentino,
University of Naples Federico II, Italy

***Correspondence:**
Regina Joice Cordy
cordyrj@wfu.edu

The big data movement has led to major advances in our ability to assess vast and complex datasets related to the host and parasite during malaria infection. While host and parasite genomics and transcriptomics are often the focus of many computational efforts in malaria research, metabolomics represents another big data type that has great promise for aiding our understanding of complex host-parasite interactions that lead to the transmission of malaria. Recent analyses of the complement of metabolites present in human blood, skin and breath suggest that host metabolites play a critical role in the transmission cycle of malaria. Volatile compounds released through breath and skin serve as attractants to mosquitoes, with malaria-infected hosts appearing to have unique profiles that further increase host attractiveness. Inside the host, fluctuations in the levels of certain metabolites in blood may trigger increased production of transmission-competent sexual stages (gametocytes), setting the stage for enhanced transmission of malaria from human to mosquito. Together, these recent discoveries suggest that metabolites of human blood, skin and breath play critical roles in malaria transmission. This review discusses recent advances in this area, with a focus on metabolites that have been identified to play a role in malaria transmission and methods that may lead to an improved understanding of malaria transmission.

Keywords: plasmodium, malaria, gametocyte, metabolomics, mass spectrometry, transmission, mosquito

INTRODUCTION

Technological advancements have been made in recent years in sequencing-based (genomics, transcriptomics, epigenomics) and mass spectrometry-based approaches (proteomics, lipidomics, and metabolomics). These so called 'omics technologies have enabled researchers to explore various biological contexts at multiple levels, and the integration of these technologies is being used to improve our understanding of a range of human diseases (Hasin et al., 2017). An exciting area in which 'omics technology has been applied is in the realm of host-microbe interactions, including the complex interplay between microbes and their hosts in both pathogenic (e.g., viral, bacterial, and parasitic) and commensal (e.g., microbiome) relationships. These such interactions between microbes and their human hosts are often quite complex, resulting from co-evolution over massive time scales.

A highly complex interaction exists between *Plasmodium* (the etiological agent of malaria) and its invertebrate and vertebrate hosts, resulting from tens of thousands of years of co-evolution (Loy et al., 2017). In addition to *Plasmodium's* ability to replicate asexually within the blood cells of vertebrate hosts, *Plasmodium* also undergoes complex stage conversions to successfully transmit itself to the invertebrate host (*Anopheles* mosquito), where it must again undergo a series of stage conversions to be successfully delivered to the next vertebrate host. The propagation of malaria, which is attributed to over 400,000 deaths annually (World Health Organization [WHO], 2018), is therefore highly dependent on the ability of *Plasmodium* to successfully undergo multiple complex stage conversions, and move efficiently between the invertebrate and vertebrates hosts. *Plasmodium* has evolved multiple mechanisms for manipulating its hosts in order to enhance the chances of its successful transmission (Koella, 2005; Cator et al., 2012), and the manipulation of the metabolites present in human blood, skin and breath appears to be one of these such mechanisms.

Metabolomics, the high-throughput profiling of small molecules, has been employed to investigate the role of small molecules (metabolites) in the stage conversions and host exchanges that lead to the successful transmission of malaria. Methods that have been employed to investigate such metabolites run the gamut from functional approaches (e.g., sensory attraction tests), classic metabolic approaches (e.g., fractionation and metabolic labeling), and mass spectrometry-based methods (e.g., gas and liquid chromatography). Within mass-spectrometry-based methods, untargeted big data metabolomics approaches and reference compound-based targeted approaches are both utilized.

In this review, the roles of host metabolites are discussed in the context of malaria transmission, with an emphasis on findings resulting from metabolomics-based investigations. Also discussed are the various ways in which different mass spectrometry-based techniques, computational analyses, and multi-omic modeling approaches can further our knowledge about the impact of host metabolites on malaria transmission.

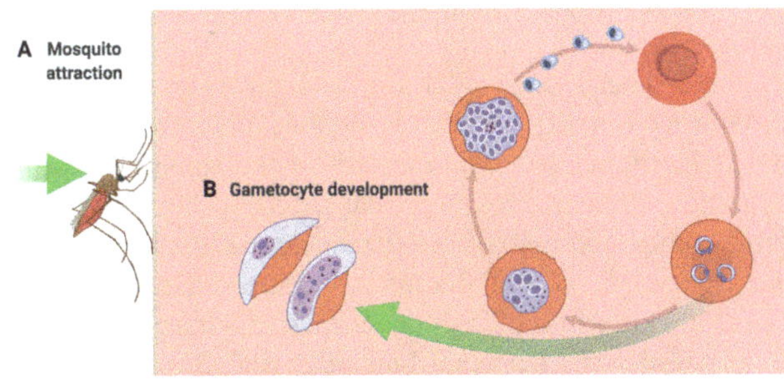

FIGURE 1 | Metabolic windows into malaria transmission. **(A)** Mosquito attraction and feeding. Malaria-infected human hosts produce volatile metabolites (e.g., terpenes and aldehydes) through their skin and/or breath that may serve as attractants for the female *Anopheles* mosquito when she takes her blood meal. **(B)** Gametocyte development. Certain metabolites undergo dynamic fluctuations in the blood plasma during the course of a malaria infection. Some specific metabolite changes have been hypothesized to be detected by parasites *in vivo* and trigger increased conversion to gametocytes (e.g., amino acids and phospholipids).

METABOLIC WINDOWS INTO MALARIA TRANSMISSION

In step with ongoing efforts worldwide to eradicate malaria, there has been an increased focus in recent years on gaining an improved understanding of malaria transmission and in developing novel ways to block and interrupt the cycle. The process of malaria transmission involves complex transitions between mosquito vector and vertebrate host, involving multiple parasite stage transitions.

Initiating a malaria infection in a human begins with the bite of a female *Anopheline* mosquito, which must locate and bite a human host in order to take a bloodmeal (**Figure 1A**). In doing so, the mosquito injects sporozoite stage parasites into the blood of the human host. Once inside the host, and following a period of development within the liver, the parasites begin to replicate asexually within red blood cells. At some point during the infection, a subset of parasites diverge down a path of sexual development, resulting in the formation of mature male and female gametocytes (**Figure 1B**). Importantly, mature gametocytes are the only stages that can be picked up by a mosquito and go on to successfully undergo fertilization and further development within the mosquito. Inside the mosquito, oocysts develop, and eventually burst, and sporozoites are released, migrating to the salivary gland, where they are now ready to be transmitted to the next human host during a subsequent bloodmeal. Adding to the complexity, recent studies suggest that metabolites present in the human host's blood, skin, and breath affect the efficacy of each of the key transition points in the parasite's life cycle, enhancing transmission. Specifically, volatile metabolites in the skin and breath of malaria-infected hosts have been shown to increase attractiveness to the mosquito vector (**Figure 1A**). And upstream of that biting event, metabolites in the host's bloodstream appear to act as signals for parasites to increase their rate of developing transmissible gametocyte stages (**Figure 1B**). The following sections focus on how metabolites in the blood, skin and breath of malaria-infected hosts play key roles in malaria transmission through modulating (a) the attractiveness of hosts to mosquitoes and (b) the rate of gametocyte development within host blood.

Metabolites Involved in Mosquito Attraction

It has been known for some time that carbon dioxide (CO_2) and other volatile chemicals help mosquitoes locate their vertebrate hosts and that certain molecules released through the skin, sweat and/or breath of vertebrates are attractive to mosquitoes (Brouwer, 1960; Takken and Kline, 1989). Some of these compounds, such as 1-Octen-3-ol, are routinely manufactured into baited mosquito traps, for example. However, a key question still remaining regarding the transmission of malaria is – *do individuals with malaria have increased attractiveness to mosquitoes, as compared to uninfected people?* (**Figure 1A**).

Gas chromatography mass spectrometry (GCMS) has been employed in efforts to answer this question. A specific type of GCMS called head space gas chromatography mass spectrometry (HS-GCMS) is used to analyze volatile organic compounds (VOCs) in the air space coming off of the subject or sample in question. Human cross-sectional studies using this method in the context of malaria have focused on analyzing VOCs from the breath of malaria-infected individuals. This work, termed "breathprinting," has demonstrated increased levels of multiple terpenes (α-pinene, limonene, and 3-carene), which are known mosquito-attractants (Nyasembe et al., 2012), in the breath of malaria-infected hosts (Kelly et al., 2015; Schaber et al., 2018) (**Table 1**). Additionally, controlled human malaria infection (CHMI) studies have also employed HS-GCMS to study the breath and skin odor composition in malaria-infected subjects (Berna et al., 2015; de Boer et al., 2017). In breath, four thioethers were found to increase in breath alongside increases in malaria parasitemia in blood: allyl methyl sulfide, 1-methylthio-propane, (*Z*)-1-methylthio-1-propene, and (*E*)-1-methylthio-1-propene (Berna et al., 2015). In skin, volatile compounds 2- and 3-methylbutanal, 3-hydroxy-2-butanone, and 6-methyl-5-hepten-2-one were all found to be present at higher levels in human skin odor during malaria infection, and also thought to attract mosquitoes (de Boer et al., 2017). In a further effort to identify VOCs derived from malaria parasites, an analysis of headspace from *in vitro Plasmodium* cultures was performed, and the headspace of the extracellular vesicles (EV) fraction also revealed an enrichment of a previously reported mosquito attractant aldehyde, hexanal (Correa et al., 2017) (**Table 1**).

Taking this concept a step further, a subset of studies have combined HS-GCMS with functional sensory tests in order to identify specific components of the metabolome that are detected by a mosquito's antenna. This approach, termed gas chromatography electroantennography (GC-EAG) involves the coupling of two approaches – chromatography-based compound analysis and an invertebrate sensory functional assessment. In short, as a compound comes off the column, it goes past a mosquito antenna. An olfactory nerve response occurs in the antenna, allowing for the determination of EAG-active metabolites. Example studies using GC-EAG include the analysis of foot odor of malaria-infected individuals, which revealed a set of aldehydes including heptanal, octanal, and nonanal produced at higher levels in malaria-infected individuals and shown to be sensed by mosquitoes (Robinson et al., 2018). Studies involving mammalian hosts including rodents have also used a combination of HS-GCMS and functional sensory tests and have demonstrated that 3-methyl butanoic acid, 2-methyl butanoic acid, hexanoic acid, and tridecane were all elevated at phases of mosquito attraction (De Moraes et al., 2014) (**Table 1**).

Olfactometers, devices used to test for host attractiveness to mosquitoes, have also been used to demonstrate that malaria-infected individuals are more attractive to mosquitoes. Of particular interest, this method has been used to demonstrate that humans carrying *Plasmodium* gametocytes have higher mosquito attractiveness than humans carrying asexual stages alone (Lacroix et al., 2005; Batista et al., 2014; Busula et al., 2017). Importantly this was seen in both *Plasmodium falciparum* and *P. vivax*. In addition, a similar approach was applied in a study of birds, which revealed that birds with chronic malaria are more attractive to mosquito vectors than those with acute malaria (Cornet et al., 2013).

While the production of specific VOCs seems to be linked to the presence of malaria parasites and particularly gametocytes

TABLE 1 | Metabolites associated with enhanced transmission of malaria.

Role	Context	Method	Metabolite	Citation
Increased mosquito attraction/feeding	mouse whole body headspace	GC	*Alkane*: tridecane *Fatty acids*: 3-methyl butanoic acid, 2-methyl butanoic acid, hexanoic acid	De Moraes et al., 2014
	In vitro Plasmodium headspace	GC	*Terpenes*: pinene, limonene	Kelly et al., 2015
	In vitro HMBPP-stimulated RBC headspace	GC	*Aldehydes*: octanal, nonanal, decanal *Terpenes*: α- and β-pinene, limonene *Oxide:* CO_2	Emami et al., 2017
	human skin (foot) headspace	GC	*Aldehyde*: 3-methylbutanal *Ketones*: 6-methyl-5-hepten-2-one, 2- and 3-hydroxy-2-butanone	de Boer et al., 2017
	In vitro Plasmodium headspace	GC	*Aldehyde*: hexanal	Correa et al., 2017
	human skin (foot) headspace	GC-EAG	*Aldehydes:* heptanal, octanal, nonanal	Robinson et al., 2018
	human breath	GC	*Terpenes:* α-pinene and 3-carene	Schaber et al., 2018
	human skin (foot) headspace	GC-EAG	*Aldehydes:* hexanal, nonanal *Aromatic hydrocarbon*: toluene	Stanczyk et al., 2019
Increased gametocyte development	*In vitro Plasmodium*	LC	*α-amino acid:* homocysteine	Beri et al., 2017
	in vitro Plasmodium, human blood	LC	*Phospholipid:* lysophosphotidylcholine	Brancucci et al., 2017; Usui et al., 2019
	In vitro Plasmodium	LC	*Phospholipids:* polyunsaturated fatty acid-containing phospholipids	Tanaka et al., 2019

within the mammalian hosts, the attraction by mosquitoes toward those hosts similarly appears to be affected by the infection status of the *mosquito*. Using olfactometers and neurophysiological assays, mosquitoes of the genus *Anopheles* were found to have a higher attractiveness toward human odors when they were infected with and carrying *Plasmodium* sporozoites than mosquitoes that were uninfected or were infected with those stages of the parasite that were not infectious yet (e.g., oocysts) (Cator et al., 2013; Smallegange et al., 2013). A recent study using GC-EAG to assess this question identified multiple compounds that infected mosquitoes responded to at a higher rate than uninfected mosquitoes, including some of the aldehydes identified in previous studies: hexanal and nonanal (Stanczyk et al., 2019) (**Table 1**). Further work combining olfactory tests with metabolomics approaches are likely to shed light on the full set of volatile chemicals that emanate from malaria-infected individuals, and can lead to broader characterization of compounds that increase host attractiveness to the mosquito vector.

Metabolites Involved in Gametocyte Development

While the attraction of mosquitoes to human hosts is a major part of malaria transmission, another key aspect is the production of gametocytes, which need to be present in the bloodstream of the human host in order to successfully transmit the parasite to the mosquito vector. The process by which asexually reproducing malaria parasites switch to sexual development is called gametocytogenesis and appears to involve both genetic and environmental cues. Specific transcriptional cascades are turned on during the transition from asexual to sexual replication, and environmental changes in host physiology have been long thought to contribute to this process (Josling and Llinás, 2015). A combination of mass spectrometry-based metabolomics, metabolic labeling approaches, and functional assays have implicated a role for exogenous metabolites in triggering sexual development. The primary question here being - *what are the signals in host blood that trigger Plasmodium to undergo gametocytogenesis?* (**Figure 1B**).

Liquid chromatography mass spectrometry (LC-MS) has been utilized in a number of studies to identify metabolites within *in vitro* culture media that are taken up or produced by *Plasmodium* parasites. Studies have been done to investigate the metabolic needs of asexually replicating *Plasmodium* parasites *in vitro* (Olszewski et al., 2009). Additional studies have focused on metabolites in human blood that are altered during malaria infections (Basant et al., 2010; Pappa et al., 2015; Surowiec et al., 2015; Decuypere et al., 2016; Gardinassi et al., 2017; Uppal et al., 2017; Ghosh et al., 2018; Cordy et al., 2019). This body of work has demonstrated the utility of this tool for identifying a wide range of physiological changes that occur in vertebrate hosts during malaria infection.

In addition to these aforementioned studies which focus on asexual replication, a subset of investigations focus on how host metabolites affect disease transmission. For example, a combination of *in vitro* and *in vivo* studies has identified a role for homocysteine in sexual development. This α-amino acid has been shown to accumulate within *Plasmodium*-infected red blood cells *in vitro*, causing redox stress and triggering gametocytogenesis (Chaubey et al., 2014; Beri et al., 2017). Validating the role of this metabolite, homocysteine was also administered to mice with *P. berghei* and an increase in gametocytes was subsequently observed *in vivo* (Beri et al., 2017) (**Table 1**).

Another finding identified through *in vitro* studies paired with LCMS was the discovery that a decline in lysophosphotidylcholine species (lysoPC) in the media was associated with an increased rate of gametocytogenesis (Brancucci et al., 2017). This finding was also supported by LCMS and Flow Injection Analysis (FIA) data from human subjects, demonstrating that *Plasmodium* grown in serum from subjects with lower lysoPC resulted in higher rates of gametocyte development *in vitro* (Usui et al., 2019). Finally, another LCMS-based *in vitro* study examined the difference between human serum and AlbuMAX supplementation in media and found that higher levels of polyunsaturated fatty acid (PUFA)-containing phospholipids in the media were associated with higher rates of gametocyte development *in vitro* (Tanaka et al., 2019) (**Table 1**). Altogether, through the use of LCMS alongside *in vitro* and/or *in vivo* methodologies, multiple host metabolic signals (including α-amino acids and phospholipids) have been identified that appear to trigger gametocyte development, and thus could contribute to malaria transmission.

WHO MAKES WHAT? COMPLEX ORIGINS OF HOST METABOLITES DURING MALARIA INFECTION

Metabolites found in the blood, skin and breath of malaria-infected hosts do not all come from the host. The host, its infecting parasite and even its commensal microbes can all contribute to the metabolome during infection. A key question, therefore, about the metabolites identified in the aforementioned approaches is – *are these metabolites coming from the parasite or the host (or the host's microbiome)?*

Plasmodium exhibits certain metabolic pathways that are not present in the vertebrate host, and chemicals of such pathways are thus known to be produced by the parasite. One such pathway is the 2-*C*-methyl-d-erythritol 4-phosphate (MEP) pathway, and one such chemical is (*E*)-4-hydroxy-3-methyl-but-2-enyl pyrophosphate (HMBPP), a precursor of the parasite's MEP pathway. While HMBPP itself is not a mosquito attractant molecule, HMBPP plays a role in malaria transmission through a complex interaction between the parasite and the host's red blood cells. HMBPP, which is produced by the parasite, has been shown to stimulate host red blood cells to increase their production of CO_2, aldehydes and monoterpenes, thereby indirectly affecting mosquito attractiveness (Emami et al., 2017) (**Table 1**). The volatile metabolites that attract the mosquito are thus host-derived, but the signal that stimulated the metabolite production is of parasite origin.

Commensal microbes of vertebrate hosts also demonstrate complex interplays leading to the production of mosquito attractant molecules, as has been reviewed previously (Braks et al., 1999). For example, 2- and 3-methylbutanal and 3-hydroxy-2-butanone, mosquito attractants found in the skin odor of malaria-infected individuals (de Boer et al., 2017) (**Table 1**), had been shown previously to be produced by skin microbes (Verhulst et al., 2009). In this study, GCMS identified these metabolites in the headspace of skin-associated microbes which were grown *in vitro* (Verhulst et al., 2009). This work suggests that the host's commensal skin microbes may be the source of several important mosquito-attractant compounds. Future work involving parallel investigations of skin microbiota and skin headspace VOCs during malaria infection may shed light on the significance of skin commensal microbes in the context of malaria transmission.

DATA WRANGLING: BIOINFORMATICS APPROACHES FOR TACKLING THE MALARIA INFECTION METABOLOME

Bioinformatics tools are critically important in the analysis of big data that arises from 'omic technologies. Metabolomics, particularly untargeted metabolomics, can yield a large amount of data on many unique metabolic features which must be sifted out and sorted through in order to determine meaning. A key question here is – *how to find signal within the noise in a metabolomics data set?*

A combination of targeted and untargeted approaches has been used to explore the question of host metabolites in the context of malaria. The strength of untargeted analyses is that these approaches enable the analysis of an extremely large set of metabolic features, allowing for unbiased assessments without setting an *a priori* hypotheses about what may be found. Unsupervised statistical analyses can be applied to these big datasets, such as principal components analysis (PCA) and hierarchical clustering analysis (HCA), and metabolic features that are highly associated with the phenomenon of interest can be identified based on their chemical features (e.g., mass:charge ratio). From that point, computational annotation approaches can be applied to give putative identities, and pathway analysis can be performed to test for significantly perturbed metabolic pathways (Uppal et al., 2016). These approaches can be helpful in the context of exploring new and under-researched questions in the field. Ultimately, however, these approaches should be combined with targeted methods and reference compounds to confirm identities of any putative metabolites (Uppal et al., 2017; Cordy et al., 2019).

Biomarker discovery is another key area in which bioinformatic approaches are applied to metabolomics data. While often used in the context of disease pathogenesis, metabolites could also potentially be identified as biomarkers to indicate malaria transmissibility. To identify metabolite biomarkers of malaria transmission, approaches such as receiver operating curve (ROC) analysis, can be used. More advanced approaches that incorporate multivariate statistics may also be used to help identify robust biomarkers. Importantly these studies require validation in multiple cohorts, and the use of independent datasets on which to build and subsequently apply any given model. Such bioinformatics approaches are likely to lead to the discovery of new biomarkers of transmissibility, that could be highly relevant during the era of malaria eradication.

Potential biomarkers could include those metabolites which have already been found in multiple studies to be associated with enhanced transmissibility. Biomarkers for increased mosquito attraction may include elevated levels of certain terpenes (e.g., pinene) (Kelly et al., 2015; Emami et al., 2017; Schaber et al., 2018) and/or aldehydes (e.g., hexanal, octanal, nonanal) (Correa et al., 2017; Emami et al., 2017; Robinson et al., 2018; Stanczyk et al., 2019) in the headspace of malaria-infected individuals. Biomarkers for increased gametocytogenesis may include altered levels of certain phospholipids (e.g., lysoPC, PUFA-containing phospholipids) (Brancucci et al., 2017; Tanaka et al., 2019; Usui et al., 2019) in the blood of malaria-infected hosts. The utility of such biomarkers is that there may be potential to generate diagnostic tests, particularly non-invasive ones, that detect relevant biomarkers for malaria infection and/or transmissibility. Further, as demonstrated by a recent study of canines identifying malaria-infected individuals through the smell of their socks alone (Guest et al., 2019), it is apparent that volatile chemicals can be detected in a wide variety of ways, and the successful detection of these types of biomarkers may not require expensive equipment.

Finally, in trying to understand the source of these metabolites, data integration across multiple 'omic analyses derived from the same experiment can be helpful toward determining possible sources of metabolites within the complex milieu of the host-parasite-microbial system (Salinas et al., 2014). Data integration techniques can aid in sifting through big datasets to gauge which metabolites are coming from the parasite and which are coming from host (and possibly which from its commensal microbiota). Combining transcriptional data from host, parasite, and microbiota with metabolomics data from the complex host-parasite-microbe system may help to elucidate the ways in which these different components may contribute to the resulting metabolites. Metabolic flux models are particularly helpful for these such joint analyses, as they can combine transcriptional data (which is annotated and thus of known origin) with metabolomics data (from unknown origin). Putting these data together can help to illustrate the predicted activity of various metabolic pathways of either the host or parasite (Chiappino-Pepe et al., 2017; Tang et al., 2018).

CONCLUSION

Plasmodium is a highly complex pathogen which undergoes multiple stage transitions during its passage between its invertebrate and vertebrate hosts. And despite (or more likely, due to) this complexity, transmission of the pathogen results in over 200 million cases of malaria per year (World Health Organization [WHO], 2018). Host, parasite and microbial-derived metabolites, through their impacts on mosquito attractiveness and gametocytogenesis, appear to play a critical role in ensuring the successful transmission of this devastating parasitic disease. While several recent studies have greatly added to our knowledge in this area, there are still many aspects of malaria transmission biology that are not well understood. Further mining of the host metabolome may help to improve our understanding of the complexities that exist in the malaria host-pathogen system that enhance or hinder transmission.

AUTHOR CONTRIBUTIONS

RJ conceived and wrote the manuscript.

ACKNOWLEDGMENTS

Members of the Malaria Host-Pathogen Interaction Center (MaHPIC) and of the Emory University Clinical Biomarkers Lab are acknowledged for helpful discussions. Figure was created with BioRender.com.

REFERENCES

Basant, A., Rege, M., Sharma, S., and Sonawat, H. M. (2010). Alterations in urine, serum and brain metabolomic profiles exhibit sexual dimorphism during malaria disease progression. *Malar. J.* 9:110. doi: 10.1186/1475-2875-9-110

Batista, E. P., Costa, E. F., and Silva, A. A. (2014). Anopheles darlingi (Diptera: Culicidae) displays increased attractiveness to infected individuals with *Plasmodium vivax* gametocytes. *Parasit. Vectors* 7:251. doi: 10.1186/1756-3305-7-251

Beri, D., Balan, B., Chaubey, S., Subramaniam, S., Surendra, B., and Tatu, U. (2017). A disrupted transsulphuration pathway results in accumulation of redox metabolites and induction of gametocytogenesis in malaria. *Sci. Rep.* 7:40213. doi: 10.1038/srep40213

Berna, A. Z., McCarthy, J. S., Wang, R. X., Saliba, K. J., Bravo, F. G., Cassells, J., et al. (2015). Analysis of breath specimens for biomarkers of *Plasmodium falciparum* infection. *J. Infect. Dis.* 212, 1120–1128. doi: 10.1093/infdis/jiv176

Braks, M. A., Anderson, R. A., and Knols, B. G. (1999). Infochemicals in mosquito host selection: human skin microflora and *Plasmodium parasites*. *Parasitol. Today* 15, 409–413. doi: 10.1016/s0169-4758(99)01514-8

Brancucci, N. M. B., Gerdt, J. P., Wang, C., De Niz, M., Philip, N., Adapa, S. R., et al. (2017). Lysophosphatidylcholine regulates sexual stage differentiation in the human malaria parasite *Plasmodium falciparum*. *Cell* 171:1532-1544.e15. doi: 10.1016/j.cell.2017.10.020

Brouwer, R. (1960). The attraction of carbon dioxide excreted by the skin of the arm for malaria mosquitoes. *Trop. Geogr. Med.* 12, 62–66.

Busula, A. O., Bousema, T., Mweresa, C. K., Masiga, D., Logan, J. G., Sauerwein, R. W., et al. (2017). Gametocytemia and attractiveness of *Plasmodium falciparum*-infected kenyan children to anopheles gambiae mosquitoes. *J. Infect. Dis.* 216, 291–295. doi: 10.1093/infdis/jix214

Cator, L. J., George, J., Blanford, S., Murdock, C. C., Baker, T. C., Read, A. F., et al. (2013). 'Manipulation' without the parasite: altered feeding behaviour of mosquitoes is not dependent on infection with malaria parasites. *Proc. R. Soc. B* 280:20130711. doi: 10.1098/rspb.2013.0711

Cator, L. J., Lynch, P. A., Read, A. F., and Thomas, M. B. (2012). Do malaria parasites manipulate mosquitoes? *Trends Parasitol.* 28, 466–470. doi: 10.1016/j.pt.2012.08.004

Chaubey, S., Grover, M., and Tatu, U. (2014). Endoplasmic reticulum stress triggers gametocytogenesis in the malaria parasite. *J. Biol. Chem.* 289, 16662–16674. doi: 10.1074/jbc.M114.551549

Chiappino-Pepe, A., Tymoshenko, S., Ataman, M., Soldati-Favre, D., and Hatzimanikatis, V. (2017). Bioenergetics-based modeling of *Plasmodium falciparum* metabolism reveals its essential genes, nutritional requirements, and thermodynamic bottlenecks. *PLoS Comput. Biol.* 13:e1005397. doi: 10.1371/journal.pcbi.1005397

Cordy, R. J., Patrapuvich, R., Lili, L. N., Cabrera-Mora, M., Chien, J.-T., Tharp, G. K., et al. (2019). Distinct amino acid and lipid perturbations characterize acute versus chronic malaria. *JCI Insight* 4:125156. doi: 10.1172/jci.insight.125156

Cornet, S., Nicot, A., Rivero, A., and Gandon, S. (2013). Malaria infection increases bird attractiveness to uninfected mosquitoes. *Ecol. Lett.* 16, 323–329. doi: 10.1111/ele.12041

Correa, R., Coronado, L. M., Garrido, A. C., Durant-Archibold, A. A., and Spadafora, C. (2017). Volatile organic compounds associated with *Plasmodium falciparum* infection in vitro. *Parasit. Vectors* 10:215. doi: 10.1186/s13071-017-2157-x

de Boer, J. G., Robinson, A., Powers, S. J., Burgers, S. L., Caulfield, J. C., Birkett, M. A., et al. (2017). Odours of *Plasmodium falciparum*-infected participants influence mosquito-host interactions. *Sci. Rep.* 7:9283. doi: 10.1038/s41598-017-08978-9

De Moraes, C. M., Stanczyk, N. M., Betz, H. S., Pulido, H., Sim, D. G., Read, A. F., et al. (2014). Malaria-induced changes in host odors enhance mosquito attraction. *Proc. Natl. Acad. Sci. U.S.A.* 111, 11079–11084. doi: 10.1073/pnas.1405617111

Decuypere, S., Maltha, J., Deborggraeve, S., Rattray, N. J. W., Issa, G., Bérenger, K., et al. (2016). Towards improving point-of-care diagnosis of non-malaria febrile illness: a metabolomics approach. *PLoS Negl. Trop. Dis.* 10:e0004480. doi: 10.1371/journal.pntd.0004480

Emami, S. N., Lindberg, B. G., Hua, S., Hill, S. R., Mozuraitis, R., Lehmann, P., et al. (2017). A key malaria metabolite modulates vector blood seeking, feeding, and susceptibility to infection. *Science* 355, 1076–1080. doi: 10.1126/science.aah4563

Gardinassi, L. G., Cordy, R. J., Lacerda, M. V. G., Salinas, J. L., Monteiro, W. M., Melo, G. C., et al. (2017). Metabolome-wide association study of peripheral parasitemia in *Plasmodium vivax* malaria. *Int. J. Med. Microbiol.* 307, 533–541. doi: 10.1016/j.ijmm.2017.09.002

Ghosh, S., Pathak, S., Sonawat, H. M., Sharma, S., and Sengupta, A. (2018). Metabolomic changes in vertebrate host during malaria disease progression. *Cytokine* 112, 32–43. doi: 10.1016/j.cyto.2018.07.022

Guest, C., Pinder, M., Doggett, M., Squires, C., Affara, M., Kandeh, B., et al. (2019). Trained dogs identify people with malaria parasites by their odour. *Lancet Infect. Dis.* 19, 578–580. doi: 10.1016/S1473-3099(19)30220-8

Hasin, Y., Seldin, M., and Lusis, A. (2017). Multi-omics approaches to disease. *Genome Biol.* 18:83. doi: 10.1186/s13059-017-1215-1

Josling, G. A., and Llinás, M. (2015). Sexual development in *Plasmodium parasites*: knowing when it's time to commit. *Nat. Rev. Microbiol.* 13:573. doi: 10.1038/nrmicro3519

Kelly, M., Su, C.-Y., Schaber, C., Crowley, J. R., Hsu, F.-F., Carlson, J. R., et al. (2015). Malaria parasites produce volatile mosquito attractants. *mBio* 6:e00235-15. doi: 10.1128/mBio.00235-15

Koella, J. C. (2005). Malaria as a manipulator. *Behav. Process.* 68, 271–273. doi: 10.1016/j.beproc.2004.10.004

Lacroix, R., Mukabana, W. R., Gouagna, L. C., and Koella, J. C. (2005). Malaria infection increases attractiveness of humans to mosquitoes. *PLoS Biol.* 3:e298. doi: 10.1371/journal.pbio.0030298

Loy, D. E., Liu, W., Li, Y., Learn, G. H., Plenderleith, L. J., Sundararaman, S. A., et al. (2017). Out of Africa: origins and evolution of the human malaria parasites *Plasmodium falciparum* and *Plasmodium vivax*. *Int. J. Parasitol.* 47, 87–97. doi: 10.1016/j.ijpara.2016.05.008

Nyasembe, V. O., Teal, P. E. A., Mukabana, W. R., Tumlinson, J. H., and Torto, B. (2012). Behavioural response of the malaria vector *Anopheles gambiae* to host plant volatiles and synthetic blends. *Parasit. Vectors* 5:234. doi: 10.1186/1756-3305-5-234

Olszewski, K. L., Morrisey, J. M., Wilinski, D., Burns, J. M., Vaidya, A. B., Rabinowitz, J. D., et al. (2009). Host-parasite interactions revealed by *Plasmodium falciparum* metabolomics. *Cell Host Microbe* 5, 191–199. doi: 10.1016/j.chom.2009.01.004

Pappa, V., Seydel, K., Gupta, S., Feintuch, C. M., Potchen, M. J., Kampondeni, S., et al. (2015). Lipid metabolites of the phospholipase A2 pathway and inflammatory cytokines are associated with brain volume in paediatric cerebral malaria. *Malar. J.* 14, 513. doi: 10.1186/s12936-015-1036-1

Robinson, A., Busula, A. O., Voets, M. A., Beshir, K. B., Caulfield, J. C., Powers, S. J., et al. (2018). *Plasmodium*-associated changes in human odor attract mosquitoes. *Proc. Natl. Acad. Sci. U.S.A.* 115, E4209–E4218. doi: 10.1073/pnas.1721610115

Salinas, J. L., Kissinger, J. C., Jones, D. P., and Galinski, M. R. (2014). Metabolomics in the fight against malaria. *Mem. Inst. Oswaldo Cruz* 109, 589–597. doi: 10.1590/0074-0276140043

Schaber, C. L., Katta, N., Bollinger, L. B., Mwale, M., Mlotha-Mitole, R., Trehan, I., et al. (2018). Breathprinting reveals malaria-associated biomarkers and mosquito attractants. *J. Infect. Dis.* 217, 1553–1560. doi: 10.1093/infdis/jiy072

Smallegange, R. C., van Gemert, G.-J., van de Vegte-Bolmer, M., Gezan, S., Takken, W., Sauerwein, R. W., et al. (2013). Malaria infected mosquitoes express enhanced attraction to human odor. *PLoS One* 8:e63602. doi: 10.1371/journal.pone.0063602

Stanczyk, N. M., Brugman, V. A., Austin, V., Sanchez-Roman Teran, F., Gezan, S. A., Emery, M., et al. (2019). Species-specific alterations in Anopheles mosquito olfactory responses caused by *Plasmodium* infection. *Sci. Rep.* 9:3396. doi: 10.1038/s41598-019-40074-y

Surowiec, I., Orikiiriza, J., Karlsson, E., Nelson, M., Bonde, M., Kyamanwa, P., et al. (2015). Metabolic signature profiling as a diagnostic and prognostic tool in pediatric *Plasmodium falciparum* malaria. *Open Forum Infect. Dis.* 2:ofv062. doi: 10.1093/ofid/ofv062

Takken, W., and Kline, D. L. (1989). Carbon dioxide and 1-octen-3-ol as mosquito attractants. *J. Am. Mosq. Control Assoc.* 5, 311–316.

Tanaka, T. Q., Tokuoka, S. M., Nakatani, D., Hamano, F., Kawazu, S.-I., Wellems, T. E., et al. (2019). Polyunsaturated fatty acids promote *Plasmodium falciparum* gametocytogenesis. *Biol. Open* 8:bio042259. doi: 10.1242/bio.042259

Tang, Y., Gupta, A., Garimalla, S., MaHPIC Consortium, Galinski, M. R., Styczynski, M. P., et al. (2018). Metabolic modeling helps interpret transcriptomic changes during malaria. *Biochim. Biophys. Acta Mol. Basis Dis.* 1864, 2329–2340. doi: 10.1016/j.bbadis.2017.10.023

Uppal, K., Salinas, J. L., Monteiro, W. M., Val, F., Cordy, R. J., Liu, K., et al. (2017). Plasma metabolomics reveals membrane lipids, aspartate/asparagine and nucleotide metabolism pathway differences associated with chloroquine resistance in *Plasmodium vivax* malaria. *PLoS One* 12:e0182819. doi: 10.1371/journal.pone.0182819

Uppal, K., Walker, D. I., Liu, K., Li, S., Go, Y.-M., and Jones, D. P. (2016). Computational metabolomics: a framework for the million metabolome. *Chem. Res. Toxicol.* 29, 1956–1975. doi: 10.1021/acs.chemrestox.6b00179

Usui, M., Prajapati, S. K., Ayanful-Torgby, R., Acquah, F. K., Cudjoe, E., Kakaney, C., et al. (2019). *Plasmodium falciparum* sexual differentiation in malaria patients is associated with host factors and GDV1-dependent genes. *Nat. Commun.* 10:2140. doi: 10.1038/s41467-019-10172-6

Verhulst, N. O., Beijleveld, H., Knols, B. G., Takken, W., Schraa, G., Bouwmeester, H. J., et al. (2009). Cultured skin microbiota attracts malaria mosquitoes. *Malaria J.* 8:302. doi: 10.1186/1475-2875-8-302

World Health Organization [WHO], (2018). *World Malaria Report 2018*. Geneva: WHO.

5

Cytokines and Chemokines in Cerebral Malaria Pathogenesis

Josefine Dunst[1,2,3*], *Faustin Kamena*[1,2,3] *and Kai Matuschewski*[1,2]

[1] *Parasitology Unit, Max Planck Institute for Infection Biology, Berlin, Germany,* [2] *Institute of Chemistry and Biochemistry, Free University, Berlin, Germany,* [3] *Molecular Parasitology, Institute of Biology, Humboldt University, Berlin, Germany*

Edited by:
Slobodan Paessler, University of Texas Medical Branch, United States

Reviewed by:
Tracey Lamb, University of Utah, United States
Teresa Carvalho, La Trobe University, Australia

***Correspondence:**
Josefine Dunst
dunstj@zedat.fu-berlin.de

Cerebral malaria is among the major causes of malaria-associated mortality and effective adjunctive therapeutic strategies are currently lacking. Central pathophysiological processes involved in the development of cerebral malaria include an imbalance of pro- and anti-inflammatory responses to *Plasmodium* infection, endothelial cell activation, and loss of blood-brain barrier integrity. However, the sequence of events, which initiates these pathophysiological processes as well as the contribution of their complex interplay to the development of cerebral malaria remain incompletely understood. Several cytokines and chemokines have repeatedly been associated with cerebral malaria severity. Increased levels of these inflammatory mediators could account for the sequestration of leukocytes in the cerebral microvasculature present during cerebral malaria, thereby contributing to an amplification of local inflammation and promoting cerebral malaria pathogenesis. Herein, we highlight the current knowledge on the contribution of cytokines and chemokines to the pathogenesis of cerebral malaria with particular emphasis on their roles in endothelial activation and leukocyte recruitment, as well as their implication in the progression to blood-brain barrier permeability and neuroinflammation, in both human cerebral malaria and in the murine experimental cerebral malaria model. A better molecular understanding of these processes could provide the basis for evidence-based development of adjunct therapies and the definition of diagnostic markers of disease progression.

Keywords: malaria, *Plasmodium*, cerebral malaria, cytokines, chemokines, endothelial activation, blood-brain barrier, neuroinflammation

INTRODUCTION

Malaria is one of the most prevalent infectious diseases worldwide and contributes considerably to the global disease burden. With ~200 million new cases and an estimated 430,000 deaths annually (WHO, 2016), malaria remains the most important vector-borne infectious disease. The human-adapted *Plasmodium* species *P. falciparum* and *P. vivax* account for the majority of malaria cases and are transmitted by the bite of an infective *Anopheles* mosquito. Despite considerable progress in malaria eradication over the past 15 years (WHO, 2016),

---

Abbreviations: CD, cluster of differentiation; CM, cerebral malaria; CSF, cerebrospinal fluid; DAMP, danger-associated molecular patterns; DC, dendritic cell; ECM, experimental cerebral malaria; EPCR, endothelial protein C receptor; GPI, glycosylphosphatidylinositol; ICAM, intercellular adhesion molecule; IFN, interferon; IL, interleukin; IP-10, IFN-γ-inducible protein 10; KC, keratinocyte chemoattractant; LPS, lipopolysaccharide; LT, lymphotoxin; MCP-1, monocyte chemoattractant protein 1; MIG, monokine induced by IFN-γ; MIP, macrophage inflammatory protein; NK, natural killer; NLR, NOD-like receptors, PAMP, pathogen-associated molecular pattern; PF4, platelet factor 4; *Pf*EMP1, *Plasmodium falciparum* erythrocyte membrane protein 1; PRR, pattern recognition receptor; TLR, Toll-like receptor; TNF, tumor necrosis factor; VCAM, vascular cell adhesion molecule; ZO-1, zonula occludens 1.

efforts are hampered by emerging *Plasmodium* resistance to commonly used anti-malaria drugs (Cui et al., 2015) and limited efficacy of the currently most advanced vaccine candidate (White et al., 2015; Olotu et al., 2016).

Among infections by human host-adapted *Plasmodium* species, *P. falciparum* infections are most likely to progress to organ-related pathology and severe malaria, and thereby account for the vast majority of malaria-associated fatalities. Along with severe anemia and respiratory distress, cerebral malaria (CM) is one of the major manifestations of severe malaria (Haldar et al., 2007). CM manifests with impaired consciousness and coma in both children and adults (Idro et al., 2010), while other clinical features differ. In addition to the characteristic diffuse encephalopathy, retinal abnormalities are frequent in children and less common in adults with CM (Beare et al., 2006; Idro et al., 2010). In contrast, CM in adults is accompanied by multi-organ disorder including renal failure and pulmonary edema, which are less frequently observed in children suffering from CM (Idro et al., 2010). Although anti-malaria treatment using artesunate was reported to improve CM outcome in children and adults (Dondorp et al., 2005, 2010), the case-fatality rate of pediatric CM is approximately 20% (Haldar et al., 2007) and sustained cognitive and/or neurological impairment may occur (John et al., 2008a). Consequently, treatment strategies, which not only target the parasite but also other mechanisms underlying CM pathogenesis, need to be developed. Since the pathogenesis of CM is still incompletely understood, further investigations are an important medical research priority, especially in the context of adjunctive therapies. Since accumulating evidence indicates that an imbalance in pro- and anti-inflammatory immune responses partially contributes to CM pathogenesis, such therapeutic approaches could target cytokines and chemokines associated with CM severity. Cytokines are polypeptides, which mediate and generate inflammatory responses. Along with their contribution to disease pathogenesis in general, cytokines also exert physiological roles at lower concentrations (Clark and Vissel, 2017). Chemokines are chemotactic cytokines, which recruit lymphocytes and monocytes to the site of pathogen encounter by binding to their respective chemokine receptor (Griffith et al., 2014). Given that leukocytes were found to sequester in the microvasculature of the brain in human CM and murine ECM (Hunt and Grau, 2003), local chemokine gradients may mediate leukocyte recruitment and thus promote CM pathogenesis. Chemokines exert their function through binding to their respective G protein-coupled chemokine receptors (**Table 1**), which induces activation of phosphatidylinositol 3-kinase (PI3K) and Rho GTPase signaling pathways, thus leading to F-actin polymerization and migration (Viola and Luster, 2008).

In this review, we highlight findings from both experimental murine models and natural human infections, and assess the current knowledge on the role of host cytokine and chemokine responses in the severe malaria complication of cerebral malaria. We also emphasize the potential inflammatory cascade resulting from *Plasmodium* life cycle progression after sporozoite inoculation and ultimately culminating in cerebral malaria pathology (**Figure 1**).

CURRENT CONCEPTS IN CEREBRAL MALARIA PATHOGENESIS

Two central concepts to explain CM pathogenesis have evolved and they are likely mutually dependent- the vascular occlusion hypothesis and the inflammation hypothesis (Storm and Craig, 2014).

The concept of vascular occlusion leading to CM is based on the ability of mature *P. falciparum*-infected erythrocytes to sequester in the microvasculature through binding of *P. falciparum* erythrocyte membrane protein 1 (*Pf*EMP1) present on the erythrocyte surface to endothelial cell surface proteins, such as intercellular adhesion molecule 1 (ICAM-1), vascular cell adhesion molecule 1 (VCAM-1), cluster of differentiation 36 (CD36), or endothelial protein C receptor (EPCR) (Pasloske and Howard, 1994; Chen et al., 2000; Rowe et al., 2009; Smith et al., 2013; Turner et al., 2013; Lennartz et al., 2017). Sequestration occurs in various organs and, along with increased rigidity of erythrocytes, is believed to cause vascular occlusion (Dondorp et al., 2004). Additionally, microvascular obstruction during *P. falciparum* infection may be worsened by the formation of rosettes and clumps (Chen et al., 2000; Rowe et al., 2009; Adams et al., 2014), i.e., the binding of uninfected erythrocytes by infected erythrocytes (Handunnetti et al., 1989), and aggregation of infected erythrocytes and platelets (Pain et al., 2001), respectively. These events may cause a reduction in microvascular blood flow, ischemia, and tissue hypoxia (Medana and Turner, 2006), thereby accounting for cerebral pathology. Reduced vessel perfusion and occlusion was indeed observed by fluorescein angiography of the retina in pediatric CM cases (Beare et al., 2009) and by *in vivo* imaging of the microcirculation in adult patients with CM or other manifestations of severe malaria (Dondorp et al., 2008), although further studies are needed to determine the underlying cause of these observations. Additionally, sequestration of *P. falciparum*-infected erythrocytes was observed in the cerebral microvasculature of CM patients in *post mortem* brain histology studies (Ponsford et al., 2012; Milner et al., 2014, 2015).

Despite accumulating evidence, the relevance of sequestration in the development of CM is still incompletely understood, since the degree of sequestration in brains of non-fatal CM cases cannot be investigated non-invasively and is, thus, unspecified (Miller et al., 2002). Occasionally, fatal CM cases present little sequestration and vessel occlusion similar to non-CM severe malaria cases (Ponsford et al., 2012). Moreover, isolated CM cases were reported in children and adults with confirmed *P. vivax* mono-infections in India (Kochar et al., 2009), although *P. vivax* is unlikely to sequester in the microvasculature since late-stage *P. vivax*-infected erythrocytes are present in peripheral blood (Anstey et al., 2009). Together, cerebral malaria occasionally develops in a few *P. vivax* infections without obvious signs of sequestration *in vivo* or microvascular obstruction.

Given the unresolved role of sequestration in the pathogenesis of CM, additional factors may determine disease severity. Notably, other infectious diseases that result in systemic inflammation and fever also progress to severe forms,

TABLE 1 | Selected human and murine chemokines and their receptors[a].

Chemokine	Other names	Gene		Receptors	Key function
		Human	Mouse		
CCL2	MCP-1 JE (mouse)	*CCL2*	*Ccl2*	CCR2	Inflammatory monocyte trafficking
CCL3	MIP-1α	*CCL3*	*Ccl3*	CCR1, CCR5	Macrophage and NK cell migration, T cell-DC interactions
CCL4	MIP-1β	*CCL4*	*Ccl4*	CCR5	
CCL5	RANTES	*CCL5*	*Ccl5*	CCR1, CCR3, CCR5	
CCL11	Eotaxin	*CCL11*	*Ccl11*	CCR3, CCR5	Eosinophil and basophil migration
CCL20	MIP-3α	*CCL20*	*Ccl20*	CCR6	Th17 responses, B cell and DC homing
CXCL1	GROα Gm1960 (mouse)	*CXCL1*	*Cxcl3*	CXCR2	Neutrophil trafficking
CXCL3	GROγ KC (mouse)	*CXCL3*	*Cxcl1*	CXCR2	
CXCL4	PF4	*PF4*	–	CXCR3-B	Procoagulant
CXCL4L1	PF4V1	*PF4V1*	*Pf4*	CXCR3-B	
CXCL8	IL-8	*IL-8*	–	CXCR1, CXCR2	Neutrophil trafficking
CXCL9	MIG	*CXCL9*	*Cxcl9*	CXCR3	T cell and NK cell trafficking
CXCL10	IP-10	*CXCL10*	*Cxcl10*	CXCR3	

[a]*Modified from Zlotnik and Yoshie (2012) and Griffith et al. (2014).*

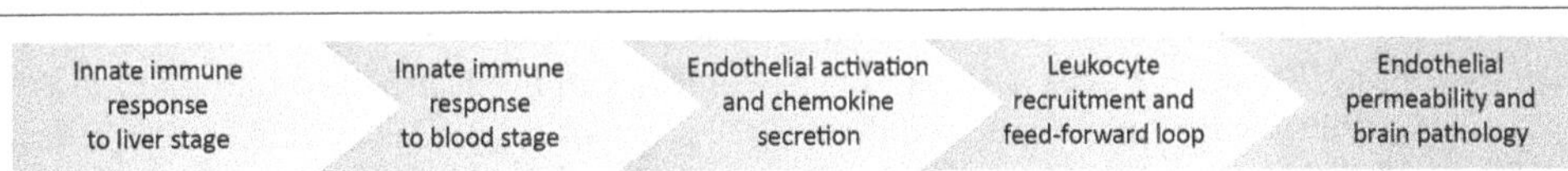

FIGURE 1 | Overview of a potential inflammatory cascade culminating in cerebral malaria pathology. Five consecutive events shape the outcome of a *Plasmodium* infection and contribute to cerebral malaria. During *Plasmodium* infection of the mammalian host, two consecutive parasite replication phases in the liver and red blood cells lead to distinct innate responses, which modulate downstream parasite/host cell interactions. Upon parasite accumulation in the microvasculature, endothelial cells become activated, leading to enhanced chemokine secretion, which in turn enhances leukocyte recruitment. Acute pathology is caused by permeabilization of the endothelial barrier. See **Figures 2–6** for the central roles of chemokines and cytokines in the individual events.

including neurological complications such as sepsis-associated encephalopathy (De Backer et al., 2002; Clark et al., 2004). Strikingly, systemic cytokine levels have been described to correlate with disease severity in malaria as well as sepsis (Prakash et al., 2006; Bozza et al., 2007). These findings corroborate an earlier proposal that an imbalance in pro- and anti-inflammatory immune responses triggers immune-induced pathology and might be a leading cause of CM pathogenesis, which may be further amplified by sequestration (Clark and Rockett, 1994). In addition to inflammation and sequestration, CM is associated with endothelial activation and increased blood-brain barrier permeability, and these processes might act reciprocally and have synergistic effects (van der Heyde et al., 2006). In line with this notion, certain *Pf*EMP1 variants, which are associated with CM, were described to compete with activated protein C in binding to EPCR (Turner et al., 2013; Bernabeu et al., 2016). Therefore, the anti-coagulant, anti-inflammatory, cytoprotective properties, which are induced upon interaction of protein C with EPCR, might be impeded by *Pf*EMP1-EPCR interaction and consequently, disease mechanisms may be further exacerbated (Bernabeu and Smith, 2017; Wassmer and Grau, 2017). However, the impact of the interaction between *Pf*EMP1 and EPCR on inflammation and coagulation remains to be demonstrated.

Insights into the mechanisms underlying CM in humans are limited and mostly based on *post mortem* histopathology or correlations of serum parameters with disease outcome (Hunt and Grau, 2003). Despite potential differences in human and murine CM pathogenesis (Riley et al., 2010; Craig et al., 2012), *P. berghei* (strain ANKA) infection reliably causes signature symptoms of CM in susceptible C57BL/6 mice (de Souza and Riley, 2002; Hunt and Grau, 2003). This host-parasite combination is a widely used and well-established murine model for CM, termed experimental cerebral malaria (ECM), which permits mechanistic studies (Craig et al., 2012). Consequently, studies highlighted in this review include reports on human cerebral malaria cases combined with mechanistic insights based on the murine ECM model and *in vitro* studies.

INNATE IMMUNE ACTIVATION DURING LIVER STAGE DEVELOPMENT

Upon transmission by the bite of an infective *Anopheles* mosquito, *Plasmodium* sporozoites rapidly migrate to the liver, invade hepatocytes and develop into thousands of merozoites. Since this developmental stage of *Plasmodium* parasites is clinically silent, the immune response mounted by the host in order to limit parasite expansion during liver stage development remains largely unexplored (Hafalla et al., 2011). However, it seems likely that sporozoite and liver stage recognition primes the innate immune system locally and well below the pyrogenic threshold. In fact, innate immune cells have occasionally been observed to surround *P. berghei*-infected hepatocytes, indicating that *Plasmodium* does not remain undetected during liver stage development (Liehl and Mota, 2012). Additionally, a type I interferon (IFN) response is induced in livers of mice infected with *P. yoelii* or *P. berghei* (Liehl et al., 2014; Miller et al., 2014). Such an initial type I IFN response might induce chemokines, including IFN-γ-inducible protein 10 (IP-10)/CXCL10, which in turn could recruit cells expressing the corresponding chemokine receptor CXCR3, such as T, natural killer (NK), and NKT cells, to the site of infection, which might contribute to the local immune response by IFN-γ secretion (**Figure 2**; Liehl et al., 2014; Miller et al., 2014). In good agreement, an increase in IFN-γ plasma concentration prior to onset of detectable blood-stage infection was reported in controlled human *P. falciparum* infection (Hermsen et al., 2003). Clearly, the initial cytokine response fails to arrest liver stage development and, thus, does not curtail the proceeding to erythrocyte infection. Interestingly, *P. berghei* sporozoite and blood stage infections result in ECM symptoms in a similar time frame (Kordes et al., 2011), suggesting that immune responses against liver stages might not modulate CM pathogenesis. Whether this first immune response reduces the initial parasite number released into the blood stream and thereby influences the magnitude of early blood stage-induced immune responses remains to be tested.

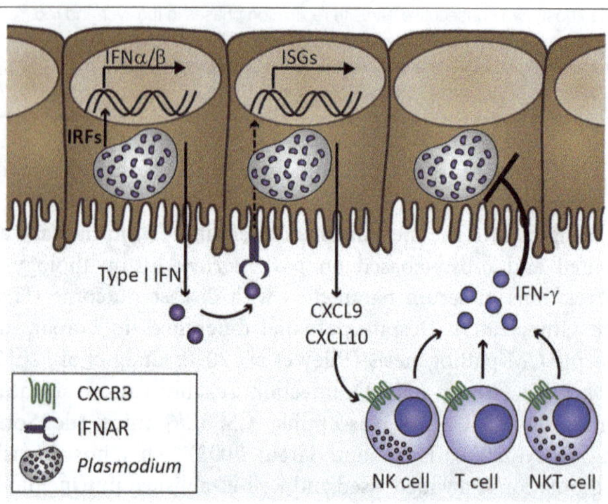

FIGURE 2 | Innate immune response to *Plasmodium* liver stage infection. *Plasmodium* infection of hepatocytes activates interferon regulatory factors (IRF), which induce transcription of type I interferons (IFN) IFNα and IFNβ. Secretion of type I IFNs activates IFNα/β receptor IFNAR in an autocrine or paracrine manner. IFNAR signaling results in transcription of IFN-stimulated genes (ISGs), which includes chemokines, such as CXCL9 and CXCL10. Upon secretion from hepatocytes, these chemokines might recruit cells expressing the corresponding chemokine receptor CXCR3, including natural killer (NK), T, and NKT cells. Upon activation by type I IFN at the site of infection, these cell types could contribute to limiting *Plasmodium* liver stage expansion by IFN-γ secretion. Based on Liehl et al. (2014) and Miller et al. (2014).

BLOOD STAGE-INDUCED INNATE IMMUNE RESPONSES

Concomitant with the release of merozoites into the bloodstream and infection of erythrocytes, a *Plasmodium* infection progresses from the clinically silent liver stage to the symptomatic blood stage. Merozoites are only very briefly (~60 s) exposed to the immune system before they rapidly enter new erythrocytes (Gilson and Crabb, 2009; Beeson et al., 2016), and blood stage infection is the exclusive cause of malaria symptoms, which is associated with systemic inflammation and fever. Fever is a common and effective host defense against microbial pathogens and swiftly initiated upon the first host-pathogen interaction. The febrile response is likely triggered through a universal mechanism, in which pyrogens, such as the pro-inflammatory cytokines interleukin 1α (IL-1α), IL-1β, IL-6, or tumor necrosis factor (TNF), are secreted by innate immune cells upon recognition of pathogen-associated molecular patterns (PAMPs) or host-derived danger-associated molecular patterns (DAMPs) by pattern recognition receptors (PRRs) (Evans et al., 2015). In *Plasmodium* infection, the characteristic recurrent fever coincides with synchronized rupture of infected erythrocytes in the schizont stage (Oakley et al., 2011). Release of parasite- and host-derived molecules due to erythrocyte rupture was described to induce TNF *in vitro* (Kwiatkowski et al., 1989; Bate and Kwiatkowski, 1994), and peaks in TNF serum concentration were found to coincide with elevated body temperature during *P. vivax* infection (Karunaweera et al., 1992), indicating that malaria fever is elicited by repeated release of PAMPs and DAMPs. Although an increase in core body temperature is associated with resolution of infection (Oakley et al., 2011), such a pro-inflammatory immune response needs to be counterbalanced by anti-inflammatory mechanisms in order to avoid a dysregulated immune response, which might lead to complications such as cerebral malaria.

The innate immune system represents the first line of defense against pathogens and mediates recognition and clearance of *Plasmodium* parasites (**Figure 3**). Cells of the innate immune system such as macrophages and dendritic cells (DCs) as well as non-professional immune cells such as endothelial cells and fibroblasts express PRR. These include Toll-like receptors (TLR), C-type lectin receptors (CLR), Retinoic acid-inducible gene (RIG)-I-like receptors, and NOD-like receptors (NLR), which recognize PAMPs and host-derived DAMPs (Takeuchi and Akira, 2010). Most malaria PAMPs and DAMPs known so far are apparently recognized by TLR. Activation of TLR initiates a signaling cascade including the adaptor protein MyD88 and the transcription factors NF-κB, AP-1, and interferon regulatory factor (IRF). As a consequence, expression of genes encoding pro-inflammatory cytokines such as type I IFN, IFN-γ, IL-6, IL-12, and TNF, is induced (Eriksson et al., 2013; Gazzinelli et al., 2014).

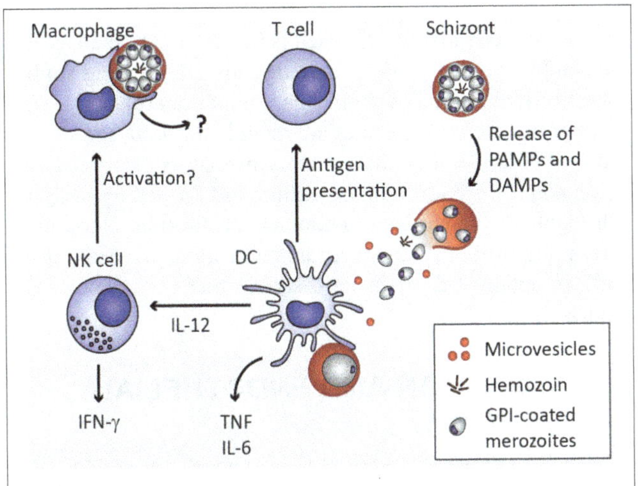

FIGURE 3 | Innate immune response to *Plasmodium* blood stage infection in the spleen. Macrophages as well as dendritic cells (DC) remove infected erythrocytes from the circulation by phagocytosis. In macrophages, uptake of infected erythrocytes might not lead to secretion of pro-inflammatory cytokines due to phagosomal acidification (Wu et al., 2015). Upon rupture of infected erythrocytes, pathogen-associated molecular patterns (PAMPs) and danger-associated molecular patterns (DAMPs) are released, including microvesicles, hemozoin, and glycosylphosphatidylinositols (GPI). These potential PAMPs and DAMPs might be recognized by DC through pattern recognition receptors, resulting in the secretion of interleukin 12 (IL-12), tumor necrosis factor (TNF), and IL-6 (Wu et al., 2015). DC-derived IL-12 might activate natural killer (NK) cells, which in turn secrete interferon γ (IFN-γ) and could thereby activate macrophages (Stevenson and Riley, 2004).

Several *Plasmodium*-derived molecules have been recognized as malaria PAMPs based on their ability to induce cytokine responses *in vitro* (**Figure 3**). One of the candidate malaria PAMPs are glycosylphosphatidylinositols (GPI). Although GPI are present in all eukaryotic cells where they serve as membrane anchors for certain cell surface proteins, *Plasmodium* GPI are structurally distinct from human GPI (Gowda, 2007). Consequently, *Plasmodium* GPI moieties may be recognized by the host immune system. Indeed, *P. falciparum* GPI were reported to induce the pro-inflammatory cytokines TNF and IL-1β in murine macrophages *in vitro* (Schofield and Hackett, 1993; Tachado et al., 1996). Moreover, purified GPI immobilized on gold particles elicited pronounced TNF responses from murine macrophages *in vitro* (Krishnegowda et al., 2005; Zhu et al., 2009, 2011), which was attributed to recognition of *P. falciparum* GPI through TLR2 or heterodimers of TLR2/1 and TLR2/6 (Krishnegowda et al., 2005; Zhu et al., 2011). However, given that TLR-deficiency did not impair immune responses elicited by *P. berghei* ANKA *in vivo* and did not protect mice from ECM (Togbe et al., 2007; Lepenies et al., 2008), the mechanism of GPI-induced innate immune activation *in vivo* remains to be determined.

Another potential malaria PAMP is hemozoin, an insoluble polymer formed inside the digestive vacuole to detoxify heme and its conjugated redox-active iron, which is released during hemoglobin proteolysis (Francis et al., 1997; Sigala and Goldberg, 2014). Hemozoin becomes accessible during erythrocyte rupture and upon phagocytosis of infected erythrocytes, and has been described to induce expression of pro-inflammatory cytokines, such as TNF and IL-1β, as well as chemokines from human monocytes, murine macrophages (Olivier et al., 2014), and human monocyte-derived DCs (Bujila et al., 2016). Hemozoin or hemozoin-bound nucleic acids are recognized by endosomal TLR9 (Coban et al., 2005; Parroche et al., 2007), cytoplasmic inflammasomes, or cytoplasmic sensors (Kalantari et al., 2014). However, it remains unresolved whether hemozoin itself or molecules bound to hemozoin, such as DNA, activate TLR9 (Liehl and Mota, 2012). In fact, the AT-rich *Plasmodium* genomic DNA, a feature shared by many pathogens including *Schistosoma*, was described to be immunomodulatory *in vitro*, but this response is apparently TLR9-independent (McCutchan et al., 1984; Sharma et al., 2011).

In addition to inducing pro-inflammatory responses, recognition of parasites and *Plasmodium*-infected erythrocytes is crucial for the phagocytic uptake and thus removal of parasites from the circulation by macrophages and DCs (McGilvray et al., 2000; Stevenson and Riley, 2004; **Figure 3**). Interestingly, although macrophages and DCs may both contribute to early pro-inflammatory cytokine responses *via* activation of PRR-mediated signaling, a recent study suggests that macrophage responsiveness is strongly compromised upon phagocytosis of *P. falciparum*- or *P. berghei*-infected erythrocytes or free merozoites due to pronounced phagosomal acidification (Wu et al., 2015). Instead, DCs contribute to increased serum levels of pro-inflammatory cytokines early during *P. berghei* infection, including IL-6, IL-12p40, and TNF (Wu et al., 2015).

Apart from parasite-derived stimuli, host-derived DAMPs such as urate crystals, heme, and microvesicles released from damaged host cells may activate the innate immune system, although so far this has only been demonstrated for microvesicles (Gazzinelli et al., 2014). *Plasmodium falciparum*-infected erythrocyte-derived microvesicles have been reported to induce TNF and IL-10 from monocyte-derived human macrophages *in vitro*, potentially through phagocytic uptake of microvesicles (Mantel et al., 2013). In line with this observation, plasma microparticles derived from *P. berghei* -infected mice stimulated bone marrow-derived macrophages to secrete TNF *in vitro*, and TNF induction was reported to be TLR4-dependent (Couper et al., 2010). In humans, increased numbers of plasma microparticles have been detected during *P. falciparum* and *P. vivax* infection, and microparticle numbers were higher in severe malaria cases, including CM, than in uncomplicated *P. falciparum* infections (Campos et al., 2010; Nantakomol et al., 2011; Sahu et al., 2013). Furthermore, two studies point toward infection-induced alterations in the microvesicle cargo, suggesting that not only microvesicle frequency but also content are relevant in inducing pro-inflammatory responses (Couper et al., 2010; Tiberti et al., 2016). Together, these studies indicate that microvesicles might contribute to CM pathogenesis and to other manifestations of severe malaria, and the association with pro-inflammatory immune responses warrants further investigations.

Although parasite-derived stimuli have been repeatedly reported to induce pro-inflammatory responses, the real qualitative and quantitative nature of the stimuli remains inadequately understood and may point toward a complex synergistic effect of multiple stimuli. Pro-inflammatory cytokines such as TNF, IL-1α (Kwiatkowski et al., 1990; Tchinda et al., 2007), IFN-γ and IL-12p40 (Hermsen et al., 2003), as well as chemokines, including IL-8/CXCL8 (Hermsen et al., 2003), platelet factor 4 (PF4)/CXCL4, and IP-10/CXCL10 (Wilson et al., 2011), are clearly elevated during *P. falciparum* infection. Several cytokines and chemokines, including TNF and CXCL10, have been found to be associated with CM severity (Kwiatkowski et al., 1990; Wilson et al., 2011), while a more recent study reported that neither plasma nor cerebrospinal fluid (CSF) TNF concentration were indicative of CM-associated mortality, yet elevated levels of TNF in CSF of pediatric CM cases were associated with long-term neurologic and cognitive deficits (Shabani et al., 2017). Consequently, it remains to be conclusively determined which cytokines and/or chemokines present suitable prognostic signatures of disease progression.

While many early studies focused on the identification of single inflammatory cytokines critically involved in malaria pathology, it is likely that numerous immune players are modulated during the course of a *Plasmodium* infection - sequentially and/or simultaneously. Accordingly, it is conceivable that a complex interplay of immune mediators contributes to the development of severe malaria in general, and to CM pathogenesis in particular. Several studies have addressed this issue by systematically analyzing pro- and anti-inflammatory markers. Since these studies included patients from different study sites of varying age and at various time points of infection, the cytokines identified to be associated with disease severity varied substantially, and the combination of selected analytes was heterogenous between studies (Prakash et al., 2006; Jain et al., 2008; Thuma et al., 2011). An early study reported two clusters of cytokines associated with mild and cerebral malaria, respectively, in *P. falciparum*-infected adults (Prakash et al., 2006). According to this study, IFN-γ, IL-2, IL-5, IL-6 and IL-12 were increased in mild malaria whereas TGF-β, TNF, IL-10 and IL-1β were particularly elevated in CM. In a study cohort of *P. falciparum*-infected children and adults, serum TNF levels did not correlate with disease severity, and instead IP-10/CXCL10, sTNF-R2, and sFas were proposed as biomarkers of CM severity and mortality (Jain et al., 2008). Additional cytokines were elevated in malaria cases compared to healthy controls and included IL-1ra, IL-10, IL-8/CXCL8, and macrophage inflammatory protein 1β (MIP-1β)/CCL4 (Jain et al., 2008). In two cohorts of *P. falciparum*-infected children, TNF concentration was slightly, albeit non-significantly, elevated in CM compared to severe anemia cases (Thuma et al., 2011; Mandala et al., 2017). In the study by Thuma et al. (2011) conducted in Zambia, IL-10, IL-1α, IL-6, and IP-10/CXCL10 plasma levels were higher in children suffering from CM than in children with severe anemia (Thuma et al., 2011). In line with these findings, Mandala et al. (2017) found higher IL-10 and IL-6 serum levels in Malawian children suffering from CM compared to those with severe anemia, while IFN-γ and IL-8/CXCL-8 were also elevated in pediatric CM cases.

In summary, cytokine profiling continues to aid in identifying distinct patterns of pro- and anti-inflammatory cytokines and chemokines in CM patients. Although a common cytokine/chemokine signature associated with CM severity has not yet been identified, which is in part due to the fact that the combination of markers investigated varies among studies, collectively, these studies point toward important roles for certain immunoregulatory molecules in modulating CM severity. In order to describe how inflammatory mediators associated with *Plasmodium* infection may contribute to CM pathogenesis, we will highlight their roles in endothelial activation, blood-brain barrier permeability, and neuroinflammation, by drawing on findings obtained from *in vitro* studies and the murine ECM model.

INFLAMMATION AND ENDOTHELIAL ACTIVATION

Functions of healthy endothelium include anti-coagulant properties through inhibiting platelet adhesion and aggregation, regulation of blood flow by releasing nitric oxide, controlling endothelial permeability, preventing extravasation of plasma proteins to tissue, and preventing leukocyte adhesion through suppressing adhesion molecule expression and sequestering chemokines within Weibel-Palade-bodies (Pober and Sessa, 2007). Under inflammatory conditions such as systemic inflammation during *Plasmodium* infection, endothelial activation may seriously impair endothelial function (**Figure 4**). A hallmark of endothelial activation is the expression of adhesion molecules such as VCAM-1 and ICAM-1 on the endothelial cell surface. Systemic endothelial activation was reported in *P. falciparum*-infected and in sepsis patients based on plasma levels of soluble adhesion molecules (Turner et al., 1998). Moreover, immunohistochemical analysis of fatal *P. falciparum* -infected CM cases revealed that expression of ICAM-1 was

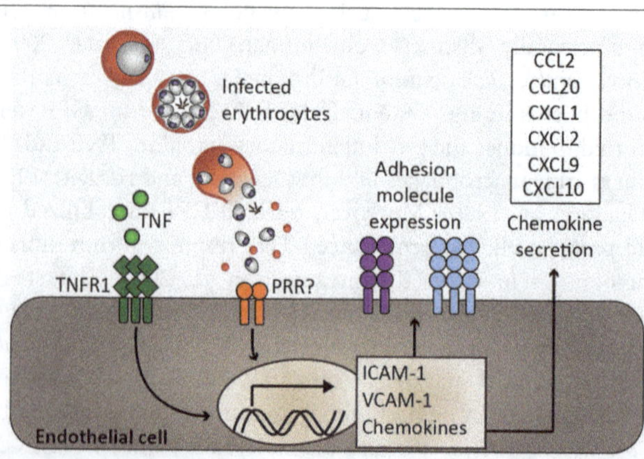

FIGURE 4 | Endothelial activation and chemokine secretion. A characteristic feature of *Plasmodium* infection is endothelial activation, which is likely induced by elevated serum tumor necrosis factor (TNF) levels. Binding of TNF to its receptor (TNFR1) induces transcription of adhesion molecules, including ICAM-1 and VCAM-1, as well as chemokines (Pober and Sessa, 2007). Endothelial activation might be directly induced by infected erythrocytes, possibly through activation of pattern recognition receptors (PRR), resulting in elevated expression of ICAM-1 and chemokine secretion (Viebig et al., 2005; Tripathi et al., 2006, 2009; Chakravorty et al., 2007).

most pronounced in the brain microvasculature compared to other organs and biopsies from non-malaria cases (Turner et al., 1994). In good agreement, ICAM-1 staining was described to be more pronounced on brain endothelial cells from *P. berghei* (strain ANKA)-infected mice during ECM than in those isolated from *P. yoelii*-infected (non-ECM) mice (Grau et al., 1991). Accordingly, *Icam1*-deficiency protected mice from *P. berghei*-induced ECM (Favre et al., 1999). Considering that adhesion molecules are thought to promote binding of infected erythrocytes and leukocytes to endothelial cells, and that human as well as murine CM is associated with intravascular accumulation of leukocytes in the brain (Hunt and Grau, 2003), these findings signify a critical role for endothelial activation in CM pathogenesis.

Among other factors, endothelial activation may be induced by inflammatory cytokines. TNF and lymphotoxin α (LTα) activate human endothelial cells *in vitro* (Cavender et al., 1989; Pober and Cotran, 1990). Similarly, IFN-γ, IL-1α, and IL-1β function in endothelial activation (Pober and Cotran, 1990; Bauer et al., 2002). These pro-inflammatory cytokines have been found to be elevated in serum or plasma of *P. falciparum*-infected patients and TNF as well as IL-1α and IL-1β were described to be associated with CM severity (Prakash et al., 2006; Thuma et al., 2011). Consequently, endothelial activation observed in *P. falciparum* infection might in part be mediated by these cytokines. In accordance with a proposed role for endothelial activation in CM, the pathology observed in murine ECM is associated with a T helper 1 (Th 1) immune response, and cytokines, such as IFN-γ, TNF, and LTα, and immune cells, e.g., $CD4^+$ and $CD8^+$ T cells together with NK cells are involved in ECM (Yanez et al., 1996; Lucas et al., 1997; Engwerda et al., 2002; Hunt and Grau, 2003; Schofield and Grau, 2005; Langhorne et al., 2008). Of note, despite an association of TNF with disease severity in CM, *Tnf*-deficient mice were not protected from ECM (Engwerda et al., 2002), and blocking of TNF by anti-TNF antibodies or pentoxifylline did not improve survival in human CM (Di Perri et al., 1995; van Hensbroek et al., 1996). Consequently, blocking TNF was demonstrated to be insufficient to prevent fatal CM, and, therefore, additional mechanisms are likely to critically contribute to CM pathogenesis. Moreover, these early therapeutic interventions highlight the complexity of this malaria syndrome, indicating that single serum cytokines associated with CM severity do not necessarily translate into therapeutic approaches. Notably, elevated serum TNF in particular may represent a secondary immune response, which might further amplify severity while not being critical in initiating CM pathogenesis.

Apart from the induction of endothelial activation by pro-inflammatory cytokines, endothelial cells are an important part of the innate immune response since they recognize PAMPs through expression of PRR such as TLR and NLR. Endothelial cells were found to secrete pro-inflammatory cytokines, including IL-1α, IL-1β, or IL-6, as well as immunomodulatory cytokines, namely IL-10 and TGF-β, and chemokines, e.g., monocyte chemoattractant protein 1 (MCP-1)/CCL2, RANTES/CCL5, and IL-8/CXCL8, upon stimulation by pro-inflammatory cytokines or lipopolysaccharide (LPS) *in vitro* (Mai et al., 2013). Notably, microvascular endothelial cells derived from subcutaneous adipose tissue of patients with uncomplicated malaria and fatal CM were demonstrated to differ in their endothelial inflammatory response to TNF stimulation *ex vivo* in that MCP-1/CCL2 and IL-6 were induced to a larger extent in endothelial cells derived from CM patients. Consequently, it was proposed that inter-individual differences in the endothelial response to inflammation might account for CM severity (Wassmer et al., 2011). These results support the notion that the pro-inflammatory microvascular environment during *P. falciparum* infection might be enhanced by endothelial cells. Interestingly, human brain microvascular endothelial cells have been described to phagocytose *P. berghei* merozoites *in vitro* (Howland et al., 2015b). Furthermore, upon co-culture with *P. falciparum*-infected erythrocytes, human endothelial cell lines were reported to upregulate ICAM-1 expression (Viebig et al., 2005; Tripathi et al., 2006), to increase transcription of *CCL20*, *CXCL1*, *CXCL2*, *CXCL8*, and *IL6* (Tripathi et al., 2009), and to secrete MCP-1/CCL2, MIP-3α/CCL20, and IL-8/CXCL8 (Viebig et al., 2005; Chakravorty et al., 2007) (**Figure 4**). Together, these *in vitro* observations suggest that endothelial cells are potentially directly involved in the immune response to *Plasmodium* infection. Since leukocyte sequestration in the microvasculature of the brain was described in human CM and murine ECM (Hunt and Grau, 2003), local chemokine gradients originating from brain endothelial cells might orchestrate leukocyte migration and thus promote local inflammation, thereby contributing to the development of CM.

Although the extent of the contribution of endothelial cell-derived chemokines in the process of leukocyte accumulation in brains of patients suffering from CM and of ECM mice remains to be established, a number of clinical studies reported that several chemokines are elevated in serum and CSF of CM patients, thereby providing a potential link between serum or CSF chemokine levels and progression from mild malaria to CM. Chemokines that were elevated in human CM cases included MCP-1/CCL2, MIP-1β/CCL4, PF4/CXCL4, IL-8/CXCL8, and IP-10/CXCL10 (Jain et al., 2008; Wilson et al., 2011). Particularly, MCP-1/CCL2, Eotaxin/CCL11, and IP-10/CXLC10 were reported to be indicative of disease severity (Armah et al., 2007; Jain et al., 2008; Thuma et al., 2011; Wilson et al., 2011). Moreover, *post mortem* MIP-1β/CCL4, IL-8/CXCL8, and IP-10/CXCL10 levels were significantly elevated in cerebrospinal fluid (CSF) of fatal *P. falciparum*-induced CM cases when compared to fatal severe malarial anemia cases and non-malaria deaths (Armah et al., 2007). In another study, IL-8/CXCL8 was elevated in CSF of non-fatal CM cases of *P. falciparum*-infected children (John et al., 2008b), while MCP-1/CCL2, MIP-1α/CCL3, MIP-1β/CCL4, and RANTES/CCL5 levels were comparable to malaria-free controls. The relevance of certain chemokines in cerebral malaria pathogenesis was demonstrated in the murine ECM model, in which *Cxcl4*-, *Cxcl9*-, or *Cxcl10*-deficiency resulted in reduced ECM-associated mortality (Campanella et al., 2008; Srivastava et al., 2008; Nie et al., 2009). Notably, PF4/CXCL4 was elevated in plasma of *P. berghei* ANKA-infected mice and demonstrated to induce TNF secretion from peritoneal macrophages and T cells *in vitro*, and *Cxcl4*-deficiency resulted in reduced serum TNF and IFN-γ levels during *P. berghei* ANKA-infection (Srivastava et al., 2008), indicating that PF4/CXCL4 contributes to establishing a pro-inflammatory environment, which might amplify further immune responses and could thereby promote CM pathogenesis. Furthermore, protection from ECM in *Cxcl10*-deficient mice was associated with a decrease in leukocyte sequestration in brains of *P. berghei* ANKA-infected mice, while parasite-specific $CXCR3^+$ T cells were increased in spleens of *Cxcl10*-deficient compared to WT mice (Nie et al., 2009), suggesting that IP-10/CXCL10-mediated recruitment of $CXCR3^+$ T cells to the brain might contribute to the development of ECM. A similar phenomenon might account for a decrease in ECM-associated mortality described for *Cxcl9*-deficient mice (Campanella et al., 2008), since recruitment of CXCR3-expressing cells can also be initiated by monokine induced by IFN-γ (MIG)/CXCL9. However, the precise mechanism by which MIG/CXCL9 contributes to ECM pathogenesis is yet to be determined. Apart from studies using specific gene deletions, chemokine transcripts were found to be induced to a higher extent in brains of ECM- compared to non-ECM mice. These transcripts included *Ccl2*, *Ccl3*, *Ccl4*, *Ccl5*, *Cxcl1*, *Cxcl9*, and *Cxcl10* (Miu et al., 2008; Van den Steen et al., 2008), supporting the finding that apart from NK and T cells, monocytes and neutrophils also sequester in the microvasculature (Renia et al., 2012), e.g., through recruitment by MCP-1/CCL2 and keratinocyte chemoattractant (KC)/*Cxcl1*, respectively. Nevertheless, studies to identify the cell types producing these chemokines in the brain are very limited. For instance, CXCL9 was demonstrated to be expressed by endothelial cells, while the source(s) of CXCL10 in the brain during *P. berghei* infection remain to be conclusively determined, and could include neurons, astrocytes, or endothelial cells (Campanella et al., 2008; Miu et al., 2008) as well as recruited monocytes (Ioannidis et al., 2016).

Together, activated endothelial cells likely contribute to local inflammation by secreting cytokines and chemokines, thereby recruiting leukocytes, including monocytes, macrophages, neutrophils and T cells, which accumulate in brains of mice and humans during ECM and CM, respectively (Renia et al., 2012; Storm and Craig, 2014). Since these cell types might secrete cytokines and chemokines themselves, local inflammation and endothelial activation could be further exacerbated (**Figure 5**). For instance, potential endothelial cell-induced recruitment of neutrophils and monocytes expressing IP-10/CXCL10 may promote further recruitment of $CXCR3^+$ cells such as NK and T cells to the brain (Ioannidis et al., 2016).

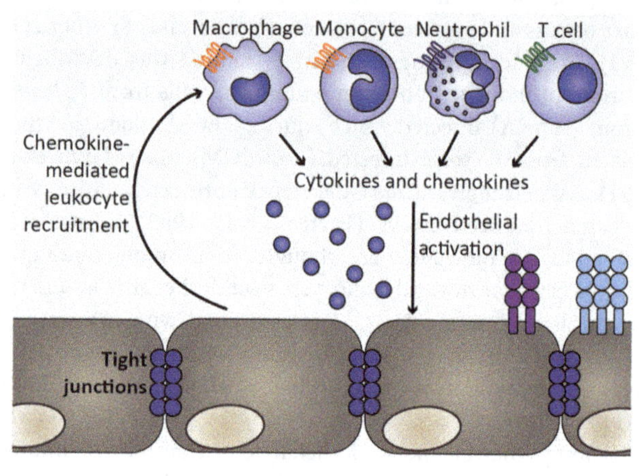

FIGURE 5 | Chemokine-mediated leukocyte recruitment and progression of local inflammation. As a consequence of endothelial activation by pro-inflammatory cytokines, such as TNF, and infected erythrocytes, chemokines are secreted from endothelial cells, which initiate recruitment of leukocytes expressing the respective chemokine receptors, including macrophages, monocytes, neutrophils, and T cell. These cell types were also found to sequester in the microvasculature during human CM as well as murine ECM (Hunt and Grau, 2003; Renia et al., 2012). Upon arrival at the site of the inflammatory insult, these leukocyte subsets may in turn secrete cytokines as well as chemokines, thereby further promoting endothelial activation and leukocyte recruitment. Thus, a feed-forward loop is initiated which exacerbates local inflammation in the brain.

ENDOTHELIAL ACTIVATION AND BLOOD-BRAIN BARRIER INTEGRITY

The blood-brain barrier is comprised of endothelial cells forming a continuous barrier through tight junctions, a basement membrane and astrocytes, which are in direct contact with neurons and microglia. This composition is critical to minimize local inflammation and neuronal damage (Obermeier et al., 2013). In the course of *Plasmodium* infection, endothelial activation may progress to vascular permeability and loss of blood-brain barrier integrity, as indicated by hemorrhages in brains of CM patients and extravasation of dyes or antibodies into the brain parenchyma in ECM (Renia et al., 2012). Although the extent of pathological events related to blood-brain barrier function in human CM is variable, dysfunction of the blood-brain barrier appears to be associated with progression of cerebral disease (Medana and Turner, 2006). Histology of brain sections from fatal human CM cases revealed a redistribution of the tight junction proteins occludin, vinculin, and zonula occludens 1 (ZO-1), which are central to blood-brain barrier integrity (Brown et al., 1999). Moreover, immunohistochemistry of brain sections derived from pediatric fatal CM cases indicated blood-brain barrier impairment in areas containing sequestered *P. falciparum*-infected erythrocytes, where they were associated with focal loss of endothelial intercellular junctions (Brown et al., 2001). Additionally, *in vitro* studies have demonstrated a decrease in endothelial resistance upon addition of *P. falciparum*-infected erythrocytes to endothelial cells (Tripathi et al., 2007; Jambou et al., 2010). This model, however, only partially reflects the response at the blood-brain barrier due to lack of barrier components such as astrocytes and pericytes (Medana and Turner, 2007).

Interestingly, MCP-1/CCL2 induces redistribution of tight junction proteins and increases endothelial permeability *in vitro* (Stamatovic et al., 2003; Song and Pachter, 2004; Yao and Tsirka, 2011). Thus, chemokines may contribute to organ-specific inflammation by inducing signals that promote endothelial permeability (**Figure 6**). The roles of the respective chemokine receptors are less clear in this context. This is exemplified in the

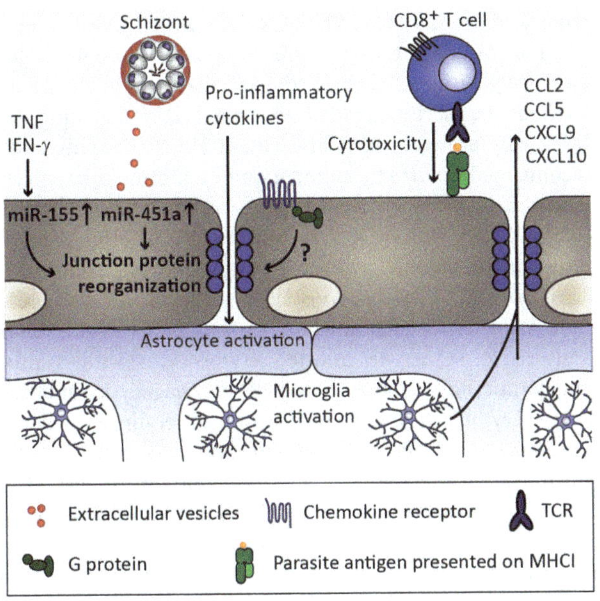

FIGURE 6 | Endothelial permeability and neuroinflammation. Through continued inflammatory insults toward endothelial cells by, for instance, circulating tumor necrosis factor (TNF) and interferon γ (IFN-γ), miR-155 might be upregulated in endothelial cells. Along with uptake of miR-451a from *P. falciparum*-infected erythrocyte-derived extracellular vesicles, reorganization of tight junction proteins such as zonula occludens 1 (ZO-1) is induced and could contribute to endothelial permeability during cerebral malaria (Lopez-Ramirez et al., 2014; Mantel et al., 2016). Additionally, chemokine receptors might induce redistribution of tight junction proteins in a G protein-dependent manner (Stamatovic et al., 2003; Song and Pachter, 2004; Yao and Tsirka, 2011), while the contribution of chemokine-induced opening of tight junctions is less clear in the context of cerebral malaria. $CD8^+$ T cell-mediated cytotoxity toward endothelial cells through recognition of parasite antigen presented on MHC class I molecules on endothelial cells likely contributes substantially to blood-brain barrier permeability during cerebral malaria (Howland et al., 2015a,b). Consequently, pro-inflammatory cytokines enter the brain parenchyma and could thereby activate astrocytes and microglia, which in turn could secrete chemokines (Capuccini et al., 2016) and thus promote leukocyte recruitment and local inflammation.

MCP-1/CCL2 receptor CCR2. *Ccr2*-deficiency abrogated CCL2-induced endothelial permeability *in vitro* (Stamatovic et al., 2003), but did not protect against ECM (Belnoue et al., 2003), indicating that other chemokines and/or additional mechanisms induce blood-brain barrier permeability.

Along with the observed redistribution of endothelial tight junction proteins and loss of intercellular junctions, growing evidence from the murine ECM model suggests that $CD8^+$ T cells are primary mediators in CM disease pathogenesis by contributing considerably to the loss of blood-brain barrier integrity (Howland et al., 2015a). Indeed, the accumulation of $CD8^+$ T cells in brains of *P. berghei* ANKA-infected mice appears to be critical for the development of ECM (Villegas-Mendez et al., 2012), and blood-brain barrier disruption was proposed to be a consequence of $CD8^+$ T cell-mediated cytotoxicity toward endothelial cells cross-presenting parasite antigen (Howland et al., 2015b) (**Figure 6**). Recruitment of $CD8^+$ T cells to the brain of infected mice has been described to be partly mediated by expression of the chemokine receptor CXCR3 and its IFN-γ-inducible ligands MIG/CXCL9 as well as IP-10/CXCL10 (Hansen et al., 2007; Villegas-Mendez et al., 2012). Indeed, NK cell-derived IFN-γ has been demonstrated to be crucial for the induction of CXCR3 expression on T cells and subsequent T-cell migration to the brain of *P. berghei* ANKA-infected mice (Hansen et al., 2007). In line with these findings, brain transcripts of *Cxcr3* were reduced in mice deficient for IFN-γR1 in comparison to wild type mice infected with *P. berghei* ANKA. Additionally, while expression of MIG/CXCL9 and IP-10/CXCL10 is induced in brains of *P. berghei* ANKA-infected wild type mice, expression levels of these chemokines in *Ifngr1*-deficient mice were similar to those of uninfected mice (Palomo et al., 2013). Collectively, these findings suggest that IFN-γ-induced signaling is crucial for chemokine-mediated leukocyte recruitment to the brain during ECM, while it remains to be established to which extent activated endothelium might contribute to this chemokine response.

Importantly, *Cxcr3*-deficient mice were less likely to succumb to ECM (Campanella et al., 2008; Miu et al., 2008), and numbers of $CD4^+$ and $CD8^+$ T cells in brains of *Cxcr3*-deficient mice were reported to be reduced compared to wild type mice during *P. berghei* ANKA infection. However, the extent of $CD8^+$ T cell recruitment was similar in *Cxcr3*-deficient mice which were either resistant or susceptible to ECM (Miu et al., 2008). These results indicate that the quantity of $CD8^+$ T cells in brains of *P. berghei* ANKA-infected mice is not critical for the development of ECM. Rather, additional aspects such as $CD8^+$ T-cell specificity toward parasite antigen presented on endothelium, expression levels of key cytotoxic effector molecules perforin and granzyme B by $CD8^+$ T cells, and localization of these $CD8^+$ T cells within the brain might play a substantial role in the development of ECM (Miu et al., 2008; Haque et al., 2011; Howland et al., 2015b; Huggins et al., 2017). Nevertheless, it remains to be determined why susceptibility to ECM among *Cxcr3*-deficient mice is variable. Moreover, these findings indicate that additional mechanisms other than $CD8^+$ T cell-mediated cytotoxicity might be involved in the loss of blood-brain barrier integrity.

In fact, in addition to $CD8^+$ T cells and chemokines, extracellular vesicles derived from *P. falciparum*-infected erythrocytes were recently implicated in blood-brain barrier permeability *in vitro* (Mantel et al., 2016; **Figure 6**). These extracellular vesicles contained miRNA miR-451a, which, upon endocytosis by endothelial cells, correlated with reduced endothelial caveolin-1 expression. Interestingly, MCP-1/CCL2-induced redistribution of tight junction proteins and concomitant endothelial permeability (Stamatovic et al., 2003) was also accompanied by a decrease in caveolin-1 protein (Song and Pachter, 2004), thus pointing toward a common underlying mechanism in the induction of endothelial permeability by CCL2 and extracellular vesicles derived from *P. falciparum*-infected erythrocytes. Since sequestration of infected erythrocytes in the microvasculature is likely promoted by expression of adhesion molecules upon endothelial activation, locally increased release of *P. falciparum*-infected erythrocyte-derived extracellular vesicles carrying miRNA miR-451a might be an additional mechanism involved in blood-brain barrier permeability in CM.

In addition to miR-451a, another miRNA, miR-155, was implicated in inflammation-associated blood-brain barrier permeability. Upon stimulation of human brain endothelial cells with pro-inflammatory cytokines TNF and IFN-γ *in vitro*, miR-155 was found to be upregulated. The tight junction protein claudin-1 was reported to be among the candidate targets of miR-155, and cytokine stimulation or miR-155 overexpression resulted in reorganization of the tight junction protein ZO-1 along with increased endothelial permeability (Lopez-Ramirez et al., 2014), indicating that cytokines such as TNF and IFN-γ might directly contribute to blood-brain barrier permeability through induction of regulatory miRNAs. Interestingly, levels of miR-155 were recently reported to be elevated in extracellular vesicles in the circulation of *P. berghei* ANKA-infected mice, and *miR-155*-deficiency resulted in preservation of blood-brain barrier integrity and reduced ECM-associated mortality (Barker et al., 2017). Notably, plasma concentrations of IL-6, IFN-γ, and MCP-1/CCL2 were significantly elevated in *P. berghei* ANKA-infected *miR-155*-deficient compared to wild type mice in this study, suggesting that miR-155 might have additional targets other than tight junction proteins. Importantly, whether miR-155-carrying extracellular vesicles are derived from activated endothelium, and their impact on tight junction reorganization in the context of ECM, remain to be determined. Nevertheless, inhibition of the function of miR-155 might present a useful target for therapeutic approaches (Barker et al., 2017). These processes of chemokine induction, microvascular sequestration of infected erythrocytes and leukocytes, and release of extracellular vesicles carrying regulatory miRNAs are most likely not exclusive to the brain. However, endothelial permeability is likely more detrimental in the brain than in other organs and, hence, cerebral malaria may be the most severe manifestation of these processes. Additionally, brain endothelial cells have been described to express comparably low levels of thrombin-binding thrombomodulin, and excess of unbound thrombin may further promote local endothelial activation by inducing further expression of adhesion molecules (Clark et al., 2006).

Together, cytokine- or *Plasmodium*-induced endothelial activation may lead to chemokine induction and leukocyte recruitment as well as sequestration of infected erythrocytes, which may act synergistically in promoting endothelial permeability. Nevertheless, the precise molecular mechanisms that trigger loss of blood-brain barrier integrity in CM are incompletely understood and need to be further investigated.

NEUROINFLAMMATION

Upon disruption of the blood-brain barrier, cytokines, chemokines, and soluble parasite products might enter the brain parenchyma and, thereby, activate astrocytes and microglia, and result in symptoms of neuroinflammation in the absence of extravasation of infected erythrocytes or leukocytes into the brain parenchyma (Combes et al., 2010). Indeed, activation of microglia and astrocytes has been observed in murine and human CM (Hunt et al., 2006; Combes et al., 2010). For instance, transcriptome analysis of microglia isolated from *P. berghei*-infected mice revealed that several chemokines as well as transcripts related to type I IFN signaling were differentially upregulated (Capuccini et al., 2016). This finding was confirmed *in vitro* by stimulation of a murine microglia cell line with IFN-β, which resulted in secretion of MCP-1/CCL2, RANTES/CCL5, MIG/CXCL9, and IP-10/CXCL10. Moreover, stimulation of human primary astrocytes with a combination of IFN-γ and LTα synergistically induced IP-10/CXCL10 secretion *in vitro* (Bakmiwewa et al., 2016). Additionally, co-culture of *P. berghei*-infected erythrocytes with a mixed astrocyte-microglia culture resulted in phagocytic uptake of infected erythrocytes and of parasitized erythrocyte-derived microvesicles by microglia and astrocytes, respectively, which in turn was associated with an induction in IP-10/CXCL10 secretion (Shrivastava et al., 2017). Furthermore, astrocytes and microglia may secrete various cytokines and chemokines upon activation (Dong and Benveniste, 2001; Medana et al., 2001). Consequently, loss of blood-brain barrier integrity and subsequent activation of microglia and astrocytes might result in further chemokine-mediated recruitment of leukocytes to the brain and subsequent amplification of inflammation (**Figure 6**). Additionally, activation of microglia might induce expression of FasL, which, upon binding to Fas expressed on astrocytes, could induce astrocyte damage (Hunt et al., 2006). However, to our knowledge, this has so far not been demonstrated in the context of CM. Since astrocytes are critically involved in maintaining blood-brain barrier properties and survival of neurons (Combes et al., 2010), their functional impairment might disrupt neuronal activity and could thereby account for the neurological impairment observed in some CM cases (Hunt et al., 2006).

SUMMARY AND PERSPECTIVES

The human and murine immune system are in part strikingly different (Stevenson and Riley, 2004). For instance, IL-8/CXCL8 was reported to be associated with cerebral malaria (Armah et al., 2007; John et al., 2008b), while this chemokine is not expressed in mice (Viola and Luster, 2008). However, KC/*Cxcl1* is considered a functional homolog of IL-8/CXCL8 in mice (Hol et al., 2010), which mediates neutrophil recruitment, and *Cxcl1* transcripts were reported to be elevated in brains of ECM compared to non-ECM mice (Miu et al., 2008), suggesting that KC/*Cxcl1* might be similarly involved in ECM pathogenesis. Yet, the precise contribution of IL-8/CXCL8 and KC/*Cxcl1* to human CM and murine ECM, respectively, needs to be further investigated. Moreover, the murine ECM model shares several features with human CM, including aspects of histopathology and inflammatory responses. Importantly, mechanistic insights can only be gained from the murine ECM model, and many observations are in remarkably good agreement with clinical data obtained from *P. falciparum*-induced CM. Although a comprehensive representation of the events leading to CM pathogenesis remains elusive, a working model of an inflammatory cascade leading to CM is conceivable (**Figure 1**).

Upon establishing liver stage infection, a first type I IFN response is mounted by hepatocytes, leading to a primary activation of IFN-γ-producing NK cells (Liehl et al., 2014; Miller et al., 2014; **Figure 2**) and, consequently, induction of MIG/CXCL9 and IP-10/CXCL10 secretion, potentially from endothelial cells (Campanella et al., 2008; Miu et al., 2008). Upon progression of the *Plasmodium* infection to the blood stages, infected erythrocytes are recognized by DCs and induce the secretion of IL-12 and TNF (Wu et al., 2015; **Figure 3**). IL-12 contributes to further activation of NK and differentiation of Th1 cells (Stevenson and Riley, 2004), while TNF and IFN-γ activate chemokine transcription and adhesion molecule expression on endothelial cells (Pober and Sessa, 2007; Miu et al., 2008; Griffith et al., 2014). As the infection progresses further, *Plasmodium*-infected erythrocytes are recognized by endothelial cells and induce expression of chemokines, such as MCP-1/CCL2 and IL-8/CXCL8 (Viebig et al., 2005; Chakravorty et al., 2007; Tripathi et al., 2009; **Figure 4**). As a result, leukocytes are recruited, including monocytes, macrophages, neutrophils, as well as T cells, and initiate a local inflammatory response (Renia et al., 2012; Storm and Craig, 2014; **Figure 5**). These cell types secrete chemokines, thereby amplifying the response leading to further leukocyte recruitment and intensifying local inflammation. Additionally, endothelial cells phagocytose merozoites and parasite material released during schizont rupture and present parasite antigens to $CD8^+$ T cells (Howland et al., 2015b; **Figure 6**), which may result in targeted elimination of antigen-presenting endothelial cells and, thus, cause damages to the endothelial lining of the blood-brain barrier. This process can be further exacerbated by openings of tight junctions mediated by chemokines and extracellular vesicle-derived miRNAs (Song and Pachter, 2004; Mantel et al., 2016). As a result, small molecules can enter the brain parenchyma and potentially activate brain-resident microglia and astrocytes, further amplifying local inflammation through cytokine secretion and leukocyte recruitment and impairing neuronal functionality (Hunt et al., 2006; Combes et al., 2010).

Even though the febrile response elicited during *Plasmodium* blood stage infection together with the concomitant inflammatory cytokine responses limit parasite growth and mediate the resolution of infection, imbalances in pro-inflammatory and anti-inflammatory cytokines cause progression of malaria disease to manifestations of severe malaria, such as CM, and death. Adjunctive therapies that prevent adverse effects of the immune response to *Plasmodium* infection are therefore urgently needed. Although immunomodulation is a promising approach to alleviate immune-mediated pathology, such therapies need to be designed carefully in order to maintain efficient control of parasite growth. Notably, adjunct therapies modulating chemokine responses may have fewer side-effects compared to therapies based on neutralizing cytokines (Ioannidis et al., 2014). Indeed, antibody-mediated targeting of IP-10/CXCL10 was demonstrated to result in reduced ECM-induced mortality and parasite burden in mice, which was likely mediated by retention and expansion of parasite-specific T cells in the spleen (Nie et al., 2009). Such treatments may be relevant in other contexts as well: murine *Toxoplasma* encephalitis has been described to be associated with constant expression of *Ccl2*, *Ccl3*, *Ccl4*, *Ccl5*, and *Cxcl10* in brains of infected mice concomitant with continuous recruitment of $CD4^+$ and $CD8^+$ T cells, which was not the case for mice in which the infection developed into chronic latency (Strack et al., 2002). Furthermore, targeted neutralization of single chemokines, including MCP-1/CCL2, MIP-1α/CCL3, RANTES/CCL5, or IP-10/CXCL10, resulted in protection of mice from experimental autoimmune encephalomyelitis, a murine model for multiple sclerosis (Karin and Wildbaum, 2015). These findings from other neuroinflammatory diseases highlight that chemokines might present a valuable target for intervention strategies in several diseases. However, efforts to design chemokine-based therapies are challenged by the complexity of the chemokine system as well as properties such as redundancy, pleiotropy, and speciation (Viola and Luster, 2008). In fact, most cell populations express several different chemokine receptors and thus single chemokine or chemokine receptor blockade may not affect disease outcome in certain pathological conditions.

Together, reliable biomarkers which predict disease outcome and allow for potential prophylactic measures are yet to be identified. Several clinical studies have reported potential diagnostic and prognostic biomarkers for CM, which apart from chemokines such as IP-10/CXCL10 and PF4/CXCL4 also include *P. falciparum* histidine-rich protein 2 (*Pf*HRP2), a protein which correlates with parasite biomass, as well as regulators of endothelial activation angiopoietin-1 and -2 (summarized in Sahu et al., 2015). Still, comprehensive studies with defined clinical parameters and systematic assessment of plasma levels of multiple inflammatory mediators need to be performed to determine whether distinct clusters of markers can be associated with disease severity in order to identify patients at risk of developing CM early during infection. Such studies will inform future investigations into mechanisms underlying disease pathogenesis in order to develop novel evidence-based malaria intervention strategies.

AUTHOR CONTRIBUTIONS

All authors listed have made a substantial, direct and intellectual contribution to the work, and approved it for publication.

ACKNOWLEDGMENTS

Work on chemokines and cytokines in murine malaria models is funded by the Deutsche Forschungsgemeinschaft (KA 3347/4-1) and partly by the Max Planck Society.

REFERENCES

Adams, Y., Kuhnrae, P., Higgins, M. K., Ghumra, A., and Rowe, J. A. (2014). Rosetting *Plasmodium falciparum*-infected erythrocytes bind to human brain microvascular endothelial cells *in vitro*, demonstrating a dual adhesion phenotype mediated by distinct *P. falciparum* erythrocyte membrane protein 1 domains. *Infect. Immun.* 82, 949–959. doi: 10.1128/IAI.01233-13

Anstey, N. M., Russell, B., Yeo, T. W., and Price, R. N. (2009). The pathophysiology of *vivax* malaria. *Trends Parasitol.* 25, 220–227. doi: 10.1016/j.pt.2009.02.003

Armah, H. B., Wilson, N. O., Sarfo, B. Y., Powell, M. D., Bond, V. C., Anderson, W., et al. (2007). Cerebrospinal fluid and serum biomarkers of cerebral malaria mortality in Ghanaian children. *Malar. J.* 6:147. doi: 10.1186/1475-2875-6-147

Bakmiwewa, S. M., Weiser, S., Grey, M., Heng, B., Guillemin, G. J., Ball, H. J., et al. (2016). Synergistic induction of CXCL10 by interferon-gamma and lymphotoxin-alpha in astrocytes: possible role in cerebral malaria. *Cytokine* 78, 79–86. doi: 10.1016/j.cyto.2015.11.024

Barker, K. R., Lu, Z., Kim, H., Zheng, Y., Chen, J., Conroy, A. L., et al. (2017). miR-155 modifies inflammation, endothelial activation and blood-brain barrier dysfunction in cerebral malaria. *Mol. Med.* 23, 24–33. doi: 10.2119/molmed.2016.00139

Bate, C. A., and Kwiatkowski, D. P. (1994). Stimulators of tumour necrosis factor production released by damaged erythrocytes. *Immunology* 83, 256–261.

Bauer, P. R., Van Der Heyde, H. C., Sun, G., Specian, R. D., and Granger, D. N. (2002). Regulation of endothelial cell adhesion molecule expression in an experimental model of cerebral malaria. *Microcirculation* 9, 463–470. doi: 10.1038/sj.mn.7800159

Beare, N. A., Harding, S. P., Taylor, T. E., Lewallen, S., and Molyneux, M. E. (2009). Perfusion abnormalities in children with cerebral malaria and malarial retinopathy. *J. Infect. Dis.* 199, 263–271. doi: 10.1086/595735

Beare, N. A., Taylor, T. E., Harding, S. P., Lewallen, S., and Molyneux, M. E. (2006). Malarial retinopathy: a newly established diagnostic sign in severe malaria. *Am. J. Trop. Med. Hyg.* 75, 790–797. doi: 10.4269/ajtmh.2006.75.790

Beeson, J. G., Drew, D. R., Boyle, M. J., Feng, G., Fowkes, F. J., and Richards, J. S. (2016). Merozoite surface proteins in red blood cell invasion, immunity and vaccines against malaria. *FEMS Microbiol. Rev.* 40, 343–372. doi: 10.1093/femsre/fuw001

Belnoue, E., Costa, F. T., Vigario, A. M., Voza, T., Gonnet, F., Landau, I., et al. (2003). Chemokine receptor CCR2 is not essential for the development of experimental cerebral malaria. *Infect. Immun.* 71, 3648–3651. doi: 10.1128/IAI.71.6.3648-3651.2003

Bernabeu, M., Danziger, S. A., Avril, M., Vaz, M., Babar, P. H., Brazier, A. J., et al. (2016). Severe adult malaria is associated with specific PfEMP1 adhesion types and high parasite biomass. *Proc. Natl. Acad. Sci. U.S.A.* 113, E3270–E3279. doi: 10.1073/pnas.1524294113

Bernabeu, M., and Smith, J.D. (2017). EPCR and malaria severity: the center of a perfect storm. *Trends Parasitol.* 33, 295–308. doi: 10.1016/j.pt.2016.11.004

Bozza, F. A., Salluh, J. I., Japiassu, A. M., Soares, M., Assis, E. F., Gomes, R. N., et al. (2007). Cytokine profiles as markers of disease severity in sepsis: a multiplex analysis. *Crit. Care* 11, R49. doi: 10.1186/cc5783

Brown, H., Hien, T. T., Day, N., Mai, N. T., Chuong, L. V., Chau, T. T., et al. (1999). Evidence of blood-brain barrier dysfunction in human cerebral malaria. *Neuropathol. Appl. Neurobiol.* 25, 331–340. doi: 10.1046/j.1365-2990.1999.00188.x

Brown, H., Rogerson, S., Taylor, T., Tembo, M., Mwenechanya, J., Molyneux, M., et al. (2001). Blood-brain barrier function in cerebral malaria in Malawian children. *Am. J. Trop. Med. Hyg.* 64, 207–213. doi: 10.4269/ajtmh.2001.64.207

Bujila, I., Schwarzer, E., Skorokhod, O., Weidner, J. M., Troye-Blomberg, M., and Ostlund Farrants, A. K. (2016). Malaria-derived hemozoin exerts early modulatory effects on the phenotype and maturation of human dendritic cells. *Cell. Microbiol.* 18, 413–423. doi: 10.1111/cmi.12521

Campanella, G. S., Tager, A. M., El Khoury, J. K., Thomas, S. Y., Abrazinski, T. A., Manice, L. A., et al. (2008). Chemokine receptor CXCR3 and its ligands CXCL9 and CXCL10 are required for the development of murine cerebral malaria. *Proc. Natl. Acad. Sci. U.S.A.* 105, 4814–4819. doi: 10.1073/pnas.0801544105

Campos, F. M., Franklin, B. S., Teixeira-Carvalho, A., Filho, A. L., De Paula, S. C., Fontes, C. J., et al. (2010). Augmented plasma microparticles during acute *Plasmodium vivax* infection. *Malar. J.* 9:327. doi: 10.1186/1475-2875-9-327

Capuccini, B., Lin, J., Talavera-Lopez, C., Khan, S. M., Sodenkamp, J., Spaccapelo, R., et al. (2016). Transcriptomic profiling of microglia reveals signatures of cell activation and immune response, during experimental cerebral malaria. *Sci. Rep.* 6:39258. doi: 10.1038/srep39258

Cavender, D. E., Edelbaum, D., and Ziff, M. (1989). Endothelial cell activation induced by tumor necrosis factor and lymphotoxin. *Am. J. Pathol.* 134, 551–560.

Chakravorty, S. J., Carret, C., Nash, G. B., Ivens, A., Szestak, T., and Craig, A. G. (2007). Altered phenotype and gene transcription in endothelial cells, induced by *Plasmodium falciparum*-infected red blood cells: pathogenic or protective? *Int. J. Parasitol.* 37, 975–987. doi: 10.1016/j.ijpara.2007.02.006

Chen, Q., Schlichtherle, M., and Wahlgren, M. (2000). Molecular aspects of severe malaria. *Clin. Microbiol. Rev.* 13, 439–450. doi: 10.1128/CMR.13.3.439-450.2000

Clark, I. A., Alleva, L. M., Mills, A. C., and Cowden, W. B. (2004). Pathogenesis of malaria and clinically similar conditions. *Clin. Microbiol. Rev.* 17, 509–539. doi: 10.1128/CMR.17.3.509-539.2004

Clark, I. A., Budd, A. C., Alleva, L. M., and Cowden, W. B. (2006). Human malarial disease: a consequence of inflammatory cytokine release. *Malar. J.* 5:85. doi: 10.1186/1475-2875-5-85

Clark, I. A., and Rockett, K. A. (1994). The cytokine theory of human cerebral malaria. *Parasitol. Today* 10, 410–412. doi: 10.1016/0169-4758(94)90237-2

Clark, I.A., and Vissel, B. (2017). The meteorology of cytokine storms, and the clinical usefulness of this knowledge. *Semin. Immunopathol.* 39, 505–516. doi: 10.1007/s00281-017-0628-y

Coban, C., Ishii, K. J., Kawai, T., Hemmi, H., Sato, S., Uematsu, S., et al. (2005). Toll-like receptor 9 mediates innate immune activation by the malaria pigment hemozoin. *J. Exp. Med.* 201, 19–25. doi: 10.1084/jem.20041836

Combes, V., El-Assaad, F., Faille, D., Jambou, R., Hunt, N. H., and Grau, G. E. (2010). Microvesiculation and cell interactions at the brain-endothelial interface in cerebral malaria pathogenesis. *Prog. Neurobiol.* 91, 140–151. doi: 10.1016/j.pneurobio.2010.01.007

Couper, K. N., Barnes, T., Hafalla, J. C., Combes, V., Ryffel, B., Secher, T., et al. (2010). Parasite-derived plasma microparticles contribute significantly to malaria infection-induced inflammation through potent macrophage stimulation. *PLoS Pathog.* 6:e1000744. doi: 10.1371/journal.ppat.1000744

Craig, A. G., Grau, G. E., Janse, C., Kazura, J. W., Milner, D., Barnwell, J. W., et al. (2012). The role of animal models for research on severe malaria. *PLoS Pathog.* 8:e1002401. doi: 10.1371/journal.ppat.1002401

Cui, L., Mharakurwa, S., Ndiaye, D., Rathod, P. K., and Rosenthal, P. J. (2015). Antimalarial drug resistance: literature review and activities and findings of the ICEMR network. *Am. J. Trop. Med. Hyg.* 93, 57–68. doi: 10.4269/ajtmh.15-0007

De Backer, D., Creteur, J., Preiser, J. C., Dubois, M. J., and Vincent, J. L. (2002). Microvascular blood flow is altered in patients with sepsis. *Am. J. Respir. Crit. Care Med.* 166, 98–104. doi: 10.1164/rccm.200109-016OC

de Souza, J. B., and Riley, E. M. (2002). Cerebral malaria: the contribution of studies in animal models to our understanding of immunopathogenesis. *Microbes Infect.* 4, 291–300. doi: 10.1016/S1286-4579(02)01541-1

Di Perri, G., Di Perri, I. G., Monteiro, G. B., Bonora, S., Hennig, C., Cassatella, M., et al. (1995). Pentoxifylline as a supportive agent in the treatment of cerebral malaria in children. *J. Infect. Dis.* 171, 1317–1322. doi: 10.1093/infdis/171.5.1317

Dondorp, A. M., Fanello, C. I., Hendriksen, I. C., Gomes, E., Seni, A., Chhaganlal, K. D., et al. (2010). Artesunate versus quinine in the treatment of severe *falciparum* malaria in African children (AQUAMAT): an open-label, randomised trial. *Lancet* 376, 1647–1657. doi: 10.1016/S0140-6736(10)61924-1

Dondorp, A. M., Ince, C., Charunwatthana, P., Hanson, J., Van Kuijen, A., Faiz, M. A., et al. (2008). Direct *in vivo* assessment of microcirculatory dysfunction in severe *falciparum* malaria. *J. Infect. Dis.* 197, 79–84. doi: 10.1086/523762

Dondorp, A. M., Pongponratn, E., and White, N. J. (2004). Reduced microcirculatory flow in severe *falciparum* malaria: pathophysiology and electron-microscopic pathology. *Acta Trop.* 89, 309–317. doi: 10.1016/j.actatropica.2003.10.004

Dondorp, A., Nosten, F., Stepniewska, K., Day, N., White, N., and South East Asian Quinine Artesunate Malaria Trial, G. (2005). Artesunate versus quinine for treatment of severe *falciparum* malaria: a randomised trial. *Lancet* 366, 717–725. doi: 10.1016/S0140-6736(05)67176-0

Dong, Y., and Benveniste, E. N. (2001). Immune function of astrocytes. *Glia* 36, 180–190. doi: 10.1002/glia.1107

Engwerda, C. R., Mynott, T. L., Sawhney, S., De Souza, J. B., Bickle, Q. D., and Kaye, P. M. (2002). Locally up-regulated lymphotoxin alpha, not systemic tumor necrosis factor alpha, is the principle mediator of murine cerebral malaria. *J. Exp. Med.* 195, 1371–1377. doi: 10.1084/jem.20020128

Eriksson, E. M., Sampaio, N. G., and Schofield, L. (2013). Toll-like Receptors and malaria: sensing and susceptibility. *J. Trop. Dis.* 2:126. doi: 10.4172/2329-891X.1000126

Evans, S. S., Repasky, E. A., and Fisher, D. T. (2015). Fever and the thermal regulation of immunity: the immune system feels the heat. *Nat. Rev. Immunol.* 15, 335–349. doi: 10.1038/nri3843

Favre, N., Da Laperousaz, C., Ryffel, B., Weiss, N. A., Imhof, B. A., Rudin, W., et al. (1999). Role of ICAM-1 (CD54) in the development of murine cerebral malaria. *Microbes Infect.* 1, 961–968. doi: 10.1016/S1286-4579(99)80513-9

Francis, S. E., Sullivan, D. J. Jr., and Goldberg, D.E. (1997). Hemoglobin metabolism in the malaria parasite *Plasmodium falciparum*. *Annu. Rev. Microbiol.* 51, 97–123. doi: 10.1146/annurev.micro.51.1.97

Gazzinelli, R. T., Kalantari, P., Fitzgerald, K. A., and Golenbock, D. T. (2014). Innate sensing of malaria parasites. *Nat. Rev. Immunol.* 14, 744–757. doi: 10.1038/nri3742

Gilson, P. R., and Crabb, B. S. (2009). Morphology and kinetics of the three distinct phases of red blood cell invasion by *Plasmodium falciparum* merozoites. *Int. J. Parasitol.* 39, 91–96. doi: 10.1016/j.ijpara.2008.09.007

Gowda, D. C. (2007). TLR-mediated cell signaling by malaria GPIs. *Trends Parasitol.* 23, 596–604. doi: 10.1016/j.pt.2007.09.003

Grau, G. E., Pointaire, P., Piguet, P. F., Vesin, C., Rosen, H., Stamenkovic, I., et al. (1991). Late administration of monoclonal antibody to leukocyte function-antigen 1 abrogates incipient murine cerebral malaria. *Eur. J. Immunol.* 21, 2265–2267. doi: 10.1002/eji.1830210939

Griffith, J. W., Sokol, C. L., and Luster, A. D. (2014). Chemokines and chemokine receptors: positioning cells for host defense and immunity. *Annu. Rev. Immunol.* 32, 659–702. doi: 10.1146/annurev-immunol-032713-120145

Hafalla, J. C., Silvie, O., and Matuschewski, K. (2011). Cell biology and immunology of malaria. *Immunol. Rev.* 240, 297–316. doi: 10.1111/j.1600-065X.2010.00988.x

Haldar, K., Murphy, S. C., Milner, D. A., and Taylor, T. E. (2007). Malaria: mechanisms of erythrocytic infection and pathological correlates of severe disease. *Annu. Rev. Pathol.* 2, 217–249. doi: 10.1146/annurev.pathol.2.010506.091913

Handunnetti, S. M., David, P. H., Perera, K. L., and Mendis, K. N. (1989). Uninfected erythrocytes form "rosettes" around *Plasmodium falciparum* infected erythrocytes. *Am. J. Trop. Med. Hyg.* 40, 115–118. doi: 10.4269/ajtmh.1989.40.115

Hansen, D. S., Bernard, N. J., Nie, C. Q., and Schofield, L. (2007). NK cells stimulate recruitment of CXCR3+ T cells to the brain during *Plasmodium berghei*-mediated cerebral malaria. *J. Immunol.* 178, 5779–5788. doi: 10.4049/jimmunol.178.9.5779

Haque, A., Best, S. E., Unosson, K., Amante, F. H., De Labastida, F., Anstey, N. M., et al. (2011). Granzyme B expression by CD8+ T cells is required for the development of experimental cerebral malaria. *J. Immunol.* 186, 6148–6156. doi: 10.4049/jimmunol.1003955

Hermsen, C. C., Konijnenberg, Y., Mulder, L., Loe, C., Van Deuren, M., Van Der Meer, J. W., et al. (2003). Circulating concentrations of soluble granzyme A and B increase during natural and experimental *Plasmodium falciparum* infections. *Clin. Exp. Immunol.* 132, 467–472. doi: 10.1046/j.1365-2249.2003.02160.x

Hol, J., Wilhelmsen, L., and Haraldsen, G. (2010). The murine IL-8 homologues KC, MIP-2, and LIX are found in endothelial cytoplasmic granules but not in Weibel-Palade bodies. *J. Leukoc. Biol.* 87, 501–508. doi: 10.1189/jlb.0809532

Howland, S. W., Claser, C., Poh, C. M., Gun, S. Y., and Renia, L. (2015a). Pathogenic CD8+ T cells in experimental cerebral malaria. *Semin. Immunopathol.* 37, 221–231. doi: 10.1007/s00281-015-0476-6

Howland, S. W., Poh, C. M., and Renia, L. (2015b). Activated brain endothelial cells cross-present malaria antigen. *PLoS Pathog.* 11:e1004963. doi: 10.1371/journal.ppat.1004963

Huggins, M. A., Johnson, H. L., Jin, F., N'Songo A., Hanson, L. M., Lafrance, S. J., et al. (2017). Perforin expression by CD8 T cells Is sufficient to cause fatal brain edema during experimental cerebral malaria. *Infect. Immun.* 85, e00985–e00916. doi: 10.1128/IAI.00985-16

Hunt, N. H., Golenser, J., Chan-Ling, T., Parekh, S., Rae, C., Potter, S., et al. (2006). Immunopathogenesis of cerebral malaria. *Int. J. Parasitol.* 36, 569–582. doi: 10.1016/j.ijpara.2006.02.016

Hunt, N. H., and Grau, G. E. (2003). Cytokines: accelerators and brakes in the pathogenesis of cerebral malaria. *Trends Immunol.* 24, 491–499. doi: 10.1016/S1471-4906(03)00229-1

Idro, R., Marsh, K., John, C. C., and Newton, C. R. (2010). Cerebral malaria: mechanisms of brain injury and strategies for improved neurocognitive outcome. *Pediatr. Res.* 68, 267–274. doi: 10.1203/PDR.0b013e3181eee738

Ioannidis, L. J., Nie, C. Q., and Hansen, D. S. (2014). The role of chemokines in severe malaria: more than meets the eye. *Parasitology* 141, 602–613. doi: 10.1017/S0031182013001984

Ioannidis, L. J., Nie, C. Q., Ly, A., Ryg-Cornejo, V., Chiu, C. Y., and Hansen, D. S. (2016). Monocyte- and neutrophil-derived CXCL10 impairs efficient control of blood-stage malaria infection and promotes severe disease. *J. Immunol.* 196, 1227–1238. doi: 10.4049/jimmunol.1501562

Jain, V., Armah, H. B., Tongren, J. E., Ned, R. M., Wilson, N. O., Crawford, S., et al. (2008). Plasma IP-10, apoptotic and angiogenic factors associated with fatal cerebral malaria in India. *Malar. J.* 7:83. doi: 10.1186/1475-2875-7-83

Jambou, R., Combes, V., Jambou, M. J., Weksler, B. B., Couraud, P. O., and Grau, G. E. (2010). *Plasmodium falciparum* adhesion on human brain microvascular endothelial cells involves transmigration-like cup formation and induces opening of intercellular junctions. *PLoS Pathog.* 6:e1001021. doi: 10.1371/journal.ppat.1001021

John, C. C., Bangirana, P., Byarugaba, J., Opoka, R. O., Idro, R., Jurek, A. M., et al. (2008a). Cerebral malaria in children is associated with long-term cognitive impairment. *Pediatrics* 122, e92–e99. doi: 10.1542/peds.2007-3709

John, C. C., Panoskaltsis-Mortari, A., Opoka, R. O., Park, G. S., Orchard, P. J., Jurek, A. M., et al. (2008b). Cerebrospinal fluid cytokine levels and cognitive impairment in cerebral malaria. *Am. J. Trop. Med. Hyg.* 78, 198–205. doi: 10.4269/ajtmh.2008.78.198

Kalantari, P., Deoliveira, R. B., Chan, J., Corbett, Y., Rathinam, V., Stutz, A., et al. (2014). Dual engagement of the NLRP3 and AIM2 inflammasomes by *plasmodium*-derived hemozoin and DNA during malaria. *Cell Rep.* 6, 196–210. doi: 10.1016/j.celrep.2013.12.014

Karin, N., and Wildbaum, G. (2015). The role of chemokines in shaping the balance between CD4(+) T cell subsets and its therapeutic implications in autoimmune and cancer diseases. *Front. Immunol.* 6:609. doi: 10.3389/fimmu.2015.00609

Karunaweera, N. D., Grau, G. E., Gamage, P., Carter, R., and Mendis, K. N. (1992). Dynamics of fever and serum levels of tumor necrosis factor are closely associated during clinical paroxysms in *Plasmodium vivax* malaria. *Proc. Natl. Acad. Sci. U.S.A.* 89, 3200–3203. doi: 10.1073/pnas.89.8.3200

Kochar, D. K., Das, A., Kochar, S. K., Saxena, V., Sirohi, P., Garg, S., et al. (2009). Severe *Plasmodium vivax* malaria: a report on serial cases from Bikaner in northwestern India. *Am. J. Trop. Med. Hyg.* 80, 194–198. doi: 10.3410/f.1161230.621714

Kordes, M., Matuschewski, K., and Hafalla, J.C. (2011). Caspase-1 activation of interleukin-1beta (IL-1beta) and IL-18 is dispensable for induction of experimental cerebral malaria. *Infect. Immun.* 79, 3633–3641. doi: 10.1128/IAI.05459-11

Krishnegowda, G., Hajjar, A. M., Zhu, J., Douglass, E. J., Uematsu, S., Akira, S., et al. (2005). Induction of proinflammatory responses in macrophages by the glycosylphosphatidylinositols of *Plasmodium falciparum*: cell signaling receptors, glycosylphosphatidylinositol (GPI) structural requirement, and regulation of GPI activity. *J. Biol. Chem.* 280, 8606–8616. doi: 10.1074/jbc.M413541200

Kwiatkowski, D., Cannon, J. G., Manogue, K. R., Cerami, A., Dinarello, C. A., and Greenwood, B. M. (1989). Tumour necrosis factor production in Falciparum malaria and its association with schizont rupture. *Clin. Exp. Immunol.* 77, 361–366.

Kwiatkowski, D., Hill, A. V., Sambou, I., Twumasi, P., Castracane, J., Manogue, K. R., et al. (1990). TNF concentration in fatal cerebral, non-fatal cerebral, and uncomplicated Plasmodium falciparum malaria. *Lancet* 336, 1201–1204. doi: 10.1016/0140-6736(90)92827-5

Langhorne, J., Ndungu, F. M., Sponaas, A. M., and Marsh, K. (2008). Immunity to malaria: more questions than answers. *Nat. Immunol.* 9, 725–732. doi: 10.1038/ni.f.205

Lennartz, F., Adams, Y., Bengtsson, A., Olsen, R. W., Turner, L., Ndam, N. T., et al. (2017). Structure-guided identification of a family of dual receptor-binding PfEMP1 that is associated with cerebral malaria. *Cell Host Microbe* 21, 403–414. doi: 10.1016/j.chom.2017.02.009

Lepenies, B., Cramer, J. P., Burchard, G. D., Wagner, H., Kirschning, C. J., and Jacobs, T. (2008). Induction of experimental cerebral malaria is independent of TLR2/4/9. *Med. Microbiol. Immunol.* 197, 39–44. doi: 10.1007/s00430-007-0057-y

Liehl, P., and Mota, M. M. (2012). Innate recognition of malarial parasites by mammalian hosts. *Int. J. Parasitol.* 42, 557–566. doi: 10.1016/j.ijpara.2012.04.006

Liehl, P., Zuzarte-Luis, V., Chan, J., Zillinger, T., Baptista, F., Carapau, D., et al. (2014). Host-cell sensors for *Plasmodium* activate innate immunity against liver-stage infection. *Nat. Med.* 20, 47–53. doi: 10.1038/nm.3424

Lopez-Ramirez, M. A., Wu, D., Pryce, G., Simpson, J. E., Reijerkerk, A., King-Robson, J., et al. (2014). MicroRNA-155 negatively affects blood-brain barrier function during neuroinflammation. *FASEB J.* 28, 2551–2565. doi: 10.1096/fj.13-248880

Lucas, R., Juillard, P., Decoster, E., Redard, M., Burger, D., Donati, Y., et al. (1997). Crucial role of tumor necrosis factor (TNF) receptor 2 and membrane-bound TNF in experimental cerebral malaria. *Eur. J. Immunol.* 27, 1719–1725. doi: 10.1002/eji.1830270719

Mai, J., Virtue, A., Shen, J., Wang, H., and Yang, X. F. (2013). An evolving new paradigm: endothelial cells–conditional innate immune cells. *J. Hematol. Oncol.* 6:61. doi: 10.1186/1756-8722-6-61

Mandala, W. L., Msefula, C. L., Gondwe, E. N., Drayson, M. T., Molyneux, M. E., and Maclennan, C. A. (2017). Cytokine profiles in Malawian children presenting with uncomplicated malaria, severe malarial anemia and cerebral malaria. *Clin. Vaccine Immunol.* 24:e00533-16. doi: 10.1128/CVI.00533-16

Mantel, P. Y., Hjelmqvist, D., Walch, M., Kharoubi-Hess, S., Nilsson, S., Ravel, D., et al. (2016). Infected erythrocyte-derived extracellular vesicles alter vascular function via regulatory Ago2-miRNA complexes in malaria. *Nat. Commun.* 7:12727. doi: 10.1038/ncomms12727

Mantel, P. Y., Hoang, A. N., Goldowitz, I., Potashnikova, D., Hamza, B., Vorobjev, I., et al. (2013). Malaria-infected erythrocyte-derived microvesicles mediate cellular communication within the parasite population and with the host immune system. *Cell Host Microbe* 13, 521–534. doi: 10.1016/j.chom.2013.04.009

McCutchan, T. F., Dame, J. B., Miller, L. H., and Barnwell, J. (1984). Evolutionary relatedness of *Plasmodium* species as determined by the structure of DNA. *Science* 225, 808–811. doi: 10.1126/science.6382604

McGilvray, I. D., Serghides, L., Kapus, A., Rotstein, O. D., and Kain, K. C. (2000). Nonopsonic monocyte/macrophage phagocytosis of *Plasmodium falciparum*-parasitized erythrocytes: a role for CD36 in malarial clearance. *Blood* 96, 3231–3240. Available online at: http://www.bloodjournal.org/content/96/9/3231

Medana, I. M., Chaudhri, G., Chan-Ling, T., and Hunt, N. H. (2001). Central nervous system in cerebral malaria: 'Innocent bystander' or active participant in the induction of immunopathology? *Immunol. Cell Biol.* 79, 101–120. doi: 10.1046/j.1440-1711.2001.00995.x

Medana, I. M., and Turner, G. D. (2006). Human cerebral malaria and the blood-brain barrier. *Int. J. Parasitol.* 36, 555–568. doi: 10.1016/j.ijpara.2006.02.004

Medana, I. M., and Turner, G. D. (2007). *Plasmodium falciparum* and the blood-brain barrier–contacts and consequences. *J. Infect. Dis.* 195, 921–923. doi: 10.1086/512089

Miller, J. L., Sack, B. K., Baldwin, M., Vaughan, A. M., and Kappe, S. H. (2014). Interferon-mediated innate immune responses against malaria parasite liver stages. *Cell Rep.* 7, 436–447. doi: 10.1016/j.celrep.2014.03.018

Miller, L. H., Baruch, D. I., Marsh, K., and Doumbo, O. K. (2002). The pathogenic basis of malaria. *Nature* 415, 673–679. doi: 10.1038/415673a

Milner, D. A. Jr., Lee, J. J., Frantzreb, C., Whitten, R. O., Kamiza, S., Carr, R. A., et al. (2015). Quantitative assessment of multiorgan sequestration of parasites in fatal pediatric cerebral malaria. *J. Infect. Dis.* 212, 1317–1321. doi: 10.1093/infdis/jiv205

Milner, D. A. Jr., Whitten, R. O., Kamiza, S., Carr, R., Liomba, G., Dzamalala, C., et al. (2014). The systemic pathology of cerebral malaria in African children. *Front. Cell. Infect. Microbiol.* 4:104. doi: 10.3389/fcimb.2014.00104

Miu, J., Mitchell, A. J., Muller, M., Carter, S. L., Manders, P. M., Mcquillan, J. A., et al. (2008). Chemokine gene expression during fatal murine cerebral malaria and protection due to CXCR3 deficiency. *J. Immunol.* 180, 1217–1230. doi: 10.4049/jimmunol.180.2.1217

Nantakomol, D., Dondorp, A. M., Krudsood, S., Udomsangpetch, R., Pattanapanyasat, K., Combes, V., et al. (2011). Circulating red cell-derived microparticles in human malaria. *J. Infect. Dis.* 203, 700–706. doi: 10.1093/infdis/jiq104

Nie, C. Q., Bernard, N. J., Norman, M. U., Amante, F. H., Lundie, R. J., Crabb, B. S., et al. (2009). IP-10-mediated T cell homing promotes cerebral inflammation over splenic immunity to malaria infection. *PLoS Pathog.* 5:e1000369. doi: 10.1371/journal.ppat.1000369

Oakley, M. S., Gerald, N., Mccutchan, T. F., Aravind, L., and Kumar, S. (2011). Clinical and molecular aspects of malaria fever. *Trends Parasitol.* 27, 442–449. doi: 10.1016/j.pt.2011.06.004

Obermeier, B., Daneman, R., and Ransohoff, R. M. (2013). Development, maintenance and disruption of the blood-brain barrier. *Nat. Med.* 19, 1584–1596. doi: 10.1038/nm.3407

Olivier, M., Van Den Ham, K., Shio, M. T., Kassa, F. A., and Fougeray, S. (2014). Malarial pigment hemozoin and the innate inflammatory response. *Front. Immunol.* 5:25. doi: 10.3389/fimmu.2014.00025

Olotu, A., Fegan, G., Wambua, J., Nyangweso, G., Leach, A., Lievens, M., et al. (2016). Seven-Year efficacy of RTS,S/AS01 malaria vaccine among young African children. *N. Engl. J. Med.* 374, 2519–2529. doi: 10.1056/NEJMoa1515257

Pain, A., Ferguson, D. J., Kai, O., Urban, B. C., Lowe, B., Marsh, K., et al. (2001). Platelet-mediated clumping of *Plasmodium falciparum*-infected erythrocytes is a common adhesive phenotype and is associated with severe malaria. *Proc. Natl. Acad. Sci. U.S.A.* 98, 1805–1810. doi: 10.1073/pnas.98.4.1805

Palomo, J., Fauconnier, M., Coquard, L., Gilles, M., Meme, S., Szeremeta, F., et al. (2013). Type I interferons contribute to experimental cerebral malaria development in response to sporozoite or blood-stage *Plasmodium berghei* ANKA. *Eur. J. Immunol.* 43, 2683–2695. doi: 10.1002/eji.201343327

Parroche, P., Lauw, F. N., Goutagny, N., Latz, E., Monks, B. G., Visintin, A., et al. (2007). Malaria hemozoin is immunologically inert but radically enhances innate responses by presenting malaria DNA to Toll-like receptor 9. *Proc. Natl. Acad. Sci. U.S.A.* 104, 1919–1924. doi: 10.1073/pnas.0608745104

Pasloske, B. L., and Howard, R. J. (1994). Malaria, the red cell, and the endothelium. *Annu. Rev. Med.* 45, 283–295. doi: 10.1146/annurev.med.45.1.283

Pober, J. S., and Cotran, R. S. (1990). Cytokines and endothelial cell biology. *Physiol. Rev.* 70, 427–451.

Pober, J. S., and Sessa, W. C. (2007). Evolving functions of endothelial cells in inflammation. *Nat. Rev. Immunol.* 7, 803–815. doi: 10.1038/nri2171

Ponsford, M. J., Medana, I. M., Prapansilp, P., Hien, T. T., Lee, S. J., Dondorp, A. M., et al. (2012). Sequestration and microvascular congestion are associated with coma in human cerebral malaria. *J. Infect. Dis.* 205, 663–671. doi: 10.1093/infdis/jir812

Prakash, D., Fesel, C., Jain, R., Cazenave, P. A., Mishra, G. C., and Pied, S. (2006). Clusters of cytokines determine malaria severity in *Plasmodium falciparum*-infected patients from endemic areas of central India. *J. Infect. Dis.* 194, 198–207. doi: 10.1086/504720

Renia, L., Howland, S. W., Claser, C., Charlotte Gruner, A., Suwanarusk, R., Hui Teo, T., et al. (2012). Cerebral malaria: mysteries at the blood-brain barrier. *Virulence* 3, 193–201. doi: 10.4161/viru.19013

Riley, E. M., Couper, K. N., Helmby, H., Hafalla, J. C., De Souza, J. B., Langhorne, J., et al. (2010). Neuropathogenesis of human and murine malaria. *Trends Parasitol.* 26, 277–278. doi: 10.1016/j.pt.2010.03.002

Rowe, J. A., Claessens, A., Corrigan, R. A., and Arman, M. (2009). Adhesion of *Plasmodium falciparum*-infected erythrocytes to human cells: molecular mechanisms and therapeutic implications. *Expert Rev. Mol. Med.* 11:e16. doi: 10.1017/S1462399409001082

Sahu, P. K., Satpathi, S., Behera, P. K., Mishra, S. K., Mohanty, S., and Wassmer, S. C. (2015). Pathogenesis of cerebral malaria: new diagnostic tools, biomarkers, and therapeutic approaches. *Front. Cell. Infect. Microbiol.* 5:75. doi: 10.3389/fcimb.2015.00075

Sahu, U., Sahoo, P. K., Kar, S. K., Mohapatra, B. N., and Ranjit, M. (2013). Association of TNF level with production of circulating cellular microparticles during clinical manifestation of human cerebral malaria. *Hum. Immunol.* 74, 713–721. doi: 10.1016/j.humimm.2013.02.006

Schofield, L., and Grau, G. E. (2005). Immunological processes in malaria pathogenesis. *Nat. Rev. Immunol.* 5, 722–735. doi: 10.1038/nri1686

Schofield, L., and Hackett, F. (1993). Signal transduction in host cells by a glycosylphosphatidylinositol toxin of malaria parasites. *J. Exp. Med.* 177, 145–153. doi: 10.1084/jem.177.1.145

Shabani, E., Ouma, B. J., Idro, R., Bangirana, P., Opoka, R. O., Park, G. S., et al. (2017). Elevated cerebrospinal fluid tumour necrosis factor is associated with acute and long-term neurocognitive impairment in cerebral malaria. *Parasite Immunol.* 39:e12438. doi: 10.1111/pim.12438

Sharma, S., Deoliveira, R. B., Kalantari, P., Parroche, P., Goutagny, N., Jiang, Z., et al. (2011). Innate immune recognition of an AT-rich stem-loop DNA motif in the *Plasmodium falciparum* genome. *Immunity* 35, 194–207. doi: 10.1016/j.immuni.2011.05.016

Shrivastava, S. K., Dalko, E., Delcroix-Genete, D., Herbert, F., Cazenave, P. A., and Pied, S. (2017). Uptake of parasite-derived vesicles by astrocytes and microglial phagocytosis of infected erythrocytes may drive neuroinflammation in cerebral malaria. *Glia* 65, 75–92. doi: 10.1002/glia.23075

Sigala, P. A., and Goldberg, D. E. (2014). The peculiarities and paradoxes of *Plasmodium* heme metabolism. *Annu. Rev. Microbiol.* 68, 259–278. doi: 10.1146/annurev-micro-091313-103537

Smith, J. D., Rowe, J. A., Higgins, M. K., and Lavstsen, T. (2013). Malaria's deadly grip: cytoadhesion of *Plasmodium falciparum*-infected erythrocytes. *Cell. Microbiol.* 15, 1976–1983. doi: 10.1111/cmi.12183

Song, L., and Pachter, J. S. (2004). Monocyte chemoattractant protein-1 alters expression of tight junction-associated proteins in brain microvascular endothelial cells. *Microvasc. Res.* 67, 78–89. doi: 10.1016/j.mvr.2003.07.001

Srivastava, K., Cockburn, I. A., Swaim, A., Thompson, L. E., Tripathi, A., Fletcher, C. A., et al. (2008). Platelet factor 4 mediates inflammation in experimental cerebral malaria. *Cell Host Microbe* 4, 179–187. doi: 10.1016/j.chom.2008.07.003

Stamatovic, S. M., Keep, R. F., Kunkel, S. L., and Andjelkovic, A. V. (2003). Potential role of MCP-1 in endothelial cell tight junction 'opening': signaling via Rho and Rho kinase. *J. Cell Sci.* 116, 4615–4628. doi: 10.1242/jcs.00755

Stevenson, M. M., and Riley, E. M. (2004). Innate immunity to malaria. *Nat. Rev. Immunol.* 4, 169–180. doi: 10.1038/nri1311

Storm, J., and Craig, A. G. (2014). Pathogenesis of cerebral malaria–inflammation and cytoadherence. *Front. Cell. Infect. Microbiol.* 4:100. doi: 10.3389/fcimb.2014.00100

Strack, A., Schlüter, D., Asensio, V.C., Campbell, I. L., and Deckert, M. (2002). Regulation of the kinetics of intracerebral chemokine gene expression in murine *Toxoplasma* encephalitis: impact of host genetic factors. *Glia* 40, 372–377. doi: 10.1002/glia.10104

Tachado, S. D., Gerold, P., Mcconville, M. J., Baldwin, T., Quilici, D., Schwarz, R. T., et al. (1996). Glycosylphosphatidylinositol toxin of *Plasmodium* induces nitric oxide synthase expression in macrophages and vascular endothelial cells by a protein tyrosine kinase-dependent and protein kinase C-dependent signaling pathway. *J. Immunol.* 156, 1897–1907.

Takeuchi, O., and Akira, S. (2010). Pattern recognition receptors and inflammation. *Cell* 140, 805–820. doi: 10.1016/j.cell.2010.01.022

Tchinda, V. H., Tadem, A. D., Tako, E. A., Tene, G., Fogako, J., Nyonglema, P., et al. (2007). Severe malaria in Cameroonian children: correlation between plasma levels of three soluble inducible adhesion molecules and TNF-alpha. *Acta Trop.* 102, 20–28. doi: 10.1016/j.actatropica.2007.02.011

Thuma, P. E., Van Dijk, J., Bucala, R., Debebe, Z., Nekhai, S., Kuddo, T., et al. (2011). Distinct clinical and immunologic profiles in severe malarial anemia and cerebral malaria in Zambia. *J. Infect. Dis.* 203, 211–219. doi: 10.1093/infdis/jiq041

Tiberti, N., Latham, S. L., Bush, S., Cohen, A., Opoka, R. O., John, C. C., et al. (2016). Exploring experimental cerebral malaria pathogenesis through the characterisation of host-derived plasma microparticle protein content. *Sci. Rep.* 6:37871. doi: 10.1038/srep37871

Togbe, D., Schofield, L., Grau, G. E., Schnyder, B., Boissay, V., Charron, S., et al. (2007). Murine cerebral malaria development is independent of toll-like receptor signaling. *Am. J. Pathol.* 170, 1640–1648. doi: 10.2353/ajpath.2007.060889

Tripathi, A. K., Sha, W., Shulaev, V., Stins, M. F., and Sullivan, D. J. Jr., (2009). *Plasmodium falciparum*-infected erythrocytes induce NF-kappaB regulated inflammatory pathways in human cerebral endothelium. *Blood* 114, 4243–4252. doi: 10.1182/blood-2009-06-226415

Tripathi, A. K., Sullivan, D. J., and Stins, M. F. (2006). *Plasmodium falciparum*-infected erythrocytes increase intercellular adhesion molecule 1 expression on brain endothelium through NF-kappaB. *Infect. Immun.* 74, 3262–3270. doi: 10.1128/IAI.01625-05

Tripathi, A. K., Sullivan, D. J., and Stins, M. F. (2007). *Plasmodium falciparum*-infected erythrocytes decrease the integrity of human blood-brain barrier endothelial cell monolayers. *J. Infect. Dis.* 195, 942–950. doi: 10.1086/512083

Turner, G. D., Ly, V. C., Nguyen, T. H., Tran, T. H., Nguyen, H. P., Bethell, D., et al. (1998). Systemic endothelial activation occurs in both mild and severe malaria. Correlating dermal microvascular endothelial cell phenotype and soluble cell adhesion molecules with disease severity. *Am. J. Pathol.* 152, 1477–1487.

Turner, G. D., Morrison, H., Jones, M., Davis, T. M., Looareesuwan, S., Buley, I. D., et al. (1994). An immunohistochemical study of the pathology of fatal malaria. Evidence for widespread endothelial activation and a potential role for intercellular adhesion molecule-1 in cerebral sequestration. *Am. J. Pathol.* 145, 1057–1069.

Turner, L., Lavstsen, T., Berger, S. S., Wang, C. W., Petersen, J. E., Avril, M., et al. (2013). Severe malaria is associated with parasite binding to endothelial protein C receptor. *Nature* 498, 502–505. doi: 10.1038/nature12216

Van den Steen, P. E., Deroost, K., Van Aelst, I., Geurts, N., Martens, E., Struyf, S., et al. (2008). CXCR3 determines strain susceptibility to murine cerebral malaria by mediating T lymphocyte migration toward IFN-gamma-induced chemokines. *Eur. J. Immunol.* 38, 1082–1095. doi: 10.1002/eji.200737906

van der Heyde, H. C., Nolan, J., Combes, V., Gramaglia, I., and Grau, G. E. (2006). A unified hypothesis for the genesis of cerebral malaria: sequestration, inflammation and hemostasis leading to microcirculatory dysfunction. *Trends Parasitol.* 22, 503–508. doi: 10.1016/j.pt.2006.09.002

van Hensbroek, M. B., Palmer, A., Onyiorah, E., Schneider, G., Jaffar, S., Dolan, G., et al. (1996). The effect of a monoclonal antibody to tumor necrosis factor on survival from childhood cerebral malaria. *J. Infect. Dis.* 174, 1091–1097. doi: 10.1093/infdis/174.5.1091

Viebig, N. K., Wulbrand, U., Forster, R., Andrews, K. T., Lanzer, M., and Knolle, P. A. (2005). Direct activation of human endothelial cells by *Plasmodium falciparum*-infected erythrocytes. *Infect. Immun.* 73, 3271–3277. doi: 10.1128/IAI.73.6.3271-3277.2005

Villegas-Mendez, A., Greig, R., Shaw, T. N., De Souza, J. B., Gwyer Findlay, E., Stumhofer, J. S., et al. (2012). IFN-gamma-producing CD4+ T cells promote experimental cerebral malaria by modulating CD8+ T cell accumulation within the brain. *J. Immunol.* 189, 968–979. doi: 10.4049/jimmunol.1200688

Viola, A., and Luster, A. D. (2008). Chemokines and their receptors: drug targets in immunity and inflammation. *Annu. Rev. Pharmacol. Toxicol.* 48, 171–197. doi: 10.1146/annurev.pharmtox.48.121806.154841

Wassmer, S. C., and Grau, G. E. (2017). Severe malaria: what's new on the pathogenesis front? *Int. J. Parasitol.* 47, 145–152. doi: 10.1016/j.ijpara.2016.08.002

Wassmer, S. C., Moxon, C. A., Taylor, T., Grau, G. E., Molyneux, M. E., and Craig, A. G. (2011). Vascular endothelial cells cultured from patients with cerebral or uncomplicated malaria exhibit differential reactivity to TNF. *Cell. Microbiol.* 13, 198–209. doi: 10.1111/j.1462-5822.2010.01528.x

WHO (2016). *World Malaria Report 2016.* Geneva: World Health Organisation.

White, M. T., Verity, R., Griffin, J. T., Asante, K. P., Owusu-Agyei, S., Greenwood, B., et al. (2015). Immunogenicity of the RTS,S/AS01 malaria vaccine and implications for duration of vaccine efficacy: secondary analysis of data from a phase 3 randomised controlled trial. *Lancet Infect. Dis.* 15, 1450–1458. doi: 10.1016/S1473-3099(15)00239-X

Wilson, N. O., Jain, V., Roberts, C. E., Lucchi, N., Joel, P. K., Singh, M. P., et al. (2011). CXCL4 and CXCL10 predict risk of fatal cerebral malaria. *Dis. Markers* 30, 39–49. doi: 10.1155/2011/828256

Wu, X., Gowda, N. M., and Gowda, D. C. (2015). Phagosomal acidification prevents macrophage inflammatory cytokine production to malaria, and dendritic cells are the major source at the early stages of infection: implication for malaria protective immunity development. *J. Biol. Chem.* 290, 23135–23147. doi: 10.1074/jbc.M115.671065

Yanez, D. M., Manning, D. D., Cooley, A. J., Weidanz, W. P., and Van Der Heyde, H. C. (1996). Participation of lymphocyte subpopulations in the pathogenesis of experimental murine cerebral malaria. *J. Immunol.* 157, 1620–1624.

Yao, Y., and Tsirka, S. E. (2011). Truncation of monocyte chemoattractant protein 1 by plasmin promotes blood-brain barrier disruption. *J. Cell Sci.* 124, 1486–1495. doi: 10.1242/jcs.082834

Zhu, J., Krishnegowda, G., Li, G., and Gowda, D. C. (2011). Proinflammatory responses by glycosylphosphatidylinositols (GPIs) of *Plasmodium falciparum* are mainly mediated through the recognition of TLR2/TLR1. *Exp. Parasitol.* 128, 205–211. doi: 10.1016/j.exppara.2011.03.010

Zhu, J., Wu, X., Goel, S., Gowda, N. M., Kumar, S., Krishnegowda, G., et al. (2009). MAPK-activated protein kinase 2 differentially regulates plasmodium falciparum glycosylphosphatidylinositol-induced production of tumor necrosis factor-{alpha} and interleukin-12 in macrophages. *J. Biol. Chem.* 284, 15750–15761. doi: 10.1074/jbc.M901111200

Zlotnik, A., and Yoshie, O. (2012). The chemokine superfamily revisited. *Immunity* 36, 705–716. doi: 10.1016/j.immuni.2012.05.008

6

Elimination of Falciparum Malaria and Emergence of Severe Dengue: An Independent or Interdependent Phenomenon?

Ib C. Bygbjerg[1], Lone Simonsen[2] and Karin L. Schiøler[1]*

[1] Department of Public Health, University of Copenhagen, Copenhagen, Denmark, [2] Department of Science and Environment, Roskilde University, Roskilde, Denmark

Edited by:
Leonard Peruski,
Centers for Disease Control and Prevention, United States

Reviewed by:
V. Ann Stewart,
Uniformed Services University of the Health Sciences, United States
Tonya Michelle Colpitts,
Boston University, United States

****Correspondence:***
Ib C. Bygbjerg
lby@sund.ku.dk

The global malaria burden, including falciparum malaria, has been reduced by 50% since 2000, though less so in Sub-Saharan Africa. Regional malaria elimination campaigns beginning in the 1940s, up-scaled in the 1950s, succeeded in the 1970s in eliminating malaria from Europe, North America, the Caribbean (except Haiti), and parts of Asia and South- and Central America. Dengue has grown dramatically throughout the pantropical regions since the 1950s, first in Southeast Asia in the form of large-scale epidemics including severe dengue, though mostly sparing Sub-Saharan Africa. Globally, the WHO estimates 50 million dengue infections every year, while others estimate almost 400 million infections, including 100 million clinical cases. Curiously, despite wide geographic overlap between malaria and dengue-endemic areas, published reports of co-infections have been scarce until recently. Superimposed acute dengue infection might be expected to result in more severe combined disease because both pathogens can induce shock and hemorrhage. However, a recent review found no reports on more severe morbidity or higher mortality associated with co-infections. Cases of severe dual infections have almost exclusively been reported from South America, and predominantly in persons infected by *Plasmodium vivax*. We hypothesize that malaria infection may partially protect against dengue – in particular falciparum malaria against severe dengue – and that this inter-species cross-protection may explain the near absence of severe dengue from the Sub-Saharan region and parts of South Asia until recently. We speculate that malaria infection elicits cross-reactive antibodies or other immune responses that infer cross-protection, or at least partial cross-protection, against symptomatic and severe dengue. *Plasmodia* have been shown to give rise to polyclonal B-cell activation and to heterophilic antibodies, while some anti-dengue IgM tests have high degree of cross-reactivity with sera from malaria patients. In the following, the historical evolution of falciparum malaria and dengue is briefly reviewed, and we explore early evidence of subclinical dengue in high-transmission malaria areas as well as conflicting reports on severity of co-morbidity. We also discuss examples of other interspecies interactions.

Keywords: dengue, falciparum malaria, co-morbidity, cross-protection, heterologous immunity, interaction

PRESENT AND PAST PREVALENCE OF MALARIA, DENGUE, AND POPULATION-LEVEL PROTECTION AGAINST EACH DISEASE

Origin, Spread, and Burden of Falciparum Malaria

Plasmodium falciparum malaria parasites probably emerged as a human pathogen from its enzootic origin in West Africa about 5,000–10,000 years ago (Carter and Mendis, 2002). This coincides with the point in time when humans began living in large agricultural communities, and when African *Anopheles* mosquitoes adapted to the novel agrarian environment breeding in man-made water collections and feeding almost exclusively on humans. The parasite accompanied man to Asia and Melanesia around 4,000 years ago and to the Americas with the slave trade 500 years ago (Curtin, 1993).

According to Carter and Mendis (2002), malaria reached its apex during the 19th century, when more than half of the global population was at risk of infection, and case fatality rates reached above 10%. Declines in malaria incidence were noted by the turn of the 20th century. The halving of the global malaria mortality burden since 2000 has been attributed to a combination of malaria interventions such as the use of insecticide-treated nets (Beiersmann et al., 2011; Kramer et al., 2017), indoor residual spraying, and artemisinin combination therapy (Streatfield et al., 2014), as well as the effect of development, such as increasing urbanization (Tatem et al., 2013) and poverty reduction (Teklehaimanot and Mejia, 2008). Still, each year more than 200 million cases and almost 0.5 million deaths occur due to malaria; these deaths are mainly in children in Sub-Saharan Africa and largely from *Plasmodium falciparum* transmitted by nocturnal *Anopheles* species (Streatfield et al., 2014). Transmission in urban areas is generally of lower intensity than in rural areas but can be surprisingly elevated in some urban environments (Wilson et al., 2015).

No effective vaccine exists for malaria, and natural immunity takes years of repeated exposure to develop. Residents of malaria-endemic areas eventually develop some immunity to the infection (Tomson, 1933), but immunity wanes after a single year without exposure (Hoffman, 1986). The difficulties in developing long lasting immunity, including the mechanism by which partial protection is finally achieved, remain largely unexplained. Two main hypotheses, not mutually exclusive, have been put forward (Greenwood and Targett, 2011). The first suggests that adaptive immunity is especially challenged in the case of *P. falciparum* malaria, as the key parasite protein family, PfEMP1, has more than 60 variants (Gardner et al., 2002). The second postulates that repeated exposure to malaria antigens is needed to drive an effective immune response, perhaps accompanied by a maturation of the immune system with increasing age. Studying inflammatory cytokine responses in individuals with malaria from areas of different transmission intensities have shown that levels of pro-inflammatory cytokines decreased with increasing transmission intensity (Ademolue et al., 2017).

Origin, Spread, and Burden of Dengue

There is no consensus regarding the enzootic origin of dengue virus (DENV); some suggest an African origin, others an Asian, given the presence of sylvatic ("jungle") viruses in both regions (Rudnick et al., 1967; Gubler, 1987; Halstead, 1990). Irrespective, the virus probably evolved into four distinct serotypes about 1,000 years ago within sylvatic cycles involving mosquitoes and primates. Phylogenetic evidence suggests that each of the four serotypes entered a cycle of stable transmission between humans and mosquito vectors only 125–320 years ago, coinciding with the out-of-Africa migration of the anthropophilic vector *Aedes aegypti* (Crawford et al., 2017) and historical accounts of local outbreaks and general pandemics of dengue-like disease from the 17th seventeenth century and onwards (Gubler, 1998; Twiddy et al., 2003).

The global pattern of spread of the four dengue serotypes since the early 1940s – when DENV was first isolated – has been highlighted by Messina et al. (2014). These show consistent dispersal of each serotype from South Asia over Southeast Asia to the Pacific and the Americas, with relatively few reported occurrences in sub-Saharan Africa, tribal areas of Papua New-Guinea, North-East India and inner parts of South America. This recently intensified transmission and spread of the DENVs is largely attributed to massive urbanization and globalized travel and trade that characterize the latter half of the 20th century. Importantly, the urban ecology in the tropics has enabled the proliferation of the "domestic" vector *Ae. aegypti*, while travel and trade have helped widen the global range of both vector and virus (Gubler, 1998; Li et al., 2014).

Today, an estimated 3.9 billion people live at risk of infection in at least 128 countries (Brady et al., 2012). Dengue presents a continuously expanding global disease burden, with a suggested doubling or more in the number of symptomatic infections, every 10 years – between 1990 and 2013 (Stanaway et al., 2016). There is, however, wide variation and substantial uncertainty in estimates of the dengue disease burden (Shepard et al., 2014) given both under-recognition and under-reporting of dengue, in general. Notably, only three WHO regions provide regular reports of annual case numbers (WHO, 2017a). In 2015, WHO recoded 3.2 million illness episodes (WHO, 2017a), yet the true figure is probably far higher, with current estimates based on comprehensive risk models ranging between 96 million (Bhatt et al., 2013) in 2010 and 58.4 million in 2013 (Stanaway et al., 2016).

Major challenges for understanding and controlling dengue through the use of preventive or therapeutic interventions include lack of a laboratory correlate and animal models to investigate protective immunity; continued DENV evolution due to major clade replacements and genetic shifts (Holmes and Twiddy, 2003; Rico-Hesse, 2003; Endy, 2014); and not least the complex viral-host pathogenesis that ranges from mild unspecific manifestations to severe and potentially fatal disease (Endy, 2014). A tetravalent vaccine (Capeding et al., 2014; Hadinegoro et al., 2015; Villar et al., 2015) has been licensed for use in several endemic countries in South America and Asia. However, recent data indicate increased risk of severe dengue among vaccinees without previous exposure to DENV (WHO, 2017b) suggesting that – in spite of its tetravalent properties – the vaccine may induce severe manifestations on secondary exposure, through mechanisms of immuno-enhancement (Deen, 2016). Current recommendations by the WHO/GACVS are that individuals who have not been previously infected with wild DENV should not be administered the vaccine (WHO, 2016, 2017b). In addition, the long term effectiveness of this vaccine remains uncertain (López-Gatell et al., 2016). As such, vector control remains the principal dengue prevention option. The primary vectors of DENV, *Ae. aegypti* and *Aedes albopictus,* are both diurnal, rendering insecticide-treated nets of less use for dengue than for malaria control. Public health efforts currently focus on environmental management for elimination of vector breeding sites and on various insecticide applications targeting either larvae or adult stages in the peri-domestic environment (Chu et al., 2013).

The Emergence of Severe Dengue as an Epidemic Entity

The global emergence of severe DENV infection in the latter half of the 20th century is closely aligned with the intensified transmission and spread of the four serotypes, and the occurrence of sequential transmission or actual co-circulation of two or more serotypes (hyperendemicity) in a given population. Dengue epidemics involving severe disease with mortality rates as high as 10% were first noted in Manila and Bangkok in 1954 (Hammon et al., 1960; Hammon and Sather, 1964), but were soon followed by similar epidemics in several other Southeast Asian cities (Rudnick, 1967; Chambers et al., 1990; Endy, 2014). Urban Southeast Asia remained the focus of intense epidemics of severe dengue throughout the 1960s and 1970s, and by the 1970s severe dengue was recorded as a leading cause of pediatric hospitalization and death in many Southeast Asian countries (WHO, 1997).

Whereas the Pacific islands experienced their first outbreaks with severe dengue in the 1970s, the phenomenon was not reported in the Americas before 1981, when Cuba reported a large-scale epidemic with tens of thousands of severe dengue cases (Guzman and Kouri, 2003). The subsequent pattern of intensified transmission with frequent large-scale epidemics in the urban centers of the Pacific and Americas has largely mimicked that of Southeast Asia, albeit two to three decades later. Thus, in the Americas, dengue has doubled every decade, with increasing severity and mortality particularly in children and young adults (San Martín et al., 2010). Interestingly, Halstead et al. (2001) noted the absence of severe dengue despite hyperendemic DENV transmission in Haiti.

For Sub-Saharan Africa, evidence of dengue disease – not least that of severe disease – has been relatively sparse, even though the disease is likely to have been present for centuries (Amarasinghe et al., 2011). Notably, in 1970, Geser et al. (1970) reported the presence of *Ae. aegypti* in the coastal area of Kenya. In addition, 47% of the population presented with hemagglutinin inhibiting (HI) dengue antibodies, although no outbreaks of dengue had been reported. In 1977, Fagbami et al. found that 45% of tested adults in Nigeria were seropositive for anti-DENV-2 antibodies, as evidenced by neutralizing antibodies (Fagbami et al., 1977). In several African countries DENV transmission has been recognized primarily through diagnosis of travelers or stationed military personnel or through sero-prevalence population studies (de Araújo Lobo et al., 2016; Onoja et al., 2016). It is mainly on the basis of such evidence that dengue is considered endemic to both East and West Africa (Brady et al., 2012).

Recent reviews have cataloged multiple small-scale outbreaks of the 1980s and 1990s, across Sub-Saharan Africa (Messina et al., 2014; Baba et al., 2016). Interestingly, the frequency and scale of outbreaks appear to have increased – as have the numbers of deaths – since the turn of this century (Massangaie et al., 2016). Most notable are: the 2009 outbreak in Cape Verde, with 21,304 reported cases and four deaths; the 2010 outbreak in Sudan involving 3,765 cases and 12 deaths; and the 2011 outbreak in Kenya with 5,000 reported cases and four deaths (Baba et al., 2016). Tanzania has experienced no less than four recurrent outbreaks in 2010, 2012, 2013, and 2014, the latter of which included more than 3,000 reported cases and four deaths (Mboera et al., 2016) (**Figure 1D**).

It is generally argued that dengue and severe dengue have been subject to under-diagnosis in Africa given a lack of index of suspicion and little access to laboratory diagnostics (Amarasinghe et al., 2011). However, awareness is typically high in this region regarding hemorrhagic fevers and shock syndromes due to the recurrent outbreaks of yellow fever, Lassa, Marburg, Ebola and Crimean-Congo hemorrhagic fevers (Parkes-Ratanshi et al., 2014). As such, one would expect that outbreaks involving severe dengue would be subject to substantial levels of scrutiny. In spite of the potential under-diagnosis of dengue, the apparent escalation in dengue epidemic activity in Sub-Saharan Africa (Stanaway et al., 2016) might suggest that the region is on the verge of experiencing the emergence of severe dengue as an epidemic entity, similar to the experience of South and Southeast Asia in the 1950s, the Pacific in the 1970s, and the Americas in the 1980s.

Risk Factors for Severe Dengue

Several factors have been shown to modulate the clinical response to DENV infection. Notable risk factors for severe manifestations include previous heterotypic DENV infection; viral virulence, co-morbidities such as diabetes and hypertension; as well as host genetic factors (Carabali et al., 2015; Halstead, 2015).

Immuno Pathogenesis

The groups of (Halstead, 1980, 1988, 2012), Rothman and Ennis (1999), and Rothman et al. (2014) have both been crucial in detailing different aspects of the immuno-pathological mechanisms of severe disease that arise in response to sequential heterotypic DENV infections. These mechanisms implicate the development of heterotypic, cross-reactive but non-neutralizing antibodies and T cells during primary infection and their subsequent activation upon secondary infections with a heterotypic serotype (Endy, 2014). Cross reactive IgG DENV-antibodies have been shown (*in vitro*) to enhance viral uptake and proliferation in target cells, a mechanism known as antibody dependent enhancement (ADE) of infection with

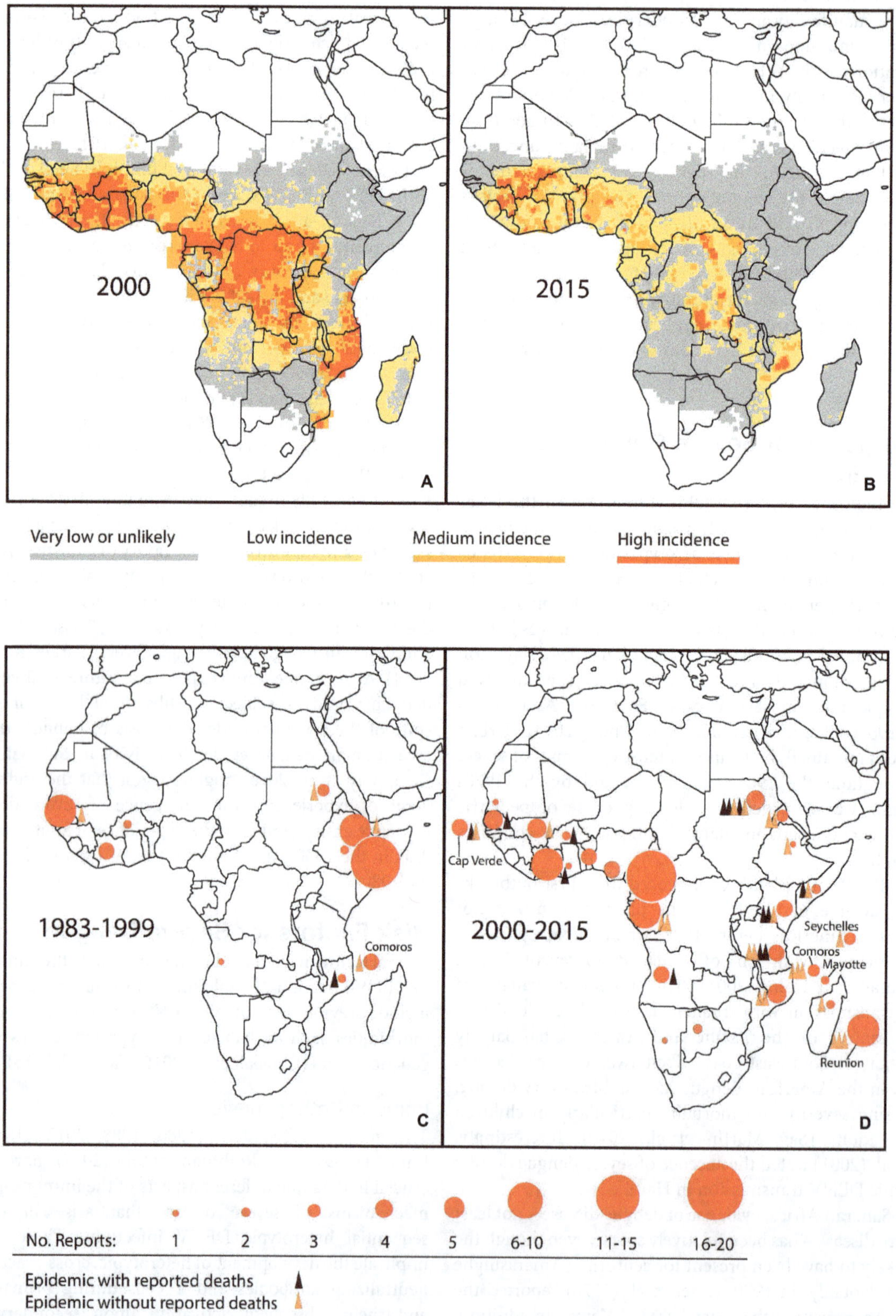

FIGURE 1 | Noted changes in malaria and dengue activity in Sub-Saharan Africa. **(A,B)** Estimated *Plasmodium falciparum* incidence (cases per 100,000) in 2000 and 2015. Modified from original MAP (Source: MAP, 2018). **(C,D)** Accumulated reports of dengue activity and reported dengue epidemics for the periods 1983–1999 and 2000–2015. (Source: Messina et al., 2014; Gideon, 2018).

a second dengue serotype. Notably, recent studies suggest that IgG DENV-antibodies may also be linked to thrombocytopenia as observed in severe dengue (Wang et al., 2017). In addition, cross reactive T-cells may unleash a cascade of cytokines and chemical mediators linked to various severity outcomes including endothelial permeability (Pang et al., 2007). New insights in the immunopathology of dengue were recently reviewed by Screaton et al. (2015).

A key point is that the risk of experiencing immune-mediated pathogenesis increases if a population is subject to consecutive infections by heterotypic serotypes. The emergence of severe dengue throughout large parts of the world is thus aligned with the increased global spread of each serotype. Co-circulation of DENV types has been increasingly documented, even in malarious areas of Sub-Saharan Africa (Messina et al., 2014). Although the true extent of DENV co-circulation in Sub-Saharan Africa remains unclear, it is notable that recent outbreaks, as detailed above, have occurred predominantly in areas with reported co-circulation of DENVs (Saluzzo et al., 1986; Caron et al., 2013; Ridde et al., 2016).

Virulence

Rapid molecular evolution and genetic diversity is a common feature among RNA viruses and may explain why certain strains and genotypes of the four DENVs display greater epidemic potential and pathogenicity than others. Gubler and Trent (1994) were among the first to argue that increased circulation of DENVs as observed in hyperendemic areas, increases the likelihood of virulent strains, as viral competition intensifies the evolutionary pressure on each serotype.

Co-morbidity With Other Than Malaria

A recent review of comorbidity with dengue identified - in addition to old age - several non-communicable diseases of importance for the development of severe manifestations including: cardiovascular disease, diabetes, respiratory disease, and renal disease (Toledo et al., 2016). However, due to heterogeneity among studies, the real estimate effect of comorbidities as modifiers of dengue severity could not be established. Bacterial co-infection with dengue is also increasingly described (Trunfio et al., 2017).

Host Genetic Factors

It has been reported that people of African descent are less prone to suffer severe dengue than other ethnic groups, such as Hispanics and Caucasians in Cuba (Guzman and Kouri, 2003), Haiti (Halstead et al., 2001), Brazil (Blanton et al., 2008), and Colombia (Palacios et al., 2016). This observation has offered a plausible explanation for the absence of severe disease from Sub-Saharan Africa - at least up until the recent outbreaks, where severe dengue apparently has increased also among native Africans, as indicated in the following. Furthermore, the study by Moraes et al. (2013) did not confirm that Afro-Americans have lower risks of severe dengue; on the contrary the risk was higher, except when corrected for socio-economic risk factors. HLA and other gene associations have also been linked with dengue disease severity (Stephens, 2010).

EVIDENCE THAT ELIMINATION OF FALCIPARUM MALARIA COINCIDES WITH THE EMERGENCE OF SEVERE DENGUE

In a review of the malaria elimination history, Tanner and de Savigny (2008) noticed how regional malaria elimination campaigns conducted in the late 1940s paved the way for the Global Malaria Eradication Program in 1955. As part of this campaign malaria was eliminated from Europe, North America, the Caribbean (except Haiti) (Agarwal et al., 2012) and parts of Asia and South and Central America during the 1960s and by the early 1970s (Bruce-Chwatt, 1986).

After a temporary setback, in part due to the development of insecticide- and drug-resistance, reduction of malaria by 50–75% was eventually obtained in most of Asia and South and Central America (WHO, 2013). However, no major success was obtained in Sub-Saharan Africa until recent decades. As indicated by **Figures 1A,B**, malaria is now on the retreat in several parts of sub-Saharan Africa. Since 2000, a historically unprecedented decline has been observed (Snow et al., 2017, the Malaria Atlas Project - MAP). For example, malaria has virtually disappeared even in children in Dar es Salaam, Tanzania (Strøm et al., 2013). At the same time, major outbreaks of dengue have been reported in Dar es Salaam, including the 2014 DENV2 outbreak registering a case fatality rate of 4% (Vairo et al., 2016). Dengue epidemics have also been reported from other parts of Tanzania (Mboera et al., 2016), neighboring Kenya (Brady et al., 2012), Mozambique (Massangaie et al., 2016), as well as Angola (Sharp et al., 2015), Sierra Leone (de Araújo Lobo et al., 2016), Burkina Faso (Ridde et al., 2016), and Nigeria (Onoja et al., 2016) and several other parts of Sub-Saharan Africa (L'Azou et al., 2015). Notably, in 2017, dengue outbreaks were reported from eight Sub-Saharan countries reaching an excess of 21,000 total cases. Burkina Faso recorded more than half of these cases (13,135) including 28 deaths (Gideon, 2018). Details for accumulated reports of dengue including epidemic activity in Sub-Saharan Africa from 1983 to 2015 are provided in **Figures 1B,C**.

CO-MORBIDITY OF DENGUE AND MALARIA

So far, we have discussed concurrent phenomena of dengue emergence and malaria decline at population-level. Another way to consider the hypothesis of mutual exclusion or interdependence of the two pathogens comes from evidence of co-infections at the patient-level. Clinical diagnosis and distinction of malaria and dengue is difficult due to overlapping symptoms. Either disease may induce similar general symptoms as well as severe manifestations in terms of thrombocytopenia, central nervous symptoms, "cytokine-storm" (Clark, 2007), shock and even bleeding. Manifestations of concurrent infection in a patient would be expected to have severe consequences (Hati et al., 2012). However, as noticed by Mohapatra et al. (2012)

reports on co-infection are relatively scarce in literature and those of severe manifestations even more so.

The first patient with falciparum malaria and dengue co-infection was reported by Charrel et al. (2005). Our own search from 2005 to 2017 revealed 55 reports of co-infections, including more than 360 cases of acute co-infections as confirmed by malaria RDT and/or microcopy and DENV virology, antigen tests and/or seroconversion (for details please refer to Supplementary Material). The malaria-immune status was not reported for most co-infections neither were parasitaemia levels which could otherwise be used as a proxy for immunity (with high parasitaemia indicating low immunity). Instead, we suggest that malaria incidence in the countries from where co-infections were reported may be used to assume the general level of malaria immunity. With the exception of Sub-Saharan Africa, most areas reported low or medium transmission of *P. falciparum* malaria during the period of interest.

Table 1 includes only cases of *P. falciparum* in acute dengue confirmed by DENV RT-PCR, NS1 test, or seroconversion. Of 74 identified co-infections, severe symptoms were only recorded in three cases of which one was acquired in West Africa as reported by Charrel et al. (2005). This case involved a traveler, assumed to be non-malaria immune, who after returning to France developed disseminated intravascular coagulation, which may be a manifestation of either disease (*ibid*). Alam and Dm (2013) reported a single case of cerebral malaria and dengue co-infection in a military personnel located in Patna, India. Again, the level of parasitaemia was not reported; however, cerebral malaria would indicate low or absence of malaria immunity, in line with the low incidence level reported for the area. Finally, Yong et al. (2012) reported severe manifestations in a local Indonesian adult male with 4% falciparum parasitaemia and dengue co-infection. This case was complicated by rhabdomyolysis and acute renal insufficiency, which may both be induced by malaria and dengue.

Lack of reporting of dual infection in the field could result from testing positive for either malaria or dengue infection with no further testing being done, given low index of suspicion for co-infections (i.e., case considered diagnosed after one positive test). Yet, some argue that severity could also prompt testing for dual disease, and thereby potentially bias reporting. Notably, studies that have actively investigated the clinical picture of mono-infections as compared to that of dengue and malaria co-infections disagree with respect to observed differences in severity levels. Epelboin et al. (2012) reported that among local resident in French Guyana, the clinical picture of dual infections was more severe than in either dengue or malaria alone. It is notable that *P. vivax* was identified in the majority of cases (~80%) and that only 50% of the dual infected reported previous malaria. Unfortunately, the report did not stratify between *P. vivax* or *P. falciparum* co-infections, nor did it report on parasitaemia levels.

TABLE 1 | Reported cases of acute dengue virus and *P. falciparum* co-infections by global region, 2005–2017.

Region	Total cases	Mild symptoms	Severe symptoms	Severity not reported
Sub-Saharan Africa	5	1	1[1]	3
Americas	28	7	0	21
South Asia	39	38	1[2]	0
Southeast Asia	2	1	1[3]	0
Total	74	47	3	24

Method of confirmation of acute dengue: RT-PCR, NS1 test and/or IgM/IgG seroconversion. Categorization of severity based on case description by source authors. Sources for severe cases: [1]Charrel et al., 2005 (returning traveller); [2]Alam and Dm, 2013 (military personnel; [3]Yong et al., 2012 (local resident). For additional sources please refer to Supplementary Table 1).

In contrast, Halsey et al. (2016) found similar severity levels between mono and co-infected individuals among local populations in Peru. As for Epelboin et al. (2012) the majority of cases were reported as *P. vivax*. In India, Mohapatra et al. (2012) reported generally benign manifestations among co-infections as compared with malaria mono-infections. In this study the majority of cases (~90%) were reported as *P. falciparum* infections. Notably, lower parasitic counts were observed among co-infected than for mono-infected patient, although reported as non-significant. In line with these findings, Ahmad reported that the presentation and severity of co-infections appeared "to be milder and outcomes comparable (if not better) to mono-infections" during a dengue outbreak in Uttarakhand, India. While co-infections occurred with both *P. falciparum* and *P. vivax* these were not clearly distinguished in the report.

Stoler et al. (2015) reported dengue-specific IgG antibodies in 22% of urban Ghanaian children with *P. falciparum* parasitaemia, suggesting previous exposure, and dengue IgM antibodies in 3%, indicating probable acute co-infection. While co-infection was indicated, co-morbidity or increased severity was not. None of the children appeared to have severe disease; but IgM dengue positive children had (non-significantly) higher levels of *P. falciparum* parasitaemia, which could indicate they were only partially immune to falciparum malaria at the time of DENV infection. Unfortunately, levels of malaria antibodies were not reported. Specificity of the anti-dengue Ig tests used was 97% for multisite pooled sera, though cross-reactivity with other flavivira was high (30% and 60% for IgM and IgG, respectively).

Cross-Reactivity and "False-Positivity" in Tests for Dengue and Malaria

Malaria infection gives rise to polyclonal B-cell activation (Greenwood, 1974) and to heterophilic antibodies (Houba et al., 1974), which may react to host antigens as well as to other pathogens (Ribeiro, 1988). Some anti-dengue IgM tests have shown a high degree of cross-reactivity (10–70%) with sera from malaria patients, and with other flavivira (Hunsperger et al., 2009; WHO, 2009). Hunsperger et al. (2009), when evaluating four anti-DENV IgM kits and five micro-plate ELISAs found between 5 and 70% false-positive results for patients with malaria or past dengue infections. Knowing the true population prevalence of dengue as well as malaria infections is hampered by the lack of representative population-based studies, and also by false-positive test results or cross-reactivity that are a problem in many serological assays including rapid diagnostic tests (RDTs) for dengue and malaria. In other words, a positive DENV IgM test may signify current or recent primary infection, secondary or tertiary infection (often lower titers, though primary infection responses also vary), or cross-reactivity with other virus or even malaria (current or past infection). Thus, with current laboratory assays available in countries with limited resources, it is very difficult to tease apart the possibility of malaria and dengue together in an area or a patient, wherefore low-cost antigen tests and viral and plasmodia gene detection kits are needed.

Possible Co-protection of Malaria Infection Against Severe Dengue?

Repeated exposure to falciparum malaria is followed by development of protective antibodies, decline of pro-inflammatory host-responses (Ademolue et al., 2017) and decreasing severity (Reyburn et al., 2005), whereas sequential exposure to heterogeneous DENVs - and related viruses, e.g., Zika virus - may lead to enhanced host immune responses (Cohen, 2017). However, on the basis of the presented clinical, epidemiological, immunological and laboratory-based reports, we speculate whether cross-reactivity observed between tests for dengue and malaria pathogens could also be an indicator of some level of cross-protection between two potentially severe diseases. In other words, could dengue-induced antibody-dependent enhancement of infection (ADE) (de Alwis et al., 2014) be "de-hanced" by malaria induced antibodies? Or could alleviated cytokine responses among clinically malaria immune individuals (Ademolue et al., 2017) similarly reduce "over"-reaction to dengue (re-)infection?

Proof of concept of cross-protection from malaria to dengue in man would require exposing malaria immune humans to dengue in controlled experiments. As reviewed by Sabin (1952), research on dengue during World War II did include research on human volunteers exposed to DENV and the development of immunity to the homologues strain. Unfortunately, the level of immunity to malaria was not reported in these volunteers. A human model of dengue exposure is currently being re-introduced (Larsen et al., 2015; Royer, 2015).

Examples of Interspecies Interactions

In the literature, there are certainly important examples of interaction between infections of unrelated pathogens leading to more severe outcomes, such as HIV infection leading to latent tuberculosis reactivation (Pitchenik et al., 1983), and severe outcomes of pneumococcal disease following influenza infection, the so-called lethal synergy (McCullers, 2014). And most recently, Zika virus infection has been found to be enhanced in recent dengue cases, much like ADE among the four DENV types (Kawiecki and Christofferson, 2016). But examples in which co- or sequential infection may decrease severity of either or both diseases have been less investigated. An interesting, historical example is the now obsolete treatment of syphilis with malaria (Moore, 1930), and the possible sharp reduction in tuberculosis in the US population immediately following the 1918 severe pandemic influenza outbreak (Noymer, 2011). More recently, it has been shown that *P. falciparum* infection may protect partly against severe Ebola outcomes (Rosenke et al., 2016).

CONCLUSION

In summary, we conclude that at the population level the evidence of interaction between dengue and malaria is perhaps already there: when comparing time trends in the two diseases at continent level, a suggestive pattern emerges. We have discussed the striking coincidence of the emergence of dengue in recent years (**Figure 1D**), with the reduction in incidence of malaria (**Figure 1B**), suggesting that declining malaria exposure due to successful control programs or other environmental factors may have inadvertently led to the cessation of protection against clinically apparent and severe dengue infections, especially in Sub-Saharan Africa. However, individual-level studies would be the best way to determine if co-protection exists between falciparum malaria and dengue. Available individual-level studies reviewed here are only suggestive and interpretation hampered by non-specificity of used tests. Also, they present a risk of bias in favor of our hypothesis, in that more severe patients are more likely to be tested for several pathogens and subsequently reported, and vice versa that lack of reporting of dual infection in the field could result from testing positive for either malaria or dengue infection and then no further testing being done.

Evidently, more research is required to investigate whether there is a causal link between declining falciparum malaria and increased dengue in recent years. We suggest *in vitro* experiments such as exposing *in vitro* cultures of DENV to malaria antibodies, and vice versa as a proxy to evidence (or not) of cross-protection. Other modern *in vitro* technologies including epigenetic silencing or activation of regulatory genes implicated in immunity and susceptibility of disease (Kirchner et al., 2016) or development of animal models may also help, while acknowledging that suitable animal models are still not available for either infection. It would be interesting - if considered ethically acceptable - to include malaria-immune individuals in the ongoing dengue human exposure model. Further studies of the potential role of unspecific sides of acquired immunity (Muraille, 2016), and studies of cross-kingdom interaction (Luckhart et al., 2015) could be rewarding as well. Especially, if combined with integrated epidemiology and surveillance for vector-borne diseases and by integrating layers of data from both malaria and dengue (Wardrop, 2016). These studies could be complemented by large-scale prospective studies e.g. through the INDEPTH-network of health and demographic surveillance systems in low- and middle-income countries (INDEPTH, 2018).

Finally, we believe it is important to broaden considerations across pathogens and diseases in order to explain the striking associations in temporal patterns of malaria and dengue globally observed since the 1950s and in Africa, specifically, after the Millennium. More broadly, we suggest that considering non-specific effects of inter-species interaction and interdependences may be a critical aspect of recognizing possible outcomes beyond those of the target pathogen and to understand the broader consequences of global health intervention programs designed to eliminate a given disease.

AUTHOR CONTRIBUTIONS

IB conceived the hypothesis of potential interaction between malaria and dengue, and drafted the first version of the manuscript, and wrote the subsequent versions in close collaboration with KS and LS. KS contributed in particular to the sections of dengue and malaria epidemiology mapping, and to **Table 1** and to the Supplementary Material, and contributed to all sections and versions of the manuscript. LS contributed in particular to the sections on historic epidemiology and interspecies interaction and to other sections and versions of the manuscript. All authors read and approved the submitted version.

ACKNOWLEDGMENTS

We wish to thank Mr. Casper Nielsen, COBL University of Copenhagen, and Ms. Ditte Frisk Hansen for graphic support.

REFERENCES

Ademolue, T. W., Aniweh, Y., Kusi, K. A., and Awandare, G. A. (2017). Patterns of inflammatory responses and parasite tolerance vary with malaria transmission intensity. *Malar. J.* 16:145. doi: 10.1186/s12936-017-1796-x

Agarwal, A., McMorrow, M., Arguin, P. M. (2012). The increase of imported malaria acquired in Haiti among US travelers in 2010. *Am. J. Trop. Med. Hyg.* 86, 9–10. doi: 10.4269/ajtmh.2012.11-0394

Alam, A., and Dm, M. (2013). A case of cerebral malaria and dengue concurrent infection. *Asian Pac. J. Trop. Biomed.* 3, 416–417. doi: 10.1016/S2221-1691(13)60087-8

Amarasinghe, A., Kuritsk, J. N., Letson, G. W., and Margolis, H. S. (2011). Dengue virus infection in Africa. *Emerg. Infect. Dis.* 17, 1349–1354. doi: 10.3201/eid1708.101515

Baba, M., Villinger, J., and Masiga, D. K. (2016). Repetitive dengue outbreaks in East Africa: a proposed phased mitigation approach may reduce its impact. *Rev. Med. Virol.* 26, 183–196. doi: 10.1002/rmv.1877

Beiersmann, C., Bountogo, M., Tiendrébeogo, J., De Allegri, M., Louis, V. R., Coulibaly, B., et al. (2011). Falciparum malaria in young children of rural Burkina Faso: comparison of survey data in 1999 with 2009. *Malar. J.* 10:296. doi: 10.1186/1475-2875-10-296

Bhatt, S., Gething, P. W., Brady, O. J., Messina, J. P., Farlow, A. W., et al. (2013).The global distribution and burden of dengue. *Nature* 496, 504–507. doi: 10.1038/nature12060

Blanton, R. E., Silva, L. K., Morato, V. G., Parrado, A. R., Dias, J. P., Melo, P. R., et al. (2008). Genetic ancestry and income are associated with dengue hemorrhagic fever in a highly admixed population. *Eur. J. Hum. Genet.* 16, 762–765. doi: 10.1038/ejhg.2008.4

Brady, O. J., Gething, P. W., Bhatt, S., Messina, J. P., Brownstein, J. S., and Hoen, A. G. et al. (2012). Refining the global spatial limits of dengue virus transmission by evidence-based consensus. *PLoS Negl. Trop. Dis.* 12:e1760. doi: 10.1371/journal.pntd.0001760

Bruce-Chwatt, L. S. (1986). *Essential Malariology*. London: Heinemann, 285.

Capeding, M. R., Tran, N. H., Hadinegoro, S. R., Ismail, H. I., Chotpitayasunondh, T., and Chua, M. N., et al. (2014). Clinical efficacy and safety of a novel tetravalent dengue vaccine in healthy children in Asia: a phase 3, randomized, observer-masked, placebo-controlled trial. *Lancet* 384, 1358–1365. doi: 10.1016/S0140-6736(14)61060-6

Carabali, M., Hernandez, L. M., Arauz, M. J., Villar, L. A., and Ridde, V. (2015). Why are people with dengue dying? A scoping review of determinants for dengue mortality. *BMC Infect. Dis.* 15:301. doi: 10.1186/s12879-015-1058-x

Caron, M., Grard, G., Paupy, C., Mombo, I. M., Bi Nso, B., Kassa Kassa, F. R., Nkoghe, D., et al. (2013). First evidence of simultaneous circulation of three different dengue virus serotypes in Africa. *PLoS One* 8:e78030. doi: 10.1371/journal.pone.0078030

Carter, R., and Mendis, K. N. (2002). Evolutionary and historical aspects of the burden of malaria. *Clin. Microbiol. Rev.* 15, 564–594. doi: 10.1128/CMR.15.4.564-594.2002

Chambers, T., Hahn, C., Galle, R., and Rice, C. (1990). Flavivirus genome organization, expression, and replication. *Annu. Rev. Microbiol.* 44, 649–688. doi: 10.1146/annurev.mi.44.100190.003245

Charrel, R. N., Brouqui, P., Foucault, C., and de Lamballerie, X. (2005). Concurrent dengue and malaria. *Emerg. Infect. Dis.* 11, 1153–1154. doi: 10.3201/eid1107.041352

Chu, H. J., Chan, T. C., and Jao, F. J. (2013). GIS-aided planning of insecticide spraying to control dengue transmission. *Int. J. Health. Geogr.* 12:42. doi: 10.1186/1476-072X-12-42

Clark, I. A. (2007). The advent of the cytokine storm. *Immunol. Cell Biol.* 85, 271–273. doi: 10.1038/sj.icb.7100062

Cohen, J. (2017). Dengue may bring out the worst in Zika. *Science* 355:1362. doi: 10.1126/science.355.6332.1362

Crawford, J. E., Alves, J. M., Palmer, W. J., Day, J. P., Sylla, M., and Ramasamy, R., et al. (2017). Population genomics reveals that an anthropophilic population of *Aedes aegypti* mosquitoes in West Africa recently gave rise to American and Asian populations of this major disease vector. *BMC Biol.* 15:16. doi: 10.1186/s12915-017-0351-0

Curtin, P. D. (1993). Disease exchange across the tropical Atlantic. *Hist. Philos. Life Sci.* 15, 329–356.

de Alwis, R., Williams, K. L., Schmid, M. A., Lai, C.-Y., Patel, B., and Smith, S. A., et al. (2014). Dengue viruses are enhanced by distinct populations of serotype cross-reactive antibodies in human immune sera. *PLoS Pathog.* 10:e1004386. doi: 10.1371/journal.ppat.1004386

de Araújo Lobo, J. M., Mores, C. N., Bausch, D. G., and Christofferson, R. C. (2016). Short report: serological evidence of under-reported dengue circulation in Sierra Leone. *PLoS Negl. Trop. Dis.* 10:e0004613. doi: 10.1371/journal.pntd.0004613

Endy, T. P. (2014). Human immune responses to dengue virus infection: lessons learned from prospective cohort studies. *Front. Immunol.* 5:183. doi: 10.3389/fimmu.2014.00183

Epelboin, L., Hanf, M., Dussart, P., Ouar-Epelboin, S., Djossou, F., Nacher, M., et al. (2012). Is dengue and malaria co-infection more severe than single infections? A retrospective matched-pair study in French Guiana. *Malar. J.* 11:142. doi: 10.1186/1475-2875-11-142

Fagbami, A. H., Monath, T. P, and Fabiyi, A. (1977). Dengue virus infections in Nigeria: a survey for antibodies in monkeys and humans. *Trans. R. Soc. Trop. Med. Hyg.* 71, 60–65. doi: 10.1016/0035-9203(77)90210-3

Gardner, M. J., Hall, N., Fung, E., White, O., Berriman, M., and Hyman, R. W. et al. (2002). Genome sequence of the human malaria parasite *Plasmodium falciparum*. *Nature* 419, 498–511. doi: 10.1038/nature01097

Geser, A., Henderson, B. E., and Christensen, S. (1970). A multipurpose serological survey in Kenya. 2. Results of arbovirus serological tests. *Bull. World Health Organ.* 43, 539–552.

Gideon (2018). *The World's Premier Global Infectious Diseases Database*. Available at: www.gideononline.com [accessed May 13, 2018].

Greenwood, B. M. (1974). Possible role of a B-cell mitogen in hypergammaglobulinaemia in malaria and trypanosomiasis. *Lancet* 16,

435–436. doi: 10.1016/S0140-6736(74)92386-1

Greenwood, B. M., and Targett, G. A. (2011). Malaria vaccines and the new malaria agenda. *Clin. Microbiol. Infect.* 17, 1600–1607. doi: 10.1111/j.1469-0691.2011.03612.x

Gubler, D. J., and Trent, D. W. (1994). Emergence of epidemic dengue/dengue hemorrhagic fever as a public health problem in the Americas. *Infect. Agents Dis.* 2, 83–393.

Gubler, D. J. (1987). Dengue and dengue hemorrhagic fever in the Americas. *P. R. Health Sci. J.* 6, 107–111.

Gubler, D. J. (1998). Dengue and dengue hemorrhagic fever. *Clin. Microbiol. Rev.* 11, 480–496.

Guzman, M. G., and Kouri, G. (2003). Dengue and dengue hemorrhagic fever in the Americas: lessons and challenges. *J. Clin. Virol.* 27, 1–13. doi: 10.1016/S1386-6532(03)00010-6

Hadinegoro, S. R., Arredondo-García, J. L., Capeding, M. R., Deseda, C., Chotpitayasunondh, T., Dietze, R., et al. (2015). Efficacy and long-term safety of a dengue vaccine in regions of endemic disease. *N. Engl. J. Med.* 373, 1195–1206. doi: 10.1056/NEJMoa1506223

Halsey, E. S., Baldeviano, G. C., Edgel, K. A., Vilcarromero, S., Sihuincha, M., and Lescano, A. G. (2016). Symptoms and immune markers in plasmodium/dengue virus co-infection compared with mono-infection with either in Peru. *PLoS Negl. Trop. Dis.* 10:e0004646. doi: 10.1371/journal.pntd.0004646

Halstead, S. B. (1980). Dengue haemorrhagic fever- a public health problem and a field for research. *Bull. World Health Organ.* 58, 1–21.

Halstead, S. B. (1988). Pathogenesis of dengue: challenges to molecular biology. *Science* 239, 476–481. doi: 10.1126/science.239.4839.476

Halstead, S. B. (1990). Global epidemiology of dengue hemorrhagic fever. *Southeast Asian J. Trop. Med. Public Health* 21, 636–641.

Halstead, S. B. (2012). Controversies in dengue pathogenesis. *Paediatr. Int. Child Health* 32(Suppl. 1), 5–9. doi: 10.1179/2046904712Z.00000000045

Halstead, S. B. (2015). Pathogenesis of dengue: dawn of a new Era. *F1000Res.* 4:F1000 Faculty Rev-476. doi: 10.12688/f1000research.7024.1

Halstead, S. B., Streit, T. G., Lafontant, J. G., Putvatana, R., Russell, K., Sun, W., et al. (2001). Haiti: absence of dengue hemorrhagic fever despite hyperendemic dengue virus transmission. *Am. J. Trop. Med. Hyg.* 65, 180–183. doi: 10.4269/ajtmh.2001.65.180

Hammon, W. M., and Sather, G. E. (1964). Virological findings in the 1960 hemorrhagic fever epidemic (Dengue) in Thailand. *Am. J. Trop. Med. Hyg.* 13, 629–641. doi: 10.4269/ajtmh.1964.13.629

Hammon, W. M., Rudnic, A., and Sather, G. E. (1960). Viruses associated with epidemic hemorrhagic fevers of the Philippines and Thailand. *Science* 131, 1102–1103. doi: 10.1126/science.131.3407.1102

Hati, A. K., Bhattacharjee, I., Mukherjee, H., Bandyopadhayay, B., Bandyopadhyay, D., De, R., et al. (2012). Concurrent dengue and malaria in an area in Kolkata. *Asian Pac. J. Trop. Med.* 5, 315–317. doi: 10.1016/S1995-7645(12)60046-7

Hoffman, S. L. (1986). "Treatment of malaria," in *Malaria Clinics in Tropical Medicine and Communicable Diseases*, Vol. 1, ed. G. T. Strickland (London: WB Saunders Company), 214.

Holmes, E. C., and Twiddy, S. (2003). The origin, emergence and evolutionary genetics of dengue virus. *Infect. Genet. Evol.* 3, 19–28. doi: 10.1016/S1567-1348(03)00004-2

Houba, V., Faulk, W. P., and Matola, Y. G. (1974). Heterophilic antibodies in relation to malarial infection: population and experimental studies. *Clin. Exp. Immunol.* 18, 89–93.

Hunsperger, E. A., Yoksan, S., Buchy, P., Nguyen, V. C., Sekaran, S. D., Enria, D. A., et al. (2009). Evaluation of commercially available anti-dengue virus immunoglobulin M tests. *Emerg. Infect. Dis.* 15, 436–440. doi: 10.3201/eid1503.080923

INDEPTH (2018). *INDEPTH Network.* Available at: http://www.indepth-network.org/ [accessed February 17, 2018].

Kawiecki, A. B. and Christofferson, R. C. (2016). Zika virus-induced antibody response enhances dengue virus serotype 2 replication in vitro. *J. Infect. Dis* 214, 1357–1360. doi: 10.1093/infdis/jiw377

Kirchner, S., Power, B. J., and Waters, A. P. (2016). Recent advances in malaria genomics and epigenomics. *Genome Med.* 8:92. doi: 10.1186/s13073-016-0343-7

Kramer, K., Mandike, R., Nathan, R., Mohamed, A., Lynch, M., Brown, N., et al. (2017). Effectiveness and equity of the Tanzania National Voucher Scheme for mosquito nets over 10 years of implementation. *Malar. J.* 16:255. doi: 10.1186/s12936-017-1902-0

Larsen, C. P., Whitehead, S. S., and Durbin, A. P. (2015). Dengue human infection models to advance dengue vaccine development. *Vaccine* 33, 7075–7082. doi: 10.1016/j.vaccine.2015.09.052

L'Azou, M., Succo, T., Kamagaté, M., Ouattara, A., Gilbernair, E., Adjogoua, E., et al. (2015).Dengue: etiology of acute febrile illness in Abidjan, Côte d'Ivoire, in 2011-2012. *Trans. R. Soc. Trop. Med. Hyg.* 109, 717–722. doi: 10.1093/trstmh/trv076

Li, Y., Kamara, F., Zhou, G., Puthiyakunnon, S., Li, C., Liu, Y., et al. (2014). Urbanization increases *Aedes albopictus* larval habitats and accelerates mosquito development and survivorship. *PLoS Negl. Trop. Dis.* 8:e3301. doi: 10.1371/journal.pntd.0003301

López-Gatell, H., Alpuche-Aranda, C. M., Santos-Preciado, J. I., and Hernández-Ávila, M. (2016).Dengue vaccines: local decision, global consequences. *Bull. World Health Organ.* 94, 850–855. doi: 10.2471/BLT.15.168765

Luckhart, S., Pakpour, N., and Giulivi, C. (2015). Host-pathogen interactions in malaria: cross-kingdom signaling and mitochondrial regulation. *Curr. Opin. Immunol.* 36, 73–79. doi: 10.1016/j.coi.2015.07.002

MAP (2018). *Malaria Atlas Project.* Available at: https://map.ox.ac.uk [accessed February 17, 2018].

Massangaie, M., Pinto, G., Padama, F., Chambe, G., da Silva, M., Mate, I., et al. (2016). Clinical and epidemiological characterization of the first recognized outbreak of dengue virus-type 2 in Mozambique, 2014. *Am. J. Trop. Med. Hyg.* 94, 413–441 doi: 10.4269/ajtmh.15-0543

Mboera, L. E., Mweya, C. N., Rumisha, S. F., Tungu, P. K., Stanley, G., Makange, M. R., et al. (2016). The Risk of Dengue Virus Transmission in Dar es Salaam, Tanzania during an epidemic period of 2014. *PLoS Negl. Trop. Dis.* 10:e0004313. doi: 10.1371/journal.pntd.0004313

McCullers, J. A. (2014). The co-pathogenesis of influenza viruses with bacteria in the lung. *Nat. Rev. Microbiol.* 12, 252–262. doi: 10.1038/nrmicro3231

Messina, J. P., Brady, O. J., Scott, T. W., Zou, C., Pigott, D. M., Duda, K. A., et al. (2014). Global spread of dengue virus types: mapping the 70 year history. *Trends Microbiol.* 22, 138–146. doi: 10.1016/j.tim.2013.12.011

Mohapatra, M. K., Patra, P., and Agrawala, R. (2012). Manifestation and outcome of concurrent malaria and dengue infection. *J. Vector Borne Dis.* 49, 262–265.

Moore, R. (1930). Late syphilis-treatment with a single strain of malaria: analytical evaluation of therapeutic results in four hundred cases. *Cal. West. Med.* 33, 796–798.

Moraes, G. H., de Fátima Duarte, E., and Duarte, E. C. (2013). Determinants of mortality from severe dengue in Brazil: a population-based case-control study. *Am. J. Trop. Med. Hyg.* 88, 670–676. doi: 10.4269/ajtmh.11-0774

Muraille, E. (2016). The unspecific side of acquired immunity against infectious disease: causes and consequences. *Front. Microbiol.* 6:1525. doi: 10.3389/fmicb.2015.01525

Noymer, A. (2011). The 1918 influenza pandemic hastened the decline of tuberculosis in the United States: an age, period, cohort analysis. *Vaccine.* 22, 29 Suppl 2:B38-41. doi: 10.1016/j.vaccine.2011.02.053.

Onoja, A. B., and Adeniji, J. A., Olaleye, O. D. (2016). High rate of unrecognized dengue virus infection in parts of the rainforest region of Nigeria. *Acta Trop.* 160, 39–43. doi: 10.1016/j.actatropica.2016.04.007

Palacios, J. H. R., Alzate, A., Romero H. J. M., Concha-Eastman, A. I. (2016). Afro Colombian ethnicity, a paradoxical protective factor against Dengue. *Colomb. Med.* 47, 133–141.

Pang, T., Cardosa, M. J., and Guzman, M. G. (2007). Of cascades and perfect storms: the immunopathogenesis of dengue haemorrhagic fever-dengueshock syndrome (DHF/DSS). *Immunol. Cell Biol.* 85, 43–45. doi: 10.1038/sj.icb.7100008

Parkes-Ratanshi, R., Elbireer, A., Mbambu, B., Mayanja, F., Coutinho, A., and Merry, C. (2014). Ebola outbreak response; experience and development of screening tools for viral haemorrhagic fever (VHF) in a HIV center of excellence near to VHF epicentres. *PLoS One* 9:e100333. doi: 10.1371/journal.pone.0100333

Pitchenik, A. E., Fischl, M. A., Dickinson, G. M., Becker, D. M., Fournier, A. M., O'Connell, M. T., et al. (1983). Opportunistic infections and Kaposi's sarcoma among Haitians: evidence of a new acquired immunodeficiency state. *Ann. Intern. Med.* 98, 277–284. doi: 10.7326/0003-4819-98-3-277

Reyburn, H., Mbatia, R., Drakeley, C., Bruce, J., Carneiro, I., Olomi, R., et al. (2005). Association of transmission intensity and age with clinical manifestations and case fatality of severe *Plasmodium falciparum* malaria. *JAMA* 293, 1461–1470. doi: 10.1001/jama.293.12.1461

Ribeiro, C. D. (1988). Polyclonal B-cell activation (PBA). What have we learned from the study of malaria? *Mem. Inst. Oswaldo Cruz* 83(Suppl. 1), 633–648. doi: 10.1590/S0074-02761988000500076

Rico-Hesse, R. (2003). Microevolution and virulence of dengue viruses. *Adv. Virus Res.* 59, 315–341. doi: 10.1016/S0065-3527(03)59009-1

Ridde, V., Agier, I., Bonnet, E., Carabali, M., Dabiré, K. R., Fournet, F., et al. (2016). Presence of three dengue serotypes in Ouagadougou (Burkina Faso): research and public health implications. *Infect. Dis. Poverty* 5:23. doi: 10.1186/s40249-016-0120-2

Rosenke, K., Adjemian, J., Munster, V. J., Marzi, A., Falzarano, D., Onyango, C. O., et al. (2016). Plasmodium Parasitemia associated with increased survival in Ebola virus-infected patients. *Clin. Infect. Dis.* 63, 1026–1033. doi: 10.1093/cid/ciw452

Rothman, A. L., and Ennis, F. A. (1999). Immunopathogenesis of Dengue hemorrhagic fever. *Virology* 257, 1–6. doi: 10.1006/viro.1999.9656

Rothman, A. L., Medin, C. L., Friberg, H., and Currier, J. R. (2014). Immunopathogenesis versus protection in dengue virus infections. *Curr. Trop. Med. Rep.* 1, 13–20. doi: 10.1007/s40475-013-0009-0

Royer, D. (2015). *Upstate Medical University*. Available at: www.upstate.edu/news/article.php?title=8993

Rudnick, A. (1967). *Aedes aegypti* and haemorrhagic fever. *Bull. World Health Organ.* 36, 528–532.

Rudnick, A., Marchette, N. J., Garcia, R. (1967). Possible jungle dengue- recent studies and hypotheses. *Jpn. J. Med. Sci. Biol.* 20 Suppl, 69–74.

Sabin, A. B. (1952). Research on dengue during World War II. *Am. J. Trop. Med. Hyg.* 1, 30–50.. doi: 10.4269/ajtmh.1952.1.30

Saluzzo, J. F., Cornet, M., Castagnet, P., Rey, C., Digoutte, J. P. (1986). Isolation of dengue 2 and dengue 4 viruses from patients in Senegal. *Trans. R. Soc. Trop. Med. Hyg.* 80:5. doi: 10.1016/0035-9203(86)90182-3

San Martín, J. S., Brathwaite, O., Zambrano, B., Solórzano, J. O., Bouckenooghe, A., Dayan, G. H., et al. (2010). The epidemiology of dengue in the Americas over the last three decades: a worrisome reality. *Am. J. Trop. Med. Hyg.* 82, 128–135. doi: 10.4269/ajtmh.2010.09-0346

Screaton, G., Mongkolsapaya, J., Yacoub, S., and Roberts, C. (2015). New insights into the immunopathology and control of dengue virus infection. *Nat. Rev. Immunol.* 15, 745–759. doi: 10.1038/nri3916

Sharp, T. M., Moreira, R., Soares, M. J., Miguel da Costa, L., Mann, J., DeLorey, M., et al. (2015). Underrecognition of Dengue during 2013 Epidemic in Luanda, Angola. *Emerg. Infect. Dis.* 21, 1311–1316. doi: 10.3201/eid2108.150368

Shepard, D. S., Undurraga, E. A., Betancourt-Cravioto, M., Guzmán, M. G., Halstead, S. B., Harris, E., et al. (2014). Approaches to refining estimates of global burden and economics of dengue. *PLoS Negl. Trop. Dis.* 8:e3306. doi: 10.1371/journal.pntd.0003306

Snow, R. W., Sartorius, B., Kyalo, D., Maina, J., Amratia, P., and Mundia, C. W., et al. (2017). The prevalence of *Plasmodium falciparum* in sub-Saharan Africa since 1900. *Nature* 550, 515–518. doi: 10.1038/nature24059

Stanaway, J. D., Shepard, D. S, Undurraga, E. A., Halasa, Y. A., Coffeng, L. E., Brady, O. J., et al. (2016). The global burden of dengue: an analysis from the Global Burden of Diseases Study 2013. *Lancet Infect. Dis.* 16, 712–723. doi: 10.1016/S1473-3099(16)00026-8

Stephens, H. A. (2010). HLA and other gene associations with dengue disease severity. *Curr. Top. Microbiol. Immunol.* 338, 99–114. doi: 10.1007/978-3-642-02215-9_8

Stoler, J., Delimini, R. K., Bonney, J. H., Oduro, A. R., Owusu-Agyei, S., Fobil, J. N., Awandare, G. A. (2015). Evidence of recent dengue exposure among malaria parasite-positive children in three urban centers in Ghana. *Am. J. Trop. Med. Hyg.* 92, 497–500. doi: 10.4269/ajtmh.14-0678

Streatfield, P. K., Khan, W. A., Bhuiya, A., Hanifi, S. M., Alam, N., and Diboulo, E., et al. (2014). Malaria mortality in Africa and Asia: evidence from INDEPTH health and demographic surveillance system sites. *Glob. Health Action* 7:25369. doi: 10.3402/gha.v7.25369

Strøm, G. E. A., Haanshuus, C. G., Fataki, M., Langeland, N., and Blomberg, B. (2013). Challenges in diagnosing paediatric malaria in Dar es Salaam, Tanzania. *Malar. J.* 12:228. doi: 10.1186/1475-2875-12-228

Tanner, M., and de Savigny, D. (2008). Malaria eradication back on the table. *Bull. World Health Organ.* 86:82. doi: 10.2471/BLT.07.050633

Tatem, A. J., Gething, P. W., Smith, D. L., and Hay, S. I. (2013). Urbanization and the global malaria recession. *Malar. J.* 12:133. doi: 10.1186/1475-2875-12-133

Teklehaimanot, A., and Mejia, P. (2008). Malaria and poverty. *Ann. N. Y. Acad. Sci.* 1136, 32–37.

Toledo, J., George, L., Martinez, E., Lazaro, A., Han, W. W., Coelho, G. E., et al. (2016). Relevance of non-communicable comorbidities for the development of the severe forms of dengue: a systematic literature review. *PLoS Negl. Trop. Dis.* 10:e0004284. doi: 10.1371/journal.pntd.0004284

Tomson, G. (1933). Immunity in malaria. *Trans. R. Soc. Trop. Med. Hyg.* 26, 483–503. doi: 10.1016/S0035-9203(33)90123-6

Trunfio, M., Savoldi, A., Viganò, O., and d'Arminio Monforte, A. (2017). Bacterial coinfections in dengue virus disease: what we know and what is still obscure about an emerging concern. *Infection* 45, 1–10. doi: 10.1007/s15010-016-0927-6

Twiddy, S. S., Holmes, E. C., and Rambaut, A. (2003). Inferring the rate and time-scale of dengue virus evolution. *Mol. Biol. Evol.* 20, 122–129. doi: 10.1093/molbev/msg010

Vairo, F., Mboera, L. E. G., De Nardo, P., Oriyo, N. M., Meschi, S., Rumisha, S. F., et al. (2016). Clinical, virologic, and epidemiologic characteristics of dengue outbreak, Dar es Salaam, Tanzania, 2014. *Emerg. Infect. Dis.* 22, 895–899. doi: 10.3201/eid2205.151462

Villar, L., Dayab, G. H., Aredono-Garcia, J. L., Rivera, D. M., Cunha, R., Deseda, C., et al. (2015) Efficacy of a tetravalent dengue vaccine in children in Latin America. *N. Engl. J. Med.* 372, 113–123. doi: 10.1056/NEJMoa1411037

Wang, T. T., Sewatanon, J., Memoli, M. J., Wrammert, J., Bournazos, S., Bhaumik, S. K., et al. (2017). IgG antibodies to dengue enhanced for FcγRIIIA binding determine disease severity. *Science* 355, 395–398. doi: 10.1126/science.aai8128

Wardrop, N. A. (2016). Integrated epidemiology for vector-borne zoonoses. *Trans. R. Soc. Trop. Med. Hyg.* 110, 87–89. doi: 10.1093/trstmh/trv115

WHO (2013). Malaria Policy Advisory Committee to the WHO: conclusions and recommendations of September 2013 meeting. *Malar. J.* 12:456. doi: 10.1186/1475-2875-12-456

WHO (1997). *Dengue Haemorrhagic Fever: Diagnosis, Treatment, Prevention and Control*, 2nd edn. Geneva: WHO

WHO (2009). *Evaluation of Commercially Available Anti-Dengue Virus Immunoglobulin M Tests*. Available at: http://www.who.int/tdr/publications/documents/diagnostics-evaluation-3.pdf?ua=1 [accessed February 18, 2017].

WHO (2016). *Dengue Vaccine: WHO Position Paper - July 2016*. Available at: http://www.who.int/wer/2016/wer9130.pdf?ua=1 [accessed February 18, 2017].

WHO (2017a). *Dengue and Severe Dengue. Fact sheet, Updated April 2017*. Available at: http://www.who.int/mediacentre/factsheets/fs117/en/ [accessed February 18, 2017].

WHO (2017b). *GACVS Statement on Dengvaxia® (CYD-TDV)*. Available at: http://www.who.int/vaccine_safety/committee/GACVS-StatementonDengvaxia-CYD-TDV/en/ [accessed February 18, 2017].

Wilson, M. L. Krogstad, D. J., Arinaitwe, E., Arevalo-Herrera, M., Chery, L., Marcelo, U. et al. (2015). Urban Malaria: understanding its epidemiology, ecology, and transmission across seven diverse ICEMR network sites. *Am. J. Trop. Med. Hyg.* 93(3 Suppl), 110–123. doi: 10.4269/ajtmh.14-0834

Yong, K. P., Tan, B. H., and Low, C. Y. (2012). Severe falciparum malaria with dengue coinfection complicated by rhabdomyolysis and acute kidney injury: an unusual case with myoglobinemia, myoglobinuria but normal serum creatine kinase. *BMC Infect. Dis.* 12:364. doi: 10.1186/1471-2334-12-364.

7

Dendritic Cell Responses and Function in Malaria

Xi Zen Yap [1,2*†‡], *Rachel J. Lundie* [1,3*†‡], *James G. Beeson* [1,2,4] *and Meredith O'Keeffe* [1,3]

[1] Burnet Institute, Melbourne, VIC, Australia, [2] Department of Medicine, Dentistry, and Health Sciences, The University of Melbourne, Parkville, VIC, Australia, [3] Department of Biochemistry and Molecular Biology, Biomedicine Discovery Institute, Monash University, Clayton, VIC, Australia, [4] Department of Microbiology and Central Clinical School, Monash University, Clayton, VIC, Australia

Edited by:
Noah Butler,
The University of Iowa, United States

Reviewed by:
Silvia Beatriz Boscardin,
University of São Paulo, Brazil
Michelle N. Wykes,
QIMR Berghofer Medical Research Institute, Australia
Anton Goetz,
National Institutes of Health (NIH), United States

***Correspondence:**
Xi Zen Yap
zen.yap@radboudumc.nl
Rachel J. Lundie
lundie.r@wehi.edu.au

† These authors have contributed equally to this work

‡Present Address:
Xi Zen Yap,
Radboud University Medical Centre, Nijmegen, Netherlands
Rachel J. Lundie,
The Walter and Eliza Hall Institute of Medical Research, Parkville, VIC, Australia

Malaria remains a serious threat to global health. Sustained malaria control and, eventually, eradication will only be achieved with a broadly effective malaria vaccine. Yet a fundamental lack of knowledge about how antimalarial immunity is acquired has hindered vaccine development efforts to date. Understanding how malaria-causing parasites modulate the host immune system, specifically dendritic cells (DCs), key initiators of adaptive and vaccine antigen-based immune responses, is vital for effective vaccine design. This review comprehensively summarizes how exposure to *Plasmodium* spp. impacts human DC function *in vivo* and *in vitro*. We have highlighted the heterogeneity of the data observed in these studies, compared and critiqued the models used to generate our current understanding of DC function in malaria, and examined the mechanisms by which *Plasmodium* spp. mediate these effects. This review highlights potential research directions which could lead to improved efficacy of existing vaccines, and outlines novel targets for next-generation vaccine strategies to target malaria.

Keywords: dendritic cells, malaria, *Plasmodium falciparum*, *Plasmodium vivax*, vaccines

INTRODUCTION: MALARIA

Malaria remains one of the greatest challenges to public health in the developing world. It is caused by infection with the *Plasmodium* species of Apicomplexans, which have a complex life cycle spanning multiple organ sites (**Figure 1**), facilitated by multiple morphologically and antigenically distinct life stages, and expression of multiple antigens (1–5).

The *Plasmodium* life cycle bridges two hosts: mosquitoes, where sexual replication occurs, and humans, where the parasite undergoes asexual replication. The latter begins when an infected mosquito injects sporozoite-stage parasites from mosquito salivary glands into the skin (**Figure 1**). A small fraction of sporozoites will travel to the liver, where the sporozoite will traverse hepatic tissue until it locates a suitable hepatocyte. The subsequent exoerythrocytic form will release merozoites into the bloodstream upon rupture (6). *Plasmodium vivax* can also enter a dormant liver stage known as the hypnozoite, which can mature and produce merozoites weeks to years after the initial infection (7, 8). Despite being only 1 μm in size, the merozoite expresses a range of parasite proteins that ligate host red blood cell (RBC) ligands to drive invasion. After invasion the merozoite forms a parasitophorous vacuole in host cells, where it begins to mature into a trophozoite (9).

From 18 to 32 h post-invasion, the trophozoite increases DNA replication and metabolic activity. The mid-trophozoite stage exports various parasite proteins, including those crucial to host pathology, such as the *P. falciparum* erythrocyte membrane protein 1 (*Pf*EMP1) (10). At 34 h post-invasion, the parasite becomes a

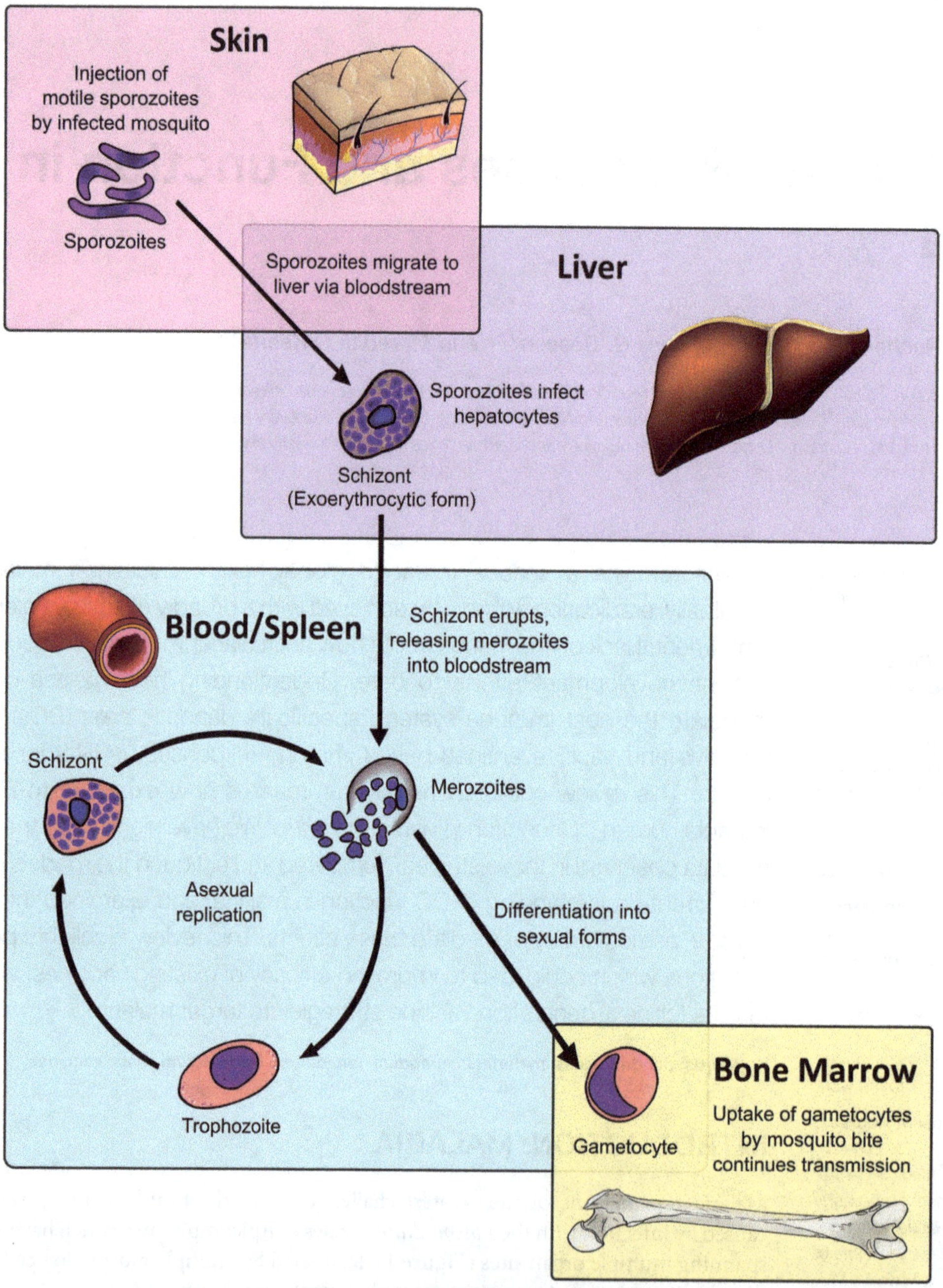

FIGURE 1 | Dendritic cells, located throughout the body at various stages of maturity, interact with all stages of the malaria parasite life cycle within the human host. The *Plasmodium* life cycle encompasses multiple life stages across a range of tissues. The asexual life cycle in the human host begins when mosquitoes inject sporozoites, the highly motile infectious life stage, into the host's skin. The sporozoite migrates to the liver, where it traverses multiple host cells before entering into an exoerythrocytic form. The exoerythrocytic form matures into a multinucleate schizont, which releases merozoites into the bloodstream upon lysis. Merozoites infect host red blood cells and mature into intraerythrocytic life stages known as trophozoites, which are highly metabolically active. After DNA replication the trophozoite will become a blood-stage schizont, which will lyse and release daughter merozoites into the bloodstream, resuming the process. Instead of becoming trophozoites, a fraction of merozoites will instead differentiate into sexual stages known as gametocytes, which sequester in the bone marrow. Only at the end of their maturation process do gametocytes re-enter the bloodstream, where they are taken up by mosquito bite to commence sexual replication in the mosquito host and continue the cycle.

multinucleate, segmented stage known as the schizont. After 48 h of intracellular maturation and replication, the schizont ruptures, destroying the erythrocyte and releasing parasite metabolites, waste products, and between 16 to 32 daughter merozoites are released into the bloodstream (9), where the cycle will begin afresh.

After 7–15 days in circulation, a small proportion of *P. falciparum* trophozoites will commit to sexual replication, where the process of schizogony is replaced by the formation of sexual stages known as gametocytes (11, 12). Generation of *P. vivax* gametocytes is much faster, with gametocytes being detectable in circulation from 3 days post-infection (13, 14). Gametocytes undergo five maturation stages: stages I-IV preferentially sequester in the bone marrow (BM) and spleen (15–17) while stage V gametocytes re-enter the circulation, where they can be taken up by the bite of infected mosquitoes (18).

The effect of each malaria life stage on host immune function is not well understood, nor are the broader underlying mechanisms of antimalarial immunity. It is frequently observed that individuals living in highly endemic regions develop clinical immunity against symptomatic disease, but generally do not develop sterilizing immunity that completely protects against infection. Antibodies are a crucial component of naturally acquired clinical immunity, as passive transfer of immunoglobulins from malaria immune to non-immune individuals is sufficient to reduce parasitaemia and resolve symptoms (19). Furthermore, clinical immunity appears in most cases to be relatively short-lived and broadly declines in the absence of boosting [reviewed in (20)]. An improved understanding of antimalarial immunity will enable development of future vaccines which can accelerate acquisition of clinical immunity, or better yet, induce sterile immunity.

Malaria Vaccines

The most advanced malaria vaccine candidate to date is RTS,S, which targets the circumsporozoite protein (CSP) of *P. falciparum*. RTS,S has shown modest efficacy in Phase III clinical trials, with 29 and 36% efficacy in young infants and young children, respectively over 3–4 years, with a booster dose given at 20 months (21). The sub-optimal efficacy of RTS,S and its failure to elicit protective immunity in many recipients is poorly understood (21–23). To elucidate the immunological responses that future malaria vaccines should aim to induce or improve upon, it is vital to understand how different parasite life stages modulate the host immune system. This review focuses specifically on the interactions between malaria parasites and dendritic cells (DCs), sentinel antigen presenting cells of the immune system that are crucial for generating effective immune responses and immunological memory.

Dendritic Cells

DCs function as a crucial bridge between innate and adaptive immunity. In a healthy individual, DCs constitute only 1% of all peripheral blood mononuclear cells (PBMC) (24–26), yet they exert potent regulatory effects on both the innate and adaptive immune system (**Figure 2**). Upon encountering foreign antigens in the presence of pathogen associated molecular patterns (PAMPs), DCs undergo a process of maturation and migrate to the spleen and draining lymph nodes where they interact with pathogen-specific T cells. In addition to presenting antigen via major histocompatibility complex (MHC) surface molecules, DCs express co-stimulatory molecules required for naïve T cell proliferation and differentiation into effector cells, including CD40, CD80 (B7-1), and CD86 (B7-2). Through secretion of cytokines and chemokines, DCs recruit other immune cells and influence the nature of the adaptive T and B cell response, ultimately leading to clearance of infected cells and extracellular pathogens (**Figure 2**). Crucially, DCs are present at all clinically relevant sites for the development of *Plasmodium* life stages, namely the skin, blood, bone marrow, spleen, and liver (**Figure 1**).

Based on the expression of CD11c and CD123, human DCs can be broadly classified into plasmacytoid DCs (pDC; $Lin^-HLA\text{-}DR^+CD11c^-CD123^+$) and conventional DCs (cDC; $Lin^-HLA\text{-}DR^+CD11c^+CD123^-$) populations. The pDCs are the body's major producers of the anti-viral interferon (IFN)-α, though they constitute only 0.35% of PBMCs (25, 26). These cells are crucial in antiviral responses. The cDCs specialize in priming and presenting antigen to T cells (27), and constitute 0.6% of PBMCs (25, 26). Using the blood dendritic cell antigen (BDCA) markers, it is possible to further differentiate cDC populations into cDC1 ($BDCA\text{-}3^+/CD141^+$) and cDC2 ($BDCA\text{-}1^+/CD1c^+$) subsets, while pDCs express BDCA-2 (CD303) and BDCA-4 (CD304) (28–30).

Given the central role of DCs in sensing infection and orchestrating immune responses, it is not surprising that many pathogens have evolved immune evasion strategies which specifically target DCs in order to interfere with innate and adaptive immune responses (31–34). Thus, understanding how DCs initiate and maintain effective immune responses against malaria parasites, whilst minimizing detrimental and life-threatening immunopathology, is imperative for vaccine development.

AT THE MEETING POINTS: SITES OF DC AND *PLASMODIUM* SPP. INTERACTION

Interactions between DCs and *Plasmodium* parasites occur at every stage of the parasite life cycle within the human host: skin (35), liver (36), and most importantly within the blood and spleen (37), where the majority of host pathology occurs. Recent studies have also revealed that the bone marrow (BM) compartment is a major tissue reservoir for gametocyte development and proliferation of malaria parasites (38–41). Tissue-resident DCs in each of these sites have the potential to endocytose parasite components and initiate the development of specific adaptive immune responses to *Plasmodium* infection. Importantly, DCs in these tissues exist in different maturation states and thus vary in their ability to influence adaptive and innate immune responses and induce inflammatory responses. Within the liver, DCs are thought to induce tolerogenic responses to prevent induction of harmful immunopathology (42, 43), whilst in spleen, DCs propagate strong immune responses, and blood DCs have an intermediate phenotype with a lower capacity for inducing inflammation compared to their splenic counterparts (44).

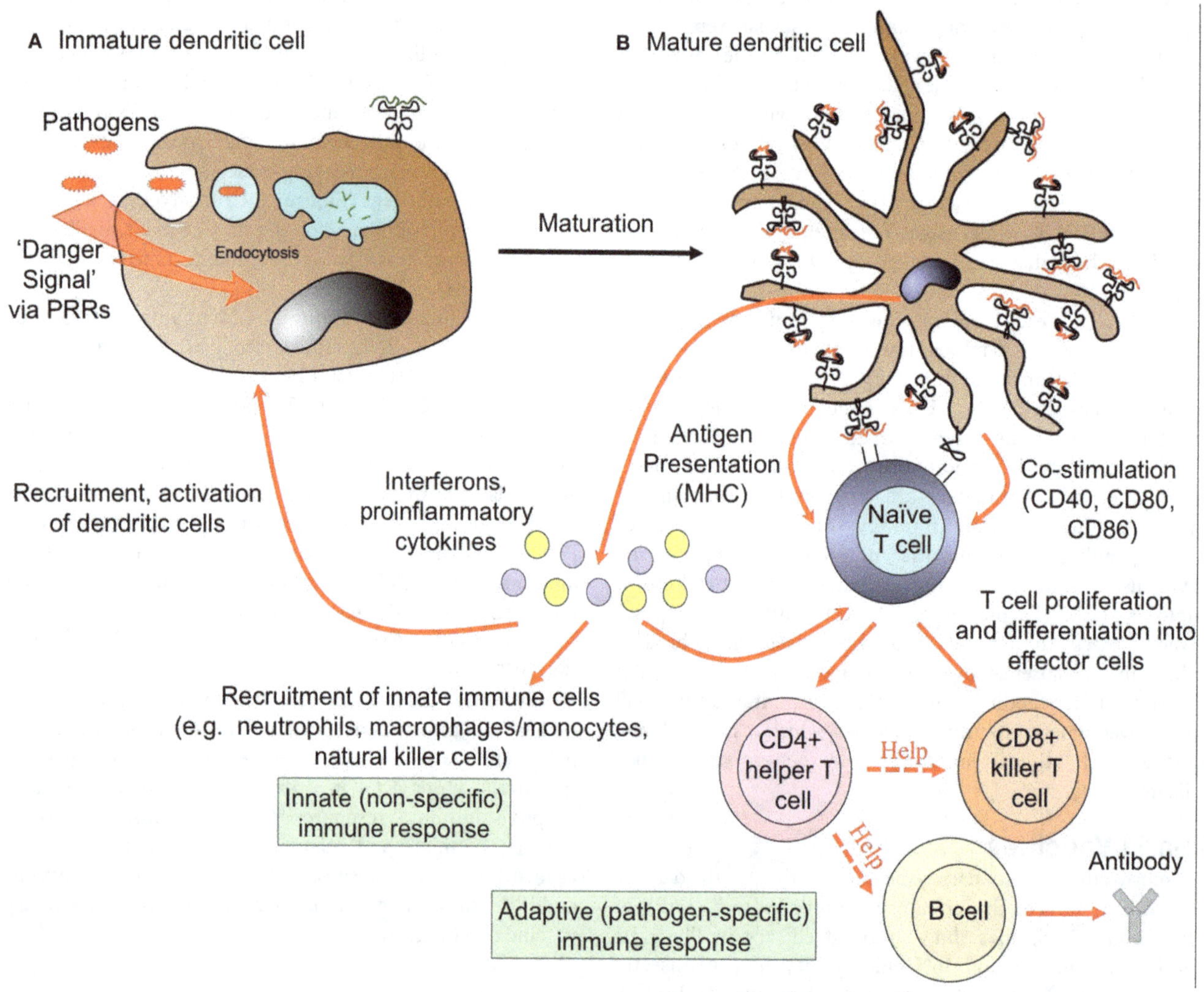

FIGURE 2 | Dendritic cells link innate and adaptive arms of the immune system. **(A)** Uptake of pathogens and recognition of pathogen-associated "danger signals" by pattern recognition receptors (PRRs) triggers dramatic morphological and functional changes in DCs, termed maturation. These changes involve the formation of dendrites, down-regulation of antigen uptake, and redistribution of major histocompatibility complex (MHC) molecules from intracellular endocytic compartments to the cell surface. **(B)** Mature DCs migrate to draining lymph nodes and present information about the invading pathogen in the form of processed peptides loaded onto MHC molecules to naïve T cells. Upregulation of MHC and co-stimulation molecules enables activated DCs to initiate adaptive T and B cell immune responses, the nature of which are determined by the cytokine milieu. This initiates the cascade to an adaptive immune response, leading to clearance of infected cells, and extracellular pathogens. Activated mature DCs also secrete interferons and proinflammatory cytokines that recruit circulating innate immune cells to provide rapid defense against infection.

Skin and Liver DC Interactions With Sporozoites: Lessons From Murine Models

The skin is the site of first contact between DCs and *Plasmodium* spp. Studies in mice have demonstrated that sporozoites remain in the skin for up to 60 min prior to entering the circulation, after which they lose motility (45). Remarkably, up to 50% of sporozoites become trapped in the dermis, while 30% of those that succeed in entering the circulation enter lymphatic rather than blood vessels (45). Thus, the majority of sporozoites fail to reach the bloodstream and are instead phagocytosed by DCs in the skin-draining lymph nodes, which prime protective $CD4^+$ (46–48) and $CD8^+$ T cell responses (49, 50). It is likely that a substantial proportion of immunity to sporozoite stages arises predominantly in response to these "failed" sporozoites.

Interestingly, there is some evidence that sporozoites which arrest within the liver may promote induction of limited liver-stage immunity. A murine study demonstrated that apoptosing hepatocytes infected by irradiated sporozoites triggered recruitment of circulating blood DCs to the liver (51). These DCs phagocytosed apoptotic hepatocytes and migrated to lymph nodes, where they induced protective IFN-γ-producing $CD8^+$ T cell responses (50).

Importantly, in the above study, infiltrating DCs from the cutaneous lymph nodes initiated immune responses, not liver-resident DCs (50). In humans (52) and mice (53), tissue-resident liver DCs are reportedly less mature than blood DCs, as they are poor at antigen processing and express only low levels of costimulatory markers. While liver DCs in humans are capable of inducing allogeneic T cell responses, they are less effective at this than their blood counterparts, and therefore promote a T cell phenotype that is less responsive to subsequent stimulation (52, 54). When considered in conjunction with their high capacity for IL-10 secretion (52), the liver DC phenotype may be one that promotes a more tolerogenic environment, favorable to sporozoite survival. This could partly explain why sterile immunity rarely occurs in response to natural infection, with tolerogenic liver-resident DCs acting to suppress inflammatory responses which would induce protection. Studies using mouse models with humanized livers have shown promise for investigating *Plasmodium* spp. skin-to-liver transfer (55, 56). In combination with FMS-like tyrosine kinase 3 ligand (Flt3-L)-treated cord blood engrafted humanized mice, which produce large quantities of human DCs similar to those seen in blood (57), combined liver-immune system humanized mice could be a useful avenue to investigate DC involvement in liver-stage immunity.

The Bone Marrow As a Reservoir for Gametocytes

A similar phenomenon of immune tolerance may occur in the BM, which emerging evidence suggests is a privileged developmental niche for the transmission stages of *Plasmodium*. Autopsy studies have indicated that both *P. vivax* and *P. falciparum* (15, 58–61) gametocytes sequester in the BM, the latter of which is supported by the presence of a *Pf*EMP1 type capable of binding BM endothelium (62). Poor immune responses to parasites in this milieu may be due to tolerogenic potential of the BM microenvironment. There is very little data on BM DCs. One non-human primate study indicated that BM-derived CD123$^+$HLA-DR$^+$ pDCs had a decreased capacity to express co-stimulatory molecules in response to pathogens relative to blood DCs (63), while CD11c$^+$ BM cells in a murine study had a similar capacity for T cell stimulation relative to their blood and spleen counterparts (64). However, it is not clear whether the CD11c$^+$ population in the latter study was comprised solely of DCs.

No studies to date have examined how DCs in the BM respond to sequestered parasites, although one murine study has reported that pDCs, present in the BM at frequencies 20 times higher than in the blood or spleen, are the major producers of IFN α during *P. yoelii 17X YM* infection (65). If the BM is indeed a reservoir for infection, as is suggested by recent primate studies (41), studying whether BM DCs are capable of initiating antimalarial immune responses will be important for achieving elimination.

Blood and Spleen DC Interactions With Malaria Blood-Stages

Blood-stage parasitaemia provides multiple opportunities for blood and splenic DCs to interact with parasites. The parasite spends the majority of the asexual blood-stage cycle within the host RBC. While *P. vivax* exclusively infects reticulocytes, which express surface MHC and can therefore be cleared by CD8$^+$ T cells (66), *P. falciparum* also infects mature RBCs, which do not express surface MHC molecules, thus enabling host immune evasion. Despite this, the blood-stage is an antigenically rich phase of the *Plasmodium* life cycle [reviewed in (67, 68)], affecting a large proportion of host cells and triggering potent inflammatory immune responses that cause most of the symptoms of malaria. Maturation of parasitized RBCs (pRBCs) culminates in lysis of the host RBC, releasing merozoites into the circulation. Merozoites that fail to invade a new RBC will remain in the circulation where they are directly phagocytosed (69) or circulate to the spleen for clearance. The *Pf*EMP1 molecule, which is expressed on the pRBC surface, may play a dual role in this life stage. While it is a prime target for antibodies in naturally acquired immunity (70), one report suggests it may also modulate immune function via binding to CD36 on APCs, including DCs (71). Furthermore, *Pf*EMP1-mediated sequestration in the periphery is long held to be a parasite adaptation aimed at avoiding splenic clearance (72).

DCs play a vital role in initiating and regulating adaptive immunity to blood-stage malaria (73–75). However, there is strong evidence that *Plasmodium* parasites modulate DC maturation and function to interfere with the development of protective immune responses. Data from mouse models indicate that blood-stage infection suppresses both existing and developing liver-stage immunity by inhibiting DC activation (76), and inhibits DCs from responding to subsequently encountered pathogens (77–79). Importantly, murine studies suggest that DCs also play a role in the induction of immune-mediated pathology, including the life-threatening syndrome of cerebral malaria (80, 81). Thus, it is of vital importance that we understand the factors governing the ability of DCs to alter the balance between protection and pathology.

DCs, Malaria, and Unanswered Questions

The majority of DC-*Plasmodium* interactions in humans have been studied in two ways: (1) studying peripheral blood DCs from currently or previously infected individuals, or (2) measuring DC responses to parasite stimuli *in vitro*. In the first method, DCs were isolated from the blood of individuals who were naturally or experimentally infected with malaria. The surface phenotype and function of these DCs was compared to uninfected controls, either the same individuals prior to or post-infection, or a matched control group (82–102). In the second method, DCs from malaria-naïve individuals were stimulated with *Plasmodium* products to assess the resulting phenotype. The majority of reports which used the latter generated DCs from monocytes *in vitro* using GM-CSF and IL-4 (71, 103–106), while a minority reported responses from *bona fide* DCs from blood (83, 85, 107, 108).

As such, there is limited knowledge about how naïve DC subsets resident in different human tissues and blood respond to *Plasmodium*, and what factors influence this response. This knowledge is vitally important for designing vaccine strategies which specifically enhance the ability of DCs to induce protective responses while limiting induction of immunopathology. Understanding how naïve DC function is altered by *Plasmodium* exposure will provide insight into how DCs are affected in infected individuals, and therefore what vaccine strategies will be required to overcome this altered phenotype.

PERIPHERAL BLOOD DC RESPONSES TO NATURAL OR EXPERIMENTAL *PLASMODIUM* INFECTION

A total of 24 *ex vivo* studies to date have examined how natural or experimental exposure to *Plasmodium* spp. affects the activation phenotype and function of human peripheral blood DCs, in both acute infection and after prior exposure (summarized in **Table 1**). The following sections analyse these studies in detail, according to species infection.

DC Phenotypes and Responses During *P. falciparum* Infection

Plasmodium falciparum is responsible for a high burden of morbidity and mortality in pregnant women and children, and can cause severe and fatal disease outcomes including cerebral malaria, miscarriage, and multiple organ failure (110). Infected persons typically present to hospital when blood-stage infection becomes symptomatic, which can occur nine to 30 days after the initial infection (111). Classifying malaria cases as mild/uncomplicated vs. severe is based on specific clinical features, including but not limited to coma, haemoglobinuria, vital organ dysfunction, or respiratory distress (110). The majority of *ex vivo* studies have been carried out in settings of high *P. falciparum* transmission, focusing on the phenotype and function of DCs in high-risk groups including children and pregnant women (**Table 1**).

DCs and *P. Falciparum* in Children in High-Transmission Settings

In a DC study comparing infected children to non-infected controls in a holoendemic setting, Kenyan children hospitalized with mild vs. severe malaria exhibited decreased HLA-DR expression on DCs and reduced DC numbers in circulating blood, regardless of disease severity (82). A subsequent study which followed children during malaria and after treatment showed that malaria specifically decreased HLA-DR expression on cDC but not pDC subsets, and reduced the ability of DCs to induce allogeneic T cell proliferation in mixed leucocyte reactions (MLR) (96). Furthermore, infection correlated to an increase in absolute numbers of circulating BDCA-3$^+$ cDC1s. Importantly, these effects of *P. falciparum* on DC phenotype and function were still observed 14 days after hospital discharge and curative treatment (96), suggesting that malaria-induced immunosuppression can persist for some time after parasite clearance.

A subsequent study was conducted in Mali, another holoendemic setting, where DC function was compared between infected and non-infected children from the Fulani and Dogon ethnic groups. DCs from children aged 2–10 years displayed reduced HLA-DR expression after malaria exposure (100). Infection was also associated with increased proportions of circulating BDCA-2$^+$ pDC and BDCA-3$^+$ cDC1 populations, with reduced CD86 expression in the former (100). In this study genetic differences were proposed to play a role in clinical outcomes of *P. falciparum* infection due to differences in cytokine production between the 2 ethnic groups, with PBMCs from Dogon children displaying significantly impaired cytokine production, correlating with more severe fever and higher parasitaemia (100). These responses could be attributed in part to reduced DC function, including a reduction of pDC-derived IFN-α production in response to TLR9 ligands.

More recently, Guermonprez et al. reported that children with malaria, regardless of disease severity, had an increased frequency of the BDCA-3$^+$ cDC1 population (102). This correlated with increased serum concentrations of the DC growth factor Flt3-L that preferentially increases pDC and cDC1 *in vivo* (112, 113). During malaria, Flt3-L is produced by mast cells in response to uric acid metabolism by *Plasmodium* parasites (102).

Together, these studies suggest that malaria in children in high-transmission settings negatively impacts DC activation marker expression and modulates DC function. The low activation status of peripheral DCs may be due to sequestration of activated DCs in affected tissues. Moreover, an increased number of circulating BDCA-3$^+$ cDC1s appears to be a common feature of malaria in this setting. Urban et al. also showed that DC dysfunction persisted after the resolution of malaria (96), leaving these individuals vulnerable to co-infections. The apparent contradiction between reduced DC numbers in the first study (82) and elevated numbers of BDCA-3$^+$ cDC1s in the second study (96) is likely due to more sophisticated gating strategies in the latter, enabling discrimination of individual DC subsets (96), rather than classifying all HLA-DR$^+$ cells as DCs (82). Rigorous and well-defined flow cytometry gating strategies that use an appropriate combination of antibodies to DC subset-specific surface markers are imperative for DC research and may help to resolve some of the apparent discrepancies in the literature.

DCs and *P. Falciparum* in Pregnancy in High-Transmission Settings

Four studies evaluating changes in DC populations in infection during pregnancy have yielded conflicting results. Two studies, one from Gabon (94) and one from Benin and Tanzania (101), observed that overall DC numbers were decreased in pregnant women infected with *P. falciparum* compared to uninfected matched pregnant controls, while a study from Senegal (97) reported a decrease in the pDC population only relative to non-pregnant uninfected controls. Another study from Benin (109) did not observe any difference in DC numbers between infected and non-infected pregnant women. Changes in surface activation marker expression varied across studies (**Table 1**).

Again, different gating strategies may underlie some of the differences observed between these studies. Simply gating on CD123$^+$ or CD11c$^+$ populations may run a risk of false positives if isolation and lineage staining is not extensive enough. Use of cord blood (94, 97) or placenta-derived (97) DCs may also

TABLE 1 | *In vivo* exposure to *Plasmodium* species modulates human DC responses.

References	Cohort demographic	Transmission intensity (country)	DC subset gating strategy (phenotype)	Changes in surface molecule expression	Serum /plasma cytokines	Other effects
P. falciparum						
Urban et al. (82)	Children	Holoendemic (Kenya)	HLA-DR$^+$, CD83$^+$	Decreased: HLA-DR No change: CD83	Increased: TNF-α IL-10	Decreased DC numbers
Pichyangkul et al. (83)	Hospitalized adults	Mesoendemic (Thailand)	cDC (HLA-DR$^+$CD11c$^+$) pDC (HLA-DR$^+$CD123$^+$)		Increased: IFN-α	Reduced numbers of circulating pDC
Breitling et al. (94)	Pregnant women	Holoendemic (Gabon)	cDC (BDCA1$^+$) pDC (BDCA2$^+$)	No change: HLA-DR*		Decrease in overall DC numbers
Urban et al. (96)	Children	Holoendemic (Kenya)	cDC (CD11c$^+$BDCA1$^+$, CD11c$^+$BDCA3$^+$) pDC (CD123$^+$BDCA2$^+$)	Decreased: HLA-DR (cDC)	Increased: TNF-α IL-10 IL-12	Elevated number of BDCA-3$^+$ cDC1 in circulating blood during and after malaria infection Decreased cDC ability to induce allogeneic T cell proliferation
Diallo et al. (97)	Pregnant women	Hypoendemic (Senegal)	cDC (CD11c$^+$CD123^{lo}) pDC (CD11c$^-$CD123^{hi}) Less differentiated DC (CD11c$^-$CD123^{lo})	No change: CD83* Decreased: HLA-DR*	Increased: TNF-α IFN-γ IL-10	Women who have had malaria have higher percentages of less differentiated DC Decreased circulating pDC in infected pregnant women
Loharungsikul et al. (98)	Hospitalized adults	Mesoendemic (Thailand)	cDC (BDCA1$^+$, BDCA3$^+$) pDC (BDCA2$^+$)	Increased: TLR2 (cDC) Decreased: TLR9 (pDC) No change: TLR4 (cDC)		Decreased fraction of TLR2$^+$ cDC in peripheral blood during infection
Fievet et al. (109)	Pregnant women	Mesoendemic (Benin)	cDC (BDCA1$^+$, BDCA3$^+$) pDC (BDCA2$^+$)	Increased: HLA-DR (BDCA1, BDCA2) No change: CD86* HLA-DR (BDCA3)	No change: TNF-α IFN-γ IL-10 IL-12 IL-6 MIP-1α	Increased percentage of HLA-DR positive BDCA2$^+$ cells during infection Decreased absolute number of all DCs from women with $\geq$3 pregnancies Increased pDC number in women with $\geq$3 pregnancies
Gonçalves et al. (99)	Clinic admission	Hypo- to mesoendemic (Brazil)	cDC (HLA-DR$^+$CD11c$^+$) pDC (HLA-DR$^+$CD123$^+$)	No change: CD86*	Increased: IFN-γ TNF-α IL-10	Decreased cDC number Decreased total DC number

(Continued)

TABLE 1 | Continued

References	Cohort demographic	Transmission intensity (country)	DC subset gating strategy (phenotype)	Changes in surface molecule expression	Serum /plasma cytokines	Other effects
Arama et al. (100)	Children	Mesoendemic (Mali)	cDC (HLA-DR$^+$BDCA1$^+$, HLA-DR$^+$BDCA3$^+$, HLA-DR$^+$CD16$^+$) pDC (HLA-DR$^+$BDCA2$^+$)	Decreased: HLA-DR* CD86 (pDC)	Decreased: IFN-γ	Increased BDCA-2$^+$ pDC and BDCA-3$^+$ cDC1 populations in peripheral blood Impairment of TLR signaling in DC during malaria results in more severe clinical symptoms
Ibitokou et al. (101)	Pregnant women	Mesoendemic (Benin) Holoendemic (Tanzania)	cDC (HLA-DR$^+$BDCA1$^+$) pDC (HLA-DR$^+$BDCA2$^+$)	Decreased: HLA-DR (cDC) Increased: CD86 (pDC)		Decreased pDC and cDC fraction in peripheral blood
Guermonprez et al. (102)	Children	Holoendemic (Kenya)	cDC (CD11c$^+$BDCA1$^+$, CD11c$^+$BDCA3$^+$) pDC (CD123$^+$BDCA2$^+$)		Increased: Flt3L	Increased BDCA-3$^+$ cDC1 fraction in peripheral blood Increased CD8$^+$ T cell activation in peripheral blood
Pinzon-Charry et al. (84)	Infected adults	Holoendemic (Papua)	cDC (HLA-DR$^+$CD11c$^+$) pDC (HLA-DR$^+$CD123$^+$) iDC (HLA-DR$^+$CD123$^-$CD11c$^-$)	Decreased: HLA-DR CD83 CD86	Increased: TNF-α IFN-γ IL-2 IL-4 IL-6 IL-10	Decreased pDC and cDC fractions Increased fraction of immature DC Increased DC apoptosis Decreased ability to induce T cell proliferation Decreased antigen uptake
Restimulation of DCs from naturally *P. falciparum*-infected individuals[†]						
Fievet et al. (109)	Pregnant women	Mesoendemic (Benin)	cDC (BDCA1$^+$, BDCA3$^+$) pDC (BDCA2$^+$)	No change: HLA-DR (cDC)	Increased: IFN-γ TNF-α IL-10 No change: IFN-α IL-6 IL-12 MIP-1α	Increased production of proinflammatory cytokines by women ≤25 years independent of gravidity
Götz et al. (85)	Adults	Holoendemic (Mali)	cDC (HLA-DR$^+$BDCA1$^+$, HLA-DR$^+$BDCA3$^+$, HLA-DR$^+$CD16$^+$)	Increased: HLA-DR CD86 No change: CD40 CD80	Increased: CCL2 CXCL9 CXCL10 No change: IL-1β IL-6 IL-10 TNF-α CCL5	

(*Continued*)

TABLE 1 | Continued

References	Cohort demographic	Transmission intensity (country)	DC subset gating strategy (phenotype)	Changes in surface molecule expression	Serum /plasma cytokines	Other effects
P. vivax						
Jangpatarapongsa et al. (86)	Hospitalized adults	Mesoendemic (Thailand)	cDC ($HLA\text{-}DR^+CD11c^+$) pDC ($HLA\text{-}DR^+CD123^+$)		Increased: IL-10	Decreased fraction of cDC and pDC during infection Increased numbers of $FOXP3^+$ T_{REG} during infection
Gonçalves et al. (99)	Clinic admission	Hypo- to mesoendemic (Brazil)	cDC ($HLA\text{-}DR^+CD11c^+$) pDC ($HLA\text{-}DR^+CD123^+$)	*Decreased*: CD86*	Increased: TNF-α IL-10	Increased pDC fraction Decreased cDC number Decreased total DC number
Pinzon-Charry et al. (84)	Infected adults	Holoendemic (Papua)	cDC ($HLA\text{-}DR^+CD11c^+$) pDC ($HLA\text{-}DR^+CD123^+$) iDC ($HLA\text{-}DR^+CD123^-CD11c^-$)	Decreased: HLA-DR CD83 CD86	Increased: TNF-α IFN-γ IL-2 IL-4 IL-6 IL-10	Decreased pDC and cDC fractions Increased fraction of immature DC Increased DC apoptosis Decreased T cell proliferation Decreased antigen uptake
***P. falciparum* and *P. vivax* coinfection**						
Gonçalves et al. (99)	Clinic admission	Hypo- to mesoendemic (Brazil)	cDC ($HLA\text{-}DR^+CD11c^+$) pDC ($HLA\text{-}DR^+CD123^+$)	No change: CD86*	Increased: TNF-α IL-10	Decreased cDC fraction Increased pDC fraction
Kho et al. (87)	Children, adults, hospitalized children, and adults	Holoendemic (Papua)	cDC ($HLA\text{-}DR^+BDCA1^+$, $HLA\text{-}DR^+BDCA3^+$) pDC ($HLA\text{-}DR^+BDCA2^+$)	Increased: HLA-DR* Decreased: HLA-DR (cDC)		Increased pDC fraction during asymptomatic *P. vivax* but not *P. falciparum* infection Decrease in $BDCA\text{-}1^+$ cDC2 fraction during asymptomatic infection with either species or during uncomplicated malaria
Kho et al. (88)	Adults	Holoendemic (Papua)	cDC ($HLA\text{-}DR^+BDCA1^+$, $HLA\text{-}DR^+BDCA3^+$) pDC ($HLA\text{-}DR^+BDCA2^+$)	Decreased: HLA-DR		Decreased numbers of circulating pDC and $BDCA\text{-}1^+$ cDC2 during symptomatic infections but not during subpatent infections Reduced $CD4^+$ T cell proportion Decreased proportion of activated and resting T_{REG}
Controlled human malaria infection with *P. falciparum*						
Woodberry et al. (89)	Healthy adult males	N/A (CHMI)	cDC ($HLA\text{-}DR^+CD11c^+$) pDC ($HLA\text{-}DR^+CD123^+$)	Decreased: HLA-DR (pDC)	No change: TNF-α IL-6 IL-10 IL-12	Increased DC apoptosis Decreased overall DC numbers Decreased phagocytic activity

(Continued)

TABLE 1 | Continued

References	Cohort demographic	Transmission intensity (country)	DC subset gating strategy (phenotype)	Changes in surface molecule expression	Serum /plasma cytokines	Other effects
Teirlinck et al. (90)	Healthy adults	N/A (CHMI)	cDC (HLA-DR$^+$BDCA1$^+$, HLA-DR$^+$BDCA3$^+$) pDC (HLA-DR+BDCA2$^+$) CD16$^+$ DC (HLA-DR$^+$CD16$^+$ CD14$^-$)	Increased: HLA-DR (CD16$^+$, pDC) CD86 (CD16$^+$) CD16 (CD16$^+$, BDCA-1$^+$, pDC) CD1c (CD16$^+$, BDCA-1$^+$, pDC) No change: HLA-DR (cDC) CD86 (cDC, pDC)		Increased expression of BDCA-1 and CD16 on all subsets except BDCA-3$^+$ cDC1 Increased CD1c/BDCA-1 and CD16 expression on monocytes after treatment
Loughland et al. (91)	Healthy adults	N/A (CHMI)	cDC (HLA-DR$^+$CD11c$^+$ BDCA-1$^+$)	Decreased: HLA-DR CD86	Increased: TNF-α No change: IL-12	Increased DC apoptosis Decreased antigen uptake Decreased overall DC numbers
Loughland et al. (92)	Healthy adults	N/A (CHMI)	pDC (HLA-DR$^+$CD11c$^-$CD123$^+$)	Decreased: HLA-DR No change: HLA Class I	No change: TNF-α Increased: IFN-α	Reduced circulating pDC at and 24 h after peak parasitaemia Increased caspase-3 expression in pDCs Increased expression of *NLRC5*, *C14orf119* and *TSG101* Decreased expression of *DMBT1*, *AREGB*, *RNF139*, *CRYM*, and *BAG3*
Loughland et al. (93)	Healthy adults	N/A (CHMI)	CD16$^+$ DC (HLA-DR$^+$CD14$^-$CD11c$^+$BDCA-1$^-$CD16$^+$CD86$^+$)	Decreased: CD16 Increased: HLA-DR CD86	Increased: TNF-α IL-10	Increased proportion of CD16$^+$ DCs among all CD11c$^+$ DCs Non-parasite-specific loss of CD16 when DCs are in culture
Controlled human malaria infection with *P. vivax*						
Woodberry et al. (95)	Healthy adults	N/A (CHMI)	cDC (HLA-DR$^+$CD11c$^+$ BDCA1$^+$, HLA-DR$^+$CD11c$^+$ BDCA3$^+$) pDC (HLA-DR$^+$CD123$^+$) CD16$^+$ DC (HLA-DR$^+$CD11c$^+$ CD16$^+$)	Decreased: HLA-DR (cDC) CD123* No change: HLA-DR (pDC)	Increased: IFN-γ	Reduced circulating pDC, BDCA-1$^+$ and BDCA-3$^+$ DC Increased caspase-3 expression in pDC, CD16$^+$, and BDCA-1$^+$ cDC Increased numbers of activated T_{REG} during infection Increased indoleamine 2,3-dioxygenase metabolism drives T_{REG} differentiation

*Transmission intensity, reported intensity of transmission in the catchment area at the time of sample collection; DC subset gating strategy, subsets and markers used to define the subsets which were examined in the study; changes in surface molecule expression, change in activation marker expression after exposure to Plasmodium, relative to healthy controls; serum/plasma cytokines, cytokines assayed for in serum or plasma, change measured relative to healthy controls (no stimulation/no exposure); other effects, other observed changes in cell populations, numbers, or function. *All DC subsets affected. †Surface molecule expression and cytokine secretion for DCs in these studies were measured in supernatants of purified DC cultures after restimulation with pRBCs (85) or TLR ligands (109), as opposed to direct measurement of DC phenotypes from whole blood.*

contribute to phenotypic differences between these DCs and peripheral blood DCs, due to the unique microenvironments of these pregnancy-associated tissues. Gravidity can also be an important contributing factor. Since primigravid women are at the highest risk of severe inflammatory disease [reviewed in (114)], the proportion of women in their first pregnancy should always be accounted for in immunological studies. Inclusion of pregnant non-infected controls is also imperative to determine whether pregnancy itself is a confounding factor affecting DC function during malaria.

Function of DCs From Naturally Exposed Individuals

Three studies of adults with symptomatic malaria carried out in Thailand (98), Brazil (99), and Papua (84) provide insights into how *P. falciparum* immunity develops in lower-transmission settings. Within the Thailand cohort, activation marker expression was not assessed, but circulating numbers of pDCs were significantly reduced in both mild and severe malaria compared to healthy controls. IFN-α levels in the serum increased (83), but it was not established whether this directly correlated with pDC function. The percentage of immature HLA-DR$^+$CD11c$^-$CD123$^-$ cells in circulation increased, while the fractions of circulating CD11c$^+$ cDCs and CD123$^+$ pDCs were decreased. DCs from infected participants were apoptotic (upregulated the apoptotic marker Annexin-V) and were defective at antigen uptake and induction of naïve T cell proliferation in allogeneic T cell activation assays (84). All three cohorts were recruited via clinical admissions, which self-selects for individuals with lower pre-existing immunity and perhaps a more naïve phenotype.

In short, it appears that while impairment is more pronounced in high-transmission settings due to frequent re-infection and higher overall parasite burden, downregulation of DC function is a common feature of malaria. Considering that malaria induces potent inflammation, this DC phenotype may therefore be comparable to what is seen in other inflammatory diseases such as bacterial sepsis (115), HIV (116), or HCV (117). In these patients it is also common to observe reductions in circulating DC numbers (115, 116) and reduced HLA-DR (117) or CD86 (115, 117) expression. Persistent systemic inflammation may therefore explain this reduction in DC function in naturally malaria-infected persons. Again, more rigorous classification of cDC1, cDC2, and pDCs may clarify some of the discrepancies amongst different reports.

Stimulation of DCs From Naturally Exposed Individuals

In a study examining DC responses to TLR stimulation after natural *P. falciparum* infection, DCs from naturally exposed pregnant women in Benin were collected from cord blood (109). Whole PBMC cultures were stimulated with TLR4 ligand LPS, TLR3 ligand polyinosinic:polycytidylic acid (polyI:C), or TLR9 ligand CpG-A ODN to stimulate BDCA-1$^+$ cDC2, BDCA-3$^+$ cDC1, or pDCs, respectively, due to the high expression of each TLR on these specific DC subsets (118). Synthetic hemozoin prepared from haemin chloride was also used for DC stimulation. There was no difference in HLA-DR expression between infected and non-infected women upon stimulation with either TLR ligands or hemozoin. PBMCs from infected women produced more TNF-α and IL-10 in response to CpG-A stimulation, more IFN-γ in response to polyI:C, and more TNF-α in response to hemozoin relative to non-infected women (109).

Only one study to date has stimulated DCs from naturally exposed individuals using pRBCs (85). DCs were purified from the blood of adults from a highly endemic region in Mali at the end of the transmission season and DC activation was compared to that in naïve controls. All exposed individuals were PCR-negative for infection at the time of enrolment (85). When stimulated with pRBCs at a ratio of 3 pRBCs per DC, DCs from these individuals upregulated expression of HLA-DR and CD86 and expressed CCL2, CXCL9, and CXCL10, but did not produce any IL-1β, IL-6, IL-10, or TNF-α (85). In Section 4, this review outlines how a lack of cytokine secretion is commonly observed in *in vitro* studies of *bona fide* DC, and therefore should not necessarily be considered a sign of DC suppression. However, it is interesting that when DCs isolated from malaria-exposed individuals were stimulated with pRBCs following cessation of high malaria transmission (85), DCs could express an activatory surface phenotype in response to stimulation. Thus, it may be that sustained reductions in transmission allow restoration of DC function.

TLR Modulation in DCs by *P. falciparum*

Only one study to date has investigated the ability of *P. falciparum* to modulate TLR expression on DCs as a potential mechanism of immune suppression (98). In this study, individuals with severe or mild *P. falciparum* infection exhibited increased TLR2 expression on cDCs but decreased TLR9 expression on pDCs, with no observable change in TLR4 expression (98) compared to healthy controls. The severity of infection did not impact these changes in TLR expression. Moreover, the fraction of TLR2$^+$ DCs in the periphery decreased during infection (98). TLR2, TLR4, and TLR9 have all been implicated in sensing of *Plasmodium*-derived "danger signals." Namely, TLR2 and TLR4 recognize glycophospholipid (GPI) anchors for merozoite surface proteins (119), and TLR9 detects *Plasmodium* DNA (120). As this is the only study to assess TLR expression profiles during *Plasmodium* infection, it is unclear whether this effect is a common feature of malaria. Nevertheless, it suggests that even low-level *Plasmodium* infections can modulate host responses by downregulating the signals required for APC activation.

The Effects of Natural *P. vivax* Infection on DC Phenotype and Function

Plasmodium vivax is the second major malaria pathogen. It inhabits a broader geographical range than *P. falciparum*, posing a risk to more than 3.2 billion individuals worldwide (121). Its pathogenic potential is enhanced by its ability to become a latent hypnozoite in the liver (7), but as it exclusively infects reticulocytes (122), it is difficult to maintain in culture and remains relatively understudied. Immunity to *P. vivax* has primarily been studied in symptomatic persons who present to healthcare. As the geographical ranges of *P. vivax* and *P. falciparum* transmission overlap, it is often difficult to exclude the immunological impact of prior *P. falciparum* exposure. Nonetheless, it is possible to describe the acute effects of *P. vivax* single-species infection, even though an individual's infection history may be unclear, if diagnosis is sufficiently rigorous. The gold standard for species-specific diagnosis is PCR. However, in resource-poor settings rapid diagnostic tests are typically used.

Due to the paucity of studies from *P. vivax*-exposed individuals it is difficult to conclude the effects of *P. vivax* malaria on DC function. DC numbers decreased during infection, both as a fraction (84, 86) and as total numbers (99). In the latter study, the pDC fraction was increased while cDC numbers decreased (99). Another study observed a decrease in both pDC and cDC fractions, as well as increased DC apoptosis (84). *Plasmodium vivax* malaria has also been reported to down-regulate CD86 expression on DCs (84, 99).

The Effect of Mixed *Plasmodium* Infections on DC Function

Phenotypic analyses of peripheral blood DC from individuals co-infected with two *Plasmodium* spp. support similar reductions in overall DC numbers as seen in individuals experiencing single infections (87, 88, 99). However, it is not yet known whether this correlates to impairments in DC function. A study from Gonçalves et al. in a mesoendemic area of Brazil found that asymptomatic individuals infected with both *P. falciparum* and *P. vivax* had decreased circulating cDCs but increased circulating pDCs (99). Studies in a holoendemic region of Papua found that pDC fractions increased during asymptomatic *P. vivax* but not *P. falciparum* infection, with pDC and BDCA-1$^+$ cDC2 fractions decreasing during acute infection with either species (87, 88). No changes were observed in the BDCA-3$^+$ cDC1 fraction in children or adults during acute or asymptomatic infection with either species (87, 88), in contrast to the findings in African cohorts (96, 100, 102). HLA-DR expression on DCs was increased during asymptomatic *P. vivax* infection (87), but decreased during acute mixed or single-species infections (87, 88).

It is interesting that HLA-DR expression on DCs was positively correlated with parasitaemia in children with asymptomatic *P. vivax* infection, but negatively correlated with parasitaemia in adults with asymptomatic *P. falciparum* infection (87). Thus, it may be that the two major pathogenic *Plasmodium* species polarize the immune system in different ways. This data also suggests fundamental differences in how childrens' and adults' DCs respond to *Plasmodium* exposure—an important factor to keep in mind considering the at-risk populations for either species.

Insights From Controlled Malaria Infection Models

Controlled Human Malaria Infection With *P. falciparum*

The development of a controlled human malaria infection model (CHMI) has produced valuable insights into antimalarial immunity. In one CHMI model which has been used to study DC in malaria, healthy volunteers who are typically malaria-naïve were inoculated with an ultra-low (<180) or low (1,800) dose of *P. falciparum* pRBCs thawed from a pre-prepared biobank. Atovaquone/proguanil or artemether/lumefantrine treatment was administered 6 days post-infection (ultra-low-dose group) or when parasitaemia reached 1,000 parasites per mL (low-dose group). Despite the low parasite biomass of the inoculum in the low-dose group, an estimated 20 times lower than the number of merozoites released from an infected hepatocyte after sporozoite replication (123), DC numbers were significantly decreased in the low-dose group due to increased DC apoptosis (89). Intriguingly, infection-induced apoptosis appeared to be exclusive to HLA-DR$^+$ cells, including DCs. Furthermore, the decrease in DC numbers coincided with the peak of symptomatic malaria, and while cDC numbers recovered to pre-infection levels after drug treatment, pDC numbers remained at 47% of baseline 60 h post-cure (89). HLA-DR expression on pDCs was also impaired. Importantly, DCs from the low-dose group displayed impaired phagocytosis, which persisted for 36 h after drug cure. In contrast, the ultra-low-dose group experienced no symptoms and no DC impairment (89). This study suggests that a certain parasite biomass is required for functional impairment of DCs. However, since the ultra-low-dose group were treated prior to development of symptoms, it is unclear whether an ultra-low dose is sufficient to induce immunity that can control sub-symptomatic parasitaemia, or whether immune impairment would have eventuated if parasitaemia had been allowed to develop.

Function of pDCs and BDCA-1$^+$ cDC2s during CHMI

A second controlled infection study from Loughland et al. utilized a similar low- (1800 pRBCs) and ultra-low (150 pRBCs) dose to more closely study BDCA-1$^+$ cDC2 activation (91) and pDC function (92) after controlled infection. Unlike the prior study, patients were treated upon reaching a parasitaemia of 1000 pRBCs per mL, regardless of initial parasite inoculum. Importantly, both groups experienced a decrease in HLA-DR expression on BDCA-1$^+$ cDC2s that coincided with peak parasitaemia but also persisted 24 h after drug treatment (91). However, only the high-dose group exhibited decreased DC numbers, increased DC apoptosis, and reduced phagocytic capacity relative to baseline (91, 92). A positive association was also observed between phagocytic activity and HLA-DR expression at peak parasitaemia (91).

The ability of DCs to respond to TLR stimulation after exposure to malaria was also evaluated in these studies (91) by restimulating DCs taken from participants during peak parasitaemia. Interestingly, the BDCA-1$^+$ cDC2 from individuals in the high-dose group were impaired in their capacity to upregulate HLA-DR and CD86 in response to stimulation with TLR1/2, TLR4, and TLR7 ligands or whole pRBCs. This impairment was DC-specific, as monocytes' capacity for activation marker expression was unaltered by malaria exposure (91). In contrast, pDCs restimulated with TLR7 and TLR9 ligands upregulated expression of HLA-DR, CD123, and IFN-α, and upregulated CD86 in response to TLR7 stimulation (92). The cDC1 subset was not examined in these studies. These results were similar to TLR stimulations of cord blood

DCs from pregnant women, where CpG-A stimulation of pDCs showed enhancement of cytokine production in infected individuals (109), though caution must be taken when comparing naïve CHMI participants to naturally-exposed pregnant women in Benin.

Together, these studies suggest that a single infection is sufficient to impair cDC function, while pDC function is more resilient. As discussed further on, this highlights a need to further study pDC function during malaria and the potential role of this subset in immunopathology.

CD16⁺ DC function in CHMI

The $CD16^+$ DC subset's status as a steady-state DC rather than a monocyte subset that acquires DC-like characteristics during inflammation remains unclear (27, 124, 125). Improved strategies for distinguishing "true" $CD16^+$ DCs from $CD16^+CD14^-$ monocytes have not yet been established, although a recent single-cell RNAseq study highlighted a population of BDCA-1^-BDCA-$3^-$$CD16^+$ cDCs that is transcriptomically distinct from monocytes (126). However, two studies have examined the role of $CD16^+$ "DCs" in malaria, both in CHMI. Both studies observed that relative to pre-CHMI levels HLA-DR and CD86 expression in these DCs increased after curative treatment (90, 93) and 24 h prior to peak parasitaemia (93). At peak parasitaemia $CD16^+$ DCs had an increased ability to spontaneously produce TNF-α, IL-10, and IL-12. $CD16^+$ DCs collected at peak parasitaemia and restimulated with pRBCs expressed higher levels of IL-10 relative to baseline (93). When restimulated with TLR1/2 or TLR4 ligands, these $CD16^+$ DCs produced high levels of TNF-α and moderate amounts of IL-10 and IL-12. When restimulated with TLR7 ligands, the $CD16^+$ DCs produced TNF-α only (93). While caution must be taken in ascribing *bona fide* DC status to the $CD16^+$ DCs, these studies indicate that these cells are activated during infection and in the highly inflammatory environment post-treatment. Their high production of both TNF-α and IL-10, which may aid in killing or suppression of DCs, respectively, suggest that they could be major contributors to DC modulation, including that seen many days post-treatment and clearance of infection (96).

CHMI With *P. vivax*

Due to the technical difficulty of maintaining *P. vivax* in continuous culture, to date only one CHMI has been published using *P. vivax* (95). In this study, peripheral DC numbers were significantly reduced during acute infection relative to baseline, though this was concurrent with an overall reduction in circulating PBMC (95). All subsets (BDCA-3^+ cDC1s, BDCA-1^+ cDC2s, pDCs, and $CD16^+$ cDCs) upregulated caspase-3 during acute infection and after treatment, suggesting that the reductions in DC numbers in the periphery could also be due to increased apoptosis. Overall, DC impairment by *P. vivax* CHMI was largely similar to what was observed with *P. falciparum* (89, 91); HLA-DR expression on BDCA-1^+ cDC was reduced during acute infection and 24 h after treatment (95).

Ex vivo DCs in *Plasmodium* Infection: What Do We Know?

In summary, *Plasmodium* infection can result in reduced DC numbers in the periphery, both as an absolute number (89, 91, 94, 99) and as a proportion of total leucocytes (82, 97, 101), reportedly due to increased DC apoptosis (84, 89, 91). DC capacity for phagocytosing antigen is also decreased (89, 91), which correlates with DC activation (127), yet their ability to induce T cell proliferation in allogeneic T cell stimulation assays is impaired (84, 89, 96). HLA-DR expression is generally decreased (87–89, 91, 92, 95–97, 100, 101), with some variability between DC subsets (**Table 1**). It is not clear whether the reduction in HLA-DR is due to an increase in new immature DCs in the circulation, or direct downregulation by parasites. There is little consensus regarding other markers: reports on CD83 (84, 97) and CD86 expression are contradictory, though CD86 tends to be elevated on pDCs and decreased on DCs as a total population (83, 84, 91, 100, 101).

It is also unclear whether the decrease in the number of circulating DCs is due to cell death, as suggested by the upregulation of caspase-3 (89, 91, 95) or annexin V (84), or due to increased migration to lymphoid tissues. Decreased DC numbers in both natural and experimental infection, however, coincided with increased serum levels of IL-10 (82, 84, 86, 96, 97, 99) and TNF-α (82, 84, 91, 96, 97, 99), indicating a potential cytokine-mediated mechanism of DC loss. One subset in particular defied this trend: proportions of BDCA-3^+ cDC1s were increased during *P. falciparum* infection (96, 100, 102), and remained elevated for some time after acute infection (96). The BDCA-3^+ cDC1 subset is associated with the initiation of $CD8^+$ killer T cell responses and the secretion of IL-12 (128). It is likely that increases in serum Flt3-L lead to increased numbers of these DC in the periphery during infection, but these circulating DC do not appear to be capable of inducing functional responses. Further complicating the matter, the BDCA-3^+ cDC1 subset is not elevated in single or mixed infections from Papua, where transmission intensity is comparable (87, 88).

Overall, the different methods and markers that have been used to study DCs in this variety of settings makes it difficult to clearly define universal parameters of DC loss of function. It is possible that the DC downregulation described in these studies is a feedback loop promoting regulatory mechanisms in the face of severe malaria-induced inflammation, and that DC downregulation in malaria is not necessarily detrimental to host survival. However, the presence of functional DCs is required for effective vaccine responses, and it is still not clear how malaria-induced DC downregulation affects survival to other pathogens. There is an overall need to understand how these DC phenotypes correlate to clinical outcomes, or at minimum, how malaria directly affects DC function. It will be important to clarify whether DC downregulation during natural infection translates to suppression, namely loss of generalized immune function against non-malaria pathogens or inflammatory stimuli.

In light of this, *in vitro* studies of DC function are vital for three purposes: (1) clarifying the phenotype of DC suppression, (2) determining precisely how malaria modulates DC function, and (3) identifying whether this is through direct interaction with DCs or indirectly through soluble mediators, including cytokines such as TNF-α.

DEFINING THE INTERACTIONS BETWEEN DCS AND *PLASMODIUM* SPP. *IN VITRO*

To date, relatively few studies have investigated direct interactions between *Plasmodium* spp. and human DCs *in vitro*. The majority of these studies have examined the responses of human monocyte-derived DCs (moDCs), since they can be easily generated in large numbers from $CD14^+$ PBMCs or BM monocytes by co-culture with GM-CSF ± IL-4 (129, 130). MoDC are themselves heterogeneous and contain cells with a cDC-like phenotype with high expression of MHC class I and II, BDCA-1, CD40, CD80, and CD11c (129), and macrophage-like cells (131). Transcriptomic analysis indicates that moDC are highly distinct from blood $CD16^+$, cDC2 ($BDCA\text{-}1^+$), and cDC1 ($BDCA\text{-}3^+$) cDC subsets and therefore do not accurately represent the diversity of DC populations or their functions *in vivo* (124). Other recent findings indicate that monocyte-derived inflammatory DCs in humans are more similar to macrophages than to *bona fide* DCs [reviewed in (27, 125)]. Thus, moDCs may not be a representative model for investigating *bona fide* human DC responses. These caveats must be considered when interpreting the data from *in vitro* studies (summarized in **Table 2**).

MoDCs and Intracellular *P. falciparum* Blood-Stage Parasites

Initially, *P. falciparum* pRBCs were thought to suppress moDC function *in vitro* (103) as, when co-cultured with moDCs at a concentration of 100 parasites per DC, they impaired moDC activation via contact-dependent CD36-mediated mechanisms (103). In this study, DCs co-incubated with CD36-binding parasite lines displayed decreased expression of co-stimulatory markers CD40, CD54/ICAM-1, CD80, CD83, and CD86 in response to LPS stimulation, and had a low capacity for inducing allogeneic T cell proliferation (103). Co-incubation with non-CD36 binding parasite lines did not induce the same inhibition. However, a subsequent study found that a high ratio of pRBCs to DCs (100:1) inhibited LPS-induced DC maturation, cytokine production, and allogeneic T cell stimulation regardless of whether the parasite strain had a CD36-binding phenotype, and low doses of parasite (10:1) induced modest DC maturation and autologous T cell proliferation (104). This inhibition of LPS-induced DC maturation with high doses of pRBCs was co-incident with high levels of DC death *in vitro* (104).

Another study reported that a ratio of 10 pRBCs per moDC did not trigger upregulation of HLA-DR, CD83, or CCR7 on moDCs (132), contradicting the findings of Elliott et al. (104). However, the 100:1 ratio induced secretion of IL-1β, IL-6, IL-10, TNF-α, and upregulation of the pro-migratory chemokine receptor CXCR4 (132). Another report indicated that even at a ratio of 25 pRBCs per moDC, moDCs upregulated HLA-DR, CD40, CD80, and CD83 and secreted significantly higher levels of TNF-α, IL-6, and IL-10 (105). At higher pRBC-to-DC ratios, there was a corresponding increase in DC death (105).

Addition of CD40L to pRBC-stimulated moDCs enhanced HLA-DR and CD80 expression while CD86 expression was greatly reduced relative to CD40L alone (105). Secretion of TNF-α, IL-12, and IL-6 was also enhanced, while IL-10 secretion was unchanged relative to CD40L alone (105). In another study, exposure to schizont lysate triggered moDCs to upregulate CD86 but not CD80 or HLA-DR (106). These lysate-stimulated moDCs were capable of inducing allogeneic T cell differentiation into T_H1 and regulatory T cells (T_{REG}), both of which secreted high levels of IFN-γ. T_{REG} induced in this fashion also secreted high levels of IL-10 and TGFβ. Pre-incubating moDCs with parasite lysate did not affect their ability to undergo LPS-driven maturation (106). Lastly, moDCs stimulated with whole schizonts did not upregulate HLA-DR, CD80, or CD86, nor did they express cytokines or chemokines (**Table 2**) (85).

One explanation proposed by Elliott et al. (104) for the conflicting literature on the effect of pRBCs on moDC activation is that high ratios of pRBCs suppress DC function, while low ratios activate DCs (104), though in a recent study moDCs were not activated by stimulation with 3 pRBCs per DC (85). Alternately, variations in methodology are likely to contribute to some of the differences observed: different parasite strains and co-culture periods were used across all studies (**Table 2**). Moreover, the heterogeneity of moDC preparations can vary widely amongst different laboratories. Schizont lysate is also not a proxy for pRBCs as the lytic process produces a mixture of parasite membrane proteins, metabolites, and merozoites (107). The matter is further complicated by the multiple ways of defining "inhibition": whether pRBCs truly block DC activation in response to an external stimulus, and which stimuli in particular are susceptible to this manner of inhibition. Alternatively, it must be clarified whether pRBCs induce higher levels of DC death.

In summary, while a dose-dependent relationship between pRBC dose and moDC inhibition is suggested, this relationship must be substantiated by further studies examining the individual roles that different parasite stimuli, strains, and methodological factors have on the final DC phenotype, preferably focusing on *bona fide* DCs in future studies. A more rigorous definition of moDCs and how "activation" and "inhibition" are defined in these cells, particularly given how different groups have used different activatory cytokine stimulation methods to drive DC-like cells to begin with, will be imperative to resolve existing conflicts.

Monocyte-Derived DCs and Other *Plasmodium* Life Stages

Human DC responses to other *Plasmodium* life stages have been poorly investigated. Only one study has investigated moDC responses to *P. falciparum* merozoites (105). In this study, co-incubation with merozoites resulted in moDC secretion of TNF-α, IL-16, and large amounts of IL-10, despite no changes in costimulatory marker expression (105). Co-incubating merozoites with moDCs in the presence of

TABLE 2 | DC responses after *in vitro* exposure to *P. falciparum*.

References	DC type	Parasite strains	Stimulus type	Post-stimulation phenotype	Cytokines detected	Other effects	Proposed mechanism of action
Monocyte-derived DCs*							
Urban et al. (103)	Monocyte-derived	ITO/A4 ITO/C24 MC T9/96	Whole trophozoite	Decreased: CD40 ICAM-1 CD80 CD83 CD86		Suppressed DC ability to induce T cell activation DC suppression mediated by CD36 binding	CD36 ligation by *PfEMP1*
Urban et al, (71)	Monocyte-derived	ITO/C24 MC	Whole trophozoite	Decreased: HLA-DR CD83	Increased: IL-10 TNF-α Decreased: IFN-γ IL-4 IL-12 No change: TGF-β	Suppressed DC ability to induce T cell activation Co-incubation with CD40L does not restore DC function Apoptotic, but not necrotic cells have similar suppressive function	CD36 ligation by *PfEMP1*
Elliott et al, (104)	Monocyte-derived	ItG E8B CS2 3D7/upsCSBP1-KO	Whole trophozoite	Decreased: HLA-DR CD40 CD80 CD83 CD86	Decreased: IL-10 IL-12	pRBC lysate does not suppress LPS-mediated DC activation and can activate DCs High-dose pRBCs induce DC apoptosis Both CSA- and CD36-binding pRBCs inhibit LPS-mediated T cell proliferation	Parasite-to-DC ratio; *PfEMP1*-independent
Mukherjee and Chauhan, (105)	Monocyte-derived	3D7	Whole trophozoite	Increased: HLA-DR CD80 Decreased: CD86	Increased: TNF-α IL-6 IL-12 No change: IL-10	Stimulate $CD4^+$ T cells to produce IFN-γ, IL-5, and IL-10	Phosphorylation of p38MAPK
			Free merozoite	Decreased: HLA-DR CD80 CD83 No change: CD86	Increased: IL-10 Decreased: IL-12 No change: TNF-α IL-6	Decreased phosphorylation of p38MAPK Stimulate $CD4^+$ T cells to produce IL-10, low amounts of IFN-γ	Modulation of IL-10/IL-12 secretion via altering ERK1/2 signaling
Clemente et al. (106)	Monocyte-derived	3D7	Schizont lysate	Increased: CD86 No change: HLA-DR CD80	No change: IL-10 IL-12	Malaria-exposed DCs induce naive T cell differentiation into T_H1 and T_{REG} subsets	

(Continued)

TABLE 2 | Continued

References	DC type	Parasite strains	Stimulus type	Post-stimulation phenotype	Cytokines detected	Other effects	Proposed mechanism of action
Götz et al. (85)	Monocyte-derived	3D7	Intact schizont	No change: HLA-DR CD80 CD86	No change: CCL2 CCL5 CXCL9 CXCL10 IL-1β IL-6 IL-10 TNFα		
***Bona fide* DCs**[†]							
Pichyangkul et al. (83)	Blood pDC (HLA-DR$^+$CD123$^+$)	TM267R GR MRU LA PH	Intact schizont Schizont lysate	Increased: CD86 CCR7 No change: CD40	Increased: IFN-α No change: TNF-α	Schizont-stimulated pDCs can induce γδ T-cell proliferation and IFN-γ production	
Wu et al. (107)	Blood cDC (HLA-DR$^+$BDCA1$^+$) Blood pDC (HLA-DR$^+$BDCA2$^+$)	3D7	Merozoite lysate		Increased: TNF-α IL-12p40 IFN-α	pDC-cDC cross-signaling is required for cytokine secretion by DCs	Cell-to-cell contact between DC subsets and other immune cells
Gowda et al. (108)	Blood cDC (HLA-DR$^+$BDCA1$^+$) Blood pDC (HLA-DR$^+$BDCA4$^+$)	3D7	Intact trophozoite	Increased: CD36	Increased: TNF-α No change: IL-12p40	DCs internalize CD36-binding pRBCs more efficiently	CD36 ligation by *PfEMP1*
Götz et al. (85)	Blood cDC (HLA-DR$^+$BDCA1$^+$) Blood pDC (HLA-DR$^+$BDCA4$^+$)	3D7	Intact schizont Schizont lysate	Increased: HLA-DR CD40 CD80 CD86	Increased: CCL2 CXCL9 CXCL10 IFN-α No change: CCL5 IL-1β IL-6 IL-10 TNF-α	Low ratios of pRBCs do not suppress DC activation by LPS pRBC-primed DCs induce T_H1-like responses pDC-cDC cross-signaling is required for production of IFN-α, CXCL9 and CXCL10	NFκB- and PPARγ-independent

DC type, how DCs used in this study were derived; Parasite strain(s), P. falciparum laboratory strains used for stimulation; Stimulus type, parasite life stage used in this study and whether parasites were purified or processed.
[*]Monocyte-derived DCs, induced by co-incubating adherent precursors from whole blood with IL-4 and GM-CSF for 24 h (129). [†]Bona fide DCs, DCs which have full DC function after purification from donor tissues, without requiring any cytokine maturation.

CD40L induced high CD86 expression but no increase in other costimulatory surface markers (105). CD40L also induced merozoite-stimulated moDCs to produce high levels of IL-10 (105).

Likewise, only a single study to date has assessed moDC responses to *P. vivax* sporozoites (36). Prior to co-culture, moDCs were matured with TNF-α and LPS and primed, or not, with sporozoite extract. Primed moDC were more efficient than their unprimed counterparts at eliciting IFN-γ secretion and autologous T cell proliferation in DC-T cell co-cultures, and $CD8^+$ T cells stimulated by primed moDCs had greater cytotoxic effector activity against infected HC04 hepatocyte lines (36). It is not yet known how DCs respond to other liver-stage parasites such as hypnozoites, exo-erythrocytic forms, or sexual-stage gametocytes.

Interactions Between *Bona fide* Human DCs and *P. falciparum*

Due to the technical challenges in obtaining large numbers of viable *bona fide* human DCs from peripheral blood, relatively few studies have investigated direct interactions between *ex vivo* blood DCs from healthy donors and *P. falciparum* merozoites or pRBCs (**Table 2**). To date, studies have focused on $BDCA\text{-}1^+$ cDC2 and pDC populations. None have examined the $BDCA\text{-}3^+$ cDC1 subset, likely owing to the rarity of this population. Both merozoites and pRBCs have been shown to induce blood DCs to upregulate CD40, CD80, and CD86 (83, 85), and to secrete IFN-α (83, 85, 107), indicating that *P. falciparum* is capable of activating naïve DCs. Merozoites also triggered production of IL-12p40 and TNF-α (107). Additionally, a ratio of 3 pRBCs per DC resulted in upregulation of HLA-DR and increased expression of the chemokines CCL2, CXCL9, and CXCL10 (IP-10) (85), but did not trigger production of IL-1β, IL-6, IL-10, or TNF-α. Contrary to findings in moDCs, pRBCs did not suppress cytokine responses to LPS in *bona fide* DC, although this may be attributable to the lower pRBC-to-DC ratio used in this study (85). While the authors did not assess whether high doses of pRBCs modulated the ability of *bona fide* DCs to prime naïve T cells, as was shown for moDCs, *bona fide* DCs exposed to low doses of pRBCs were fully functional in their antigen presenting ability, inducing naive T cell proliferation and polarization toward an IFN-γ-producing T_H1 phenotype (85). This does suggest, congruent with moDC studies (104, 106) and some CHMI studies (89, 91), that single, low-parasitaemia blood-stage infections of 10 pRBCs per DC or fewer, equivalent to 200 pRBCs/μL, may induce beneficial DC activation.

It is likely that cross-talk between different DC subsets plays an important role in immune responses to *P. falciparum*. Two studies that have examined this process indicate that DC cross-talk is required for production of TNF-α, IL-12p40 (107), IFN-α, CXCL9, and CXCL10 (also known as IP-10) (85) in response to pRBCs. In the context of antimalarial responses, DC activation appears to be contact-mediated and independent of IFN-α, although partially mediated by the TLR9 pathway (85, 107), expressed by just the pDC subset of human DCs. While cDCs alone are sufficient for inducing T cell activation to pRBCs, the presence of pDCs affects the ability of activated T cells to proliferate and produce cytokines (85). When a mixed culture of pDC and cDC was used in pRBC-primed autologous T cell stimulations, T cells trended toward reduced proliferation and production of IL-10, TNF-α, IFN-γ, and IL-5, but increased IL-2 secretion (85). It is possible that since the overall number of DCs for T cell stimulations was kept constant, reduced T cell activation was a consequence of the reduced proportion of cDCs.

These data highlight a need for future studies to investigate not only the individual roles of *bona fide* DC subsets in immunity to malaria, but also to consider the complexity of the immune response and the influence of cell-to-cell interactions. This should be reflected in the establishment of better *in vitro* models and cell-based systems that more realistically mimic the dynamic interactions and cell behaviors that occur over the course of an immune response *in vivo*.

DC Interactions With Parasite by-Products

The cycle of parasite reproduction is fuelled by a range of host nutrients, not least of which is intraerythrocytic hemoglobin. Hemoglobin breakdown causes accumulation of toxic heme, which the parasite neutralizes by aggregating heme crystals into hemozoin (133). Hemozoin has been proposed to have both suppressive and activatory effects on DCs.

Initial studies reported that purified hemozoin induced CD1a, CD80, and CD83 upregulation and IL-12 secretion from moDCs, whereas monomeric heme and synthetic hemozoin (β-hematin) did not (134). However, these results were contradicted by a subsequent study demonstrating impaired upregulation of HLA-DR, CD40, CD80, CD83, ICAM-1, and CD1a in moDCs pre-incubated with *P. falciparum* hemozoin (135). These conflicting results may be due to the use of different hemozoin sources. Depending on the method of purification, parasite hemozoin can be contaminated with parasite proteins, nucleic acids, and other by-products that can activate alternate pathways. It is possible for even purified hemozoin to adhere to environmental contaminants after purification (133). The altered activity of hemozoin on treatment with phospholipase D (135) and DNAse (136) indicate that contamination with nucleic acids or other parasite metabolites is a likely explanation for the observed variations, particularly since hemozoin has been shown to be a carrier for *Plasmodium* DNA (136).

Murine models have been vital in establishing how hemozoin-malaria DNA complexes activate DCs. Murine Flt3-ligand-induced DCs (137) stimulated with hemozoin chelated to *P. falciparum* DNA secreted high levels of RANTES, IL-12, and TNF-α. In this system, hemozoin assisted in trafficking parasite DNA to intracellular endosomes, and activated DCs via a TLR9- and MyD88-dependent signaling pathway (136). Hemozoin in isolation bound strongly to the murine TLR9 ectodomain while β-hematin, a synthetic form of hemozoin, was unable to activate DCs in this study (136). A subsequent study in humans did observe CD80, CD83, and CXCR4 upregulation on human moDCs after β-hematin stimulation (132), but the β-hematin-induced DCs were unable to induce allogeneic T cell proliferation (132).

Uric acid, another toxic product of *P. falciparum* metabolism, has also been found to upregulate expression of CD80, CD86, and CD11c and to downregulate HLA-DR on purified human blood DCs (138). Uric acid also reportedly stimulated mast cells to produce high levels of the DC growth factor Flt3-L in mice (102). Interestingly, DNAse treatment of uric acid abrogated its activatory effects on DCs (138), similar to what is seen with hemozoin. While uric acid is known to drive inflammation during *Plasmodium* infection through activation of the inflammasome [reviewed in (139)], the role of the inflammasome in anti-malaria DC responses and activation has not been investigated.

Together these studies highlight an important role for *P. falciparum* DNA as an activatory ligand, particularly in activating pDCs and driving production of IFN-α (107). Since only the pDC subset in humans expresses TLR9 [reviewed in (140)], ligation of TLR9 by *P. falciparum* DNA and subsequent cytokine production by pDCs may be one of the primary mechanisms by which human DCs are activated by *Plasmodium* (107, 136). Cytoplasmic pattern recognition receptors for *Plasmodium* DNA, which are expressed in all DC subsets, may also play a prominent role in anti-*Plasmodium* interferon responses (141, 142). Of particular interest are the role of STING-dependent responses in DCs and their role in anti-malaria responses. Considering the wide distribution of *Plasmodium* DNA throughout the host during infection (143), the human DC response to malarial DNA *ex vivo* and *in vitro* is one of the key gaps in knowledge that remains unaddressed.

Murine studies have identified a number of other immunostimulatory *Plasmodium* products, but their role in DC activation has not yet been investigated. Glycosylphosphatidylinositol (GPI) molecules, membrane anchors for *Plasmodium* surface proteins, are known ligands for TLR2 (144), expressed on human cDCs (118). Parasite RNA is known to induce type I IFN via TLR7/MyD88-dependent signaling (145), and TLR7 is highly expressed on human pDCs (118), the major producers of type I IFN. Finally, microvesicles are small organelles of 1 μm of less in size, derived by blebbing of the plasma membrane, which are generated in high volumes during *Plasmodium* infection (146, 147). They can contain a range of parasite material, and are able to induce cytokine secretion from murine (148) and human (149) macrophages. In summary, considering the wide range of immunostimulatory molecules produced by *Plasmodium* spp., it remains interesting that the DC response to malaria is not always activatory. While further studies should continue to identify *Plasmodium* ligands that drive DC activation, this must be studied in combination with the factors that underlie DC suppression in malaria.

DCS AND *PLASMODIUM*: OUTSTANDING QUESTIONS AND FUTURE DIRECTIONS

Immunity to *Plasmodium* is complex, and many aspects of cellular immunity remain poorly understood, particularly the impact of malaria on DC function. A better understanding of DC responses to *Plasmodium* will provide insight into the low efficacy and relative short duration of protection of the current malaria vaccine RTS,S, as well as the slow acquisition of natural immunity in malaria-exposed individuals. One of the most important unresolved questions is one of DC "suppression": namely, whether exposure to *Plasmodium* spp., particularly *P. falciparum*, inhibits the ability of DCs to initiate and orchestrate effective immune responses. Determining precisely how DCs are modulated by *P. falciparum* is crucial for understanding the development of immunity to malaria.

Some of the most interesting insights into the effects of malaria-induced DC impairment come from field studies that stratified patients by severity of infection. Studies that analyzed mild vs. severe malaria cases separately did not observe significant differences in DC phenotype between the groups (82, 102), suggesting that there may be a "tipping point" beyond which DC dysfunction is altered regardless of the severity of clinical presentation. This is underscored by the similarities in DC phenotype between natural exposure and CHMI. The latter are a naïve population, but during acute infection and for at least 24 h after treatment they exhibited similar DC phenotypes to those seen in naturally infected cohorts. Repeated infections could lead to sustained downregulation of DC function. Considering that successful induction of vaccine responses requires DC involvement, the failure of multiple malaria vaccines when transitioning from naïve populations to endemic populations (21, 150) may be due to impaired DC function in these endemic populations prior to vaccination.

Some valuable insights could be obtained by investigating differences in DC impairment between asymptomatic and symptomatic malaria cases. The systemic inflammation characteristic of symptomatic malaria undoubtedly contributes to DC dysfunction. While asymptomatic cases seem to experience similar loss of DC function short-term (87, 88, 99), it may be that they exhibit better recovery of DC function long-term. The phenotypic differences between high- and low-dose inoculation cohorts in CHMI studies (89, 91, 92) suggest that administering curative treatment while parasitaemia is still very low is also effective at limiting DC impairment. The similarities between naturally infected cohorts (**Figure 3**) also suggest that transmission intensity does not have a major impact on DC dysfunction beyond a certain threshold. Studies that follow the long-term effects of malaria exposure on DC function will be essential to clarify whether DC impairment persists after malaria elimination, especially in unstable transmission settings.

Variations in methodology have made it difficult to ascertain the effects *Plasmodium* parasites have on DCs *in vitro*. Particularly, care must be taken when stating that *P. falciparum* "suppresses" DC function *in vitro*: levels of activation lower than that seen in response to positive controls is not necessarily indicative of suppression. True suppression should be defined by an inability of DCs to become activated by known activatory stimuli, particularly pattern recognition receptor ligands. Analyses should also always account for increased cell death, which may result in false reports of suppression. Overall, the data indicates that DC function is not universally suppressed (**Figure 3**). Rather, *Plasmodium* appears to target specific pathways, among them the ones crucial for inducing

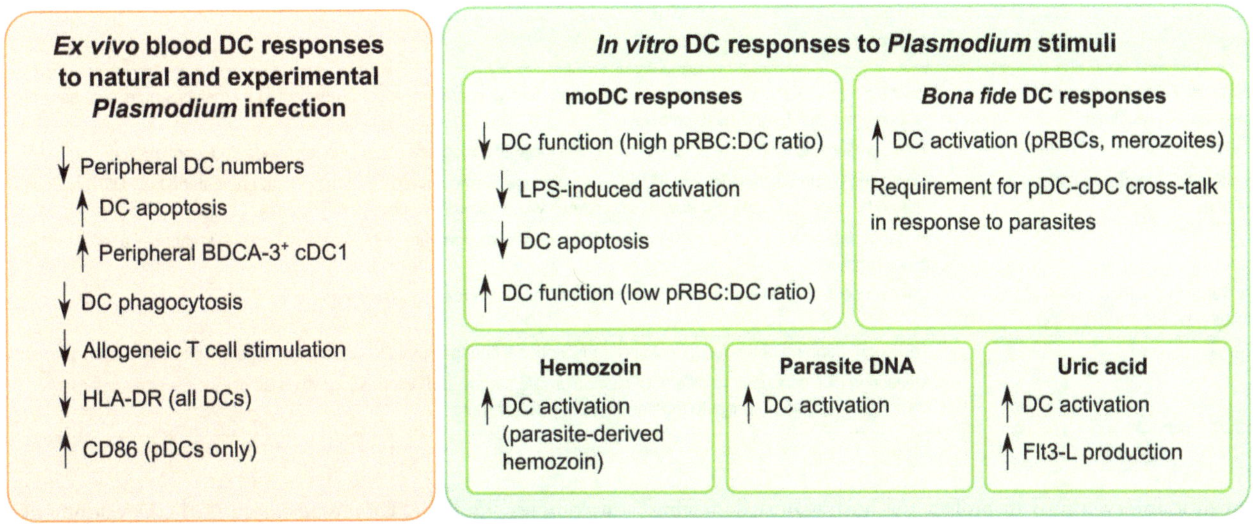

FIGURE 3 | A summary of dendritic cell responses to *Plasmodium*. While the dendritic cell response is heterogeneous, certain trends are evident when examining the entirety of the current literature. Downregulation of dendritic cell function is commonly observed in field studies of infected humans. *In vitro* studies have yielded insight into the complexities of dendritic cell activation by *Plasmodium*, particularly the types of ligands that can trigger an inflammatory response.

naïve T cell proliferation (82, 103, 104), while still allowing DCs to polarize responses toward a T_H1-like phenotype (85, 106). Research into whether the functionality of these T cells is affected relative to other pathogens which induce T_H1 polarization will be important to understand the uniquely *Plasmodium* factors that delay the development of antimalarial immunity.

There also appears to be an important role for DC cross-talk between pDC and cDC subsets (85, 107). This has two crucial implications: first, it warrants further study of how individual DC subsets respond to *Plasmodium* spp. without grouping them into a monolithic conglomeration of HLA-DR^{hi}Lin^{-} cells. In particular, elevation of the circulating BDCA-3^{+} cDC1 subset is a commonly reported phenomenon in field studies but, due to the low frequencies of this rare population, its function in malaria has not been extensively investigated. More rigorous strategies, including cell sorting, should be employed to study how purified subsets respond to malaria. Secondly, pDC cross-talk is essential for production of cytokines such as CXCL10 and IFN-α. CXCL10, also known as IP-10, is majorly implicated in malaria pathogenesis (151–153), and IFN-α has recently been shown to downregulate antimalarial immunity (154, 155). As pDC help is required for production of both of these cytokines, and pDCs are the major producers of IFN-α in malaria (65, 155), strategies to reduce pDC activation in malaria might be beneficial for the longevity of antimalarial immunity. Moreover, malarial DNA has proven to be a potent inflammatory ligand (107, 136), and since only pDCs express TLR9 in humans (118), detection of malarial DNA by pDCs may play a significant role in detrimental cytokine responses, making pDCs an ideal target for strategies to reduce pathogenicity.

Moreover, *ex vivo* and *in vitro* studies depict a complex effect of malaria on the pDC subset. Numbers of circulating pDCs were reduced during natural infection (83, 84, 86, 97, 99) and CHMI (92, 95), though it is unclear whether this is due to pDC death or sequestration. One murine study indicated that pDC could be infected with or endocytose parasites (156). Whether a similar situation exists for human pDC is not known, but it is plausible that large numbers of parasites within pDC could kill these cells, leading to lower circulating numbers. Malaria infection also triggers the upregulation of CCR7 on pDCs (83), suggesting that homing to lymphoid tissues is enhanced during infection. Thus, circulating pDCs may not be the subsets responding to infection, which could explain why pDC activation has not been reported in most field studies. Multiple other factors could also contribute to this perceived lack of pDC activation. Firstly, sustained parasitaemia in malaria-endemic regions may downregulate expression of activatory ligands on circulating pDCs. Secondly, non-conservative gating of pDCs may misrepresent the activation state of this DC population. Thirdly, no field studies to date have measured IFN-α production, which is a direct and functional read-out of pDC activation. *In vitro* studies have observed IFN-α production when pDCs were directly stimulated with parasite products (83, 85, 107). This reinforces the need to study pDC function during malaria to understand whether a loss of pDC numbers in the periphery is associated with a concomitant loss of function.

When interpreting existing literature, it must be kept in mind that the majority of studies have focused on pRBCs and only a minority have examined responses to extracellular forms of the parasite such as merozoites. Considering that DC responses change depending on the parasite life stage (85, 105, 107), even within the relatively limited scope of the blood stages, it will be vital to study the differences between responses to each life stage. Since it is unlikely that a single vaccine will be able to target the entire *Plasmodium* life cycle, understanding the type of responses induced by each life stage is essential for designing new

TABLE 3 | Research priorities in DCs and malaria.

Priority	Approach
Understanding DC functionality to improve malaria vaccines	*In vitro* assays to understand which DC signaling pathways are activated or unaffected by malaria and exploit adjuvant technologies that target these pathways
	Incorporating DC functional assays into vaccine trials as a measure of vaccine relevance and functionality
Correlating DC function in malaria to protection	Controlled human malaria infection studies in naïve and previously exposed cohorts to understand how DC responses are altered by prior exposure and how this correlates with clinical immunity
	In-depth data analyses of how changes in DC phenotypes correlate with protective immune responses and/or overall clinical immunity
Understanding the mechanism of DC modulation by *Plasmodium* spp.	Development of small animal or *in vitro* models to assess human DC responses
	Thorough mapping of the functional and transcriptional changes that DC undergo upon encountering *Plasmodium* spp.
	Measuring DC responses to different *Plasmodium* life stages and determining which life stages have the greatest immunostimulatory potential to facilitate vaccine development

therapeutic interventions to protect the host against damaging immunopathology. A two-pronged "big data" approach could be particularly informative, with the use of RNAseq or proteomics on the DC side to examine immune pathways induced by each parasite life stage, and conversely a proteomics or other—omics-based approach examining the potential immunogens expressed by each parasite life stage. In particular, understanding the pattern recognition receptor signaling pathways which are inhibited or activated by pRBCs would enable more targeted therapies to reverse their suppressive effects. This would inform functional studies, and therefore form a roadmap for vaccine strategies or other therapeutic approaches that could induce potent, long-lasting antimalarial immunity.

A primary caveat of the current literature on human DC responses to malaria, particularly in field studies of infected individuals, is that all studies have looked at circulating blood DCs. It may be that mature DCs migrate into the tissues while immature DCs remain in circulation. Therefore, care should be taken not to generalize the phenotype of these circulating DCs to the responses of liver, spleen or bone marrow tissue-resident DCs, which may have greater functional relevance. Understandably, obtaining tissue-resident cells directly from humans is difficult and ethically challenging. Thus, models such as humanized mice, which produce DCs functionally similar to those found in humans (57, 157), are a promising system to study DCs with a tissue-resident phenotype. While a humanized mouse that is able to support the entire *Plasmodium* life cycle is still out of reach, recent technological improvements have enabled development of models that allow study of immunity to specific life stages [reviewed in (158)]. For example, humanized liver mice could shed light on the elusive phenomenon of liver-stage immunity, while mice with humanized immune systems could provide better insight into cell-mediated mechanisms of protection against the blood stage. Development of a complete humanized mouse model for *Plasmodium* would be invaluable for human immunological research and vaccine development.

Organoids, miniature models of organ function, have proven useful in studying tissues such as the liver (159) and intestine (160). An intestinal organoid model has already been used to study transcriptomic regulation of another Apicomplexan with a complex life cycle, *Cryptosporidium* (161). Development of a splenic organoid could be used for development of functional tissue DCs and enable further study of blood-stage malaria, as well as other blood-borne diseases (162). Liver and skin organoids would also be invaluable for studying the pre-symptomatic phase of the life cycle, and aid development of a vaccine that confers sterile immunity.

Finally, data from *in vitro* studies using moDCs as a model may not be representative of the interactions between *Plasmodium* and steady-state DCs. Both moDCs and *bona fide* DCs show pro- and non-inflammatory responses to *Plasmodium* stimulation, but phenotypic and transcriptomic differences between them highlight that the moDC phenotype is pronouncedly different and may not necessarily be generalizable (125). It was previously thought that moDCs might be analogous to $CD16^+$ DCs. However, recent findings outline that moDCs and $CD16^+$ DCs exist as separate populations in the steady-state (124, 125), and while they may have convergent functions during inflammation, this has not yet been conclusively shown. Therefore, caution should be taken when describing DC-parasite interactions using results generated with moDCs: while it is likely that moDC-like APCs are generated during the course of *Plasmodium* infection, moDCs may not accurately reflect the behavior of steady-state DC populations.

This review has outlined many facets of DC function in malaria that are not well understood (**Table 3**). Firstly, DCs from naïve individuals appear to respond differently to each malaria life stage. These responses should be compared to those seen in exposed individuals for a better understanding of how prolonged malaria exposure affects immune recognition. Secondly, we must further develop an understanding of how the DC phenotypes we observe *ex vivo* and *in vitro* translate into effectiveness, duration, and quality of antimalarial responses. Including DC studies in vaccine trials would help to address which elements best describe a beneficial DC response. This should be supplemented by more studies of DCs in natural infection against comparable non-exposed donors. Thirdly, there is a need for better models to examine DC function in malaria. DC studies of the future should focus as much as possible upon *bona fide* DCs, and seek to develop new models that will permit a more in-depth study of how DC function is altered by the malaria parasite.

To conclude, the complexities of DCs make them a relatively understudied cell type in the context of malaria, where they have a potentially pivotal role in the regulation of antimalarial immunity. Many gaps in knowledge remain to be addressed, and there is a prominent need for novel technologies to bridge the gap. A deeper, more rigorous understanding of how *ex vivo* and *in vitro Plasmodium*-exposed DC phenotypes correlate with effective immunity, and the mechanisms that regulate DC interactions with *Plasmodium* will grant valuable insight into the acquisition of immunity, and form a basis for the development of better vaccines.

AUTHOR CONTRIBUTIONS

XZY wrote the first draft of the manuscript, which was reviewed and edited by RJL, JGB, and MOK. XZY and RJL prepared tables and figures. All authors have read and revised the manuscript.

FUNDING

Funding was provided by NHMRC (Senior Research Fellowships to JGB and MOK; Early Career Fellowship to RJL; Program Grant to JGB; Project grant to MOK). Burnet Institute was supported by the NHMRC Independent Research Institutes Support Scheme and a Victorian State Government Operational Infrastructure Grant. JGB is a member of the Australian Center for Research Excellence in Malaria Elimination (ACREME), funded by the NHMRC.

ACKNOWLEDGMENTS

We would like to thank Ms. G. Stuart for providing graphical elements for **Figure 1**.

REFERENCES

1. Laveran A. *Un Nouveau Parasite Trouvé Dans le Sang de Malades Atteints de Fièvre Palustre: Origine Parasitaire des Accidents de L'impaludisme.* Paris: Bulletins et mémoires de la Société Médicale des Hôpitaux (1881) p. 158–64.
2. Grassi B. *Studi di uno Zoologo Sulla Malaria.* Rome: R. Accademia dei Lincei. (1900). Available online at: https://archive.org/details/studidiunozoolog00gras/page/n8
3. Shortt HE, Garnham PCC. The pre-erythrocytic stage of human malaria, *Plasmodium vivax*. *Br Med J.* (1948) 1:547.
4. Shortt HE, Fairley NH, Covell G, Shute PG, Garnham PCC. Pre-erythrocytic stage of *Plasmodium falciparum*. *BMJ.* (1949) 2:1006–1008. doi: 10.1136/bmj.2.4635.1006
5. Florens L, Washburn MP, Raine JD, Anthony RM, Grainger M, Haynes JD, et al. A proteomic view of the *Plasmodium falciparum* life cycle. *Nature.* (2002) 419:520–6. doi: 10.1038/nature01107
6. Bejon P, Andrews L, Andersen RF, Dunachie S, Webster D, Walther M, et al. Calculation of liver-to-blood inocula, parasite growth rates, and preerythrocytic vaccine efficacy, from serial quantitative polymerase chain reaction studies of volunteers challenged with malaria sporozoites. *J Infect Dis.* (2005) 191:619–26. doi: 10.1086/427243
7. Krotoski W. Discovery of the hypnozoite and a new theory of malarial relapse. *Trans R Soc Trop Med Hyg.* (1985) 79:1–11.
8. Mueller I, Galinski MR, Baird JK, Carlton JM, Kochar DK, Alonso PL, et al. Key gaps in the knowledge of *Plasmodium vivax*, a neglected human malaria parasite. *Lancet Infect Dis.* (2009) 9:555–66. doi: 10.1016/S1473-3099(09)70177-X
9. Cowman AF, Crabb BS. Invasion of red blood cells by malaria parasites. *Cell.* (2006) 124:755–66. doi: 10.1016/j.cell.2006.02.006
10. McMillan PJ, Millet C, Batinovic S, Maiorca M, Hanssen E, Kenny S, et al. Spatial and temporal mapping of the PfEMP1 export pathway in *Plasmodium falciparum*. *Cell Microbiol.* (2013) 15:1401–18. doi: 10.1111/cmi.12125
11. Thomson D. I.–A research into the production, life and death of crescents in malignant tertian malaria, in treated and untreated cases, by an enumerative method. *Ann Trop Med Parasitol.* (1911) 5:57–81. doi: 10.1080/00034983.1911.11686341
12. Day KP, Hayward RE, Dyer M. The biology of *Plasmodium falciparum* transmission stages. *Parasitology.* (1998) 116(Suppl.):S95–109.
13. Boyd M, Kitchen S. On the infectiousness of patients infected with *Plasmodium vivax* and *Plasmodium falciparum*. *Am J Trop Med Hyg.* (1937) 17:253–62.
14. McKenzie FE, Jeffery GM, Collins WE. Gametocytemia and fever in human malaria infections. *J Parasitol.* (2007) 93:627–33. doi: 10.1645/GE-1052R.1
15. Smalley ME, Abdalla S, Brown J. The distribution of *Plasmodium falciparum* in the peripheral blood and bone marrow of Gambian children. *Trans R Soc Trop Med Hyg.* (1981) 75:103–5.
16. Thomson D. The origin and development of gametes (Crescents) in malignant tertian malaria: some observations on flagellation, etc. *Ann Trop Med Parasitol.* (1914) 8:85–104. doi: 10.1080/00034983.1914.11687643
17. Thomson JG, Robertson A. The structure and development of *plasmodium falciparum* gametocytes in the internal organs and peripheral circulation. *Trans R Soc Trop Med Hyg.* (1935) 29:31–40. doi: 10.1016/S0035-9203(35)90015-3
18. Lensen A, Bril A, van de Vegte M, van Gemert GJ, Eling W, Sauerwein R. *Plasmodium falciparum*: infectivity of cultured, synchronized gametocytes to mosquitoes. *Exp Parasitol.* (1999) 103:101–3. doi: 10.1006/expr.1998.4354
19. Cohen S, McGregor IA, Carrington SP. Gamma-globulin and acquired immunity to human malaria. *Nature.* (1961) 192:733–7. doi: 10.1038/192733a0
20. Fowkes FJI, Boeuf P, Beeson JG. Immunity to malaria in an era of declining malaria transmission. *Parasitology.* (2016) 143:139–53. doi: 10.1017/S0031182015001249
21. Olotu A, Fegan G, Wambua J, Nyangweso G, Leach A, Lievens M, et al. Seven-year efficacy of RTS,S/AS01 malaria vaccine among young African children. *N Engl J Med.* (2016) 374:2519–29. doi: 10.1056/NEJMoa1515257
22. Neafsey DE, Juraska M, Bedford T, Benkeser D, Valim C, Griggs A, et al. Genetic diversity and protective efficacy of the RTS,S/AS01 malaria vaccine. *N Engl J Med.* (2015) 373:2025–37. doi: 10.1056/NEJMoa1505819
23. White MT, Verity R, Griffin JT, Asante KP, Owusu-Agyei S, Greenwood B, et al. Immunogenicity of the RTS,S/AS01 malaria vaccine and implications for duration of vaccine efficacy: Secondary analysis of data from a phase 3 randomised controlled trial. *Lancet Infect Dis.* (2015) 15:1450–8. doi: 10.1016/S1473-3099(15)00239-X
24. Freudenthal PS, Steinman RM. The distinct surface of human blood dendritic cells, as observed after an improved isolation method. *Proc Natl Acad Sci USA.* (1990) 87:7698–702. doi: 10.1073/pnas.87.19.7698
25. Orsini G, Legitimo A, Failli A, Massei F, Biver P, Consolini R. Enumeration of human peripheral blood dendritic cells throughout the life. *Int Immunol.* (2012) 24:347–56. doi: 10.1093/intimm/dxs006
26. Chen XQ, Liu XF, Liu WH, Guo W, Yu Q, Wang CY. Comparative analysis of dendritic cell numbers and subsets between smoking and control subjects in the peripheral blood. *Int J Clin Exp Pathol.* (2013) 6:290–6.
27. Macri C, Pang ES, Patton T, O'Keeffe M. Dendritic cell subsets. *Semin Cell Dev Biol.* (2018) 84:11–21. doi: 10.1016/j.semcdb.2017.12.009

28. Dzionek A, Fuchs A, Schmidt P, Zysk M, Miltenyi S, Buck DW, et al. BDCA-2, BDCA-3, and BDCA-4: three markers for distinct subsets of dendritic cells in human peripheral blood. *J Immunol.* (2000) 165:6037–46. doi: 10.4049/jimmunol.165.11.6037
29. Summers KL, Hock BD, McKenzie JL, Hart DN. Phenotypic characterization of five dendritic cell subsets in human tonsils. *Am J Pathol.* (2001) 159:285–95. doi: 10.1016/S0002-9440(10)61694-X
30. MacDonald KPA, Munster DJ, Clark GJ, Dzionek A, Schmitz J, Hart DNJ, et al. Characterization of human blood dendritic cell subsets. *Blood.* (2002) 100:4512–20. doi: 10.1182/blood-2001-11-0097
31. Hambleton S, Salem S, Bustamante J, Bigley V, Boisson-Dupuis S, Azevedo J, et al. IRF8 mutations and human dendritic-cell immunodeficiency. *N Engl J Med.* (2011) 365:127–38. doi: 10.1056/NEJMoa1100066
32. Meera S, Madhuri T, Manisha G, Ramesh P. Irreversible loss of pDCs by apoptosis during early HIV infection may be a critical determinant of immune dysfunction. *Viral Immunol.* (2010) 23:241–9. doi: 10.1089/vim.2009.0112
33. Ku C-L, von Bernuth H, Picard C, Zhang S-Y, Chang H-H, Yang K, et al. Selective predisposition to bacterial infections in IRAK-4-deficient children: IRAK-4-dependent TLRs are otherwise redundant in protective immunity. *J Exp Med.* (2007) 204:2407–22. doi: 10.1084/jem.20070628
34. Bigley V, Haniffa M, Doulatov S, Wang X-N, Dickinson R, McGovern N, et al. The human syndrome of dendritic cell, monocyte, B and NK lymphoid deficiency. *J Exp Med.* (2011) 208:227–34. doi: 10.1084/jem.20101459
35. da Silva HB, Caetano SS, Monteiro I, Gómez-Conde I, Hanson K, Penha-Gonçalves C, et al. Early skin immunological disturbance after Plasmodium-infected mosquito bites. *Cell Immunol.* (2012) 277:22–32. doi: 10.1016/j.cellimm.2012.06.003
36. Vichchathorn P, Jenwithisuk R, Leelaudomlipi S, Tungpradabkul S, Hongeng S, Cui L, et al. Induction of specific immune responses against the *Plasmodium vivax* liver-stage via *in vitro* activation by dendritic cells. *Parasitol Int.* (2006) 55:187–93. doi: 10.1016/j.parint.2006.04.001
37. Menezes RG, Pant S, Kharoshah MA, Senthilkumaran S, Arun M, Nagesh KR, et al. Autopsy discoveries of death from malaria. *Leg Med.* (2012) 14:111–115. doi: 10.1016/j.legalmed.2012.01.007
38. Farfour E, Charlotte F, Settegrana C, Miyara M, Buffet P. The extravascular compartment of the bone marrow: a niche for *Plasmodium falciparum* gametocyte maturation? *Malar J.* (2012) 11:285. doi: 10.1186/1475-2875-11-285
39. Rogers NJ, Hall BS, Obiero J, Targett G a, Sutherland CJ. A model for sequestration of the transmission stages of *Plasmodium falciparum*: adhesion of gametocyte-infected erythrocytes to human bone marrow cells. *Infect Immun.* (2000) 68:3455–62. doi: 10.1128/IAI.68.6.3455-3462.2000
40. Malleret B, Li A, Zhang R, Tan KSW, Suwanarusk R, Claser C, et al. *Plasmodium vivax*: restricted tropism and rapid remodeling of CD71-positive reticulocytes. *Blood.* (2015) 125:1314–1324. doi: 10.1182/blood-2014-08-596015
41. Obaldia N, Meibalan E, Sa JM, Ma S, Clark MA, Mejia P, et al. Bone marrow is a major parasite reservoir in *Plasmodium vivax* infection. *MBio.* (2018) 9:e00625-18. doi: 10.1128/mBio.00625-18
42. Xia S, Guo Z, Xu X, Yi H, Wang Q, Cao X. Hepatic microenvironment programs hematopoietic progenitor differentiation into regulatory dendritic cells, maintaining liver tolerance. *Blood.* (2008) 112:3175–85. doi: 10.1182/blood-2008-05-159921
43. Goddard S, Youster J, Morgan E, Adams DH. Interleukin-10 secretion differentiates dendritic cells from human liver and skin. *Am J Pathol.* (2004) 164:511–9. doi: 10.1016/S0002-9440(10)63141-0
44. Mittag D, Proietto AI, Loudovaris T, Mannering SI, Vremec D, Shortman K, et al. Human dendritic cell subsets from spleen and blood are similar in phenotype and function but modified by donor health status. *J Immunol.* (2011) 186:6207–17. doi: 10.4049/jimmunol.1002632
45. Hopp CS, Chiou K, Ragheb DRT, Salman AM, Khan SM, Liu AJ, et al. Longitudinal analysis of plasmodium sporozoite motility in the dermis reveals component of blood vessel recognition. *Elife.* (2015) 4:1–21. doi: 10.7554/eLife.07789
46. Roestenberg M, Teirlinck AC, McCall MBB, Teelen K, Makamdop KN, Wiersma J, et al. Long-term protection against malaria after experimental sporozoite inoculation: an open-label follow-up study. *Lancet.* (2011) 377:1770–6. doi: 10.1016/S0140-6736(11)60360-7
47. Roestenberg M, McCall MBB, Hopman J, Wiersma J, Luty AJF, van Gemert GJ, et al. Protection against a malaria challenge by sporozoite inoculation. *N Engl J Med.* (2009) 361:468–77. doi: 10.1056/NEJMoa0805832
48. Bijker EM, Teirlinck AC, Schats R, Van Gemert GJ, Van De Vegte-Bolmer M, Van Lieshout L, et al. Cytotoxic markers associate with protection against malaria in human volunteers immunized with *plasmodium Falciparum* Sporozoites. *J Infect Dis.* (2014) 210:1605–15. doi: 10.1093/infdis/jiu293
49. Amino R, Thiberge S, Martin B, Celli S, Shorte S, Frischknecht F, et al. Quantitative imaging of Plasmodium transmission from mosquito to mammal. *Nat Med.* (2006) 12:220–4. doi: 10.1038/nm1350
50. Chakravarty S, Cockburn IA, Kuk S, Overstreet MG, Sacci JB, Zavala F. CD8+ T lymphocytes protective against malaria liver stages are primed in skin-draining lymph nodes. *Nat Med.* (2007) 13:1035–41. doi: 10.1038/nm1628
51. Leiriao P, Mota MM, Rodriguez A. Apoptotic *Plasmodium*- infected hepatocytes provide antigens to liver dendritic cells. *J Infect Dis.* (2005) 191:1576–81. doi: 10.1086/429635
52. Bamboat ZM, Stableford JA, Plitas G, Burt BM, Nguyen HM, Welles AP, et al. Human liver dendritic cells promote T cell hyporesponsiveness. *J Immunol.* (2009) 182:1901–11. doi: 10.4049/jimmunol.0803404
53. Pillarisetty VG, Shah AB, Miller G, Bleier JI, DeMatteo RP. Liver dendritic cells are less immunogenic than spleen dendritic cells because of differences in subtype composition. *J Immunol.* (2004) 172:1009–17. doi: 10.4049/jimmunol.172.2.1009
54. Bosma BM, Metselaar HJ, Mancham S, Boor PPC, Kusters JG, Kazemier G, et al. Characterization of human liver dendritic cells in liver grafts and perfusates. *Liver Transplant.* (2006) 12:384–93. doi: 10.1002/lt.20659
55. Sack BK, Mikolajczak SA, Fishbaugher M, Vaughan AM, Flannery EL, Nguyen T, et al. Humoral protection against mosquito bite-transmitted *Plasmodium falciparum* infection in humanized mice. *Npj Vaccines.* (2017) 2:27. doi: 10.1038/s41541-017-0028-2
56. Yang ASP, O'Neill MT, Jennison C, Lopaticki S, Allison CC, Armistead JS, et al. Cell traversal activity is important for *Plasmodium falciparum* liver infection in humanized mice. *Cell Rep.* (2017) 18:3105–16. doi: 10.1016/j.celrep.2017.03.017
57. Ding Y, Wilkinson A, Idris A, Fancke B, O'Keeffe M, Khalil D, et al. FLT3-ligand treatment of humanized mice results in the generation of large numbers of CD141+ and CD1c+ dendritic cells *in vivo*. *J Immunol.* (2014) 192:1982–9. doi: 10.4049/jimmunol.1302391
58. Aguilar R, Magallon-Tejada A, Achtman AH, Moraleda C, Joice R, Cisteró P, et al. Molecular evidence for the localization of *Plasmodium falciparum* immature gametocytes in bone marrow. *Blood.* (2014) 123:959–66. doi: 10.1182/blood-2013-08-520767
59. Joice R, Nilsson SK, Montgomery J, Dankwa S, Egan E, Morahan B, et al. *Plasmodium falciparum* transmission stages accumulate in the human bone marrow. *Sci Transl Med.* (2014) 6:244re5. doi: 10.1126/scitranslmed.3008882
60. Wickramasinghe SN, Phillips RE, Looareesuwan S, Warrell DA, Hughes M. The bone marrow in human cerebral malaria: parasite sequestration within sinusoids. *Br J Haematol.* (1987) 66:295–306.
61. Ru Y, Mao B-Y, Zhang F, Pang T, Zhao S, Liu J, et al. Invasion of erythroblasts by *Pasmodium vivax:* a new mechanism contributing to malarial anemia. *Ultrastruct Pathol.* (2009) 33:236–42. doi: 10.3109/01913120903251643
62. Avril M, Brazier AJ, Melcher M, Sampath S, Smith JD. DC8 and DC13 var genes associated with severe malaria bind avidly to diverse endothelial cells. *PLoS Pathog.* (2013) 9:e1003430. doi: 10.1371/journal.ppat.1003430
63. Reeves RK, Fultz PN. Characterization of plasmacytoid dendritic cells in bone marrow of pig-tailed macaques. *Clin Vaccine Immunol.* (2008) 15:35–41. doi: 10.1128/CVI.00309-07
64. Feuerer M, Beckhove P, Garbi N, Mahnke Y, Limmer A, Hommel M, et al. Bone marrow as a priming site for T-cell responses to blood-borne antigen. *Nat Med.* (2003) 9:1151–7. doi: 10.1038/nm914
65. Spaulding E, Fooksman D, Moore JM, Saidi A, Feintuch CM, Reizis B, et al. STING-licensed macrophages prime type I IFN production by plasmacytoid dendritic cells in the bone marrow during severe *Plasmodium yoelii* malaria. *PLoS Pathog.* (2016) 12:e1005975. doi: 10.1371/journal.ppat.1005975

66. Junqueira C, Barbosa CRR, Costa PAC, Teixeira-Carvalho A, Castro G, Sen Santara S, et al. Cytotoxic CD8+T cells recognize and kill *Plasmodium vivax*-infected reticulocytes. *Nat Med.* (2018) 24:1330–6. doi: 10.1038/s41591-018-0117-4
67. M Eriksson E, Sampaio NG, Schofield L. Toll-like receptors and malaria – sensing and susceptibility. *J Trop Dis.* (2013) 2:1–7. doi: 10.4172/2329-891X.1000126
68. Gazzinelli RT, Kalantari P, Fitzgerald KA, Golenbock DT. Innate sensing of malaria parasites. *Nat Rev Immunol.* (2014) 14:744–57. doi: 10.1038/nri3742
69. Trubowitz S, Masek B. *Plasmodium falciparum*: phagocytosis by polymorphonuclear leukocytes. *Science.* (1968) 162:273–4. doi: 10.1126/science.162.3850.273
70. Chan J, Howell KB, Reiling L, Ataide R, Mackintosh CL, Fowkes FJI, et al. Targets of antibodies against *Plasmodium falciparum*-infected erythrocytes in malaria immunity. *J Clin Invest.* (2012) 122:3227–38. doi: 10.1172/JCI62182
71. Urban BC, Willcox N, Roberts DJ. A role for CD36 in the regulation of dendritic cell function. *Proc Natl Acad Sci USA.* (2001) 98:8750–5. doi: 10.1073/pnas.151028698
72. Miller LH, Baruch DI, Marsh K, Doumbo OK. The pathogenic basis of malaria. *Nature.* (2002) 415:673–9. doi: 10.1038/415673a
73. Lundie RJ, de Koning-Ward TF, Davey GM, Nie CQ, Hansen DS, Lau LS, et al. Blood-stage Plasmodium infection induces CD8+ T lymphocytes to parasite-expressed antigens, largely regulated by CD8alpha+ dendritic cells. *Proc Natl Acad Sci USA.* (2008) 105:14509–14. doi: 10.1073/pnas.0806727105
74. Jung S, Unutmaz D, Wong P, Sano G-I, De los Santos K, Sparwasser T, et al. *In vivo* depletion of CD11c+ dendritic cells abrogates priming of CD8+ T cells by exogenous cell-associated antigens. *Immunity.* (2002) 17:211–20. doi: 10.1016/S1074-7613(02)00365-5
75. Voisine C, Mastelic B, Sponaas AM, Langhorne J. Classical CD11c+ dendritic cells, not plasmacytoid dendritic cells, induce T cell responses to *Plasmodium chabaudi* malaria. *Int J Parasitol.* (2010) 40:711–9. doi: 10.1016/j.ijpara.2009.11.005
76. Ocaña-Morgner C, Mota MM, Rodriguez A. Malaria blood stage suppression of liver stage immunity by dendritic cells. *J Exp Med.* (2003) 197:143–51. doi: 10.1084/jem.20021072
77. Wilson NS, Behrens GMN, Lundie RJ, Smith CM, Waithman J, Young L, et al. Systemic activation of dendritic cells by Toll-like receptor ligands or malaria infection impairs cross-presentation and antiviral immunity. *Nat Immunol.* (2006) 7:165–72. doi: 10.1038/ni1300
78. Millington OR, Gibson VB, Rush CM, Zinselmeyer BH, Phillips RS, Garside P, et al. Malaria impairs T cell clustering and immune priming despite normal signal 1 from dendritic cells. *PLoS Pathog.* (2007) 3:1380–7. doi: 10.1371/journal.ppat.0030143
79. Lundie RJ, Young LJ, Davey GM, Villadangos J a, Carbone FR, Heath WR, et al. Blood-stage *Plasmodium berghei* infection leads to short-lived parasite-associated antigen presentation by dendritic cells. *Eur J Immunol.* (2010) 40:1674–81. doi: 10.1002/eji.200939265
80. Piva L, Tetlak P, Claser C, Karjalainen K, Renia L, Ruedl C. Cutting edge: Clec9A+ dendritic cells mediate the development of experimental cerebral malaria. *J Immunol.* (2012) 189:1128–32. doi: 10.4049/jimmunol.1201171
81. deWalick S, Amante FH, McSweeney K a, Randall LM, Stanley AC, Haque A, et al. Cutting edge: conventional dendritic cells are the critical APC required for the induction of experimental cerebral malaria. *J Immunol.* (2007) 178:6033–7. doi: 10.4049/jimmunol.178.10.6033
82. Urban BC, Mwangi T, Ross A, Kinyanjui S, Mosobo M, Kai O, et al. Peripheral blood dendritic cells in children with acute *Plasmodium falciparum* malaria. *Blood.* (2001) 98:2859–61. doi: 10.1182/blood.V98.9.2859
83. Pichyangkul S, Yongvanitchit K, Kum-arb U, Hemmi H, Akira S, Krieg AM, et al. Malaria blood stage parasites activate human plasmacytoid dendritic cells and murine dendritic cells through a Toll-like receptor 9-dependent pathway. *J Immunol.* (2004) 172:4926–33. doi: 10.4049/jimmunol.172.8.4926
84. Pinzon-Charry A, Woodberry T, Kienzle V, McPhun V, Minigo G, Lampah DA, et al. Apoptosis and dysfunction of blood dendritic cells in patients with falciparum and vivax malaria. *J Exp Med.* (2013) 210:1635–46. doi: 10.1084/jem.20121972
85. Götz A, Tang MS, Ty MC, Arama C, Ongoiba A, Doumtabe D, et al. Atypical activation of dendritic cells by *Plasmodium falciparum*. *Proc Natl Acad Sci USA.* (2017) 114:E10568–77. doi: 10.1073/pnas.1708383114
86. Jangpatarapongsa K, Chootong P, Sattabongkot J, Chotivanich K, Sirichaisinthop J, Tungpradabkul S, et al. *Plasmodium vivax* parasites alter the balance of myeloid and plasmacytoid dendritic cells and the induction of regulatory T cells. *Eur J Immunol.* (2008) 38:2697–705. doi: 10.1002/eji.200838186
87. Kho S, Marfurt J, Noviyanti R, Kusuma A, Piera KA, Burdam FH, et al., Preserved dendritic cell HLA-DR expression and reduced regulatory T cell activation in asymptomatic *Plasmodium falciparum* and *P. vivax* infection. *Infect Immun.* (2015) 83:3224–32. doi: 10.1128/IAI.00226-15
88. Kho S, Marfurt J, Handayuni I, Pava Z, Noviyanti R, Kusuma A, et al. Characterization of blood dendritic and regulatory T cells in asymptomatic adults with sub-microscopic *Plasmodium falciparum* or *Plasmodium vivax* infection. *Malar J.* (2016) 15:328. doi: 10.1186/s12936-016-1382-7
89. Woodberry T, Minigo G, Piera K a, Amante FH, Pinzon-Charry A, Good MF, et al. Low-level *Plasmodium falciparum* blood-stage infection causes dendritic cell apoptosis and dysfunction in healthy volunteers. *J Infect Dis.* (2012) 206:333–40. doi: 10.1093/infdis/jis366
90. Teirlinck AC, Roestenberg M, Bijker EM, Hoffman SL, Sauerwein RW, Scholzen A. *Plasmodium falciparum* infection of human volunteers activates monocytes and CD16+ dendritic cells and induces upregulation of CD16 and CD1c expression. *Infect Immun.* (2015) 83:3732–9. doi: 10.1128/IAI.00473-15
91. Loughland JR, Minigo G, Burel J, Tipping PE, Piera KA, Amante FH, et al. Profoundly reduced CD1c + myeloid dendritic cell HLA-DR and CD86 expression and increased tumor necrosis factor production in experimental human blood-stage malaria infection. *Infect Immun.* (2016) 84:1403–12. doi: 10.1128/IAI.01522-15
92. Loughland JR, Minigo G, Sarovich DS, Field M, Tipping PE, Montes de Oca M, et al. Plasmacytoid dendritic cells appear inactive during sub-microscopic *Plasmodium falciparum* blood-stage infection, yet retain their ability to respond to TLR stimulation. *Sci Rep.* (2017) 7:2596. doi: 10.1038/s41598-017-02096-2
93. Loughland JR, Woodberry T, Boyle MJ, Tipping PE, Piera KA, Amante FH, et al. *Plasmodium falciparum* activates CD16+ dendritic cells to produce TNF and IL-10 in subpatent malaria. *J Infect Dis.* (2018) 219:660–71. doi: 10.1093/infdis/jiy555
94. Breitling LP, Fendel R, Mordmueller B, Adegnika AA, Kremsner PG, Luty AJF. Cord blood dendritic cell subsets in African newborns exposed to *Plasmodium falciparum* in utero. *Infect Immun.* (2006) 74:5725–9. doi: 10.1128/IAI.00682-06
95. Woodberry T, Loughland JR, Minigo G, Burel JG, Amante FH, Piera KA, et al. Early immune regulatory changes in a primary controlled human *Plasmodium vivax* infection: CD1c + myeloid dendritic cell maturation arrest, induction of the kynurenine pathway, and regulatory T cell activation. *Infect Immun.* (2017) 85:e00986-16. doi: 10.1128/IAI.00986-16
96. Urban BC, Cordery D, Shafi MJ, Bull PC, Newbold CI, Williams TN, et al. The frequency of BDCA3-positive dendritic cells is increased in the peripheral circulation of Kenyan children with severe malaria. *Infect Immun.* (2006) 74:6700–6. doi: 10.1128/IAI.00861-06
97. Diallo M, Aldebert D, Moreau J-C, Ndiaye M, Jambou R. Decrease of lymphoid dendritic cells in blood from malaria-infected pregnant women. *Int J Parasitol.* (2008) 38:1557–65. doi: 10.1016/j.ijpara.2008.04.013
98. Loharungsikul S, Troye-Blomberg M, Amoudruz P, Pichyangkul S, Yongvanitchit K, Looareesuwan S, et al. Expression of toll-like receptors on antigen-presenting cells in patients with falciparum malaria. *Acta Trop.* (2008) 105:10–5. doi: 10.1016/j.actatropica.2007.08.002
99. Gonçalves RM, Salmazi KC, Santos BAN, Bastos MS, Rocha SC, Boscardin SB, et al. CD4+ CD25+ Foxp3+ regulatory T cells, dendritic cells, and circulating cytokines in uncomplicated malaria: do different parasite species elicit similar host responses? *Infect Immun.* (2010) 78:4763–72. doi: 10.1128/IAI.00578-10
100. Arama C, Giusti P, Boström S, Dara V, Traore B, Dolo A, et al. Interethnic differences in antigen-presenting cell activation and TLR responses in Malian children during *Plasmodium falciparum* malaria. *PLoS ONE.* (2011) 6:e18319. doi: 10.1371/journal.pone.0018319

101. Ibitokou S, Oesterholt M, Brutus L, Borgella S, Agbowaï C, Ezinmègnon S, et al. Peripheral blood cell signatures of *Plasmodium falciparum* infection during pregnancy. *PLoS ONE.* (2012) 7:e49621. doi: 10.1371/journal.pone.0049621
102. Guermonprez P, Helft J, Claser C, Deroubaix S, Karanje H, Gazumyan A, et al. Inflammatory Flt3l is essential to mobilize dendritic cells and for T cell responses during Plasmodium infection. *Nat Med.* (2013) 19:730–8. doi: 10.1038/nm.3197
103. Urban BC, Ferguson DJ, Pain A, Willcox N, Plebanski M, Austyn JM, et al. *Plasmodium falciparum*-infected erythrocytes modulate the maturation of dendritic cells. *Nature.* (1999) 400:73–7. doi: 10.1038/21900
104. Elliott SR, Spurck TP, Dodin JM, Maier AG, Voss TS, Yosaatmadja F, et al. Inhibition of dendritic cell maturation by malaria is dose dependent and does not require *Plasmodium falciparum* erythrocyte membrane protein 1. *Infect Immun.* (2007) 75:3621–32. doi: 10.1128/IAI.00095-07
105. Mukherjee P, Chauhan VS. *Plasmodium falciparum*-free merozoites and infected RBCs distinctly affect soluble CD40 ligand-mediated maturation of immature monocyte-derived dendritic cells. *J Leukoc Biol.* (2008) 84:244–54. doi: 10.1189/jlb.0807565
106. Clemente AM, Fadigati G, Caporale R, Marchese DG, Castronovo G, Sannella AR, et al. Modulation of the immune and inflammatory responses by *Plasmodium falciparum* schizont extracts: role of myeloid dendritic cells in effector and regulatory functions of CD4+ lymphocytes. *Infect Immun.* (2013) 81:1842–51. doi: 10.1128/IAI.01226-12
107. Wu X, Gowda NM, Kumar S, Gowda DC. Protein-DNA complex is the exclusive malaria parasite component that activates dendritic cells and triggers innate immune responses. *J Immunol.* (2010) 184:4338–48. doi: 10.4049/jimmunol.0903824
108. Gowda NM, Wu X, Kumar S, Febbraio M, Gowda DC. CD36 contributes to malaria parasite-induced pro-inflammatory cytokine production and NK and T cell activation by dendritic cells. *PLoS ONE.* (2013) 8:e77604. doi: 10.1371/journal.pone.0077604
109. Fievet N, Varani S, Ibitokou S, Briand V, Louis S, Perrin RX, et al. *Plasmodium falciparum* exposure in utero, maternal age and parity influence the innate activation of foetal antigen presenting cells. *Malar J.* (2009) 8:1–12. doi: 10.1186/1475-2875-8-251
110. World Health Organisation. *Guidelines of the Treatment of Malaria.* Geneva (2010).
111. Bartoloni A, Zammarchi L. Clinical aspects of uncomplicated and severe malaria. *Mediterr J Hematol Infect Dis.* (2012) 4:e2012026. doi: 10.4084/MJHID.2012.026
112. Maraskovsky E, Brasel K, Teepe M, Roux ER, Lyman SD, Shortman K, et al. Dramatic increase in the numbers of functionally mature dendritic cells in Flt3 ligand-treated mice: multiple dendritic cell subpopulations identified. *J Exp Med.* (1996) 184:1953–62. doi: 10.1084/jem.184.5.1953
113. Waskow C, Liu K, Darrasse-Jèze G, Guermonprez P, Ginhoux F, Merad M, et al. The receptor tyrosine kinase Flt3 is required for dendritic cell development in peripheral lymphoid tissues. *Nat Immunol.* (2008) 9:676–83. doi: 10.1038/ni.1615
114. Umbers AJ, Aitken EH, Rogerson SJ. Malaria in pregnancy: small babies, big problem. *Trends Parasitol.* (2011) 27:168–75. doi: 10.1016/j.pt.2011.01.007
115. Elsayh KI, Zahran AM, Lotfy Mohamad I, Aly SS. Dendritic cells in childhood sepsis. *J Crit Care.* (2013) 28:881.e7–13. doi: 10.1016/j.jcrc.2013.05.007
116. Macatonia SE, Lau R, Patterson S, Pinching AJ, Knight SC. Dendritic cell infection, depletion and dysfunction in HIV-infected individuals. *Immunology.* (1990) 71:38–45.
117. Averill L, Lee WM, Karandikar NJ. Differential dysfunction in dendritic cell subsets during chronic HCV infection. *Clin Immunol.* (2007) 123:40–9. doi: 10.1016/j.clim.2006.12.001
118. Hémont C, Neel A, Heslan M, Braudeau C, Josien R. Human blood mDC subsets exhibit distinct TLR repertoire and responsiveness. *J Leukoc Biol.* (2013) 93:599–609. doi: 10.1189/jlb.0912452
119. Nebl T, de Veer M, Schofield L. Stimulation of innate immune responses by malarial glycosylphosphatidylinositol via pattern recognition receptors. *Parasitology.* (2005) 130(Suppl.):S45–62: doi: 10.1017/S0031182005008152
120. Coban C, Ishii KJ, Kawai T, Hemmi H, Sato S, Uematsu S, et al. Toll-like receptor 9 mediates innate immune activation by the malaria pigment hemozoin. *J Exp Med.* (2005) 201:19–25. doi: 10.1084/jem.20041836
121. World Health Organization. *World Malaria Report 2018.* Geneva (2018).
122. Kitchen S. The infection of reticulocytes by *Plasmodium vivax. Am J Trop Med Hyg.* (1938) 1–18:347–59.
123. McCarthy JS, Sekuloski S, Griffin PM, Elliott S, Douglas N, Peatey C, et al. A pilot randomised trial of induced blood-stage *Plasmodium falciparum* infections in healthy volunteers for testing efficacy of new antimalarial drugs. *PLoS ONE.* (2011) 6:e21914. doi: 10.1371/journal.pone.0021914
124. Robbins SH, Walzer T, Dembélé D, Thibault C, Defays A, Bessou G, et al. Novel insights into the relationships between dendritic cell subsets in human and mouse revealed by genome-wide expression profiling. *Genome Biol.* (2008) 9:R17. doi: 10.1186/gb-2008-9-1-r17
125. Collin M, Bigley V. Human dendritic cell subsets: an update. *Immunology.* (2018) 154:3–20. doi: 10.1111/imm.12888
126. Villani A-C, Satija R, Reynolds G, Sarkizova S, Shekhar K, Fletcher J, et al. Single-cell RNA-seq reveals new types of human blood dendritic cells, monocytes, and progenitors. *Science.* (2017) 356:eaah4573. doi: 10.1126/science.aah4573
127. Steinman RM. The Dendritic Cell System and its Role in Immunogenicity. *Annu Rev Immunol.* (1991) 9:271–96. doi: 10.1146/annurev.iy.09.040191.001415
128. Jongbloed SL, Kassianos AJ, McDonald KJ, Clark GJ, Ju X, Angel CE, et al. Human CD141+ (BDCA-3)+ dendritic cells (DCs) represent a unique myeloid DC subset that cross-presents necrotic cell antigens. *J Exp Med.* (2010) 207:1247–60. doi: 10.1084/jem.20092140
129. Sallusto F, Lanzavecchia A. Efficient presentation of soluble antigen by cultured human dendritic cells is maintained by granulocyte/macrophage colony-stimulating factor plus interleukin 4 and downregulated by tumor necrosis factor alpha. *J Exp Med.* (1994) 179:1109–18.
130. Romani N, Gruner S, Brang D, Kämpgen E, Lenz A, Trockenbacher B, et al. Proliferating dendritic cell progenitors in human blood. *J Exp Med.* (1994) 180:83–93.
131. Helft J, Böttcher J, Chakravarty P, Zelenay S, Huotari J, Schraml BU, et al. GM-CSF mouse bone marrow cultures comprise a heterogeneous population of $CD11c^{+}MHCII^{+}$ macrophages and dendritic cells. *Immunity.* (2015) 42:1197–211. doi: 10.1016/j.immuni.2015.05.018
132. Giusti P, Urban BC, Frascaroli G, Albrecht L, Tinti A, Troye-Blomberg M, et al. *Plasmodium falciparum*-infected erythrocytes and beta-hematin induce partial maturation of human dendritic cells and increase their migratory ability in response to lymphoid chemokines. *Infect Immun.* (2011) 79:2727–36. doi: 10.1128/IAI.00649-10
133. Boura M, Frita R, Góis A, Carvalho T, Hänscheid T. The hemozoin conundrum: is malaria pigment immune-activating, inhibiting, or simply a bystander? *Trends Parasitol.* (2013) 29:469–76. doi: 10.1016/j.pt.2013.07.005
134. Coban C, Ishii KJ, Sullivan DJ, Kumar N. Purified malaria pigment (Hemozoin) enhances dendritic cell maturation and modulates the isotype of antibodies induced by a DNA vaccine. *Infect Immun.* (2002) 70:3939–43. doi: 10.1128/IAI.70.7.3939-3943.2002
135. Skorokhod OA, Alessio M, Mordmüller B, Arese P, Schwarzer E. Hemozoin (malarial pigment) inhibits differentiation and maturation of human monocyte-derived dendritic cells: a peroxisome proliferator-activated receptor-gamma-mediated effect. *J Immunol.* (2004) 173:4066–74. doi: 10.4049/jimmunol.173.6.4066
136. Parroche P, Lauw FN, Goutagny N, Latz E, Monks BG, Visintin A, et al. Malaria hemozoin is immunologically inert but radically enhances innate responses by presenting malaria DNA to Toll-like receptor 9. *Proc Natl Acad Sci USA.* (2007) 104:1919–24. doi: 10.1073/pnas.0608745104
137. Brasel K, Smedt T De, Smith JL, Maliszewski CR. Generation of murine dendritic cells from flt3-ligand-supplemented bone marrow cultures. *Blood.* (2000) 96:3029–39. Available online at: http://www.bloodjournal.org/content/96/9/3029
138. van de Hoef DL, Coppens I, Holowka T, Ben Mamoun C, Branch O, Rodriguez A. *Plasmodium falciparum*-derived uric acid precipitates induce maturation of dendritic cells. *PLoS ONE.* (2013) 8:e55584. doi: 10.1371/journal.pone.0055584

139. Gallego-Delgado J, Ty M, Orengo JM, van de Hoef D, Rodriguez A. A Surprising role for uric acid: the inflammatory malaria response. *Curr Rheumatol Rep.* (2014) 16:401. doi: 10.1007/s11926-013-0401-8
140. Hochrein H, O'Keeffe M. Dendritic cell subsets and toll-like receptors. In: Bauer S, Hartmann G, editors. *Handbook of Experimental Pharmacology*. Berlin; Heidelberg: Springer (2008). p. 153–79. doi: 10.1007/978-3-540-72167-3
141. Gallego-Marin C, Schrum JE, Andrade WA, Shaffer SA, Giraldo LF, Lasso AM, et al. Cyclic GMP–AMP synthase is the cytosolic sensor of *Plasmodium falciparum* genomic DNA and activates type I IFN in malaria. *J Immunol.* (2017) 200:768–74. doi: 10.4049/jimmunol.1701048
142. Sisquella X, Ofir-Birin Y, Pimentel MA, Cheng L, Abou Karam P, Sampaio NG, et al. Malaria parasite DNA-harbouring vesicles activate cytosolic immune sensors. *Nat Commun.* (2017) 8:1985. doi: 10.1038/s41467-017-02083-1
143. Nwakanma DC, Gomez-Escobar N, Walther M, Crozier S, Dubovsky F, Malkin E, et al. Quantitative detection of *Plasmodium falciparum* DNA in saliva, blood, and urine. *J Infect Dis.* (2009) 199:1567–74. doi: 10.1086/598856
144. Krishnegowda G, Hajjar AM, Zhu J, Douglass EJ, Uematsu S, Akira S, et al. Induction of proinflammatory responses in macrophages by the glycosylphosphatidylinositols of *Plasmodium falciparum*: cell signaling receptors, glycosylphosphatidylinositol (GPI) structural requirement, and regulation of GPI activity. *J Biol Chem.* (2005) 280:8606–16. doi: 10.1074/jbc.M413541200
145. Baccarella A, Fontana MF, Chen EC, Kim CC. Toll-like receptor 7 mediates early innate immune responses to malaria. *Infect Immun.* (2013) 81:4431–42. doi: 10.1128/IAI.00923-13
146. Campos FM, Franklin BS, Teixeira-Carvalho A, Filho AL, de Paula SC, Fontes CJ, et al. Augmented plasma microparticles during acute *Plasmodium vivax* infection. *Malar J.* (2010) 9:327. doi: 10.1186/1475-2875-9-327
147. Nantakomol D, Dondorp AM, Krudsood S, Udomsangpetch R, Pattanapanyasat K, Combes V, et al. Circulating red cell-derived microparticles in human malaria. *J Infect Dis.* (2011) 203:700–6. doi: 10.1093/infdis/jiq104
148. Couper KN, Barnes T, Hafalla JCR, Combes V, Ryffel B, Secher T, et al. Parasite-derived plasma microparticles contribute significantly to malaria infection-induced inflammation through potent macrophage stimulation. *PLoS Pathog.* (2010) 6:e1000744. doi: 10.1371/journal.ppat.1000744
149. Mantel PY, Hoang AN, Goldowitz I, Potashnikova D, Hamza B, Vorobjev I, et al. Malaria-infected erythrocyte-derived microvesicles mediate cellular communication within the parasite population and with the host immune system. *Cell Host Microbe.* (2013) 13:521–34. doi: 10.1016/j.chom.2013.04.009
150. Laurens MB, Thera MA, Coulibaly D, Ouattara A, Kone AK, Guindo AB, et al. Extended safety, immunogenicity and efficacy of a blood-stage malaria vaccine in Malian children: 24-month follow-up of a randomized, double-blinded phase 2 trial. *PLoS ONE.* (2013) 8:e79323. doi: 10.1371/journal.pone.0079323
151. Wilson NO, Jain V, Roberts CE, Lucchi N, Joel PK, Singh MP, et al. CXCL4 and CXCL10 predict risk of fatal cerebral malaria. *Dis Markers.* (2011) 30:39–49. doi: 10.3233/DMA-2011-0763
152. Jain V, Singh PP, Silawat N, Patel R, Saxena A, Bharti PK, et al. A preliminary study on pro- and anti-inflammatory cytokine profiles in *Plasmodium vivax* malaria patients from central zone of India. *Acta Trop.* (2010) 113:263–8. doi: 10.1016/j.actatropica.2009.11.009
153. Herbert F, Tchitchek N, Bansal D, Jacques J, Pathak S, Bécavin C, et al. Evidence of IL-17, IP-10, and IL-10 involvement in multiple-organ dysfunction and IL-17 pathway in acute renal failure associated to *Plasmodium falciparum* malaria. *J Transl Med.* (2015) 13:369. doi: 10.1186/s12967-015-0731-6
154. Kempaiah P, Anyona SB, Raballah E, Davenport GC, Were T, Hittner JB, et al. Reduced interferon (IFN)-α conditioned by IFNA2 (−173) and IFNA8 (−884) haplotypes is associated with enhanced susceptibility to severe malarial anemia and longitudinal all-cause mortality. *Hum Genet.* (2012) 131:1375–91. doi: 10.1007/s00439-012-1175-1
155. Montes de Oca M, Kumar R, Rivera F de L, Amante FH, Sheel M, Faleiro RJ, et al. Type I interferons regulate immune responses in humans with blood-stage *Plasmodium falciparum* infection. *Cell Rep.* (2016) 17:399–412. doi: 10.1016/j.celrep.2016.09.015
156. Wykes MN, Kay JG, Manderson A, Liu XQ, Brown DL, Richard DJ, et al. Rodent blood-stage Plasmodium survive in dendritic cells that infect naive mice. *Proc Natl Acad Sci USA.* (2011) 108:11205–10. doi: 10.1073/pnas.1108579108
157. Vuckovic S, Abdul Wahid FS, Rice A, Kato M, Khalil D, Rodwell R, et al. Compartmentalization of allogeneic T-cell responses in the bone marrow and spleen of humanized NOD/SCID mice containing activated human resident myeloid dendritic cells. *Exp Hematol.* (2008) 36:1502–12. doi: 10.1016/j.exphem.2008.06.011
158. Minkah NK, Schafer C, Kappe SHI. Humanized mouse models for the study of human malaria parasite biology, pathogenesis, and immunity. *Front Immunol.* (2018) 9:807. doi: 10.3389/fimmu.2018.00807
159. Broutier L, Mastrogiovanni G, Verstegen MM, Francies HE, Gavarró LM, Bradshaw CR, et al. Human primary liver cancer–derived organoid cultures for disease modeling and drug screening. *Nat Med.* (2017) 23:1424–35. doi: 10.1038/nm.4438
160. Spence JR, Mayhew CN, Rankin SA, Kuhar MF, Vallance JE, Tolle K, et al. Directed differentiation of human pluripotent stem cells into intestinal tissue *in vitro*. *Nature.* (2011) 470:105–9. doi: 10.1038/nature09691
161. Heo I, Dutta D, Schaefer DA, Iakobachvili N, Artegiani B, Sachs N, et al. Modelling Cryptosporidium infection in human small intestinal and lung organoids. *Nat Microbiol.* (2018) 3:814–23. doi: 10.1038/s41564-018-0177-8
162. Klotz C, Aebischer T, Seeber F. Stem cell-derived cell cultures and organoids for protozoan parasite propagation and studying host-parasite interaction. *Int J Med Microbiol.* (2012) 302:203–9. doi: 10.1016/j.ijmm.2012.07.010

8

The Relative Role of Climate Variation and Control Interventions on Malaria Elimination Efforts in El Oro, Ecuador: A Modeling Study

Isabel K. Fletcher[1,2], Anna M. Stewart-Ibarra[3], Rachel Sippy[4], Gabriel Carrasco-Escobar[5,6], Mercy Silva[7], Efrain Beltran-Ayala[8], Tania Ordoñez[9], Jefferson Adrian[10], Fabián E. Sáenz[11], Chris Drakeley[12], Kate E. Jones[13] and Rachel Lowe[1,2,14]**

Edited by:
Zed Zulkafli,
University Putra Malaysia, Malaysia

Reviewed by:
Lingxin Chen,
Yantai Institute of Coastal Zone Research (CAS), China
Patricia Margaret Graves,
James Cook University, Australia
Michelle Stanton,
Liverpool School of Tropical Medicine, United Kingdom

***Correspondence:**
Isabel K. Fletcher
Isabel.Fletcher@lshtm.ac.uk
Rachel Lowe
Rachel.Lowe@lshtm.ac.uk

[1] Centre on Climate Change and Planetary Health, London School of Hygiene & Tropical Medicine, London, United Kingdom, [2] Centre for Mathematical Modelling of Infectious Diseases, London School of Hygiene & Tropical Medicine, London, United Kingdom, [3] Inter-American Institute for Global Change Research, Montevideo, Uruguay, [4] Institute for Global Health and Translational Science, SUNY Upstate Medical University, Syracuse, NY, United States, [5] Health Innovation Laboratory, Institute of Tropical Medicine "Alexander von Humboldt", Universidad Peruana Cayetano Heredia, Lima, Peru, [6] Division of Infectious Diseases and Global Public Health, Department of Medicine, University of California, San Diego, San Diego, CA, United States, [7] Hospital Teofilo Davila, Ministerio de Salud Pública, Quito, Ecuador, [8] Facultad de Medicina, Universidad Tecnica de Machala, Machala, Ecuador, [9] Distrito de Salud 07D02 del Ministerio de Salud Pública, Quito, Ecuador, [10] Departamento de Ciencias de la Computación y Electrónica, Universidad Técnica Particular de Loja, Loja, Ecuador, [11] Centro de Investigación para la Salud en América Latina, Facultad de Ciencias Exactas y Naturales, Pontificia Universidad Católica del Ecuador, Quito, Ecuador, [12] Department of Infection Biology, Faculty of Infectious and Tropical Diseases, London School of Hygiene & Tropical Medicine, London, United Kingdom, [13] Centre for Biodiversity and Environment Research, Department of Genetics, Evolution and Environment, University College London, London, United Kingdom, [14] Barcelona Institute for Global Health (ISGlobal), Barcelona, Spain

Malaria is a vector-borne disease of significant public health concern. Despite widespread success of many elimination initiatives, elimination efforts in some regions of the world have stalled. Barriers to malaria elimination include climate and land use changes, such as warming temperatures and urbanization, which can alter mosquito habitats. Socioeconomic factors, such as political instability and regional migration, also threaten elimination goals. This is particularly relevant in areas where local elimination has been achieved and consequently surveillance and control efforts are dwindling and are no longer a priority. Understanding how environmental change, impacts malaria elimination has important practical implications for vector control and disease surveillance strategies. It is important to consider climate change when monitoring the threat of malaria resurgence due to socioeconomic influences. However, there is limited assessment of how the combination of climate variation, interventions and socioeconomic pressures influence long-term trends in malaria transmission and elimination efforts. In this study, we used Bayesian hierarchical mixed models and malaria case data for a 29-year period to disentangle the impacts of climate variation and malaria control efforts on malaria risk in the Ecuadorian province of El Oro, which achieved local elimination in 2011. We found shifting patterns of malaria between rural and urban areas, with a relative increase of *Plasmodium vivax* in urbanized areas. Minimum temperature was an important driver of malaria seasonality and the association between warmer minimum temperatures and malaria incidence was greater for *Plasmodium falciparum* compared to *P. vivax* malaria. There was considerable heterogeneity in the impact of three chemical vector control measures on both *P. falciparum* and *P. vivax* malaria. We found statistically significant associations between two of the three measures [indoor residual spraying (IRS) and space spraying] and a reduction in malaria incidence, which varied between malaria type. We also found environmental suitability for malaria transmission is increasing in El Oro, which could limit future elimination efforts if malaria is allowed to re-establish. Our findings have important implications for understanding environmental obstacles to malaria elimination and highlights the importance of designing and sustaining elimination efforts in areas that remain vulnerable to resurgence.

Keywords: malaria, environmental change, elimination, vector control, climate, spatio-temporal model

INTRODUCTION

Malaria is the most important vector-borne disease worldwide, with 228 million cases reported in 2018 (WHO, 2019). Despite global elimination and eradication efforts, progress toward elimination is stalling in some endemic countries. In particular, increases in malaria incidence have been observed in some South American countries since 2014 including Venezuela, Peru, Colombia, and Ecuador, where movement of infected individuals between neighboring countries in the region can result in a resurgence of cases in local populations, threatening progress toward malaria reduction for other countries (Grillet et al., 2019; WHO, 2019). Malaria is highly sensitive to environmental conditions, including climate variability and land use practices (Moreno, 2006; Caminade et al., 2014), which along with socioeconomic influences can act as significant barriers to elimination. In addition, the lapse in control and surveillance efforts combined with global environmental changes also poses a threat to malaria elimination efforts in South America (Alimi et al., 2015; Conn et al., 2018).

Variation in meteorological conditions, particularly temperature, and rainfall, determines the spatiotemporal patterns of malaria through their effects on both the *Plasmodium* parasite and the *Anopheles* vector. Warmer temperatures can decrease the extrinsic incubation period (EIP), the time taken for the malaria parasite to complete its development inside the mosquito. A shorter EIP increases the transmission intensity of malaria by allowing mosquitoes to become infectious more quickly. The EIP for the *Plasmodium falciparum* parasite is longer (~10 days) than that for *Plasmodium vivax* (~8 days) and *P. vivax* can also develop at relatively cooler temperatures (minimum 15°C), compared to *P. falciparum* (minimum 18°C) (Patz and Olson, 2006). Temperature also impacts the mosquito vector, by affecting both larval and adult survival and longevity (Beck-Johnson et al., 2013), mosquito development (Bayoh and Lindsay, 2003), and vector population dynamics (Beck-Johnson et al., 2013). However, the effect of temperature on malaria transmission is non-linear, with the optimal temperature for malaria transmission estimated to be 25°C with transmission declining above 30°C (Paaijmans et al., 2009; Mordecai et al., 2013). Rainfall is also important for malaria transmission as it determines the availability of mosquito breeding habitat and thus mosquito abundance, although heavy and persistent rainfall can wash out larval habitats (Galardo et al., 2009; Olson et al., 2009; Prussing et al., 2019; Wolfarth-Couto et al., 2019).

Anthropogenic activities, such as urbanization and agricultural land use can also change malaria transmission patterns over longer time scales by creating more or less favorable microclimatic conditions and habitats for malaria vectors, depending on the species (Conn et al., 2002; Wayant et al., 2010; Tucker Lima et al., 2017). For example, urban development can eliminate mosquito habitat subsequently decreasing malaria incidence or in some cases increases in peri-urban malaria can occur as a result of economic migration and the creation of novel breeding habitats (Padilla et al., 2015). In addition, deforestation can facilitate malaria transmission due to the creation of new mosquito habitats on forest fringes (Vittor et al., 2006; Stefani et al., 2013). Increasing environmental suitability of malaria transmission, associated with climatic change and land use modifications, has important implications for malaria elimination efforts in South America, as these changes could compromise elimination efforts (Recht et al., 2017).

Previous studies have identified several environmental risk factors for malaria transmission that may impede elimination efforts in South America. For example, large-scale climate patterns such as the El Niño Southern Oscillation have been associated with large outbreaks of malaria in Peru, due to flooding conditions and in Colombia and Venezuela due to drought conditions (Gagnon et al., 2002). In highland areas of Colombia, warmer years were associated with an increased number of malaria cases occurring at higher altitudes (Siraj et al., 2014). Studies assessing spatial heterogeneity in malaria risk in South America have found deforestation and agricultural development have altered anopheline vector ecology in the Amazon region through creation of new *Anopheles* habitats and increased human-mosquito interactions (Moreno et al., 2007; Vittor et al., 2009; Hahn et al., 2014; Burkett-Cadena and Vittor, 2017).

When assessing the role of environmental factors on malaria incidence it is important to simultaneously consider the relative impact of control interventions, especially in elimination settings. Studies that evaluate the effectiveness of malaria control programs often consider environmental factors, most commonly rainfall and vegetation indices. Some studies used geostatistical modeling and after adjusting for climate conditions estimate the contribution and effectiveness of malaria control measures, including indoor residual spraying (IRS) in sub-Saharan Africa, relative to the impacts of climate variability (Graves et al., 2008; Giardina et al., 2014). Other studies often treat climate and environmental variables as confounders and do not apportion variation in malaria incidence due to climate (Aregawi et al., 2011; Bennett et al., 2014). There has been a limited assessment of how the combination of environmental factors, elimination efforts and socioeconomic pressures influences long-term trends in malaria and the route toward elimination. Understanding how malaria elimination efforts might be hindered by environmental changes has implications for targeting of vector control and disease surveillance, and is important especially given the possibility of shifting vector distributions and increasing climate suitability in South America (Pinault and Hunter, 2012).

According to the Pan-American Health Organization (PAHO), Ecuador is in the malaria pre-elimination phase, but has fallen short of its target to achieve elimination by 2020 (WHO, 2018). Since 2016 malaria has increased significantly in the country, mainly in the Amazon region, with more cases being detected than expected for a country on the verge of malaria elimination (PAHO, 2017; Sáenz et al., 2017). Recent surges of malaria in other South American countries, primarily Venezuela, are threatening current elimination efforts in Ecuador due to regional migration (Daniels, 2018; Grillet et al., 2019). This study focuses on Ecuador's southern province, El Oro, a high-risk region, which previously eliminated malaria but recently recorded indigenous cases, in addition to being vulnerable to the introduction of infections via imported cases due to high rates of human movement associated with its location on a strategic migration route (Jaramillo-Ochoa et al., 2019). Here we seek to identify threats to malaria elimination, with a view to prevent lapses in control efforts and the re-establishment of malaria in an area currently considered malaria-free but historically endemic for malaria. We advance the existing knowledge of the malaria elimination success in El Oro (Krisher et al., 2016) by quantifying the associations between malaria, climate and control interventions in a region vulnerable to resurgence.

MATERIALS AND METHODS

Study Area

El Oro province (latitude: 3°5′45.20″S-4°11′3.06″S, longitude:-79°43′10.92″W-80°50′37.96″W) is located in southern Ecuador on the Pacific Coast and shares a border with the Tumbes region of northern Peru (**Figure 1A**). El Oro covers 5,870 km^2 and is divided into 14 cantons, which range in size from approximately 70 km^2 up to 900 km^2. Population densities per canton range from 7 people per km^2 in rural areas and up to 760 people per km^2 in the province capital, Machala.

Plasmodium vivax and *P. falciparum* are the malaria-causing parasites in the region (WHO, 2019) and the primary mosquito vectors transmitting malaria in El Oro are *Anopheles albimanus* and *Anopheles punctimacula* (Ryan et al., 2017).

During the mid-1990s public health authorities in El Oro and neighboring Tumbes unified to implement an effective binational collaboration to tackle the surge in malaria transmission in the region (Krisher et al., 2016). El Oro has been free of locally acquired malaria infections since 2011 although malaria has been increasing elsewhere in Ecuador (WHO, 2019). In 2018 seven malaria cases were recorded in El Oro (6/7 were imported cases) during a period of elevated migration of Venezuelan citizens associated with the social and economic crisis in their country (Jaramillo-Ochoa et al., 2019). El Oro's border location, along the Pan American highway, a route used by many migrants, makes it particularly vulnerable to malaria resurgence. In addition, El Oro is one of the most hazardous coastal zones in Latin America and the Caribbean (Calil et al., 2017). Vulnerable populations are susceptible to the effects of the El Niño Southern Oscillation, which intensifies annual flooding events during the rainy season (Lowe et al., 2017; Tauzer et al., 2019). Lapses in surveillance and control efforts and reductions in funding following local elimination also means malaria resurgence is likely (PAHO, 2017; Sáenz et al., 2017).

Data Sources

Monthly counts of blood smear confirmed cases of *P. falciparum* and *P. vivax* malaria for each canton in El Oro, January 1990–December 2018, were provided by the Ecuadorian Ministry of Health, where malaria is a mandatory notifiable disease. Cases were recorded at local clinics across El Oro and collated by the Ministry of Health. Population data, available for each canton, were sourced from the national census in Ecuador, from the Instituto Nacional de Estadística y Censos (INEC[1]) for 1990, 2001, and 2010. Data for 2011–2018 were provided by INEC as annual population projections. Population values between census years 1990, 2001, and 2010 were estimated by interpolating assuming linear growth, to provide annual population estimates for each canton. To estimate the proportion of the population in poverty per canton in El Oro, we used Unmet Basic Needs (UBN) sourced from the 2010 census, an indicator based on measures including housing quality, education and access to water and sanitation. We used UBN data from 2010 as a socioeconomic covariate in all our models.

Between 2001 and 2015 an intensive period of vector control was carried out across El Oro following a resurgence of malaria cases and monthly canton-level data for three control measures were available from the Ministry of Health. Monthly estimates per canton of the number of households treated by IRS with insecticides (deltamethrin 5% concentrated suspension, deltamethrin 2.5%, malathion 50%, alphacypermethrin 10% concentrated suspension, and betacypermethrin 2.5%) were available for January 2001–September 2013. The number of neighborhoods that were treated with insecticide via ultra-low volume (ULV) fumigation, which is performed by spraying

[1]http://www.ecuadorencifras.gob.ec/institucional/home/

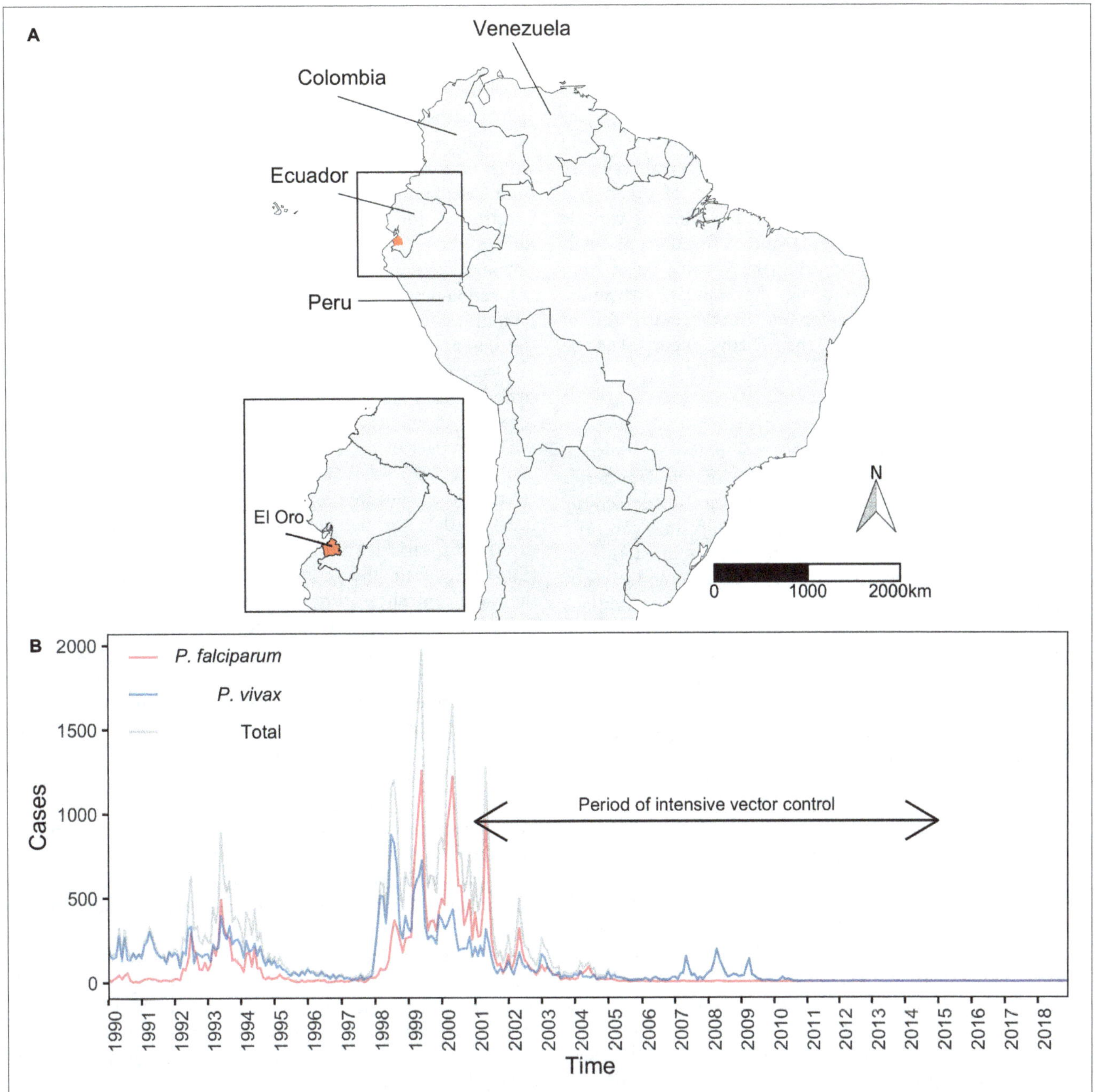

FIGURE 1 | Malaria cases in El Oro 1990–2018. **(A)** Location of El Oro province (red), Ecuador in relation to neighboring countries in South American; Colombia, Peru, and Venezuela. **(B)** Total number of malaria cases (gray), cases of *P. falciparum* (pink), and *P. vivax* malaria (blue) recorded in El Oro 1990–2018.

entire neighborhoods with 96% malathion from trucks were available between January 2004 and May 2015. Finally, the number of households space-sprayed with 2.5% deltamethrin concentrated emulsion, using a backpack fogger that creates a fog insecticide to treat both inside and outside the home, were available between January 2004 and May 2015 (**Supplementary Figure S1**). For each control measure we tested for lagged relationships, up to 3 months, in order to account for delays between implementation and impact on measurable malaria cases (**Supplementary Table S1**). Other malaria control interventions including fumigation with DDT (until banned in 1996), elimination of larval habitats, and bed net provision occurred during the study period, but no detailed data for control measures were available prior to 2001.

Monthly climate data, for temperature and precipitation, between January 1990 and December 2018 were sourced from TerraClimate, a high-spatial resolution (~4 km) dataset that uses climatically aided interpolation to produce monthly estimates (Abatzoglou et al., 2018). To obtain climate estimates for each canton in El Oro, TerraClimate variables were aggregated by taking mean grid cell values using the *raster* package in R.

Annual land cover maps at a 300 m spatial resolution generated by the European Space Agency (ESA) Climate Change Initiative (CCI) were compiled for 1990–2018[2] (European Space Agency, 2019). For each annual map, the number of grid cells in each canton that were classified in the urban category were extracted, and from this the proportion of urban grid cells per canton were calculated to give a continuous variable of urbanization (**Supplementary Figure S3**). All continuous variables were scaled by subtracting the variable mean from each value and dividing this by the standard deviation. This transformation allowed for the direct comparison of continuous variables and enabled their relative importance to be determined in the model.

Statistical Analysis

Bayesian hierarchical mixed models are powerful statistical models that can be used to estimate the marginal posterior distributions of multiple covariates whilst simultaneously accounting for multiple sources of uncertainty that can arise from disease count data. Here, spatiotemporal models were constructed, for each malaria parasite, *P. falciparum* and *P. vivax*, to explore the contributions of climate and control interventions to variations in monthly malaria incidence in El Oro between January 1990 and December 2018 (348 months).

We fitted zero-inflated negative binomial models that take into account excess zeros that cannot be explained by a standard negative binomial distribution (**Supplementary Appendix S1.1**). Where μ_{st} is the mean number of malaria cases in each canton ($s = 1,\ldots,14$) for each timestep ($t = 1,\ldots,348$), the hierarchical spatiotemporal model is defined as:

$$log(\mu_{st}) = log(P_{st}) + log(\rho_{st})$$

Annual population estimates per 1,000 inhabitants for each canton in El Oro, $\log(P_{st})$, were included as an offset in the model to account for canton-level differences in the annual parasite incidence (API). The estimated API, $\log(\rho_{st})$ is then made up of a combination of climate covariates, including mean monthly minimum temperature and precipitation for each canton. Other explanatory variables considered included socioeconomic factors (poverty rates), level of urbanization and vector control interventions (IRS, ULV fumigation and space-spraying).

To account for the seasonality in malaria incidence, a monthly random effect was introduced using a first order autoregressive prior (m_t), which allows malaria in 1 month to depend on incidence in the previous month. Independent random effects for each year (y_t), 1990–2018, were included to allow for additional sources of variation due to unobserved confounding factors such as variations in healthcare access, case reporting and diagnostics.

Spatially structured random effects, υ_s, were introduced into the model to allow for correlated heterogeneity in malaria incidence across cantons in El Oro. This spatial dependency structure was accounted for by assuming a conditional intrinsic Gaussian autoregressive (CAR) model prior distribution for the spatial effects, which takes into account the neighborhood structure of the area (Besag et al., 1991). We also included spatially unstructured random effects in the model to allow for additional uncorrelated spatial variation across cantons, ν_s, which were assigned independent diffuse Gaussian exchangeable prior distributions (Lowe et al., 2016). Separate models were constructed for both *P. falciparum* and *P. vivax* malaria due to their intrinsic differences, which include diagnostic potential, development time inside the mosquito vector (extrinsic incubation period, EIP), the differential impact of vector control on transmission, infection reservoirs of *P. vivax* hypnozoites and the presence of asymptomatic cases.

Detailed data on interventions was only available for the period January 2001–December 2015. Therefore, we formulated separate sub-models for each malaria type to investigate the relative impact of the control measures implemented between 2001 and 2015 (see **Supplementary Appendix S2**), herein referred to as "intervention models." The intervention models, fitted to data for the period 2001–2015 included the same explanatory variables and random effects as the "full" models (fitted to data for the period 1990–2018) with the addition of the three control measures. We examined differences between the random effects structures for the full models and the intervention models, to see how much variation in malaria due to interventions could be accounted for by random effects in the absence of intervention data for the entire time period.

Posterior distributions of model parameters were estimated using Integrated Nested Laplace approximations (INLA) (Rue et al., 2009). INLA provides a computationally more efficient alternative to Markov Chain Monte Carlo (MCMC) methods, by using numerical approximations of model parameters (see **Supplementary Appendix S1.2**). Covariate time lags and the most parsimonious models were selected using the deviance information criterion (DIC) (Spiegelhalter et al., 2002) and the Watanabe–Akaike information criterion (WAIC) (Watanabe, 2010), which are Bayesian methods of model comparison that trade off model adequacy against model complexity. Models with lower DIC and WAIC indicate a more parsimonious model. We also used the logarithmic score to assess model fit, which is based on the conditional predictive ordinate (CPO) leave-one-out cross-validation score, where a smaller value indicates a greater predictive power of the model (Gneiting and Raftery, 2007).

Covariates were added iteratively to the models starting with a baseline model, which included spatial and temporal structured and unstructured random effects and retained if model fit was improved, assessed through a decrease in DIC and WAIC. The most appropriate temperature variable, maximum or minimum temperature was selected using DIC and WAIC (**Supplementary Table S2**). We tested different time lags (from 0 to 3 months) to take into account the lagged effect of climate factors on malaria transmission, including development time of mosquitoes and parasites as well as the time between malaria diagnosis and case recording (**Supplementary Table S2**). We also tested non-linear functions of temperature and precipitation (**Supplementary**

[2]https://www.esa-landcover-cci.org/

Table S3). We used the root mean square error (RMSE) to assess the extent to which models of malaria incidence for 2001–2015 were improved by the inclusion of each control measure in turn. RMSE is a measure of the standard deviation of the model residuals, with smaller values indicating better model fit to the observed data.

RESULTS

Urban and Rural Malaria Incidence in El Oro

Between 1990 and 2018, 62,120 cases of malaria were recorded in El Oro, with 54% of infections resulting from *P. falciparum* malaria and 46% from *P. vivax*. Malaria transmission in El Oro was historically high, reaching up to 2,000 total annual cases in 1999 and an API of 61 cases of *P. falciparum* and 35 *P. vivax* cases per 1,000 people recorded in Huaquillas canton along the Peruvian border. Between 1998 and 2002 large outbreaks, particularly of *P. falciparum* malaria occurred across the province before declining to low levels of incidence after the period of more intensive vector control (**Figure 1B**). A small outbreak of *P. vivax* malaria occurred between 2007 and 2009 before malaria incidence was dramatically reduced and remained at a low and stable level (**Figure 1B**). The highest malaria incidence was concentrated in the western part of the province, along the Peru-Ecuador border (**Supplementary Figure S4**).

Between 1990 and 2018, outbreaks of both *P. falciparum* and *P. vivax* malaria occurred roughly at the same time. Prior to the decline in cases in 2001–2015 there was a greater difference between *P. falciparum* and *P. vivax* incidence in rural areas, compared to urbanized areas (**Supplementary Figure S5**). During the elimination phase (2001–2010) the incidence of *P. falciparum* and *P. vivax* malaria in rural areas was reduced much more than malaria in urbanized areas, where outbreaks of *P. vivax* were still observed. There was also a greater overall reduction of *P. falciparum* malaria in rural and urbanized areas.

In the models of malaria incidence in El Oro between 1990 and 2018, we found that areas that were more urbanized were associated with greater incidences of *P. falciparum* malaria (**Figure 2A**). To examine how the epidemiology of malaria in El Oro had changed with the three vector control interventions, we tested whether there was a difference in the relationship between malaria and level of urbanization in El Oro, before and after the interventions were implemented. We found a statistically significant interaction between level of urbanization in El Oro and the period the control measures were implemented (2001–2015) for *P. vivax* malaria and no significant interaction for *P. falciparum* malaria (**Supplementary Figure S6**). Prior to 2001, more urbanized areas of El Oro were associated with decreased *P. vivax* malaria and after 2001 this relationship reversed with urbanized areas associated with more *P. vivax* malaria.

During the period of malaria decline (post 2001) there was also a reduction in the seasonal pattern of both *P. falciparum* and *P. vivax* malaria in El Oro especially for *P. vivax* malaria incidence, which ceased to peak between June and July (**Supplementary Figure S7**). For *P. falciparum* a seasonal peak in incidence during this period was evident between June and July, but less distinct than before 2001.

Climate Variability and Malaria Incidence in El Oro 1990–2018

Minimum temperature was the best temperature variable in the full models (**Supplementary Table S2**) and in the 3 months prior to case reporting was an important predictor of the spatio-temporal distribution of *P. falciparum* and *P. vivax* malaria in El Oro (**Figure 2A**). Warmer temperatures in El Oro between 1990 and 2018 were associated with increases in malaria incidence and greater increases in *P. falciparum* malaria than *P. vivax* malaria (**Figure 2A**). Precipitation lagged by 3 months for *P. falciparum* and 1 month for *P. vivax* were selected as the best time lags although when included in the full model, precipitation was not significant in driving malaria incidence in El Oro (**Figure 2A**). Introducing a non-linear relationship between malaria and climatic variables improved model fit by decreasing model DIC and RMSE for *P. vivax* but not *P. falciparum* malaria incidence (**Table 1** and **Supplementary Figure S8**). We also found that higher temperatures were associated with larger increases in malaria incidence (**Figure 2B**).

We also investigated the influence of minimum temperature on the unexplained variation in *P. falciparum* and *P. vivax* incidence in El Oro between 1990 and 2018. We compared the monthly and interannual random effects of models with and without temperature to determine the extent to which temperature accounted for the seasonal pattern of malaria incidence. The monthly random effects of the model for *P. falciparum* incidence that included minimum temperature were near zero, showing that temperature accounted for all of the seasonal variation in *P. falciparum* malaria in El Oro 1990–2018 (**Figure 3A**). In contrast there was minimal reduction in the random effects for the *P. vivax* model with minimum temperature, indicating the seasonal pattern was driven by other factors (**Figure 3B**). The proportion of the variation accounted for by the yearly random effects in a model without minimum temperature was greater than the proportion of the variation accounted for by the monthly random effects in a model without minimum temperature. This suggests that temperature is the main driver of malaria seasonality and other interannual signatures as well as temperature contribute to the interannual variability of malaria in El Oro. For example, for some years the proportion of variation accounted for by the yearly random effects decreased when minimum temperature was included into models of malaria incidence 1990–2018. A reduction in the value of the random effects can be seen for 1998, when a strong El Niño event occurred (**Supplementary Figure S9**). Reductions were also particularly apparent for *P. falciparum* malaria between 2001–2004 and 2009–2011, suggesting that some additional variation was explained by minimum temperature. In contrast for some years there was no reduction for example in 2008, when an outbreak of *P. vivax* malaria occurred suggesting the outbreak was not driven by a climate event.

We explored how climate suitability for malaria transmission had changed over the time period 1990–2018 in El Oro,

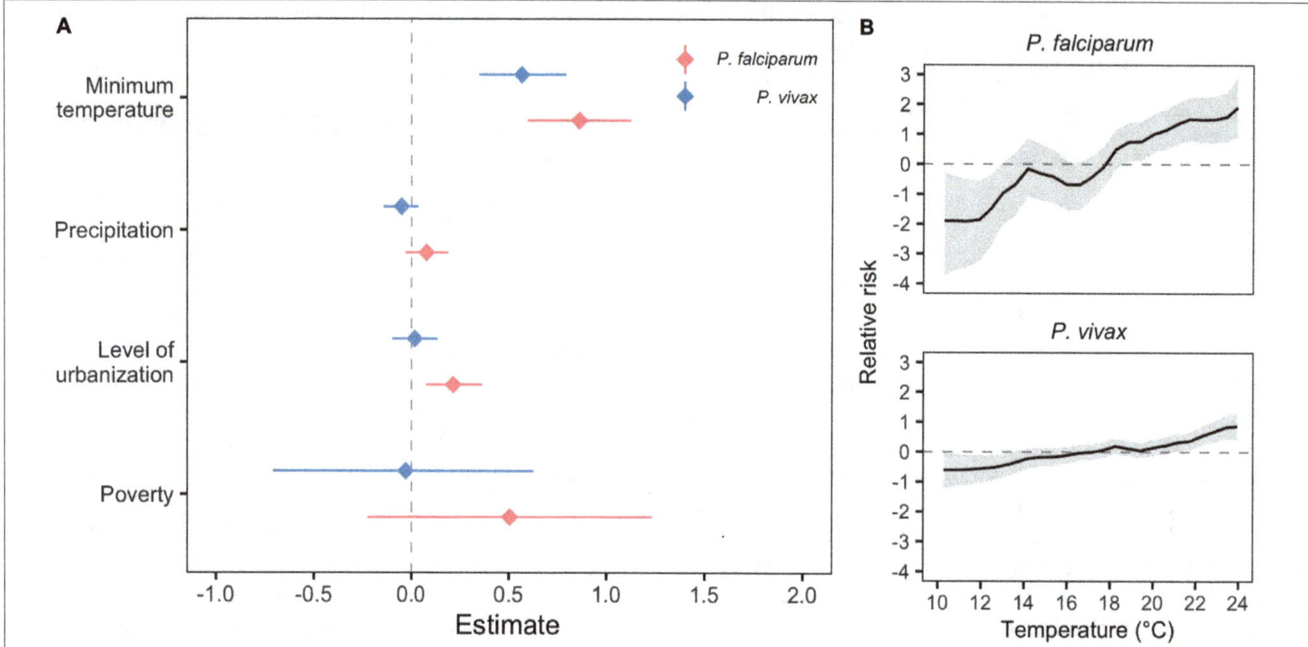

FIGURE 2 | Parameter estimates for explanatory variables of *P. falciparum* and *P. vivax* malaria in El Oro 1990–2018. **(A)** Posterior mean and 95% credible intervals for minimum temperature and precipitation, included as linear terms, level of urbanization and poverty covariates for *P. falciparum* (pink) and *P. vivax* (blue) malaria. **(B)** Relationships between *P. falciparum* and *P. vivax* relative risk, on the log scale defined as the annual parasite incidence (API), $\log(\rho_{st})$, and minimum temperature, lagged by 3 months, included in the model as a function to allow for non-linearities.

TABLE 1 | Adequacy results, deviance information criterion (DIC), Watanabe-Akaike Information Criterion (WAIC) and cross-validated log score for full models of *P. falciparum* and *P. vivax* malaria in El Oro 1990–2018.

Model	Parasite	DIC	WAIC	Log score
Baseline spatial seasonal $log\,(\rho_{st}) = \upsilon_s + \nu_s + m_t$	*P. falciparum*	12640.97	12646.73	1.38
	P. vivax	18745.44	18743.44	2.05
Unstructured yearly random effects $log\,(\rho_{st}) = \upsilon_s + \nu_s + m_t + y_t$	*P. falciparum*	11947.63	11970.4	1.31
	P. vivax	17887.75	17894.17	1.96
Socioeconomic effects $log\,(\rho_{st}) = \upsilon_s + \nu_s + m_t + y_t + x_{1s}$	*P. falciparum*	11946.75	11970.10	1.31
	P. vivax	17887.61	17893.23	1.96
Urban effects $log\,(\rho_{st}) = \upsilon_s + \nu_s + m_t + y_t + x_{1s} + x_{2st}z_i$	*P. falciparum*	11935.89	11958.12	1.31
	P. vivax	17823.38	17831.99	1.95
Temperature effects				
$log\,(\rho_{st}) = \upsilon_s + \nu_s + m_t + y_t + x_{1s} + x_{2st}z_i + x_{3st}$ (linear)	*P. falciparum*	11926.14	11941.98	1.31
$log\,(\rho_{st}) = \upsilon_s + \nu_s + m_t + y_t + x_{1s} + x_{2st}z_i + f(x_{3st})$ (non-linear)	*P. vivax*	17797.49	17806.2	1.95
Precipitation effects				
$log\,(\rho_{st}) = \upsilon_s + \nu_s + m_t + y_t + x_{1s} + x_{2st}z_i + x_{3st} + x_{4st}$ (linear)	*P. falciparum*	11924.91	11941.77	1.31
$log\,(\rho_{st}) = \upsilon_s + \nu_s + m_t + y_t + x_{1s} + x_{2st}z_i + f(x_{3st}) + f(x_{4st})$ (non-linear)	*P. vivax*	17795.36	17804.2	1.95

Covariates were added iteratively, starting with a baseline model that included structured and unstructured spatial random effects, and a seasonal term. The level of urbanization was interacted with a categorical variable indicating a decline in malaria incidence post 2001. The most parsimonious models included climate (temperature and precipitation) as linear terms for P. falciparum and as non-linear functions for P. vivax malaria.

specifically for minimum temperature since it was an important predictor. To do this, we calculated the number of months that had suitable temperature conditions for transmission of each malaria parasite. We used the lower temperature limits of the range for which the development of the malaria parasites inside the mosquito vector is considered most suitable for transmission, as an indicator of this suitability.

For *P. falciparum* a lower temperature limit of 18°C was used and for *P. vivax* 15°C (Gilles, 1999; Watts et al., 2019). Between 1990 and 2018, the number of months with

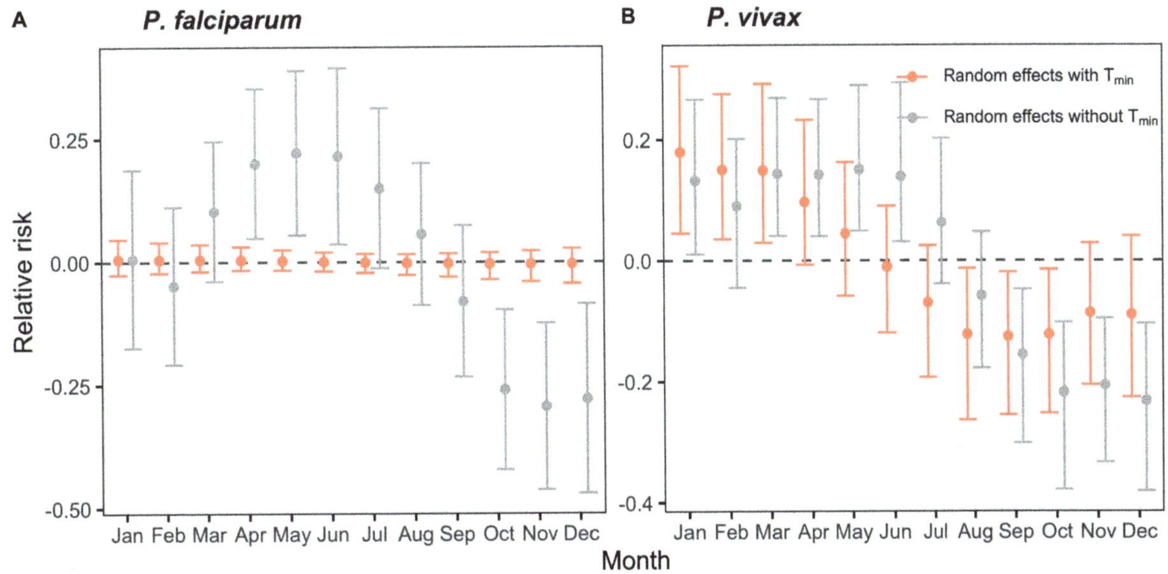

FIGURE 3 | Effect of minimum temperature (T_{min}) on the annual cycle of malaria in El Oro 1990–2018. Difference in the monthly random effect marginal posterior distributions for models of **(A)** *P. falciparum* and **(B)** *P. vivax* malaria that include minimum temperature (orange), lagged by 3 months and exclude minimum temperature (gray). Relative risk, on the log scale, is defined as the annual parasite incidence (API), $\log(\rho_{st})$.

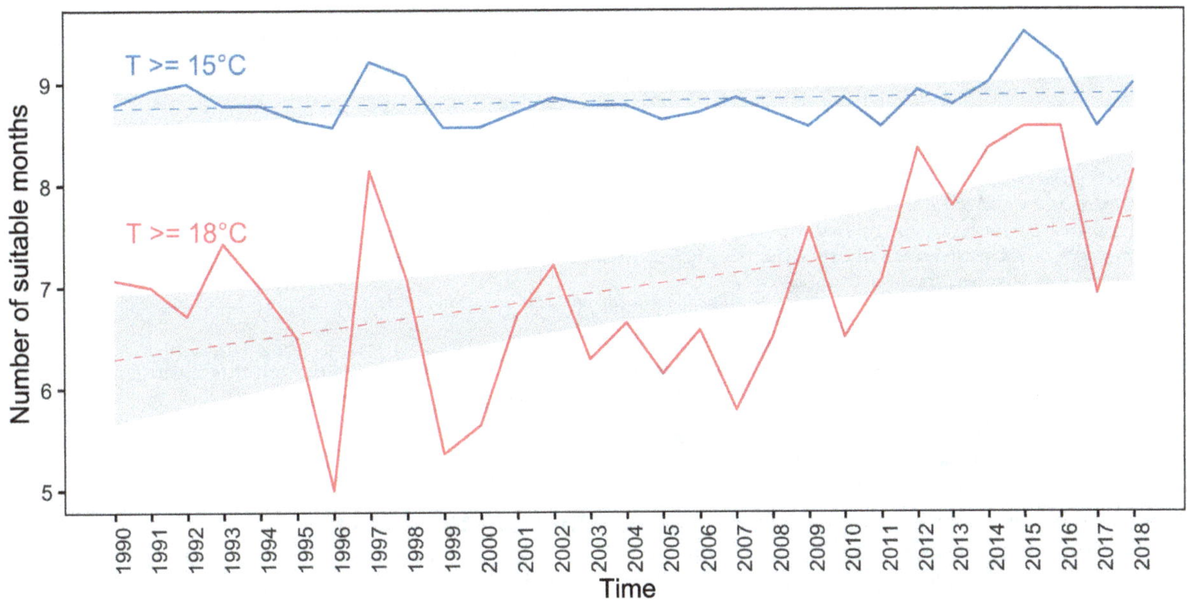

FIGURE 4 | Suitable temperature conditions for malaria transmission in El Oro 1990–2018. Mean (solid curve) number of months per year where minimum temperature exceeds 18°C (i.e., considered suitable for *P. falciparum* malaria transmission; pink) and where minimum temperature exceeds 15°C (i.e., considered suitable for *P. vivax* malaria transmission; blue), logistic regression line (dashed curve) and 95% confidence intervals (gray shading).

suitable temperatures for *P. falciparum* transmission showed an increasing trend (**Figure 4**), with noticeable peaks of around 8 months of suitable temperature conditions occurring between 1997 and 1998 and between 2014 and 2016. This trend of increasing temperatures for *P. falciparum* transmission coincides with warmer temperatures throughout the year in El Oro and increasing temperatures between 1990 and 2018 (**Supplementary Figure S10**). In contrast, temperature conditions for *P. vivax* malaria transmission showed no increasing trend in El Oro between 1990 and 2018 (**Figure 4**), although similar peaks in suitability were observed in 1997–1998 and in 2015–2016.

The most parsimonious models of malaria in El Oro 1990–2018 included minimum temperature and precipitation as

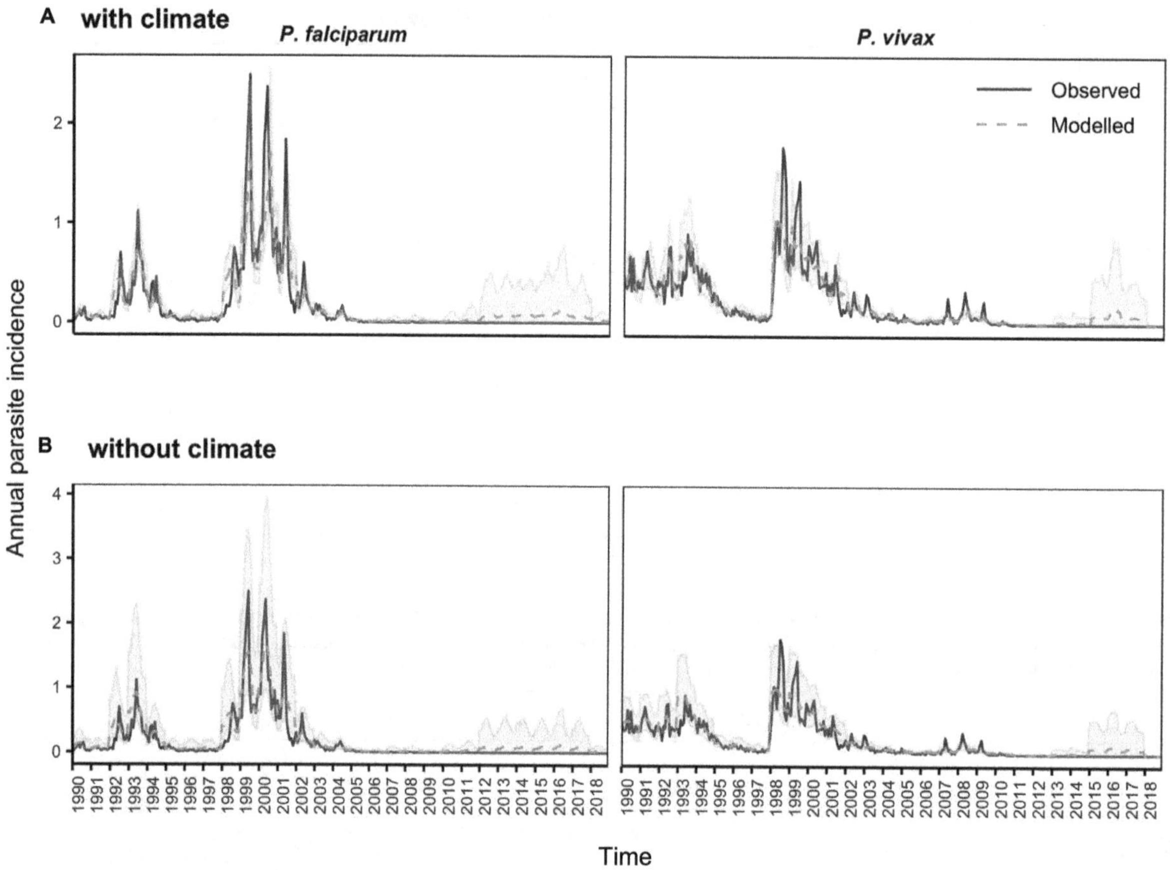

FIGURE 5 | Model posterior distributions with and without climate information for *P. falciparum* and *P. vivax* malaria in El Oro 1990–2018. Observed (gray solid line), posterior mean (blue dashed line) and 95% credible intervals (blue shading) for annual parasite incidence (API) for **(A)** models that include minimum temperature, lagged by 3 months and precipitation, lagged by 3 months for *P. falciparum* models and 1 month for *P. vivax* models and **(B)** without climate information. For models of *P. falciparum* malaria minimum temperature and precipitation were included as linear terms. For *P. vivax* malaria models, model fit improved when including non-linear functions of minimum temperature and precipitation.

linear terms for *P. falciparum* and as non-linear functions for *P. vivax* malaria, poverty rates, level of urbanization including an interaction with the period when the vector control measures were implemented, and spatial and temporal random effects (**Table 1**). Although in these models the credible intervals for precipitation and poverty rates contained zero, the addition of these covariates to the models decreased DIC values and increased model fit for *P. falciparum* and *P. vivax* malaria incidence in El Oro between 1990 and 2018. Accounting for poverty rates (socioeconomic effects) across El Oro also decreased DIC and WAIC for models of *P. falciparum* and *P. vivax* malaria. Including meteorological variables (as linear terms for *P. falciparum* and as non-linear functions for *P. vivax* malaria) decreased the uncertainty of the model posterior distributions, in comparison to distributions from models that excluded meteorological variables (**Figure 5**). In particular, model uncertainty was reduced more for *P. falciparum* malaria, especially during the large outbreaks that occurred in 1992–1994 and 1998–2002. Interestingly during the later years of the study period, model posterior distributions show an upsurge in malaria incidence, particularly for *P. vivax* incidence between 2015 and 2018 although this upsurge was not observed in case reports.

Control Interventions and Malaria Incidence in El Oro 2001–2015

We fitted separate sub-models for incidence of *P. falciparum* and *P. vivax* malaria in El Oro between 2001 and 2015, to evaluate the impact of the three vector control measures (IRS, space spraying and ULV fumigation) that were implemented during this period. These intervention models included the same covariates as the full models (linear and non-linear climate information and socioeconomic effects) and random effects but with the addition of the intervention data that were available for 2001–2015.

By comparing the differences in the covariate parameter estimates from the full models for the entire time series 1990–2018 and the intervention models for the period 2001–2015, we found that posterior mean estimates were roughly similar across the different models (**Figure 6** and **Supplementary Tables S4, S5**). However, there was more uncertainty in the

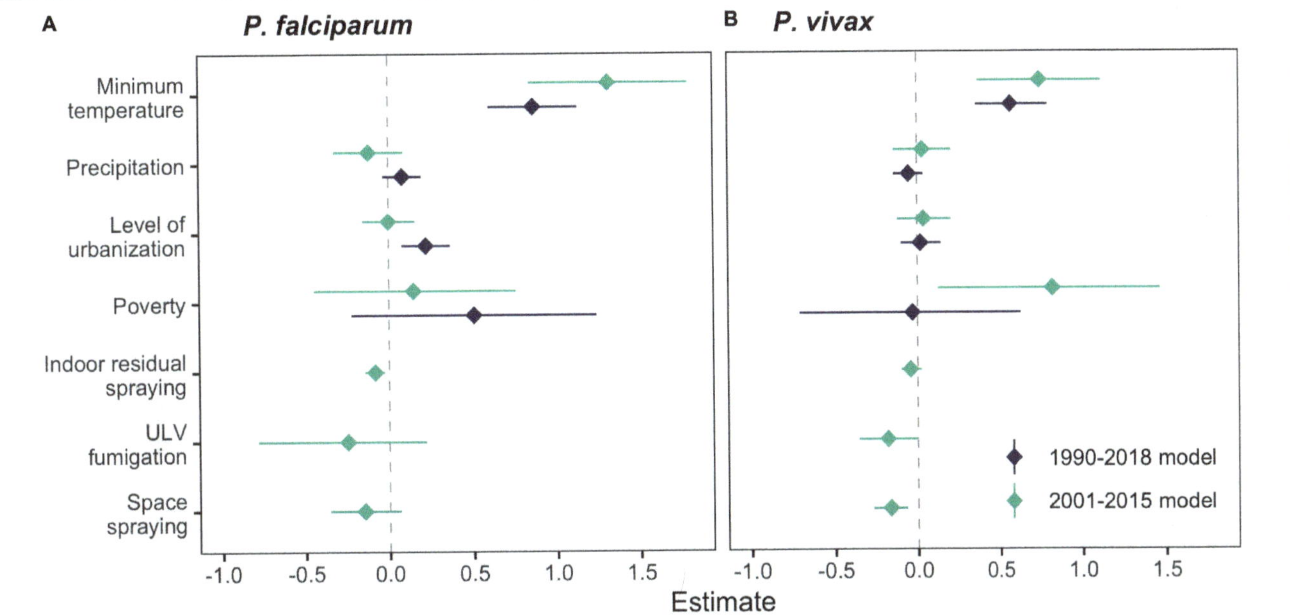

FIGURE 6 | Posterior mean estimates for environmental, socioeconomic and malaria vector control covariates for models of **(A)** *P. falciparum* and **(B)** *P. vivax* malaria from full models (dark blue) and intervention models (green). All interventions were lagged by 3 months, apart from space spraying in the *P. falciparum* model, which was lagged by 2 months.

estimates for the environmental covariates in the intervention models compared to the 1990–2018 models, particularly for minimum temperature. We also found that between 2001 and 2015 areas in El Oro with greater levels of poverty were associated with higher incidences of *P. vivax* malaria. In the intervention models, IRS implemented in El Oro 2001–2015, 3 months prior to case detection was associated with decreased incidence of *P. falciparum* malaria but was not associated with significant decreases in incidence of *P. vivax* malaria. Space spraying was associated with decreased *P. vivax* malaria incidence in the following 3 months but not *P. falciparum* malaria in the following 2 months. ULV fumigation, also lagged by 3 months was not statistically significant (i.e., the credible intervals contained zero).

We also assessed which vector control measure implemented in El Oro between 2001 and 2015 provided more valuable information to the intervention models in explaining malaria incidence across the province. We found there was considerable heterogeneity in the model improvement for each control measure, as measured by RMSE difference (**Figure 7**). IRS improved the model for *P. falciparum* malaria in the coastal northwest of El Oro and in cantons along the Ecuador-Peru border, improving the model by up to 14%. In contrast, there was little improvement in model fit for *P. vivax*. Space spraying improved models of both *P. falciparum* and *P. vivax* in the province capital, Machala, with a greater improvement for *P. vivax*. ULV fumigation provided minimal or no model improvement for either parasite.

Finally, we explored if the variation in malaria incidence in El Oro attributed to the vector control measures in the intervention model could be captured in the random effects structure of the full models. We compared the yearly random effects of the full models (fitted to data from 1990 to 2018), which did not include intervention data, to the yearly random effects of the intervention models (fitted to data from 2001 to 2015. We found that for some years (2001–2008) there was a reduction in the magnitude of the random effects for the 2001–2015 models, suggesting the control measures accounted for some of the unexplained variation in malaria incidence in the model for 1990–2018 during those years. However, a considerable portion of the random variation was likely due to other unmeasured factors. Between 2012 and 2015 the random effects of the *P. falciparum* models are close to zero, indicating that variation in malaria incidence for those years was well captured by factors included in the model (**Figure 8**). We found a similar pattern for *P. vivax* malaria, with a reduction in the value of the random effects for the intervention model, compared to the full model during the early years of the interventions 2001–2009. This reduction indicates that the control measures influenced the interannual variation of malaria risk during these years.

DISCUSSION

For regions approaching malaria elimination and where funding and disease surveillance are limited, it is important to understand the drivers of malaria incidence in order to prevent disease re-establishment and to ensure that elimination efforts are sustained. In this study, we developed a statistical modeling framework to disentangle the relative role of multiple explanatory variables in driving variation in malaria incidence, while accounting for unobserved heterogeneity. We found that minimum temperature

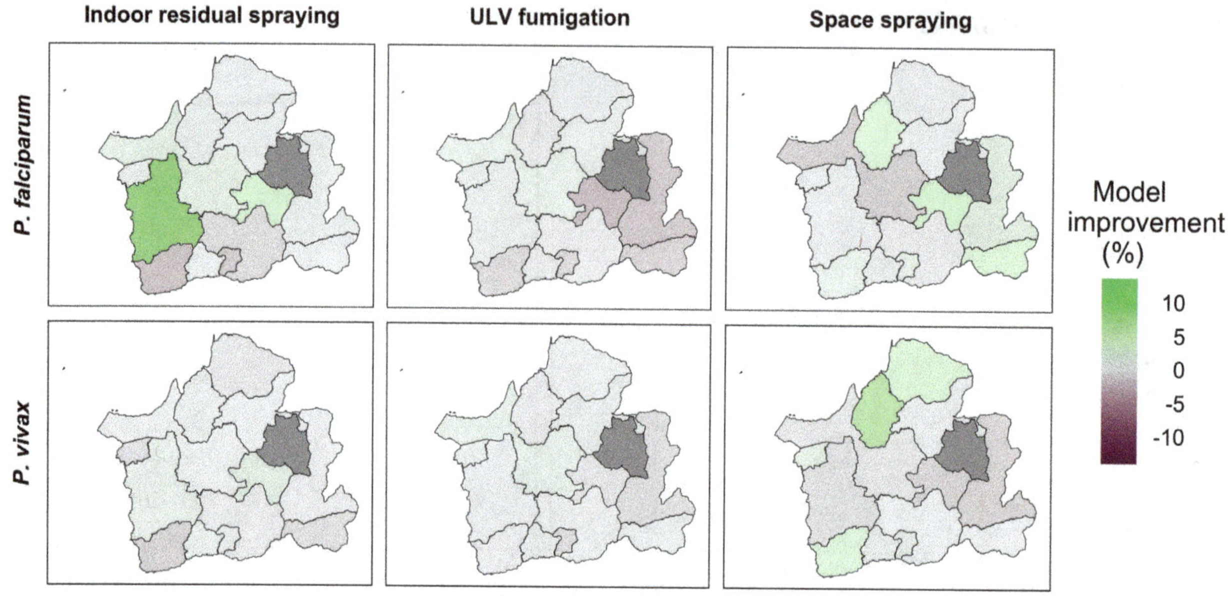

FIGURE 7 | Model improvement for each vector control measure in El Oro 2001–2015. Model improvement, calculated as percentage change in root mean square error (RMSE) between models of *P. falciparum* and *P. vivax* malaria excluding each control measure, indoor residual spraying, ULV fumigation, and space spraying, and models including each measure. Positive values (green) show where the addition of the control measure reduces RMSE and negative values (purple) show where including the intervention does not improve the model. Gray areas show missing data.

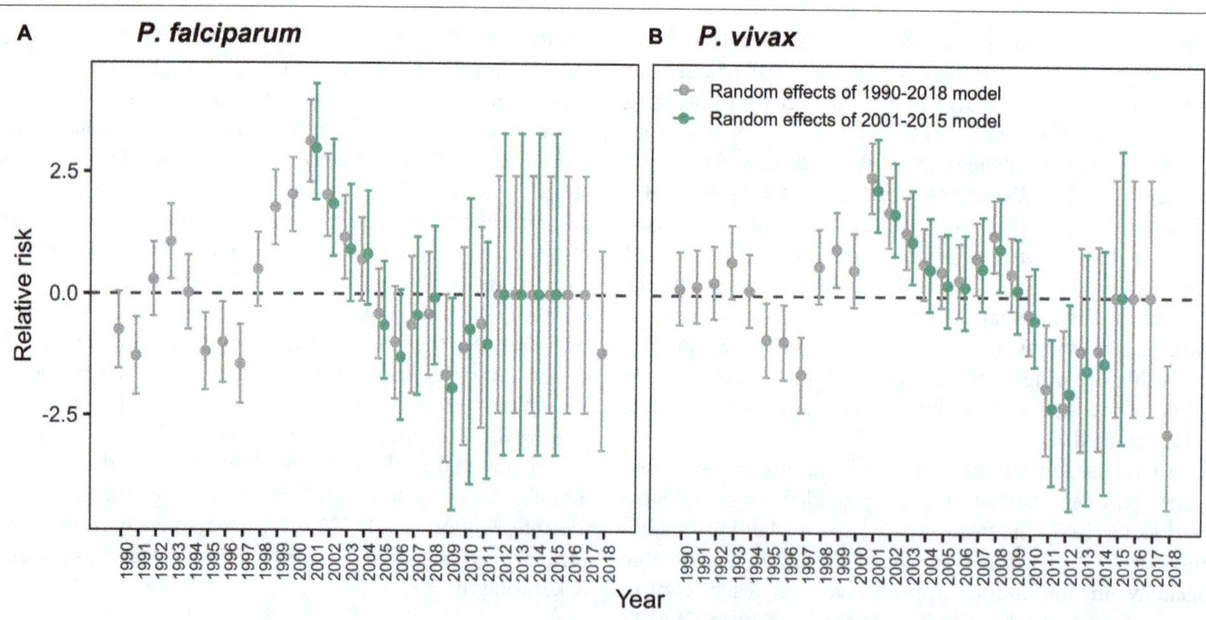

FIGURE 8 | Interannual random effects for malaria risk in El Oro 1990–2018. Difference in the interannual random effect marginal posterior distributions for **(A)** *P. falciparum* malaria models and **(B)** *P. vivax* malaria models. Distributions from the intervention model are shown in green, which include intervention data. Distributions from the full model are shown in gray, which does not include intervention data. Relative risk, on the log scale, is defined as the annual parasite incidence (API), $\log(\rho_{st})$.

was an important driver of malaria incidence in El Oro. We also found that control measures had a differential impact on the two types of malaria. After the intensive period of vector control in El Oro between 2001 and 2015 malaria incidence in rural areas declined more than malaria in urbanized areas and *P. vivax* malaria became more dominant. Incidence of *P. falciparum* malaria was also reduced more than *P. vivax* malaria and relatively more *P. vivax* cases were reported in urbanized areas during this time period. The greater reduction in *P. falciparum* malaria is expected given that malaria control measures deployed during this time, are primarily designed for use in rural settings and target mosquito vectors that are exophagic such as *An. albimanus*, a dominant malaria vector in El Oro.

Indoor residual spraying has largely been shown to be effective in reducing malaria transmission in settings with high prevalence and when applied on a large scale, especially in African countries (Pluess et al., 2010). In this study we found that IRS was effective at reducing the incidence of *P. falciparum* malaria in El Oro between 2001 and 2015, but not *P. vivax* malaria. Conventional control methods are less effective in reducing transmission of *P. vivax* compared to *P. falciparum* malaria because of the ability of *P. vivax* to cause multiple relapsing malaria episodes after the initial infection, from the activation of dormant liver stages (hypnozoites). In addition the *P. vivax* parasite develops more rapidly in the mosquito than *P. falciparum* and so control methods such as IRS deployed in El Oro, which aim to shorten the mosquito lifespan are less effective (Mendis et al., 2001; Bassat et al., 2016). The rapid development of *P. vivax* and hypnozoite stage also means that drug treatments, which are often of a longer duration are less effective in reducing transmission as mosquitoes can become infected during a pre-symptomatic period, allowing for onward transmission before drug treatment is initiated (White, 2008; McCarthy et al., 2013).

We found that IRS only reduced the incidence of *P. falciparum* malaria and in the west of the province. IRS is most effective against endophilic mosquitoes, which rest indoors following a blood meal. The two main malaria in vectors in El Oro, *A. albimanus* and *A. punctimacula*, are most commonly observed biting outdoors and mainly rest outdoors (Ryan et al., 2017). As a result, IRS and other conventional control methods may not be suitable for reducing malaria transmitted by these mosquitoes.

In contrast we found that space spraying was effective in reducing incidence of *P. vivax* in El Oro, especially in the capital, Machala and by a larger amount than IRS. Evidence for the success of space spraying is limited and it is currently only recommended during outbreaks. In our study, space-spraying is possibly targeting outdoor resting mosquitoes, such as *A. albimanus*, especially in peri-urban areas where housing conditions are poor and outdoor exposure is higher. There is evidence of a positive effect of space-spraying on malaria incidence in India, but the current evidence base is limited (Pryce et al., 2018).

The *P. vivax* malaria parasite is able to develop at lower temperatures than *P. falciparum* (Nikolaev, 1935; Moshkovsky, 1946; Olliaro et al., 2016; Ohm et al., 2018), enabling its persistence in less favorable environmental conditions (Mendis et al., 2001). We found a stronger association between minimum temperature and *P. falciparum* malaria than *P. vivax*, and all of the seasonality in *P. falciparum* malaria was explained by temperature. A greater association between minimum temperature and *P. falciparum* malaria compared to *P. vivax* has been previously identified in China (Bi et al., 2013), but to our knowledge this difference has not been previously quantified in South America. The stronger effect of temperature on *P. falciparum* malaria is due to the greater dependence of *P. falciparum* transmission on the mosquito vector, which is sensitive to climate conditions such as temperature. In contrast *P. vivax* transmission is less influenced by the mosquito vector and can be sustained by unpredictable relapsing infections, which have been suggested to be explained by other factors such as systemic illness in humans (White, 2011). Similarly, between 2001 and 2015 we found that areas in El Oro with higher levels of poverty were associated with increased incidences of *P. vivax* malaria, which suggests that socioeconomic conditions, such as limited access to healthcare, may have influenced relapsing *P. vivax* infections during this time.

Warmer minimum temperatures in El Oro were associated with increases in *P. falciparum* and *P. vivax* malaria incidence 3 months later. This finding is in agreement with other studies in South America that have found a similar relationship between higher temperatures and malaria incidence (Poveda et al., 2000; Basurko et al., 2011; Laneri et al., 2019). This relationship can be attributed to the physiological effects of temperature on both the mosquito vector and parasite that increases transmission. For example warmer temperatures shorten the development time of the parasite inside the mosquito, the EIP and increase mosquito larval reproduction thus increasing disease transmission (Bayoh and Lindsay, 2003; Blanford et al., 2013; Mordecai et al., 2013). We also found a trend of rising minimum temperatures in El Oro between 1990 and 2018, with an increase in the number of months that have suitable minimum temperature conditions for *P. falciparum* malaria transmission, which suggests a lengthening of the malaria transmission season. Large peaks in the transmission suitability of both *P. falciparum* and *P. vivax* malaria are evident between 1997–1998 and 2014–2016, when major El Niño events occurred. El Niño conditions bring warmer and wetter conditions to southern Ecuador, conditions that are favorable for malaria transmission and have previously been suggested to have caused a peak in cases observed during this time (Krisher et al., 2016). Increasingly suitable temperature conditions and large-scale climate events such as El Niño pose a real threat for the re-establishment of malaria in El Oro if cases are allowed to return, surveillance is not maintained, and interventions are not deployed appropriately. Our model posterior distributions for 2012–2018 show increases in malaria incidence despite zero or few cases being reported, which is possibly due to warmer temperatures and the large El Niño event that occurred during this time. This highlights how incidence could rise if risks, such as relaxing control efforts are not mitigated.

Rainfall is essential for providing suitable habitats for mosquito breeding (Thomson et al., 2005; Parham and Michael, 2010) and is thus considered to be a dominant factor in driving malaria transmission. Studies in the Amazon and Argentina have found that rainfall was important in determining malaria incidence (Dantur Juri et al., 2009; Olson et al., 2009). In this study, rainfall was not a statistically significant explanatory variable for malaria incidence in El Oro, possibly because ample larval habitat was already available. Two to three months prior to the peak malaria season (March–June), monthly rainfall accumulation reaches 80 mm across El Oro, which is considered to be suitable conditions for malaria transmission (Watts et al., 2019), and up to 530 mm rainfall in the southeast of the province. In addition, much of El Oro is rural with extensive mangroves in the northwest coastal regions, which provide habitat suited to *A. albimanus* mosquitoes (Pinault and Hunter, 2012). Therefore, our results suggest that rainfall is not a limiting factor for malaria transmission in El Oro.

The addition of temporal random effects for each year in the full models for 1990–2018 accounted for some of the variation in malaria incidence due to the control measures that were explicitly accounted for in the intervention model for 2001–2015, particularly for *P. falciparum* malaria, which appeared more sensitive to interventions. The use of temporal random effects also allowed us to pick up variation in malaria in El Oro due to other unobserved factors. For example, the large El Niño events mentioned previously likely caused an increased number of cases and a reduction in the unexplained yearly variation during 1997–1998 and between 2014 and 2016. However, we expect that the temperature and precipitation variables included in the models to pick up some variation to due climatic anomalies from El Niño events. The Cenepa War, a period of political instability across the Ecuador-Peru border (Krisher et al., 2016) likely hindered malaria control efforts and case reporting during 1995, and there is evidence of reduced malaria risk during this time in the interannual random effects, which is likely explained by reduced reporting. In addition we found that the outbreak of *P. vivax* in 2008 was not driven by a climatic event and may instead be driven by a political event or lapse in control efforts.

Despite the considerable length of the dataset, there are some limitations to consider. In Ecuador a high number of malaria cases are asymptomatic. Low levels of parasitemia, which act as a reservoir of transmission, are difficult to diagnose (Sáenz et al., 2017). It is likely that many cases of *P. vivax* malaria were missed and not reported during the study period. In addition, many *P. vivax* cases reported between 1990 and 2018 are likely to be relapses from the same initial infection, which could mask the true climate-malaria relationship. We also found that urban malaria was approximately 70% higher than incidence of malaria in rural areas. However, this may be a product of migration from neighboring countries and cases being imported from rural areas and subsequently recorded as originating in urban areas, as was found in Colombia (Molina Gómez et al., 2017). We could not quantify the amount of malaria variation explained by migration owing to the lack of detailed migration data for the whole time period. Due to El Oro's location on a key migratory route, including for Venezuelan refugees, it is likely that human movements are influential in driving case reporting and malaria incidence. In addition, outbreaks in northern Peru can increase the risk of malaria transmission in El Oro due to cross border human movement. Other factors that likely contributed to the spatiotemporal variation in malaria incidence in El Oro that were accounted for through the use of random effects include variations in case reporting and surveillance, as well as health seeking behavior in El Oro.

The incompleteness of the intervention data for the study period is also a limiting factor in this study. We were only able to evaluate the role of the three control measures implemented between 2001 and 2015 although there were other important elimination efforts that were carried out in El Oro between 1990 and 2018. For example, the use of DDT was widely used until 1996 and a campaign to distribute insecticide-treated bed nets (ITNs) was initiated in 2004, although no detailed data exist for this in El Oro, or for other forms of personal protection that would have contributed to local elimination. However, by examining the interannual random effects of our models we observe a reduction in *P. falciparum* malaria risk between 2004 and 2006, which could be attributed to the use of ITNs. In 2005, the Ministry of Health suspended the use of chloroquine for treatment of *P. falciparum* malaria, adopting the recommended change to artemisinin-based combination therapy (ACT) amid reports of drug resistance, which local partners reported led to a major decline in transmission (Krisher et al., 2016). The introduction of ACT in Colombia and Peru at similar times contributed to significant reductions in malaria case numbers (Rodríguez et al., 2011; Quispe et al., 2016). ACT introduction is also likely to have contributed to local malaria elimination El Oro as we observed declining malaria risk from this time through the use of interannual random effects in our models. At the same time in El Oro, a new shorter treatment regime for *P. vivax* malaria was adopted to ensure patients completed their treatment course, which was also reported to have contributed to declining transmission (Krisher et al., 2016).

In summary, we have developed a modeling framework for exploring the barriers to malaria elimination in a low-transmission setting. Accounting for unobserved interannual variation via yearly random effects is useful for investigating malaria variation in many different contexts where detailed data, such as intervention information, may not be available. Here, we used available intervention data to explore the relative impact of three vector control measures on *P. falciparum* and *P. vivax* malaria in El Oro. We also provide an assessment of where control measures improved models of *P. falciparum* and *P. vivax* incidence, which will prove useful for targeting future malaria control efforts in the region. We have shown that warmer temperatures increase incidence of *P. falciparum* malaria, which is important to consider in light of global environmental change and increasing climate suitability for malaria transmission (Laporta et al., 2015; Watts et al., 2019). In addition, with a global warming of 1.5°C above pre-industrial levels it is predicted that the western coast of South America, including southern Ecuador, will experience temperatures between 2 and 3°C warmer and precipitation could increase by up to 20% (IPCC, 2018), providing climate conditions that are highly suitable for malaria transmission. In contrast, we show that *P. vivax* malaria is less sensitive to temperature variations and shows more complex transmission patterns, making it particularly challenging to eliminate (Feachem et al., 2010). An assessment of the environmental obstacles to elimination efforts in Ecuador is timely and important. Lapses in control efforts should be avoided, especially as it becomes harder to prevent and detect cases due to limited funding for surveillance and control. Recently, indigenous cases of malaria have been detected in El Oro and re-introduction of malaria parasites along with warming temperatures threaten current elimination progress.

AUTHOR CONTRIBUTIONS

IF and RL conceived the study. IF collated the data, fitted the models, analyzed the results, and wrote the manuscript. AS-I helped conceive the study, provided information on the vector control measures, and contributed to discussion of the study results. RS provided insight on vector-borne diseases and surveillance in El Oro. GC-E helped with the environmental data sources and extraction. MS, EB-A, TO, and JA provided the malaria case data and intervention data for analysis. FS provided insight on the malaria situation in Ecuador, including treatments, and diagnostics. KJ provided input on model formulation. KJ and CD provided input on interpretation of model results. RL and AS-I edited the manuscript. All authors critically reviewed and approved the final version of the manuscript. Special recognition of MS, posthumously (1959–2020), a leader in the field of medical entomology and tireless advocate for community public health in El Oro. All authors contributed to the article and approved the submitted version.

ACKNOWLEDGMENTS

We thank all those at the Ministerio de Salud Pública, Machala, Ecuador for their kind hospitality and support for this work, Leonardo Ortega-López for his thoughtful discussion on malaria in Ecuador, members of KJ Lab Group at UCL for their discussion on data collation and analysis, and finally members of the Planetary Health and Infectious Diseases group at LSHTM for their support and discussion on this work.

REFERENCES

Abatzoglou, J. T., Dobrowski, S. Z., Parks, S. A., and Hegewisch, K. C. (2018). TerraClimate, a high-resolution global dataset of monthly climate and climatic water balance from 1958–2015. *Sci. Data* 5:170191. doi: 10.1038/sdata.2017.191

Alimi, T. O., Fuller, D. O., Qualls, W. A., Herrera, S. V., Arevalo-Herrera, M., Quinones, M. L., et al. (2015). Predicting potential ranges of primary malaria vectors and malaria in northern South America based on projected changes in climate, land cover and human population. *Paras. Vect.* 8:431. doi: 10.1186/s13071-015-1033-9

Aregawi, M. W., Ali, A. S., Al-mafazy, A., Molteni, F., Katikiti, S., Warsame, M., et al. (2011). Reductions in malaria and anaemia case and death burden at hospitals following scale-up of malaria control in Zanzibar, 1999-2008. *Malaria J.* 10:46. doi: 10.1186/1475-2875-10-46

Bassat, Q., Velarde, M., Mueller, I., Lin, J., Leslie, T., Wongsrichanalai, C., et al. (2016). Key knowledge gaps for plasmodium vivax control and elimination. *Am. J. Trop. Med. Hyg.* 95 (Suppl. 6), 62–71. doi: 10.4269/ajtmh.16-0180

Basurko, C., Hanf, M., Han-Sze, R., Rogier, S., Heritier, P., Grenier, C., et al. (2011). Influence of climate and river level on the incidence of malaria in Cacao. French Guiana. *Malaria J.* 10:26. doi: 10.1186/1475-2875-10-26

Bayoh, M. N., and Lindsay, S. W. (2003). Effect of temperature on the development of the aquatic stages of *Anopheles gambiae* sensu stricto (Diptera: Culicidae). *Bull. Entomol. Res.* 93, 375–381. doi: 10.1079/BER2003259

Beck-Johnson, L. M., Nelson, W. A., Paaijmans, K. P., Read, A. F., Thomas, M. B., and Bjørnstad, O. N. (2013). The effect of temperature on Anopheles mosquito population dynamics and the potential for malaria transmission. *PLoS One* 8:e79276. doi: 10.1371/journal.pone.0079276

Bennett, A., Yukich, J., Miller, J. M., Vounatsou, P., Hamainza, B., Ingwe, M. M., et al. (2014). A methodological framework for the improved use of routine health system data to evaluate national malaria control programs: evidence from Zambia. *Populat. Health Metrics* 12:30. doi: 10.1186/s12963-014-0030-0

Besag, J., York, J., and Mollié, A. (1991). Bayesian image restoration, with two applications in spatial statistics (with discussion). *Ann. Instit. Statist. Math.* 43, 1–59.

Bi, Y., Yu, W., Hu, W., Lin, H., Guo, Y., Zhou, X.-N., et al. (2013). Impact of climate variability on *Plasmodium vivax* and *Plasmodium falciparum* malaria in Yunnan Province, China. *Paras. Vect.* 6:357. doi: 10.1186/1756-3305-6-357

Blanford, J. I., Blanford, S., Crane, R. G., Mann, M. E., Paaijmans, K. P., Schreiber, K. V., et al. (2013). Implications of temperature variation for malaria parasite development across Africa. *Sci. Rep.* 3:1300. doi: 10.1038/srep01300

Burkett-Cadena, N. D., and Vittor, A. Y. (2017). Deforestation and vector-borne disease: forest conversion favors important mosquito vectors of human pathogens. *Basic Appl. Ecol.* 26, 101–110. doi: 10.1016/j.baae.2017.09.012

Calil, J., Reguero, B. G., Zamora, A. R., Losada, I. J., and Méndez, F. J. (2017). Comparative Coastal Risk Index (CCRI): a multidisciplinary risk index for Latin America and the Caribbean. *PLoS One* 12:e0187011. doi: 10.1371/journal.pone.0187011

Caminade, C., Kovats, S., Rocklov, J., Tompkins, A. M., Morse, A. P., Colón-González, F. J., et al. (2014). Impact of climate change on global malaria distribution. *Proc. Natl. Acad. Sci. U.S.A.* 111, 3286–3291. doi: 10.1073/pnas.1302089111

Conn, J. E., Grillet, M. E., Correa, M., and Sallum, M. A. M. (2018). *Malaria Transmission in South America—Present Status and Prospects for Elimination, Towards Malaria Elimination.* London: IntechOpen Limited.

Conn, J. E., Wilkerson, R. C., Segura, M. N. O., de Souza, R. T. L., Schlichting, C. D., Wirtz, R. A., et al. (2002). Emergence of a new neotropical malaria vector facilitated by human migration and changes in land use. *Am. J. Trop. Med. Hygiene* 66, 18–22. doi: 10.4269/ajtmh.2002.66.18

Daniels, J. P. (2018). Increasing malaria in Venezuela threatens regional progress. *Lancet Infect. Dis.* 18:257. doi: 10.1016/S1473-3099(18)30086-0

Dantur Juri, M. J., Zaidenberg, M., Claps, G. L., Santana, M., and Almiron, W. R. (2009). Malaria transmission in two localities in north-western Argentina. *Malaria J.* 8:18. doi: 10.1186/1475-2875-8-18

European Space Agency (2019). *ESA Climate Change Initiative.* Paris: European Space Agency.

Feachem, R. G. A., Phillips, A. A., Hwang, J., Cotter, C., Wielgosz, B., Greenwood, B. M., et al. (2010). Shrinking the malaria map: progress and prospects. *Lancet* 376, 1566–1578. doi: 10.1016/S0140-6736(10)61270-6

Gagnon, A. S., Smoyer-Tomic, K. E., and Bush, A. B. G. (2002). The El Niño Southern oscillation and malaria epidemics in South America. *Int. J. Biometeorol.* 46, 81–89. doi: 10.1007/s00484-001-0119-6

Galardo, A. K. R., Zimmerman, R. H., Lounibos, L. P., Young, L. J., Galardo, C. D., Arruda, M., et al. (2009). Seasonal abundance of anopheline mosquitoes and their association with rainfall and malaria along the Matapi River, Amapa, [corrected] Brazil. *Med. Veter. Entomol.* 23, 335–349. doi: 10.1111/j.1365-2915.2009.00839.x

Giardina, F., Kasasa, S., Sie, A., Utzinger, J., Tanner, M., and Vounatsou, P. (2014). Effects of vector-control interventions on changes in risk of malaria parasitaemia in sub-Saharan Africa: a spatial and temporal analysis. *Lancet Glob. Health* 2, e601–e615. doi: 10.1016/S2214-109X(14)70300-6

Gilles, H. M. (1999). *Protozoal Diseases.* London: Arnold.

Gneiting, T., and Raftery, A. E. (2007). Strictly proper scoring rules, prediction, and estimation. *J. Am. Stat. Assoc.* 102, 359–378. doi: 10.1198/016214506000001437

Graves, P., Osgood, D., Thomson, M., Sereke, K., Araia, A., Zerom, M., et al. (2008). Effectiveness of malaria control during changing climate conditions in Eritrea,

1998-2003. *Trop. Med. Int. Health* 13, 218–228. doi: 10.1111/j.1365-3156.2007.01993.x

Grillet, M. E., Hernández-Villena, J. V., Llewellyn, M. S., Paniz-Mondolfi, A. E., Tami, A., Vincenti-Gonzalez, M. F., et al. (2019). Venezuela's humanitarian crisis, resurgence of vector-borne diseases, and implications for spillover in the region. *Lancet Infect. Dis.* 19, e149–e161. doi: 10.1016/S1473-3099(18)30757-6

Hahn, M. B., Gangnon, R. E., Barcellos, C., Asner, G. P., and Patz, J. A. (2014). Influence of deforestation, logging, and fire on malaria in the Brazilian Amazon. *PLoS One* 9:e85725. doi: 10.1371/journal.pone.0085725

IPCC (2018). *Global Warming of 15°C. An IPCC Special Report on the Impacts of Global Warming of 15°C above Pre-industrial Levels and Related Global Greenhouse Gas Emission Pathways, in the Context of Strengthening the Global Response to the Threat of Climate Change.* Geneva: IPCC.

Jaramillo-Ochoa, R., Sippy, R., Farrell, D. F., Cueva-Aponte, C., Beltrán-Ayala, E., Gonzaga, J. L., et al. (2019). Effects of political instability in venezuela on malaria resurgence at Ecuador–Peru Border, 2018. *Emerg. Infect. Dis. J.* 25, 834–836. doi: 10.3201/eid2504.181355

Krisher, L. K., Krisher, J., Ambuludi, M., Arichabala, A., Beltrán-Ayala, E., Navarrete, P., et al. (2016). Successful malaria elimination in the Ecuador–Peru border region: epidemiology and lessons learned. *Malaria J.* 15:573. doi: 10.1186/s12936-016-1630-x

Laneri, K., Cabella, B., Prado, P. I., Mendes Coutinho, R., and Kraenkel, R. A. (2019). Climate drivers of malaria at its southern fringe in the Americas. *PLoS One* 14:e0219249. doi: 10.1371/journal.pone.0219249

Laporta, G. Z., Linton, Y.-M., Wilkerson, R. C., Bergo, E. S., Nagaki, S. S., Sant'Ana, D. C., et al. (2015). Malaria vectors in South America: current and future scenarios. *Paras. Vect.* 8:426. doi: 10.1186/s13071-015-1038-4

Lowe, R., Cazelles, B., Paul, R., and Rodó, X. (2016). Quantifying the added value of climate information in a spatio-temporal dengue model. *Stochas. Environ. Res. Risk Assess.* 30, 2067–2078. doi: 10.1007/s00477-015-1053-1

Lowe, R., Stewart-Ibarra, A. M., Petrova, D., García-Díez, M., Borbor-Cordova, M. J., Mejía, R., et al. (2017). Climate services for health: predicting the evolution of the 2016 dengue season in Machala, Ecuador. *Lancet Planet. Health* 1, e142–e151. doi: 10.1016/S2542-5196(17)30064-5

McCarthy, J. S., Griffin, P. M., Sekuloski, S., Bright, A. T., Rockett, R., Looke, D., et al. (2013). Experimentally induced blood-stage *Plasmodium vivax* infection in healthy volunteers. *J. Infect. Dis.* 208, 1688–1694. doi: 10.1093/infdis/jit394

Mendis, K., Sina, B. J., Marchesini, P., and Carter, R. (2001). The neglected burden of *Plasmodium vivax* malaria. *Am. J. Trop. Med. Hygiene* 64(Suppl. 1–2), 97–106. doi: 10.1179/2047772413Z.000000000179

Molina Gómez, K., Caicedo, M. A., Gaitán, A., Herrera-Varela, M., Arce, M. I., Vallejo, A. F., et al. (2017). Characterizing the malaria rural-to-urban transmission interface: the importance of reactive case detection. *PLoS Negl. Trop. Dis.* 11:e0005780. doi: 10.1371/journal.pntd.0005780

Mordecai, E. A., Paaijmans, K. P., Johnson, L. R., Balzer, C., Ben-Horin, T., de Moor, E., et al. (2013). Optimal temperature for malaria transmission is dramatically lower than previously predicted. *Ecol. Lett.* 16, 22–30. doi: 10.1111/ele.12015

Moreno, A. R. (2006). Climate change and human health in Latin America: drivers, effects, and policies. *Reg. Environ. Change* 6, 157–164. doi: 10.1007/s10113-006-0015-z

Moreno, J. E., Rubio-Palis, Y., Paez, E., Perez, E., and Sanchez, V. (2007). Abundance, biting behaviour and parous rate of anopheline mosquito species in relation to malaria incidence in gold-mining areas of southern Venezuela. *Med. Vet. Entomol.* 21, 339–349. doi: 10.1111/j.1365-2915.2007.00704.x

Moshkovsky, S. (1946). On the dependency of the speed of development of plasmodia malaria on temperature. *Med. Para Para Bol.* 15, 19–32.

Nikolaev, B. P. (1935). On the influence of temperature on the development of malaria plasmodia inside the mosquito. *Trans. Pasteur Inst. Epi. Bact. Leningrad.* 2, 1–5.

Ohm, J. R., Baldini, F., Barreaux, P., Lefevre, T., Lynch, P. A., Suh, E., et al. (2018). Rethinking the extrinsic incubation period of malaria parasites. *Paras. Vect.* 11:178. doi: 10.1186/s13071-018-2761-4

Olliaro, P. L., Barnwell, J. W., Barry, A., Mendis, K., Mueller, I., Reeder, J. C., et al. (2016). Implications of *Plasmodium vivax* biology for control, elimination, and research. *Am. J. Trop. Med. Hygiene* 95(Suppl. 6), 4–14. doi: 10.4269/ajtmh.16-0160

Olson, S. H., Gangnon, R., Elguero, E., Durieux, L., Guegan, J. F., Foley, J. A., et al. (2009). Links between climate, malaria, and wetlands in the Amazon Basin. *Emerg. Infect. Dis.* 15, 659–662. doi: 10.3201/eid1504.080822

Paaijmans, K. P., Read, A. F., and Thomas, M. B. (2009). Understanding the link between malaria risk and climate. *Proc. Natl. Acad. Sci. U.S.A.* 106, 13844–13849. doi: 10.1073/pnas.0903423106

Padilla, J. C., Chaparro, P. E., Molina, K., Arevalo-Herrera, M., and Herrera, S. (2015). Is there malaria transmission in urban settings in Colombia? *Malaria J.* 14, 453. doi: 10.1186/s12936-015-0956-0

PAHO (2017). *Epidemiological Alert: Increase in Cases of Malaria.* Washington, DC: PAHO.

Parham, P. E., and Michael, E. (2010). Modeling the effects of weather and climate change on malaria transmission. *Environ. Health Perspect.* 118, 620–626. doi: 10.1289/ehp.0901256

Patz, J. A., and Olson, S. H. (2006). Malaria risk and temperature: influences from global climate change and local land use practices. *Proc. Natl. Acad. Sci. U.S.A.* 103, 5635–5636. doi: 10.1073/pnas.0601493103

Pinault, L. L., and Hunter, F. F. (2012). Characterization of larval habitats of *Anopheles albimanus*, *Anopheles pseudopunctipennis*, *Anopheles punctimacula*, and *Anopheles oswaldoi* s.l. populations in lowland and highland Ecuador. *J. Vect. Ecol.* 37, 124–136. doi: 10.1111/j.1948-7134.2012.00209.x

Pluess, B., Tanser, F. C., Lengeler, C., and Sharp, B. L. (2010). Indoor residual spraying for preventing malaria. *Cochrane Database Syst. Rev.* 2010:CD006657. doi: 10.1002/14651858.CD006657.pub2

Poveda, G., Graham, N. E., Epstein, P. R., Rojas, W., Quiñones, M. L., Vélez, I. D., et al. (2000). "Climate and ENSO variability associated with vector-borne diseases in Colombia," in *El Niño and the Southern Oscillation: Multiscale Variability and Global and Regional Impacts*, eds H. F. Diaz and V. Markgraf (Cambridge: Cambridge University Press), 183–204. doi: 10.1017/cbo9780511573125.007

Prussing, C., Saavedra, M., Bickersmith, S., Alava, F., Guzmán, M., Manrique Valverde, E. J., et al. (2019). Malaria vector species in Amazonian Peru co-occur in larval habitats but have distinct larval microbial communities. *PLoS Negl. Trop. Dis.* 13:e0007412. doi: 10.1371/journal.pntd.0007412

Pryce, J., Choi, L., Richardson, M., and Malone, D. (2018). Insecticide space spraying for preventing malaria transmission. *Cochrane Database Syst. Rev.* 11:CD012689. doi: 10.1002/14651858.CD012689.pub2

Quispe, A. M., Llanos-Cuentas, A., Rodriguez, H., Clendenes, M., Cabezas, C., Leon, L. M., et al. (2016). Accelerating to zero: strategies to eliminate Malaria in the Peruvian Amazon. *Am. J. Trop. Med. Hygiene* 94, 1200–1207. doi: 10.4269/ajtmh.15-0369

Recht, J., Siqueira, A. M., Monteiro, W. M., Herrera, S. M., Herrera, S., and Lacerda, M. V. G. (2017). Malaria in Brazil, Colombia, Peru and Venezuela: current challenges in malaria control and elimination. *Malaria J.* 16:272. doi: 10.1186/s12936-017-1925-6

Rodríguez, J. C. P., Uribe, G. Á, Araújo, R. M., Narváez, P. C., and Valencia, S. H. (2011). Epidemiology and control of malaria in Colombia. *Memorias Instit. Oswaldo Cruz.* 106(Suppl. 1), 114–122. doi: 10.1590/s0074-02762011000900015

Rue, H., Martino, S., and Chopin, N. (2009). Approximate Bayesian inference for laten Gaussian models by using integrated nested Laplace approximations. *J. R. Stat. Soc. Ser. B* 71, 319–392. doi: 10.1111/j.1467-9868.2008.00700.x

Ryan, S. J., Lippi, C. A., Boersch-Supan, P. H., Heydari, N., Silva, M., Adrian, J., et al. (2017). Quantifying seasonal and diel variation in Anopheline and Culex human biting rates in Southern Ecuador. *Malaria J.* 16:479. doi: 10.1186/s12936-017-2121-4

Sáenz, F. E., Arévalo-Cortés, A., Valenzuela, G., Vallejo, A. F., Castellanos, A., Poveda-Loayza, A. C., et al. (2017). Malaria epidemiology in low-endemicity areas of the northern coast of Ecuador: high prevalence of asymptomatic infections. *Malaria J.* 16:300. doi: 10.1186/s12936-017-1947-0

Siraj, A. S., Santos-Vega, M., Bouma, M. J., Yadeta, D., Carrascal, D. R., and Pascual, M. (2014). Altitudinal changes in malaria incidence in highlands of Ethiopia and Colombia. *Science* 343, 1154–1158. doi: 10.1126/science.1244325

Spiegelhalter, D. J., Best, N. G., Carlin, B. P., and Van Der Linde, A. (2002). Bayesian measures of model complexity and fit. *J. R. Stat. Soc. Ser. B* 64, 583–639. doi: 10.1111/1467-9868.00353

Stefani, A., Dusfour, I., Corrêa, A. P. S. A., Cruz, M. C. B., Dessay, N., Galardo, A. K. R., et al. (2013). Land cover, land use and malaria in the Amazon: a systematic literature review of studies using remotely sensed data. *Malaria J.* 12:192. doi: 10.1186/1475-2875-12-192

Tauzer, E., Borbor-Cordova, M. J., Mendoza, J., De La Cuadra, T., Cunalata, J., and Stewart-Ibarra, A. M. (2019). A participatory community case study of periurban coastal flood vulnerability in southern Ecuador. *PLoS One* 14:e0224171. doi: 10.1371/journal.pone.0224171

Thomson, M. C., Mason, S. J., Phindela, T., and Connor, S. J. (2005). Use of rainfall and sea surface temperature monitoring for malaria early warning in Botswana. *Am. J. Trop. Med. Hygiene* 73, 214–221. doi: 10.4269/ajtmh.2005.73.214

Tucker Lima, J. M., Vittor, A., Rifai, S., and Valle, D. (2017). Does deforestation promote or inhibit malaria transmission in the Amazon? A systematic literature review and critical appraisal of current evidence. *Philos. Trans. R. Soc. Lond. Ser. B Biol. Sci.* 372:20160125. doi: 10.1098/rstb.2016.0125

Vittor, A. Y., Gilman, R. H., Tielsch, J., Glass, G., Shields, T., Lozano, W. S., et al. (2006). The effect of deforestation on the human-biting rate of *Anopheles darlingi*, the primary vector of *Falciparum malaria* in the Peruvian Amazon. *Am. J. Trop. Med. Hygiene* 74, 3–11. doi: 10.4269/ajtmh.2006.74.3

Vittor, A. Y., Pan, W., Gilman, R. H., Tielsch, J., Glass, G., Shields, T., et al. (2009). Linking deforestation to Malaria in the Amazon: characterization of the breeding habitat of the principal malaria vector, *Anopheles darlingi*. *Am. J. Trop. Med. Hygiene* 81, 5–12.

Watanabe, S. (2010). Asymptotic equivalence of bayes cross validation and widely applicable information criterion in singular learning theory. *J. Mach. Learn. Res.* 11, 3571–3594.

Watts, N., Amann, M., Arnell, N., Ayeb-Karlsson, S., Belesova, K., Boykoff, M., et al. (2019). The 2019 report of the lancet countdown on health and climate change: ensuring that the health of a child born today is not defined by a changing climate. *Lancet* 394, 1836–1878. doi: 10.1016/S0140-6736(19)32596-6

Wayant, N. M., Maldonado, D., Rojas, de Arias, A., Cousino, B., and Goodin, D. G. (2010). Correlation between normalized difference vegetation index and malaria in a subtropical rain forest undergoing rapid anthropogenic alteration. *Geospatial Health* 4, 179–190. doi: 10.4081/gh.2010.199

White, N. J. (2008). The role of anti-malarial drugs in eliminating malaria. *Malaria J.* 7:S8. doi: 10.1186/1475-2875-7-S1-S8

White, N. J. (2011). Determinants of relapse periodicity in *Plasmodium vivax* malaria. *Malaria J.* 10:297. doi: 10.1186/1475-2875-10-297

WHO (2018). *Update on the E-2020 Initiative of 21 Malaria-Eliminating Countries*. Geneva: WHO.

WHO (2019). *World Malaria Report 2019*. Geneva: WHO.

Wolfarth-Couto, B., Silva, R. A., da, and Filizola, N. (2019). Variability in malaria cases and the association with rainfall and rivers water levels in Amazonas State, Brazil. *Cad. Saúde Públ.* 35:e00020218.

9

Enlightening the Malaria Parasite Life Cycle: Bioluminescent *Plasmodium* in Fundamental and Applied Research

*Giulia Siciliano and Pietro Alano**

Dipartimento di Malattie Infettive, Parassitarie ed Immunomediate, Istituto Superiore di Sanità, Rome, Italy

Edited by:
Luca Cevenini,
University of Bologna, Italy

Reviewed by:
Lucilla Iacumin,
University of Udine, Italy
Massimo Guardigli,
University of Bologna, Italy

****Correspondence:***
Pietro Alano,
Dipartimento di Malattie Infettive,
Parassitarie ed Immunomediate,
Istituto Superiore di Sanità,
Viale Regina Elena n. 299,
00161 Rome, Italy
alano@iss.it

The unicellular protozoan parasites of the genus *Plasmodium* impose on human health worldwide the enormous burden of malaria. The possibility to genetically modify several species of malaria parasites represented a major advance in the possibility to elucidate their biology and is now turning laboratory lines of transgenic *Plasmodium* into precious weapons to fight malaria. Amongst the various genetically modified plasmodia, transgenic parasite lines expressing bioluminescent reporters have been essential to unveil mechanisms of parasite gene expression and to develop *in vivo* imaging approaches in mouse malaria models. Mainly the human malaria parasite *Plasmodium falciparum* and the rodent parasite *P. berghei* have been engineered to express bioluminescent reporters in almost all the developmental stages of the parasite along its complex life cycle between the insect and the vertebrate hosts. *Plasmodium* lines expressing conventional and improved luciferase reporters are now gaining a central role to develop cell based assays in the much needed search of new antimalarial drugs and to open innovative approaches for both fundamental and applied research in malaria.

Keywords: malaria, *Plasmodium*, bioluminescence, reporter genes, *in vivo* imaging, cell-based screening assays

Introduction

Half of the world population is at risk of malaria (World Health Organization, 2013), the most common, and severe parasitic mosquito-borne disease (White et al., 2014). Five species of the protozoan genus *Plasmodium* infect humans, with *Plasmodium falciparum* and *P. vivax* causing over 200 million cases/year and *P. falciparum* inflicting virtually all the 6–700,000 annual deaths (2013) recorded mainly in children of Sub-Saharan Africa.

The malaria parasite exhibits a complex life cycle involving an *Anopheles* mosquito and a vertebrate host (**Figure 1**). When an infected female mosquito bites a human, the *Plasmodium* sporozoites travel to the liver and invade hepatocytes, where parasites replicate as hepatic schizonts until several thousand merozoites are produced and released in the bloodstream. In *P. vivax*, but not in *P. falciparum*, some liver parasites remain instead quiescent (hypnozoites), resuming replication, and infection after several weeks or months. Upon erythrocyte invasion in the bloodstream *Plasmodium* parasites undergo asexual replication forming mature schizonts whose rupture releases merozoites that invade new erythrocytes. Some blood stage parasites differentiate instead into male and female gametocytes that, when ingested in the mosquito blood meal, are activated to produce gametes. Gamete fusion in the insect midgut produces a zygote which develops into a motile ookinete, traversing the gut wall, and transforming into an oocyst, where

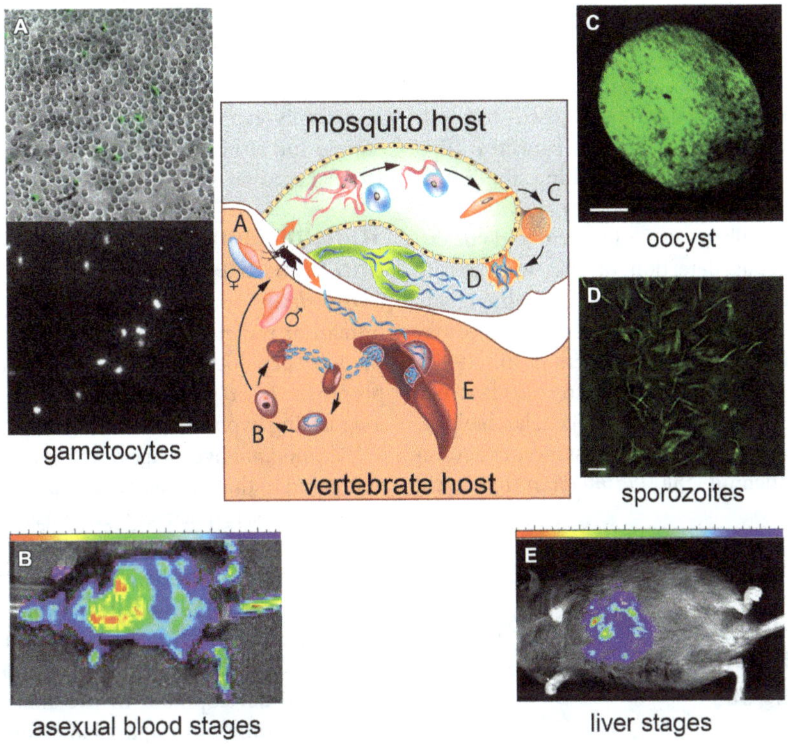

FIGURE 1 | Transgenic bioluminescent malaria parasites at different stages of their development in the vertebrate and mosquito hosts. The central diagram represents the *Plasmodium* life cycle, showing the progression through the developmental stages of the parasites in the mosquito vector and in the vertebrate host. **(A)** Bioluminescence imaging (BLI) of individual *Plasmodium falciparum* gametocytes expressing a click beetle luciferase under a sexual stage-specific promoter. The bright field image shows immobilized gametocytes, highlighted in green, amongst uninfected erythrocytes; the dark field shows the bioluminescence signal of the gametocytes incubated with D-luciferin. Magnification bar: 15 μm. (Adapted from Cevenini et al., 2014). **(B)** BLI of a mouse infected with asexual *P. berghei* parasites expressing a firefly luciferase-green fluorescent protein (GFP) fusion. Heatmap of the bioluminescent signal identifies the sites of accumulation of the parasites (Reproduced with permission from Claser et al., 2011). **(C)** Fluorescence of a firefly luciferase-GFP fusion protein expressed in *P. falciparum* sporozoites contained in a oocyst and **(D)** obtained from the dissection of infected mosquito salivary glands. Magnification bar: 5 μm. **(E)** *In vivo* bioluminescent signal obtained by transgenic *P. falciparum* liver stage parasites developing in the chimeric liver of a humanized mouse **(C–E)** are reproduced with permission from Vaughan et al. (2012).

1000s of sporozoites are produced. The life cycle is closed when sporozoites, migrated from the ruptured oocyst to the mosquito salivary glands, are injected in a new human host by the insect bite.

The pathogenesis of malaria is caused by the asexual blood stages. In the clinical manifestations of *P. falciparum* malaria, the ability of parasites to sequester in the microvasculature of several organs, including the brain, is a major cause of disease severity, and of a fatal outcome (Miller et al., 2002; Milner et al., 2014; Sack et al., 2014). Consequently, the need to cure symptomatic patients traditionally drove efforts toward finding drugs targeting the asexual blood stage parasites, often underestimating the importance of eliminating also the sporozoite, and gametocyte transmission stages or, in *P. vivax*, the hypnozoites. The recent concerning reports from South East Asia of a decreased sensitivity of some *P. falciparum* infections to frontline combination therapies based on artemisinin derivatives is now calling for renewed efforts to address this emergency in the frame of a global strategy to control malaria and eventually eradicate this deadly parasite.

It is possible to cultivate all asexual and sexual blood stages of *P. falciparum in vitro*, unlike *P. vivax*. *Plasmodium* species infecting rodents have been also intensely studied as mouse models of aspects of malaria, with *P. berghei* particularly exploited for its amenability to genetic manipulation. In contrast, transgenesis technology has been comparatively more troublesome in *P. falciparum*. This review aims to highlight the importance of *Plasmodium* transgenic parasites, particularly those engineered with bioluminescent reporters, both in the study of the fundamental biology of *Plasmodium* and in developing effective antimalarial treatments.

Luciferase enzymes catalyze the light-producing chemical reactions of bioluminescent organisms, in which a luminogenic substrate (e.g., D-luciferin) is oxidized in the presence of ATP, yielding photons. These can be accurately measured by a luminometer with a sensitivity and a virtual absence of background that made bioluminescent reporters potent and versatile tools in biology (Smale, 2010). Luciferases hold a special place in the history of *Plasmodium* transgenesis: the first plasmid construct to be successfully transfected in malaria parasites contained a firefly (*Photynus pyralis*) luciferase gene whose expression, driven by the promoter of a parasite sexual stage-specific gene, was measured in ookinetes of the bird parasite *P. gallinaceum* (Goonewardene et al., 1993). Subsequently, luciferase reporters have been used to optimize transfection techniques in *Plasmodium* parasites (Epp et al., 2008; Hasenkamp et al., 2012), including the introduction of the luciferase from the sea pansy *Renilla reniformis*, where use of different substrates (D-luciferin and coelenterazine) enabled simultaneous detection of the two parasite produced reporters (Militello and Wirth, 2003; Helm et al., 2010). Since the 1990s, with the stable genetic transformation of different species of *Plasmodium* (Waters et al., 1997), luciferase reporter genes greatly contributed to elucidate key aspects of malaria infection, from the parasite cellular biology, protein trafficking, gene function, and drug resistance, in several developmental stages throughout the *Plasmodium* life cycle (**Figure 1**).

The *Plasmodium* Life Cycle Marked by Bioluminescent Parasite Developmental Stages

Plasmodium Mosquito Stages

Parasite sexual stage development in the mosquito vector is crucial for the transmission of *Plasmodium*, and elucidating the biology of this process may therefore lead to design novel malaria transmission-blocking strategies. Some studies with bioluminescent parasites highlighted the importance of post-transcriptional regulation acting on stability and translation of several mRNAs, including those encoding major proteins of the gamete and ookinete surface (Mair et al., 2006). Assays with luciferase reporters were for instance fundamental to identify regulatory elements in the transcripts of the P25 and P28 surface proteins of *P. gallinaceum* and *P. falciparum* (Golightly et al., 2000; Oguariri et al., 2006).

Plasmodium parasites expressing luciferases also improved tool development for applied studies. A powerful bioassay to determine parasite ability to infect mosquitoes is based on feeding cultured *Plasmodium* gametocytes to mosquitoes, and it is used to measure effect of transmission blocking drugs or antibodies. This assay is, however, technically demanding and time consuming as the resulting oocysts need to be individually counted in dissected insects. After improvements by using *P. berghei* parasites expressing a green fluorescent protein (GFP) in mosquito stages (Delves and Sinden, 2010), a transgenic line of the human parasite *P. falciparum* line expressing the firefly luciferase in oocysts was developed. In the resulting luminescence-based standard membrane feeding assay (SMFA) the mean luminescence intensity of individual and pooled mosquitoes accurately quantified mean oocyst intensity, eliminating the need for mosquito dissection, and putting the basis for significant SMFA scalability (Stone et al., 2014).

Toward the end of parasite development in the mosquito, the sporozoites produced in the oocyst migrate to the insect salivary glands. Number of salivary gland sporozoites, the only mosquito stages infectious to a mammalian host, is an important index of *Plasmodium* mosquito development. The construction of a *P. berghei* line where a GFP-luciferase fusion is specifically expressed in sporozoites enabled establishment of a simple and fast assay of sporozoite loads from whole mosquitoes (Ramakrishnan et al., 2012).

Transmission from Mosquitoes: Sporozoites and Liver Stages

Plasmodium sporozoites injected from an infected mosquito to a human or rodent host start their intracellular development into the liver hepatocytes. This clinically silent stage is the target for prophylactic or vaccine strategies, particularly against *P. vivax* long lasting hypnozoites.

Plasmodium liver stage development has been poorly explored compared to that of blood stages partly because the *in vivo* and *in vitro* analyses, respectively, in mouse models and in cultured liver cells, are constrained by the necessity to sacrifice high numbers of mice or by inefficiency of sporozoite infection of cultured liver cells. Transgenic luciferase-expressing sporozoites improved detection strategies introducing bioluminescence imaging (BLI) and *in vivo* imaging system (IVIS) in the analysis of parasite liver stage development in live mice and in cultured hepatocytes. Real-time BLI requires injection of the luciferin substrate in the mouse or in the dissected organ and an intensified charge-coupled photon counting video camera to measure photon emission (Franke-Fayard et al., 2006; Braks et al., 2013). BLI and IVIS using firefly or sea pansy luciferases have been used for real-time, live monitoring of the progression of rodent parasitic infection in the whole animal or in specific organs (Ploemen et al., 2009; Annoura et al., 2013; Manzoni et al., 2014) and to test activity of drugs targeting liver stage infection, using *P. yoelii* and *P. berghei* transgenic sporozoites in human liver HepG2 or Huh-7 cells and in whole mice (Mwakingwe et al., 2009; Ramalhete et al., 2011, 2014; Derbyshire et al., 2012; Lacrue et al., 2013; Li et al., 2014; Marcsisin et al., 2014; Zuzarte-Luis et al., 2014). To improve these approaches, identification of parasite promoters specifically activated in liver development was achieved in *P. berghei*, also in this case relying on use of transgenic luciferase-promoter fusions (Helm et al., 2010).

The ability to reliably quantify parasite infection in hepatocytes is essential in the development of malaria vaccines. To overcome limitations of qRT-PCR-based quantification, *P. berghei* parasites expressing a GFP-luciferase fusion were introduced to evaluate antimalarial immunity both *in vivo*, in mice where this was induced by sporozoites unable to proliferate after irradiation or chloroquine prophylaxis, and *in vitro* in Huh-7 human liver hepatoma cells (Ploemen et al., 2011; Miller et al., 2013). Luciferase expressing *P. berghei* and *P. falciparum* sporozoites were also used to assess adequacy of sporozoite attenuation, obtained this time by genetic mutation, respectively, in *in vivo* murine malaria model and in primary human hepatocytes (Annoura et al., 2012; van Schaijk et al., 2014). These studies highlighted the role of cell mediated immunity mounting against the multiplication-deficient sporozoites. A role for antibody mediated immunity was instead shown by BLI of luciferase-expressing sporozoites of the human parasite *P. falciparum* in mice with a humanized liver, showing that infection in this organ was reduced by passive transfer of a monoclonal antibody targeting the sporozoite surface protein CSP (Sack et al., 2014). Finally, *P. berghei* and *P. yoelii* luciferase transgenic parasites were instrumental to evaluate modes of sporozoite administration, a critical bottleneck in immunization, and challenge protocols (Ploemen et al., 2013).

From the Liver to the Blood: the Asexual Erythrocytic Stages

Maturation of the liver schizont releases 1000s of merozoites that invade blood stream erythrocytes and starts the asexual, symptomatic blood stage infection. In *P. falciparum* the blood stage schizonts disappear from circulation as they adhere to host ligands on endothelial cells of the microvasculature in several organs, especially in the brain and in the placenta, through parasite proteins expressed on the infected erythrocyte surface, leading to severe pathogenesis such as cerebral malaria or adverse effects during pregnancy. As parasites are observed to accumulate in several organs, including the brain, also in the mouse malaria model, real-time BLI in whole mice or in dissected organs were conducted with *P. berghei* transgenic lines expressing luciferase under a constitutive or a schizont-specific promoter to identify the involved components of the immune system (Franke-Fayard et al., 2005; Amante et al., 2007; Spaccapelo et al., 2010; Claser et al., 2011; Pasini et al., 2013; Imai et al., 2014).

The need to elucidate the mechanisms of malaria pathogenesis directed research on the fundamental biology of parasite asexual development, one important aspect being how the parasite regulates its gene expression. The extremely high A+T content of the *Plasmodium* genomes however, prevented homology based identification of promoters, regulatory elements, and parasite transcription factors, whereas luciferase reporters proved to be of paramount importance in functionally identifying gene promoters and regulatory regions (Horrocks and Kilbey, 1996; Porter, 2002; Militello et al., 2004; Hasenkamp et al., 2013a). This work identified sequences functioning as bi-directional promoters, like the intergenic region of the *P. berghei* elongation factor-1α (*ef-1α*) gene (de Koning-Ward et al., 1999; Fernandez-Becerra et al., 2003) or the intron of the *P. falciparum var* genes (Epp et al., 2008), or evaluated whether specific promoters from one *Plasmodium* species were able (Fernandez-Becerra et al., 2003; Ozwara et al., 2003), or unable (Azevedo and del Portillo, 2007) to recruit the transcriptional machinery of a different malaria species. Importantly, luciferase expressing parasites were used to identify regulatory regions governing the expression of the *P. falciparum* polymorphic *var* genes encoding the parasite sequestration ligands, whose expression switch is responsible for parasite antigenic variation, and immune evasion (Deitsch et al., 1999; Calderwood et al., 2003; Frank et al., 2006; Muhle et al., 2009). In summary, luciferase reporters not only contributed to identify functional elements involved in parasite gene regulation (Bischoff et al., 2000; Militello et al., 2004; López-Estraño et al., 2007; Gopalakrishnan and López-Estraño, 2010; Zhang et al., 2011; Patakottu et al., 2012), but also were essential to select specific promoters in the development of *Plasmodium* inducible expression systems (de Azevedo et al., 2012; Kolevzon et al., 2014) and to test new regulatory regions in chromosomally integrated luciferase cassettes (Ekland et al., 2011; Weiwer et al., 2011; Che et al., 2012; Khan et al., 2012; Hasenkamp et al., 2013b).

A major effort in the fight against malaria, particularly *P. falciparum*, has been the screening for new antimalarial drugs, an endeavor that the appearance of artemisinin resistance in South East Asia makes dramatically urgent. In the past decades, *in vitro* methods measuring the incorporation of [^{3}H]-labeled hypoxanthine and ethanolamine or the activity of parasite Lactate Dehydrogenase have been the standard for *P. falciparum* cell based assays and used in large drug screenings (Fidock, 2010). The demand for high-throughput, non-radioactive assays prompted to exploit also in *Plasmodium* the high sensitivity and virtual absence of background of luciferase reporters, until recently used in this field only to study expression of the *P. falciparum* multidrug resistance gene *pfmdr1* in drug treated parasites (Myrick et al., 2003; Waller et al., 2003). To this aim a *P. falciparum* line expressing the firefly luciferase under the *heat shock protein 86* (*pfhsp86*) gene promoter in asexual stages enabled establishment of a cell-based luciferase drug screening assay in 96w plates (Cui et al., 2008), subsequently adapted to 384w plate using 10^5–10^6 parasites per well (Lucumi et al., 2010). Also *P. berghei* parasites expressing a firefly luciferase-GFP fusion were used for *in vitro* and *in vivo* bioluminescence drug assay, enabling use of animal models to test new drugs *in vivo* (Franke-Fayard et al., 2008; Lin et al., 2013).

Preparing Departure from the Blood: the Gametocytes

Plasmodium gametocytes are the parasite sexual stages responsible for the transmission from the vertebrate host to the mosquito. Male and female gametocytes are formed in the bloodstream and, in *P. falciparum*, they mature in 10 days through five developmental stages. Upon ingestion in the mosquito gut, mature gametocytes promptly differentiate into gametes and fertilization ensures parasite infection in the insect vector. A key priority in the present goal to globally eliminate malaria is to identify new drugs targeting in the bloodstream both the asexual and the sexual stages of the parasite. However, the non-replicative nature of gametocytes imposed to develop specific cell based screening assays, different from those used for asexual stages. One problem is for instance that of false negative signals due to the persistence of fluorescent reporter or of parasite enzyme activities in unhealthy or dying gametocytes. *P. falciparum* lines expressing a GFP-firefly luciferase gene under gametocyte specific promoters were established (Adjalley et al., 2011) and used in high-throughput screening assays of compounds with anti-asexual stage activity (Lucantoni et al., 2013). Recently, luciferase-based gametocyte assays have been improved by replacing the commonly used commercial luciferase substrates with an ATP-free, non-lysing D-luciferin formulation, yielding assay readouts that more reliably monitored viability and sensitivity to compounds of the treated gametocytes (Cevenini et al., 2014). In this work, absence of parasite cell lysis and the introduction in *P. falciparum* of the use of a potent luciferase from *Pyrophorus plagiophthalamus* under a gametocyte promoter enabled to perform for the first time BLI at the level of single parasite cells, individually distinguishing live and dead *P. falciparum* gametocytes (Cevenini et al., 2014).

Multiplexing, Subcellular Localization, Imaging: the Future in the Use of Bioluminescent Malaria Parasites

Virtually all stages of the complex life cycle of malaria parasites have been enlightened by the use in several studies of luciferase reporters. These engineered parasites provided key answers to fundamental biological questions and now represent important tools for drug screening. Novel potent reporters have already expanded the luciferase repertoire used in *P. falciparum* beyond the *P. pyralis* and Renilla enzymes (Azevedo et al., 2014; Cevenini et al., 2014), increasing sensitivity and enabling to further reduce parasite numbers in high-throughput screening assays, a non-trivial improvement when using specific stages (e.g., the gametocytes) whose cultivation is technically demanding. Nevertheless exploitation of the full potential of bioluminescent reporters in malaria research is just moving the first steps.

The possibility to tune luciferase emission properties, such as emission wavelength, kinetics or termo- and pH-stability, via random or site-directed mutagenesis or use of enzyme natural variants, led to introduce multicolor bioluminescence in antimalarial drug screening. A green and a red light emitting luciferase from *P. plagiophthalamus* were expressed in *P. falciparum* immature and mature gametocytes, providing for the first time the possibility to simultaneously measure differential, stage specific effects of drugs in a dual-color luciferase assay, and opening the possibility to apply multicolor bioluminescence to any parasite stage in fundamental and applied studies. A dual expression system with distinct luciferases would for instance be valuable in cell based high-throughput screenings to readily identify and discard compounds active against the reporter rather than the target cell (Thorne et al., 2012), as they will most likely affect only one luciferase type.

Another promising application of luciferase reporters is through their fusion to specific signals used by the parasite to traffic proteins in different extra cellular compartments of the infected erythrocyte. As protein export is uniquely regulated in the parasite and is essential for its survival, use of such fusions may be invaluable to screen for compounds targeting this process. Preliminary studies were conducted with the *P. pyralis* enzyme (Burghaus and Lingelbach, 2001) and more recent work established *P. falciparum* lines which express a brighter deep-sea shrimp luciferase equipped with sequences driving the reporter in the parasite cytoplasm or in erythrocyte compartments (Azevedo et al., 2014).

In another field of application, the achievement of single parasite cell BLI and the availability of luciferases whose red-shifted light emission is more efficiently detectable from blood and tissues are paving the road to significant progress in analyses of the host-parasite interplay. Co-cultures of different *P. falciparum* stages and human cell types *in vitro* can provide new insights of the physiology of asexual and sexual stage parasite sequestration. The increased sensitivity achieved in *in vivo* mouse imaging with a red-shifted luciferase expressed by the unicellular protozoan parasite *Trypanosoma brucei* (Van Reet et al., 2014) is promising in view of use also in *Plasmodium* infected mice. Importantly, the increasing availability of humanized mouse models for *P. falciparum* and *P. vivax* infections, supporting development of asexual, and sexual blood stages and of liver stages (Kaushansky et al., 2014) and the use of *P. falciparum* transgenic lines with a luciferase expressed constitutively (Vaughan et al., 2012) or under stage-specific promoters are expected to answer many unsolved questions.

The wealth of biological information provided by the use of engineered bioluminescent malaria parasites, not to mention those not reviewed here expressing a variety of fluorescent reporters, has been and will most likely continue to be enormous. The confined use of these whole cell biosensors in laboratory settings does not pose regulatory concerns on environmental release. From their aseptic sites of utilization, these genetically modified parasites will nevertheless have the most significant impact in the real world, contrasting the unbearable burden of a worldwide devastating disease.

Author Contribution

GS drafted and PA edited the manuscript.

Acknowledgments

Authors are indebted to Drs Luca Cevenini, Elisa Michelini, and Aldo Roda, University of Bologna, Bologna, Italy and Dr. Bruce B. Branchini, Connecticut College, New London, CT, USA, for several insightful discussions along our collaborations, and thank Mr. Cosimo M. Curianò for the figure artwork. Research in the authors' laboratory is supported from grants from the Bill & Melinda Gates Foundation and the EU EVIMalaR Network of Excellence.

References

Adjalley, S. H., Johnston, G. L., Li, T., Eastman, R. T., Ekland, E. H., Eappen, A. G., et al. (2011). Quantitative assessment of *Plasmodium falciparum* sexual development reveals potent transmission-blocking activity by methylene blue. *Proc. Natl. Acad. Sci. U.S.A.* 108, E1214–E1223. doi: 10.1073/pnas.1112037108

Amante, F. H., Stanley, A. C., Randall, L. M., Zhou, Y., Haque, A., McSweeney, K., et al. (2007). A role for natural regulatory T cells in the pathogenesis of experimental cerebral malaria. *Am. J. Pathol.* 171, 548–559. doi: 10.2353/ajpath.2007.061033

Annoura, T., Chevalley, S., Janse, C. J., Franke-Fayard, B., and Khan, S. M. (2013). Quantitative analysis of *Plasmodium berghei* liver stages by bioluminescence imaging. *Methods Mol. Biol.* 923, 429–443. doi: 10.1007/978-1-62703-026-7_30

Annoura, T., Ploemen, I. H., van Schaijk, B. C., Sajid, M., Vos, M. W., van Gemert, G. J., et al. (2012). Assessing the adequacy of attenuation of genetically modified malaria parasite vaccine candidates. *Vaccine.* 30, 2662–2670. doi: 10.1016/j.vaccine.2012.02.010

Azevedo, M. F., and del Portillo, H. A. (2007). Promoter regions of *Plasmodium vivax* are poorly or not recognized by *Plasmodium falciparum*. *Malar. J.* 6, 20. doi: 10.1186/1475-2875-6-20

Azevedo, M. F., Nie, C. Q., Elsworth, B., Charnaud, S. C., Sanders, P. R., Crabb, B. S., et al. (2014). *Plasmodium falciparum* transfected with ultra bright NanoLuc luciferase offers high sensitivity detection for the screening of growth and cellular trafficking inhibitors. *PLoS ONE* 9:e112571. doi: 10.1371/journal.pone.0112571

Bischoff, E., Guillotte, M., Mercereau-Puijalon, O., and Bonnefoy, S. (2000). A member of the *Plasmodium falciparum* Pf60 multigene family codes for a nuclear protein expressed by read through of an internal stop codon. *Mol. Microbiol.* 35, 1005–1016. doi: 10.1046/j.1365-2958.2000.01788.x

Braks, J., Aime, E., Spaccapelo, R., Klop, O., Janse, C. J., and Franke-Fayard, B. (2013). Bioluminescence imaging of *P. berghei* schizont sequestration in rodents. *Methods Mol. Biol.* 923, 353–368. doi: 10.1007/978-1-62703-026-7_25

Burghaus, P. A., and Lingelbach, K. (2001). Luciferase, when fused to an N-terminal signal peptide, is secreted from transfected *Plasmodium falciparum* and transported to the cytosol of infected erythrocytes. *J. Biol. Chem.* 276, 26838–26845. doi: 10.1074/jbc.M100111200

Calderwood, M. S., Gannoun-Zaki, L., Wellems, T. E., and Deitsch, K. W. (2003). *Plasmodium falciparum* var genes are regulated by two regions with separate promoters, one upstream of the coding region and a second within the intron. *J. Biol. Chem.* 278, 34125–34132. doi: 10.1074/jbc.M213065200

Cevenini, L., Camarda, G., Michelini, E., Siciliano, G., Calabretta, M. M., Bona, R., et al. (2014). Multicolor bioluminescence boosts malaria research: quantitative dual-color assay and single-cell imaging in *Plasmodium falciparum* parasites. *Anal. Chem.* 86, 8814–8821. doi: 10.1021/ac502098w

Che, P., Cui, L., Kutsch, O., Cui, L., and Li, Q. (2012). Validating a firefly luciferase-based high-throughput screening assay for antimalarial drug discovery. *Assay Drug Dev. Technol.* 10, 61–68. doi: 10.1089/adt.2011.0378

Claser, C., Malleret, B., Gun, S. Y., Wong, A. Y., Chang, Z. W., Teo, P., et al. (2011). CD8+ T cells and IFN-γ mediate the time-dependent accumulation of infected red blood cells in deep organs during experimental cerebral malaria. *PLoS ONE* 6:e18720. doi: 10.1371/journal.pone.0018720

Cui, L., Miao, J., Wang, J., Li, Q., and Cui, L. (2008). *Plasmodium falciparum*: development of a transgenic line for screening antimalarials using firefly luciferase as the reporter. *Exp. Parasitol.* 120, 80–87. doi: 10.1016/j.exppara.2008.05.003

de Azevedo, M. F., Gilson, P. R., Gabriel, H. B., Simões, R. F., Angrisano, F., Baum, J., et al. (2012). Systematic analysis of FKBP inducible degradation domain tagging strategies for the human malaria parasite *Plasmodium falciparum*. *PLoS ONE* 7:e40981. doi: 10.1371/journal.pone.0040981

Deitsch, K. W., del Pinal, A., and Wellems, T. E. (1999). Intra-cluster recombination and var transcription switches in the antigenic variation of *Plasmodium falciparum*. *Mol. Biochem. Parasitol.* 101, 107–116. doi: 10.1016/S0166-6851(99)00062-6

de Koning-Ward, T. F., Sperança, M. A., Waters, A. P., and Janse, C. J. (1999). Analysis of stage specificity of promoters in *Plasmodium berghei* using luciferase as a reporter. *Mol. Biochem. Parasitol.* 100, 141–146. doi: 10.1016/S0166-6851(99)00042-0

Delves, M. J., and Sinden, R. E. (2010). A semi-automated method for counting fluorescent malaria oocysts increases the throughput of transmission blocking studies. *Malar. J.* 9, 35. doi: 10.1186/1475-2875-9-35

Derbyshire, E. R., Prudêncio, M., Mota, M. M., and Clardy, J. (2012). Liver-stage malaria parasites vulnerable to diverse chemical scaffolds. *Proc. Natl. Acad. Sci. U.S.A.* 109, 8511–8516. doi: 10.1073/pnas.1118370109

Ekland, E. H., Schneider, J., and Fidock, D. A. (2011). Identifying apicoplast-targeting antimalarials using high-throughput compatible approaches. *FASEB J.* 25, 3583–3593. doi: 10.1096/fj.11-187401

Epp, C., Raskolnikov, D., and Deitsch, K. W. (2008). A regulatable transgene expression system for cultured *Plasmodium falciparum* parasites. *Malar. J.* 7, 86. doi: 10.1186/1475-2875-7-86

Fidock, D. A. (2010). Drug discovery: priming the antimalarial pipeline. *Nature* 465, 297–298. doi: 10.1038/465297a

Fernandez-Becerra, C., de Azevedo, M. F., Yamamoto, M. M., and del Portillo, H. A. (2003). *Plasmodium falciparum*: new vector with bi-directional promoter activity to stably express transgenes. *Exp. Parasitol.* 103, 88–91. doi: 10.1016/S0014-4894(03)00065-1

Frank, M., Dzikowski, R., Costantini, D., Amulic, B., Berdougo, E., and Deitsch, K. (2006). Strict pairing of var promoters and introns is required for var gene silencing in the malaria parasite *Plasmodium falciparum*. *J. Biol. Chem.* 281, 9942–9952 doi: 10.1074/jbc.M513067200

Franke-Fayard, B., Djokovic, D., Dooren, M. W., Ramesar, J., Waters, A. P., Falade, M. O., et al. (2008). Simple and sensitive antimalarial drug screening in vitro and in vivo using transgenic luciferase expressing *Plasmodium berghei* parasites. *Int. J. Parasitol.* 38, 1651–1662. doi: 10.1016/j.ijpara.2008.05.012

Franke-Fayard, B., Janse, C. J., Cunha-Rodrigues, M., Ramesar, J., Büscher, P., Que, I., et al. (2005). Murine malaria parasite sequestration: CD36 is the major receptor, but cerebral pathology is unlinked to sequestration. *Proc. Natl. Acad. Sci. U.S.A.* 102, 11468–11473. doi: 10.1073/pnas.0503386102

Franke-Fayard, B., Waters, A. P., and Janse, C. J. (2006). Real-time in vivo imaging of transgenic bioluminescent blood stages of rodent malaria parasites in mice. *Nat. Protoc.* 1, 476–485. doi: 10.1038/nprot.2006.69

Golightly, L. M., Mbacham, W., Daily, J., and Wirth, D. F. (2000). 3' UTR elements enhance expression of Pgs28, an ookinete protein of *Plasmodium gallinaceum*. *Mol. Biochem. Parasitol.* 105, 61–70. doi: 10.1016/S0166-6851(99)00165-6

Goonewardene, R., Daily, J., Kaslow, D., Sullivan, T. J., Duffy, P., Carter, R., et al. (1993). Transfection of the malaria parasite and expression of firefly luciferase. *Proc. Natl. Acad. Sci. U.S.A.* 90, 5234–5236. doi: 10.1073/pnas.90.11.5234

Gopalakrishnan, A. M., and López-Estraño, C. (2010). Role of cis-regulatory elements on the ring-specific hrp3 promoter in the human parasite *Plasmodium falciparum*. *Parasitol Res.* 106, 833–845. doi: 10.1007/s00436-010-1738-9

Hasenkamp, S., Russell, K. T., and Horrocks, P. (2012). Comparison of the absolute and relative efficiencies of electroporation-based transfection protocols for *Plasmodium falciparum*. *Malar. J.* 11, 210. doi: 10.1186/1475-2875-11-210

Hasenkamp, S., Russell, K. T., Ullah, I., and Horrocks, P. (2013a). Functional analysis of the 5' untranslated region of the phosphoglutamase 2 transcript in *Plasmodium falciparum*. *Acta Trop.* 127, 69–74. doi: 10.1016/j.actatropica.2013.03.007

Hasenkamp, S., Sidaway, A., Devine, O., Roye, R., and Horrocks, P. (2013b). Evaluation of bioluminescence-based assays of anti-malarial drug activity. *Malar. J.* 12, 58. doi: 10.1186/1475-2875-12-58

Helm, S., Lehmann, C., Nagel, A., Stanway, R. R., Horstmann, S., Llinas, M., et al. (2010). Identification and characterization of a liver stage-specific promoter region of the malaria parasite *Plasmodium*. *PLoS ONE* 5:e13653. doi: 10.1371/journal.pone.0013653

Horrocks, P., and Kilbey, B. J. (1996). Physical and functional mapping of the transcriptional start sites of *Plasmodium falciparum* proliferating cell nuclear antigen. *Mol. Biochem. Parasitol.* 82, 207–215. doi: 10.1016/0166-6851(96)02737-5

Imai, T., Iwawaki, T., Akai, R., Suzue, K., Hirai, M., Taniguchi, T., et al. (2014). Evaluating experimental cerebral malaria using oxidative stress indicator OKD48 mice. *Int. J. Parasitol.* 44, 681–685. doi: 10.1016/j.ijpara.2014.06.002

Kaushansky, A., Mikolajczak, S. A., Vignali, M., and Kappe, S. H. (2014). Of men in mice: the success and promise of humanized mouse models for human malaria parasite infections. *Cell Microbiol.* 16, 602–611. doi: 10.1111/cmi.12277

Khan, T., van Brummelen, A. C., Parkinson, C. J., and Hoppe, H. C. (2012). ATP and luciferase assays to determine the rate of drug action in in vitro cultures of *Plasmodium falciparum*. *Malar. J.* 11, 369. doi: 10.1186/1475-2875-11-369

Kolevzon, N., Nasereddin, A., Naik, S., Yavin, E., and Dzikowski, R. (2014). Use of peptide nucleic acids to manipulate gene expression in the malaria parasite *Plasmodium falciparum*. *PLoS ONE* 9:e86802. doi: 10.1371/journal.pone.0086802

Lacrue, A. N., Sáenz, F. E., Cross, R. M., Udenze, K. O., Monastyrskyi, A., Stein, S., et al. (2013). 4(1H)-Quinolones with liver stage activity against *Plasmodium berghei*. *Antimicrob. Agents. Chemother.* 57, 417–424. doi: 10.1128/AAC.00793-12

Li, Q., O'Neil, M., Xie, L., Caridha, D., Zeng, Q., Zhang, J., et al. (2014). Assessment of the prophylactic activity and pharmacokinetic profile of oral tafenoquine compared to primaquine for inhibition of liver stage malaria infections. *Malar. J.* 13, 141. doi: 10.1186/1475-2875-13141

Lin, J. W., Sajid, M., Ramesar, J., Khan, S. M., Janse, C. J., and Franke-Fayard, B. (2013). Screening inhibitors of *P. berghei* blood stages using bioluminescent reporter parasites. *Methods Mol. Biol.* 923, 507–522. doi: 10.1007/978-1-62703-026-7_35

López-Estraño, C., Gopalakrishnan, A. M., Semblat, J. P., Fergus, M. R., Mazier, D., and Haldar, K. (2007). An enhancer-like region regulates hrp3 promoter stage-specific gene expression in the human malaria parasite *Plasmodium falciparum. Biochim. Biophys. Acta* 1769, 506–513. doi: 10.1016/j.bbaexp.2007.04.009

Lucantoni, L., Duffy, S., Adjalley, S. H., Fidock, D. A., and Avery, V. M. (2013). Identification of MMV malaria box inhibitors of *Plasmodium falciparum* early-stage gametocytes using a luciferase-based high-throughput assay. *Antimicrob. Agents Chemother.* 57, 6050–6062. doi: 10.1128/AAC.00870-13

Lucumi, E., Darling, C., Jo, H., Napper, A. D., Chandramohanadas, R., Fisher, N., et al. (2010). Discovery of potent small-molecule inhibitors of multidrug-resistant *Plasmodium falciparum* using a novel miniaturized high-throughput luciferase-based assay. *Antimicrob. Agents Chemother.* 54, 3597–3604. doi: 10.1128/AAC.00431-10

Mair, G. R., Braks, J. A., Garver, L. S., Wiegant, J. C., Hall, N., Dirks, R. W., et al. (2006). Regulation of sexual development of *Plasmodium* by translational repression. *Science* 313, 667–669 doi: 10.1126/science.1125129

Manzoni, G., Briquet, S., Risco-Castillo, V., Gaultier, C., Topçu, S., Ivănescu, M. L., et al. (2014). A rapid and robust selection procedure for generating drug-selectable marker-free recombinant malaria parasites. *Sci. Rep.* 4, 4760. doi: 10.1038/srep04760

Marcsisin, S. R., Sousa, J. C., Reichard, G. A., Caridha, D., Zeng, Q., Roncal, N., et al. (2014). Tafenoquine and NPC-1161B require CYP 2D metabolism for anti-malarial activity: implications for the 8-aminoquinoline class of anti-malarial compounds. *Malar. J.* 13, 2. doi: 10.1186/1475-2875-13-2

Militello, K. T., Dodge, M., Bethke, L., and Wirth, D. F. (2004). Identification of regulatory elements in the *Plasmodium falciparum* genome. *Mol. Biochem. Parasitol.* 134, 75–88. doi: 10.1016/j.molbiopara.2003.11.004

Militello, K. T., and Wirth, D. F. (2003). A new reporter gene for transient transfection of *Plasmodium falciparum. Parasitol. Res.* 89, 154–157. doi: 10.1007/s00436-002-0721-5

Miller, J. L., Murray, S., Vaughan, A. M., Harupa, A., Sack, B., Baldwin, M., et al. (2013). Quantitative bioluminescent imaging of pre-erythrocytic malaria parasite infection using luciferase-expressing *Plasmodium yoelii. PLoS ONE* 8:e60820. doi: 10.1371/journal.pone.0060820

Miller, L. H., Baruch, D. I., Marsh, K., and Doumbo, O. K. (2002). The pathogenic basis of malaria. *Nature* 415, 673–679. doi: 10.1038/415673a

Milner, D. A. Jr., Whitten, R. O., Kamiza, S., Carr, R., Liomba, G., Dzamalala, C., et al. (2014). The systemic pathology of cerebral malaria in African children. *Front. Cell Infect Microbiol.* 4:104. doi: 10.3389/fcimb.2014.00104

Myrick, A., Munasinghe, A., Patankar, S., and Wirth, D. F. (2003). Mapping of the *Plasmodium falciparum* multidrug resistance gene 5'-upstream region, and evidence of induction of transcript levels by antimalarial drugs in chloroquine sensitive parasites. *Mol. Microbiol.* 49, 671–683. doi: 10.1046/j.1365-2958.2003.03597.x

Muhle, R. A., Adjalley, S., Falkard, B., Nkrumah, L. J., Muhle, M. E., and Fidock, D. A. (2009). A var gene promoter implicated in severe malaria nucleates silencing and is regulated by 3' untranslated region and intronic cis-elements. *Int. J. Parasitol.* 39, 1425–1439. doi: 10.1016/j.ijpara.2009.05.001

Mwakingwe, A., Ting, L. M., Hochman, S., Chen, J., Sinnis, P., and Kim, K. (2009). Non-invasive real-time monitoring of liver-stage development of bioluminescent *Plasmodium parasites. J. Infect. Dis.* 200, 1470–1478. doi: 10.1086/606115

Oguariri, R. M., Dunn, J. M., and Golightly, L. M. (2006). 3' gene regulatory elements required for expression of the *Plasmodium falciparum* developmental protein, Pfs25. *Mol. Biochem. Parasitol.* 146, 163–172. doi: 10.1016/j.molbiopara.2005.12.004

Ozwara, H., van der Wel, A., Kocken, C. H., and Thomas, A. W. (2003). Heterologous promoter activity in stable and transient *Plasmodium* knowlesi transgenes. *Mol. Biochem. Parasitol.* 130, 61–64. doi: 10.1016/S0166-6851(03)00141-5

Pasini, E. M., Braks, J. A., Fonager, J., Klop, O., Aime, E., Spaccapelo, R., et al. (2013). Proteomic and genetic analyses demonstrate that *Plasmodium berghei* blood stages export a large and diverse repertoire of proteins. *Mol. Cell. Proteomics* 12, 426–448. doi: 10.1074/mcp.M112.021238

Patakottu, B. R., Singh, P. K., Malhotra, P., Chauhan, V. S., and Patankar, S. (2012). In vivo analysis of translation initiation sites in *Plasmodium falciparum. Mol. Biol. Rep.* 39, 2225–2232. doi: 10.1007/s11033-011-0971-3

Ploemen, I., Behet, M., Nganou-Makamdop, K., van Gemert, G. J., Bijker, E., Hermsen, C., et al. (2011). Evaluation of immunity against malaria using luciferase-expressing *Plasmodium berghei* parasites. *Malar. J.* 10, 350. doi: 10.1186/1475-2875-10-350

Ploemen, I. H., Chakravarty, S., van Gemert, G. J., Annoura, T., Khan, S. M., Janse, C. J., et al. (2013). *Plasmodium* liver load following parenteral sporozoite administration in rodents. *Vaccine.* 31, 3410–3416. doi: 10.1016/j.vaccine.2012.09.080

Ploemen, I. H., Prudêncio, M., Douradinha, B. G., Ramesar, J., Fonager, J., van Gemert, G. J., et al. (2009). Visualisation and quantitative analysis of the rodent malaria liver stage by real time imaging. *PLoS ONE* 4:e7881. doi: 10.1371/journal.pone.0007881

Porter, M. E. (2002). Positive and negative effects of deletions and mutations within the 5' flanking sequences of *Plasmodium falciparum* DNA polymerase delta. *Mol. Biochem. Parasitol.* 122, 9–19. doi: 10.1016/S0166-6851(02)00064-6

Ramakrishnan, C., Rademacher, A., Soichot, J., Costa, G., Waters, A. P., Janse, C. J., et al. (2012). Salivary gland-specific P. *berghei* reporter lines enable rapid evaluation of tissue-specific sporozoite loads in mosquitoes. *PLoS ONE.* 7:e36376. doi: 10.1371/journal.pone.0036376

Ramalhete, C., da Cruz, F. P., Lopes, D., Mulhovo, S., Rosário, V. E., Prudêncio, M., et al. (2011). Triterpenoids as inhibitors of erythrocytic and liver stages of *Plasmodium* infections. *Bioorg. Med. Chem.* 19, 7474–7481. doi: 10.1016/j.bmc.2011.10.044.

Ramalhete, C., da Cruz, F. P., Mulhovo, S., Sousa, I. J., Fernandes, M. X., Prudêncio, M., et al. (2014). Dual-stage triterpenoids from an African medicinal plant targeting the malaria parasite. *Bioorg. Med. Chem.* 22, 3887–3890. doi: 10.1016/j.bmc.2014.06.019

Sack, B. K., Miller, J. L., Vaughan, A. M., Douglass, A., Kaushansky, A., Mikolajczak, S., et al. (2014). Model for in vivo assessment of humoral protection against malaria sporozoite challenge by passive transfer of monoclonal antibodies and immune serum. *Infect. Immun.* 82, 808–817. doi: 10.1128/IAI.01249-13

Smale, S. T. (2010). Luciferase assay. *Cold Spring Harb. Protoc.* 2010. doi: 10.1101/pdb.prot5421

Spaccapelo, R., Janse, C. J., Caterbi, S., Franke-Fayard, B., Bonilla, J. A., Syphard, L. M., et al. (2010). Plasmepsin 4-deficient *Plasmodium berghei* are virulence attenuated and induce protective immunity against experimental malaria. *Am. J. Pathol.* 176, 205–217. doi: 10.2353/ajpath.2010.090504

Stone, W. J., Churcher, T. S., Graumans, W., van Gemert, G. J., Vos, M. W., Lanke, K. H., et al. (2014). A scalable assessment of *Plasmodium falciparum* transmission in the standard membrane-feeding assay, using transgenic parasites expressing green fluorescent protein-luciferase. *J. Infect. Dis.* 210, 1456–1463. doi: 10.1093/infdis/jiu271

Thorne, N., Shen, M., Lea, W. A., Simeonov, A., Lovell, S., Auld, D. S., et al. (2012). Firefly luciferase in chemical biology: a compendium of inhibitors, mechanistic evaluation of chemotypes, and suggested use as a reporter. *Chem. Biol.* 19, 1060–1072. doi: 10.1016/j.chembiol.2012.07.015

Van Reet, N., Van de Vyver, H., Pyana, P. P., Van der Linden, A. M., and Büscher, P. (2014). A panel of *Trypanosoma brucei* strains tagged with blue and red-shifted luciferases for bioluminescent imaging in murine infection models. *PLoS Negl. Trop. Dis.* 8:e3054. doi: 10.1371/journal.pntd.0003054

van Schaijk, B. C., Ploemen, I. H., Annoura, T., Vos, M. W., Lander, F., van Gemert, G. J., et al. (2014). A genetically attenuated malaria vaccine candidate based on *P. falciparum b9*/slarp gene-deficient sporozoites. *Elife* 19:3. doi: 10.7554/eLife.03582

Vaughan, A. M., Mikolajczak, S. A., Camargo, N., Lakshmanan, V., Kennedy, M., Lindner, S. E., et al. (2012). A transgenic *Plasmodium falciparum* NF54 strain that expresses GFP-luciferase throughout the parasite life cycle. *Mol. Biochem. Parasitol.* 186, 143–147. doi: 10.1016/j.molbiopara.2012.10.004

Waller, K. L., Muhle, R. A., Ursos, L. M., Horrocks, P., Verdier-Pinard, D., Sidhu, A. B., et al. (2003). Chloroquine resistance modulated in vitro by expression levels of the *Plasmodium falciparum* chloroquine resistance transporter. *J. Biol. Chem.* 278, 33593–33601. doi: 10.1074/jbc.M302215200

Waters, A. P., Thomas, A. W., van Dijk, M. R., and Janse, C. J. (1997). Transfection of malaria parasites. *Methods* 13, 134–147. doi: 10.1006/meth.1997.0506

Weiwer, M., Mulrooney, C., Massi, D., Heidebrecht, R., Wiegand, R., Lukens, A. K., et al. (2011). *ML238: An Antimalarial Small Molecule of a Unique Structural Class*. Probe Reports. Bethesda, MD: NIH Molecular Libraries Program.

White, N. J., Pukrittayakamee, S., Hien, T. T., Faiz, M. A., Mokuolu, O. A., and Dondorp, A. M. (2014). Malaria. *Lancet* 383, 723–735. doi: 10.1016/S0140-6736(13)60024-0

World Health Organization. (2013). *World Malaria Report*. Available at: http://www.who.int/malaria/publications/worldmalariareport/en/

Zhang, X., Tolzmann, C. A., Melcher, M., Haas, B. J., Gardner, M. J., Smith, J. D., et al. (2011). Branch point identification and sequence requirements for intron splicing in *Plasmodium falciparum*. *Eukaryot Cell.* 10, 1422–1428. doi: 10.1128/EC.05193-11

Zuzarte-Luis, V., Sales-Dias, J., and Mota, M. M. (2014). Simple, sensitive and quantitative bioluminescence assay for determination of malaria pre-patent period. *Malar. J.* 13, 15. doi: 10.1186/1475-2875-13-15

10

Mass Drug Administration with Artemisinin-Piperaquine for the Elimination of Residual Foci of Malaria in São Tomé Island

Mingqiang Li[1†], Fei Tuo[1†], Ruixiang Tan[1], Hongying Zhang[2], Shaoqin Zheng[2], Qi Wang[1], Qin Xu[1], Xinbing Yu[3], Fangli Lu[3], Zhibing Wu[4], Jun Huang[5], Herodes Sacramento Rampao[6], Carlos Alberto Bandeira D'almeida[6], Hong Yan[2], Jianping Song[1], Wenfeng Guo[1] and Changsheng Deng[1*]*

[1] Artemisinin Research Center, Guangzhou University of Chinese Medicine, Guangzhou, China, [2] Science and Technology Park, Guangzhou University of Chinese Medicine, Guangzhou, China, [3] Department of Parasitology, Zhongshan School of Medicine, Sun Yat-Sen University, Guangzhou, China, [4] The First Affiliated Hospital of Guangzhou University of Chinese Medicine, Guangzhou, China, [5] Sino-French Hoffmann Institute, Guangzhou Medical University, Guangzhou, China, [6] Centro Nacional de Endemias, Ministry of Health, São Tomé, São Tomé and Príncipe

Edited by:
Vas Dev,
National Institute of Malaria Research (ICMR), India

Reviewed by:
Susanta Kumar Ghosh,
National Institute of Malaria Research (ICMR), India
† Surya Kant Sharma,
National Institute of Malaria Research (ICMR), India
Pradyumna Kishorr Mohapatra,
Indian Council of Medical Research (ICMR), India
Aung Pyae Phyo,
Mahidol Oxford Tropical Medicine Research Unit (MORU), Thailand

***Correspondence:**
Changsheng Deng
dcs19811202@163.com
Wenfeng Guo
guowenfeng@gzucm.edu.cn

These authors have contributed equally to this work

Background: Mass drug administration with artemisinin-piperaquine (AP-MDA) is being considered for elimination of residual foci of malaria in Democratic Republic of São Tomé and Principe.

Methods: Three monthly rounds of AP-MDA were implemented from July to October 2019. Four zones were selected. A and B were selected as a study site and a control site, respectively. C and D were located within 1.5 and 1.5 km away from the study site, respectively. Parasite prevalence, malaria incidence, and the proportion of the *Plasmodium falciparum* malaria cases were evaluated.

Results: After 3 monthly rounds of AP-MDA, the parasite prevalence and the gametocyte carriage rate of *P. falciparum* in zone A decreased from 28.29‰ to 0 and 4.99‰ to 0, respectively. Compared to zone B, the relative risk for the population with *Plasmodium falciparum* malaria in zone A was lower (RR = 0.458, 95% CI: 0.146–1.437). Malaria incidence fell from 290.49‰ (the same period of the previous year) to 15.27‰ (from the 29th week in 2019 to the 14th week in 2020), a decrease of 94.74% in zone A, and from 31.74 to 5.46‰, a decline of 82.80% in zone B. Compared to the data of the same period the previous year, the cumulative number of *P. falciparum* malaria cases were lower, decreasing from 165 to 10 in zone A and from 17 to 4 in zone B. The proportion of the *P. falciparum* malaria cases on the total malaria cases of the country decreased of 90.16% in zone A and 71.34% in zone C.

Conclusion: AP-MDA greatly curbed malaria transmission by reducing malaria incidence in the study site and simultaneously creating a knock-on effect of malaria control within 1.5 km of the study site and within the limited time interval of 38 weeks.

Keywords: mass drug administration, artemisinin-piperaquine, *P. falciparum*, elimination, malaria foci

INTRODUCTION

Malaria is one of the world's three major infectious diseases. In 2015, there were 214 million malaria cases globally, the lowest in the last decade. However, in 2016–2018, the global number of malaria cases rose from 217 million to 228 million (1, 2), an increase of more than 5%, with 90% of the cases occurring in Africa.

Situated in the Gulf of Guinea, the Democratic Republic of São Tomé and Principe (hereinafter referred to as "São Tomé and Principe") was once a malaria endemic island country (**Figure 1**). Following the implementation of comprehensive measures, such as treatment with artemisinin-based combination therapies (ACTs), long-lasting insecticide-treated nets (LLINs), intermittent preventive treatment of pregnant women (IPTp), indoor residual spraying (IRS) activities and other vector control measures, malaria incidence in São Tomé and Principe gradually reduced from 37% in 2004 to 1% in 2018. Thus, the island nation was added in the list of countries with subnational/territorial elimination program by the World Health Organization (WHO) (2). The government of São Tomé and Principe has developed a PROTOCOL FOR THE CASE MANAGEMENT OF MALARIA (revised in 2018) (3) with the objective to eliminate indigenous malaria cases by 2025.

Despite the promising outlook, the situation of malaria prevention and control in 2018 was not optimistic. In 2018, the total expenditure on malaria control and treatment in São Tomé and Principe was 16 US dollars per capita (2) equaling that of 2017. However, malaria incidence in 2018 increased by 20.54% (11.57 vs. 14.56‰).

In 2018, Água Grande and Lemba, counties in São Tomé Island, were highly endemic, malaria incidence rates were >14.56‰ in both counties, exceeding the national malaria incidence rate. Since the source of infection had not been eliminated in these counties, residual active foci (4, 5) remained. Malaria incidence in these residual active foci was high and increased the risk of malaria transmission to other surrounding villages, thus leading from time to time to malaria outbreaks.

To order to rapidly eliminate *P. falciparum* in residual active foci, block malaria transmission in surrounding villages, and accelerate the reduction of malaria incidence, we conducted 3 monthly rounds of mass artemisinin-piperaquine (AP-MDA) administration in Liberdade village from July to October 2019.

METHODS AND MATERIALS

Study Sites

Liberdade is a village located in the north-eastern part of São Tomé Island in the central part of Água Grande County. It covers an area of 66,612 m^2. The population of Liberdade in 2019 was 655 inhabitants. In 2014–2018, the yearly malaria incidence of Liberdade was within the range of 158.18–280.37‰, making Liberdade the main residual focus of the area. We thus selected Liberdade village as the MDA study site (zone A) (**Figure 2**). Budo Budo was selected as the control village (zone B), which is situated 0.8 km south-east of Liberdade and covers an area of 26,889 m^2. Its population in 2019 was 120 inhabitants. In 2014–2018, the yearly malaria incidence of Budo Budo was 191.30–342.59‰. We selected the two villages mainly for their unique geographical location; both are close to each other but with no linked land or sea borders and are separated from the sea by a main road. Furthermore, both are located in low-lying areas of gully landform of volcanic island, with similar natural microenvironments. Swamps offer breeding sites for permanent water mosquitoes (**Figure 3**).

Zone C used to observe the extended impacts of AP-MDA was the area centered on zone A and within 1.5 km. The radius of zone C was set based on the theoretical maximum flight distance (1 km) of Anopheles mosquitoes. Zone C included 13 villages: Atras Cemiterio, Bairro Hospital, Bairro Militar, Budo Budo, Campo de Milho, Cruz Mami, Oque Del Rei, Poto Poto, Gonga, Praia Lagarto, Praia Emilia, Agua Marçal, and Ferreira do Governo. The population of zone C in 2019 was 11,732 inhabitants. In 2014–2018, the yearly malaria incidence in zone C ranged from 32.88 to 56.13‰. Meanwhile, all areas beyond 1.5 km range were grouped into zone D (**Figure 2**), which represented the area completely free from AP-MDA extended impacts. The comparison of data on malaria epidemic pre- and post-AP-MDA between zone D and others can reflect the extended impacts of AP-MDA.

Ethical Review and Informed Consent

The Ethics Committee of the Centro Nacional de Endemias (CNE) of São Tomé and Principe (Approval N°2019062001) and the Ethics Committee of the Guangdong Provincial Hospital of Chinese Medicine (Approval N°BF2019-055-01) approved the implementation of the AP-MDA project in Liberdade village. The Ministry of Health of São Tomé and Principe, the CNE, the National Malaria Control Planning Commission, the health officers of Água Grande County, and the antimalarial team from Guangzhou University of Chinese Medicine (Guangzhou, China) jointly drafted the research protocol of the present study (**Figure 4**). According to the protocol approved, there would be the 3 monthly rounds of AP-MDA with an interval of 28 days between each two rounds. The first round was from July 13 to August 9, 2019, the second round was from August 10 to September 6, 2019, the third round was from September 7 to October 4, 2019.

All participants in the study were required to sign informed consent forms. Informed consent form of children (<12 years old) and adolescents (12–17 years old) were signed by their guardians. Women aged 14–60 years were required to sign an informed consent form for pregnancy test. All informed consents will be kept on record for 3 years.

Protocol of AP-MDA

Inclusion Criteria

Permanent residents of zone A and all temporary residents and foreign individuals in zone A during the AP-MDA;

Individuals aged more than 6 months;

Individuals that have signed informed consent.

Exclusion Criteria

Individuals allergic to one or more components of the drug;

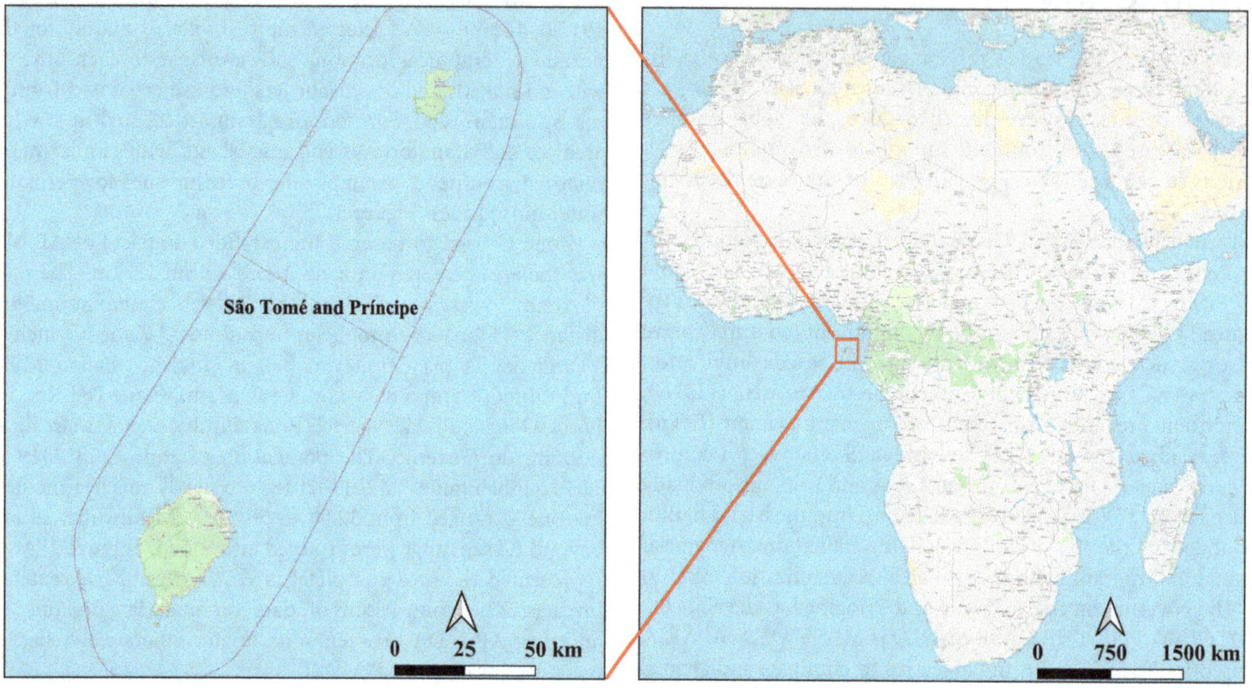

FIGURE 1 | Geographical location of SãoTomé and Principe.

Pregnant women;
Infants aged 6 months or less;
Individuals with a serious illness needing hospitalization;
Individuals with cognitive impairment.

Drug Dosage and Treatment Regimen

Each AP tablet (manufactured by Guangdong New South Artepharm CO., LTD., Meizhou, China) is composed of 62.5 mg of artemisinin and 375 mg of piperaquine. Tablets were given orally to each participant with a strictly administered dosage based on body weight (**Supplementary Table 1**). Direct observation therapy (DOT) was implemented in the 3 monthly rounds of AP-MDA.

Monitoring and Management of Adverse Drug Reactions

Community villagers were requested to report adverse drug reactions within 4 days following the drug administration. Health workers of the Hospital of Água Grande County and anti-malaria field technicians were responsible to manage and monitor the reported adverse drug reactions, and maintain data using record sheets.

Pregnancy Test

To determine the pregnancy status of women aged 14–60 years, pregnancy tests were done before each round of AP-MDA.

Blood Smear and Microscopy

Blood smears collected in the field were checked using microscopy in accordance with WHO's standard procedures (6).

Other Preventive Measures

After the third round of MDA, village anti-malaria volunteers conducted daily inspection in zone A to diagnose with RDTs all feverish individuals in a timely manner. Positive individuals were treated following PROTOCOL FOR THE CASE MANAGEMENT OF MALARIA of São Tomé and Principe. All foreign individuals entering zone A (especially those staying for the night) were subjected to temperature checks and given standard malaria treatment.

Statistical Analysis of Data

The percentage, mean and standard deviation were analyzed with SPSS 22. Counting was done using contingency tables, and the chi-square method was used for statistical analysis. Pearson's test was used when the minimum prediction frequency was higher than 5. When the minimum prediction frequency was lower than 5, Fisher's test was applied. A two-sided test $P < 0.05$ was considered to indicate statistically significant differences.

RESULTS

MDA Coverage

The coverage rates of the three rounds of AP-MDA in zone A were within the range of 92.62–95.81%. The proportion of individuals who refused to take the drug accounted for 0.42–0.74%. The main reason of refusal was concern about adverse drug reactions (**Table 1**). We further calculated the numbers of participants in each round of AP-MDA. During the first round of AP-MDA, the number of participants was 501, of which 480 individuals took the medicine. During the second round

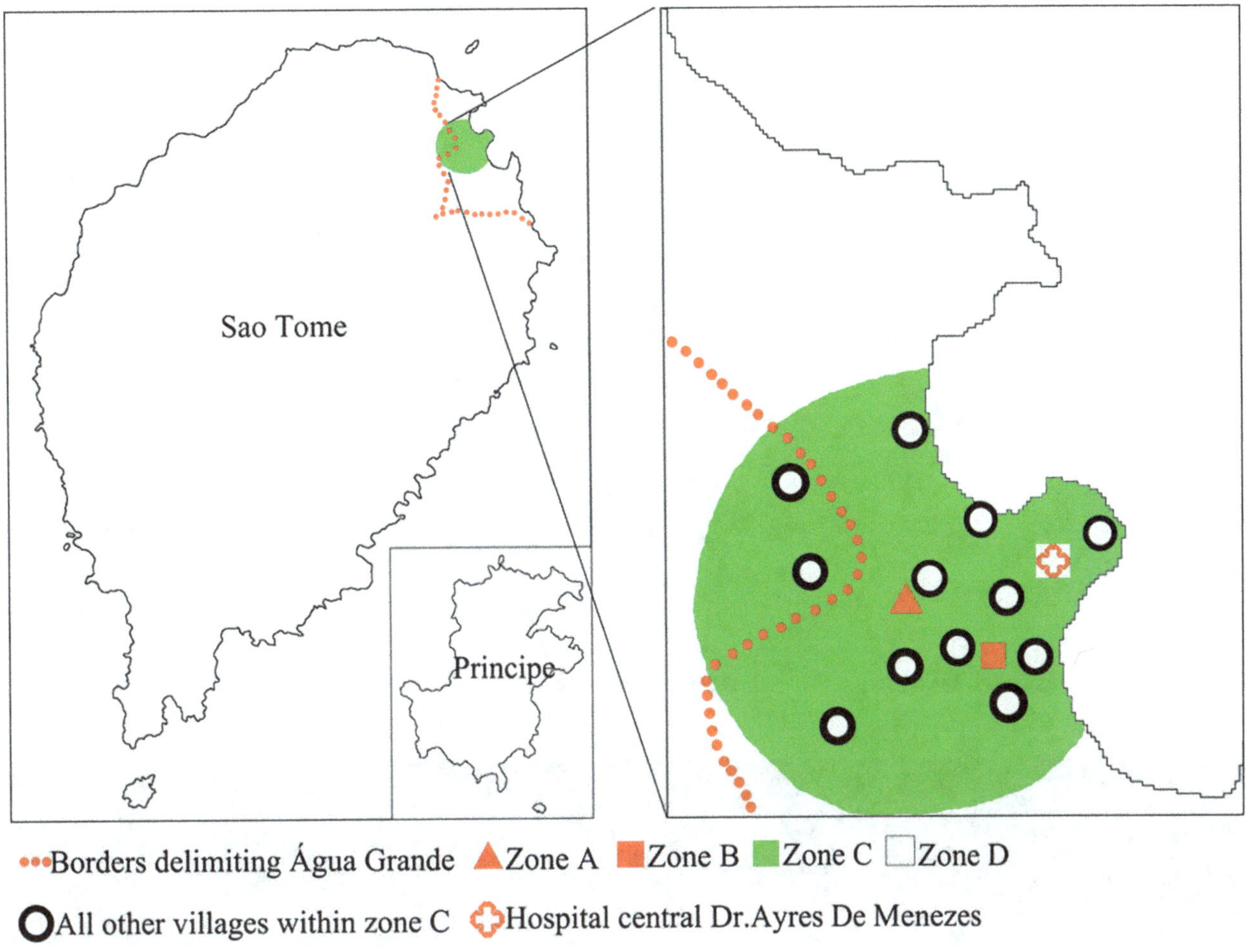

FIGURE 2 | Distribution of AP-MDA village and its surroundings.

of AP-MDA, the number of participants was 515, of which 477 individuals took the medicine, among them 423 individuals took the medicine in the first round as well as in the second round. During the third round of AP-MDA, the number of participants was 524, of which 501 individuals took the medicine, among them 429 individuals took the medicine in the first round as well as in the third round, 444 in the second round as well as in the third round. A total number of 401 individuals took the medicine in all the three rounds.

Mobile Population Monitoring

During the three rounds of AP-MDA, 320 individuals entered zone A. Except for two individuals who refused to take drugs, all remaining participants accepted the treatment in conformity with the present study protocol (**Table 2**).

Drug Safety Monitoring

During the three rounds of AP-MDA, 1,458 person-times took the drug in zone A. Thirty-five person-times reported adverse drug reactions; the occurrence rate of adverse drug reactions was 2.40%. The most common adverse reactions observed were nausea, fatigue, dizziness, and headache. Adverse drug reactions were managed by local health workers. No severe adverse drug events or deaths related to MDA were reported.

Parasite Prevalence Decreased Significantly

Before AP-MDA, 601 individuals were tested with Rapid Diagnostic Tests (RDTs), and 601 blood smear samples were collected. Nine individuals had positive RDT results and were infected with *P. falciparum* malaria. The blood smears results revealed that 14 individuals were carrying asexual *P. falciparum* and three carrying *P. falciparum* gametocytes. No other species of plasmodium and gametocytes were detected. The parasite prevalence and the gametocyte carriage rate within the population before AP-MDA were 28.29‰ (17/601) and 4.99‰ (3/601), respectively. However, the aforementioned individuals had no symptoms. At the end of AP-MDA in zone A, 534 individuals were subjected to RDT tests, the results of which were negative for all 534 individuals. In the meantime, blood smears results revealed no carriers of asexual *P. falciparum* as well as gametocytes. No other species of plasmodium and gametocytes

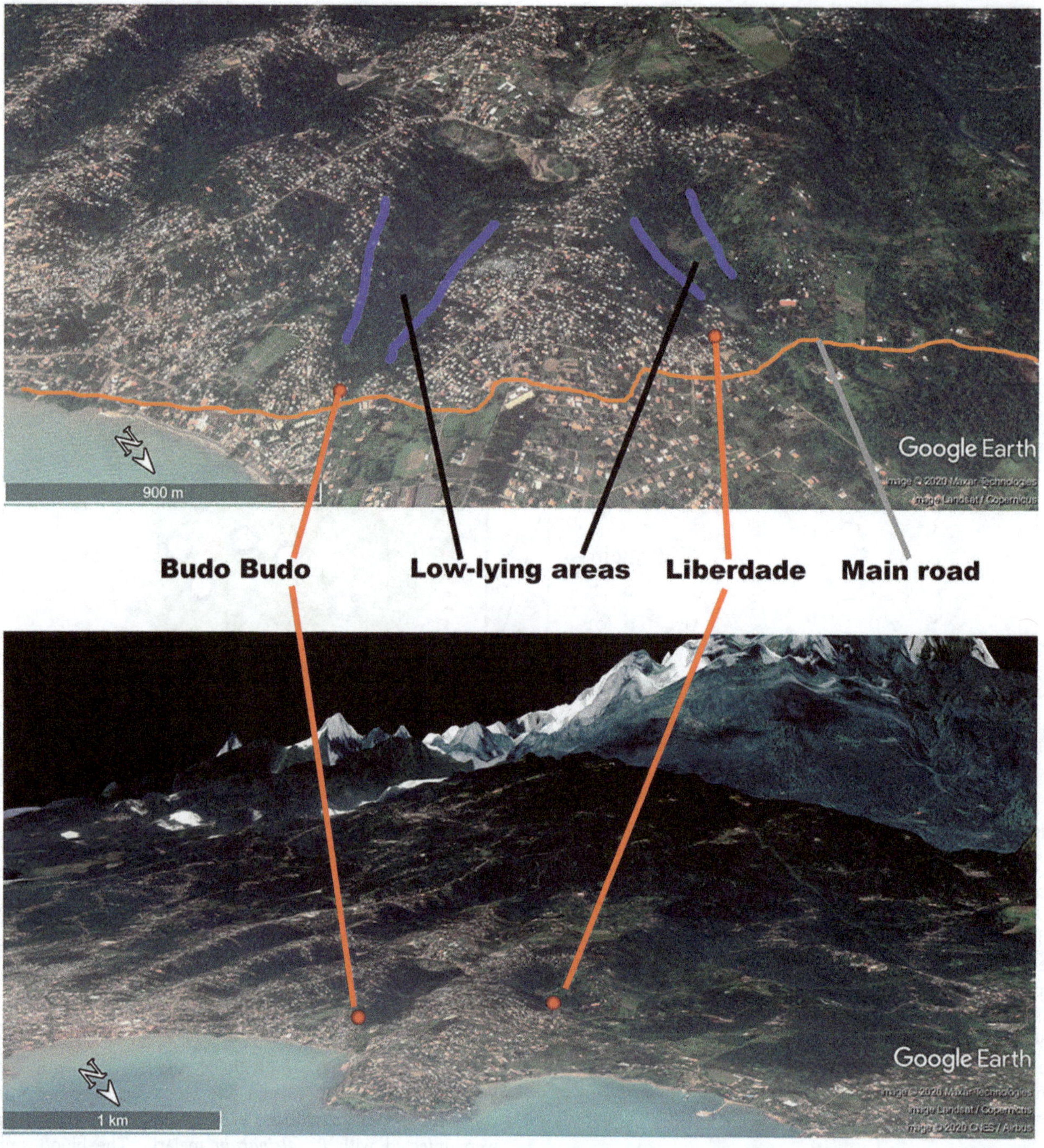

FIGURE 3 | Geographical location of Liberdade and Budo Budo.

were found. Parasite prevalence and gametocyte carriage rate within the population after AP-MDA were both nil.

After three rounds of AP-MDA, the active case detection for screening of parasitaemia was carried out once a month in zone A. 428 villagers were tested in November 2019, 329 villagers in December, 428 villagers in January 2020, 420 villagers in February, 422 villagers in March and 514 villagers in April. Microscopic examination was used to detect parasite. The results of each screening showed that both parasite prevalence and gametocyte carriage rate were zero. Follow-up screening was suspended due to the spread of COVID-19.

Malaria Incidence Decreased Significantly

In zone A, the cumulative malaria cases were reduced from 165 pre-MDA (from the 29th week in 2018 to the 14th week in 2019) to just 10 cases 38 weeks post-MDA (from the 29th week in 2019

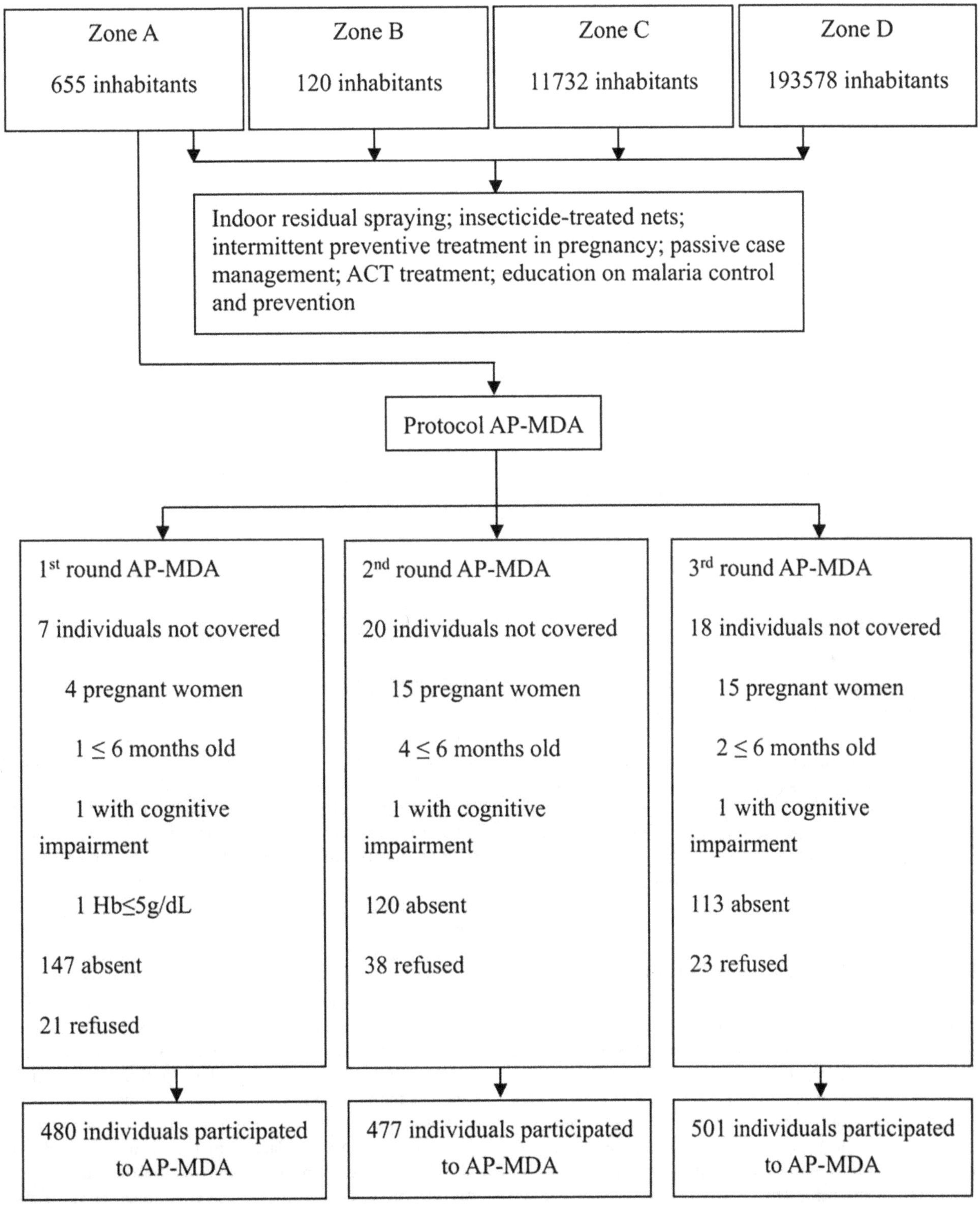

FIGURE 4 | Process of study implementation.

to the 14th week in 2020), all of which were *P. falciparum* malaria. Malaria incidence decreased from 290.49 to 15.27‰ ($P < 0.05$). During the same period in zone B, the number of cases of malaria dropped from 17 to 4, all of which were of *P. falciparum* malaria. Malaria incidence decreased from 141.67 to 32.79‰ ($P < 0.05$). Compared to zone B, the relative risk of occurrence of malaria

TABLE 1 | Artemisinin-Piperaquine-Mass Drug Administration coverage rates in zone A.

MDA round	1st	2nd	3rd
Periods of time	**July 13 to August 9, 2019**	**August 10 to September 6, 2019**	**September 7 to October 4, 2019**
Participants	501	515	524
Pregnant women	4	15	15
Infants ≤ 6 months	1	4	2
Individuals with cognitive impairment	1	1	1
Severe anemia (Hg ≤ 5g/dL)	1	0	0
Absent*	147	120	113
New arrival	0	0	0
Death	0	0	0
Participated in MDA	480	477	501
Refuse	21	38	23
MDA coverage rate	95.81% (480/501)	92.62% (477/515)	95.61% (501/524)

Any individual who was not home from the 1st day of drug administration to the next round of MDA was seen as absent.

TABLE 2 | Mobile population and compliance.

MDA round	Mobile population	Expected number of people to take the drug	Number of people taking the drug	Refuse	Drug administration coverage rate
1st	99	98*	98	0	100%
2nd	108	107*	107	0	100%
3rd	113	113	111	2	98.23%

One pregnant woman did not participate in MDA.

cases in zone A 38 weeks post-MDA was lower (RR = 0.458, CI 95%: 0.146–1.437), which was not statistically significant ($P > 0.05$; **Table 3**).

Based on data of malaria epidemic pre- and post- MDA, the degree of decline in malaria incidences among zones were different. The degree of decline in malaria incidence was 94.74% in zone A, 82.80% in zone C, 76.85% in zone B, 59.20% in São Tomé and Principe, 39.64% in Água Grande county, and 18.21% in zone D. All malaria cases were of *P. falciparum* infections.

The Proportion of Malaria Cases Dropped Significantly

The proportion of cumulative malaria cases in zone A compared to the national total cases was reduced from 9.85% the same period 1 year before MDA (from the 29th week in 2018 to the 14th week in 2019) to 0.97% 38 weeks post-MDA (from the 29th week in 2019 to the 14th week in 2020) ($P < 0.05$). During the same period, the proportion of cumulative malaria cases in zone B dropped from 1.01% 1 year before MDA to 0.39% 38 weeks post-MDA ($P > 0.05$; **Table 4**).

Based on data of malaria epidemic pre- and post- MDA, the degree of decline in the proportion of cumulative malaria cases were different among zones. The degree of decline in the proportion of cumulative malaria cases was 90.15% in zone A, 71.34% in zone C, 61.39% in zone B, 32.46% in Água Grande county. However, an increase of 26.22% was observed in zone D.

DISCUSSION

The national malaria incidences of São Tomé and Principe during 2014–2018 were 9.97–14.56‰; all malaria cases were infected with *P. falciparum* malaria (2). According to WHO epidemiological classification of malaria (7) and based on the level of malaria incidence, São Tomé and Principe is a country of low malaria incidence and is listed as a country with subnational/territorial elimination program (2), with the aim for malaria elimination by 2025. São Tomé and Principe is in the phase of transformation from malaria control to malaria pre-elimination, with a low level of malaria transmission. However, due to the differences in the natural microenvironment and population density in different counties (8), the distribution of the endemicity of malaria is uneven in São Tomé and Principe, and the presence of malaria residual foci has led to a continued epidemic in a few localities. Countries and regions aiming to eliminate residual foci of malaria transmission can plan for a selective elimination of *P. falciparum* foci in the first stage (5). Malaria incidence in Liberdade village in 2014–2018 was in the range of 158.18–280.37‰, which was 10–20 times higher than the national level of malaria incidence. Malaria was endemic the whole year in Liberdade. Vector breeding sites were available in the village that led to the formation of active foci (4, 5). Villages with residual transmission foci in countries with low malaria prevalence should use appropriate integrated interventions including the addition of new measures to further reduce the transmission

TABLE 3 | Malaria incidences (‰) *(cumulative malaria cases/population) pre- and post-MDA.

Area	3 years before MDA	2 years before MDA	1 year before MDA	38 weeks after MDA
Zone A	121.82 (67/550)	103.76 (58/559)	290.49 (165/568)**	15.27 (10/655)
Zone B	182.61 (21/113)	25.64 (3/115)	141.67 (17/117)**	32.79 (4/120)#
Zone C	26.58 (294/11,062)	10.14 (114/11,248)	31.74 (363/11,435)**	5.46 (64/11,732)
Zone D	5.11 (930/182,100)	4.92 (914/185,893)	6.04 (1,147/189,781)**	4.94 (957/193,578)
Água Grande	10.64 (795/74,720)	6.33 (481/75,974)	12.23 (950/77,689)**	4.99 (395/79,226)
Whole country	6.66 (1,291/193,712)	5.49 (1,086/197,700)	8.30 (1,675/201,784)**	5.01 (1,031/205,965)

*Malaria incidence 38 weeks post-MDA (from the 29th week in 2019 to the 14th week in 2020) compared with malaria incidence of the same period of each year in the past 3 years; **Malaria incidence 38 weeks post-MDA was compared to malaria incidence of the same period 1 year before MDA, $P < 0.05$; #Malaria incidence in zone B compared with malaria incidence in zone A 38 weeks post-MDA, $P > 0.05$.*

TABLE 4 | Proportion of cumulative malaria cases (%) *(cases of each zone/ total cases) pre- and post-MDA.

Area	3 years before MDA	2 years before MDA	1 years before MDA	38 weeks after MDA
Zone A	5.19 (67/1,291)	5.34 (58/1,086)	9.85 (165/1,675)**	0.97 (10/1,031)
Zone B	1.63 (21/1,291)	0.28 (3/1,086)	1.01 (17/1,675)#	0.39 (4/1,031)
Zone C	22.77 (294/1,291)	10.50 (114/1,086)	21.67 (363/1,675)**	6.21 (64/1,031)
Zone D	72.04 (930/1,291)	84.16 (914/1,086)	68.48 (1,147/1,675)**	92.82 (957/1,031)
Água Grande	61.58 (795/1,291)	44.29 (481/1,086)	56.72 (950/1,675)**	38.31 (395/1,031)
Whole country	100 (1,291/1,291)	100 (1,086/1,086)	100 (1,675/1,675)**	100 (1,031/1,031)

*Proportion of cumulative malaria cases 38 weeks post-MDA (from the 29th week in 2019 to the 14th week in 2020) compared with the proportion of cumulative malaria cases of the same period of each year in the past 3 years; **Proportion of cumulative malaria cases 38 weeks post-MDA was compared to proportion of cumulative malaria cases of the same period 1 year before MDA, $P < 0.05$; #Proportion of cumulative malaria cases 38 weeks post-MDA was compared to proportion of cumulative malaria cases of the same period 1 year before MDA, $P > 0.05$.*

(7). AP-MDA was never implemented in São Tomé and Principe; therefore, it was considered a new intervention in the island.

São Tomé and Principe has a seasonal climate: a heavy rain season from January to May, a dry season from June to September, and a light rainy season from October to December (9). According to the data of CNE, malaria epidemic did have seasonality in São Tomé and Principe. The malaria transmission of the whole country was in a status of lower level from the 1st week to the 13th week (January to March) and from the 28th week to the 52nd week (July to December) every year, and in a status of higher level from the 14th week to the 27th week (April to June). The number of malaria cases varies according to season; the number of cases increases in the rainy season and decreases in the dry season. As per WHO's recommendation, in an area with seasonal transmission, MDA should be implemented during the period when prevalence is the lowest (10), the reason why we conducted 3 monthly rounds of AP-MDA during the dry season (13 July 2019–5 October 2019). Each technical field team was composed of two people (6), with a total of eight field teams (seven teams responsible for entering households and administering drugs and one team responsible for the diagnosis and monitoring of the mobile population). The antimalarial drug used for MDA, artemisinin-piperaquine (AP), has a long half-life (11–13). AP has already been used in Cambodia (14), Comoros (15, 16), and Kenya (17). AP-MDA coverage rates higher than 90% were achieved mainly due to the DOT measure.

The total occurrence rate of adverse drug reactions for the 3 monthly rounds of AP-MDA was 2.40%, lower than that of the MDA study conducted in Kenya (17), with no serious adverse events. The main symptoms of adverse drug reactions resolved after stopping taking the drug, indicating that AP is clinically safe.

In this study, at the end of 3 monthly rounds of AP-MDA, the parasite prevalence of *P. falciparum* malaria in zone A dropped from 28.89‰ before MDA to zero after MDA. Additionally, the gametocyte carriage rate of *P. falciparum* dropped from 4.99‰ to zero. Our results show that AP can kill *P. falciparum* asexual parasites and gametocytes of different stages. This conclusion is in agreement with the result of a previous AP-MDA study performed in Ngodhe, Kenya (17). AP-MDA eliminated *P. falciparum* parasites in all participants and led to a significant reduction in malaria transmission in zone A. These results confirm the high efficacy and rapid effect of AP-MDA.

After AP-MDA in zone A, we continuously recorded malaria incidence in zones B, C, D, Água Grande County, and São Tomé and Principe. Compared with the same period of the previous year, malaria incidences 38 weeks post-MDA in zone A, B, C, D, Água Grande County, and São Tomé and Principe decreased by 94.73, 77.08, 82.78, 18.03, 59.35, and 39.76%, respectively. Malaria incidence reduction in each zone reflected an overall reduction of the prevalence and intensity of malaria in São Tomé and Principe (from the 29th week in 2019 to the 14th week in 2020). Obviously, the malaria incidence reduction in zone A was the highest, indicating that compared to zone B, C, D, and Água Grande County, under the existing factors, adding 3 monthly rounds of AP-MDA, can lead to a higher decrease of malaria endemicity. Interestingly, we also found that over the same period, the percentage point reduction (82.78%) of malaria incidence in zone C was greater ($P < 0.001$) than that (18.03%) in zone D, Água Grande County (59.35%), and São Tomé and Principe (39.76%), indicating that the reduction level of malaria transmission in zone C was higher than in zone D, Água Grande County, and São Tomé and Principe. Three monthly rounds of AP-MDA in zone A not only reduced malaria incidence in zone A, but also decreased malaria incidence in zone C. Meanwhile, 38 weeks post-MDA, we observed a greater reduction of the proportion of malaria cases (94.74%) in zone A than in the other zones in the same period of the previous year. In the meantime, the proportion of malaria cases in zone C declined, and the reduction level (71.34%) was second only to that in zone A.

Monitoring drug resistance is an essential component of MDA. In our research, it was the first time that artemisinin piperaquine tablets, as MDA medicines, used in São Tomé and Principe. Artemisinin piperaquine tablets were not local first-line antimalarials, and the villagers in zone A were given the full therapeutic doses, that were in accordance with the guidelines of Mass drug administration for falciparum malaria: a practical field manual. During the three rounds of AP-MDA, we were very concerned about the condition of the villagers in zone A after taking the medicine. Anti-malarial volunteers make daily inspections in zone A, conduct RDT tests on people with fever, and collect blood films. The results of passive case detection and active case detection showed that the number of new malaria cases per week was zero in zone A from the 29th week to the 50th week in 2019. It showed that the emergence of parasitaemia did not happen in all people taking the medicine in zone A, nor did it occur in the 17 parasite carriers identified prior to MDA initiation. Furthermore, our team had accomplished 3 monthly rounds artemisinin-piperaquine mass drug administration across Anjouan Island, Union of Comoros, and PfK13 Kelch-propeller gene polymorphisms were evaluated. Analysis of 52 malaria samples after MDA showed no evidence for selection of PfK13 Kelch-propeller mutations (16). In our study, the number of new malaria cases per week was zero in zone A from the 29th week to the 50th week in 2019. However, population and mosquitoes movements inevitably brought the consequence of malaria recurrence. The first new malaria case was identified by active case detection in zone A in the 51st week in 2019. From the 51st week in 2019 to the 14th week in 2020, a total number of 10 malaria cases was accumulated. Although malaria incidences greatly reduced in zone A and in zone C, there should be more efforts indeed to maintain the status. After three rounds of AP-MDA, antimalarial volunteers were assigned to identify all fever cases in zone A, and the full therapeutic doses were given to the villagers with malaria. Zone A as a malaria focus, was the one we choose in this research, there could be more malaria foci around it. The elimination of residual active foci will be an endurable work.

Above all, our findings showed that malaria transmission was curbed after 3 monthly rounds of AP-MDA implemented in Liberdade, and AP-MDA had a knock-on effect on the surrounding areas. It did not only reduce malaria incidence in the study site but also within a specific geographical space (area within 1.5 km of the study site) and within the limited time interval of 38 weeks (from the 29th week in 2019 to the 14th week in 2020).

CONCLUSION

São Tomé and Principe is a malaria endemic country, in which residual foci villages are existing in most regions of the island. In the process toward malaria elimination, the government of São Tomé and Principe shall add AP-MDA as an additional measure to other national malaria control measures to eliminate residual foci and accelerate toward malaria elimination by 2025.

AUTHOR CONTRIBUTIONS

CD, WG, JS, FT, and ML conceived and designed the experiments, SZ, RT, HY, HZ, HR, and CD'a performed the experiments, QW, ZW, QX, FL, JH, and XY analyzed the data. FT, JS, WG, and QW wrote the paper. All authors reviewed the manuscript.

design, data collection and analysis, decision to publish, or preparation of the manuscript.

ACKNOWLEDGMENTS

We would like to thank the technical staff at Centro Nacional de Endemias for technical assistance in performing mass drug administration. We also thank the medical and technical staff at Centro de Saúde de Água Grande for medical and technical service in performing mass drug administration.

REFERENCES

1. World Health Organization [WHO]. *World Malaria Report 2018* (2018). Geneva: WHO.
2. World Health Organization [WHO]. *World Malaria Report 2019* (2019). Geneva: WHO.
3. Ministério da Saúde [MS]. *PROTOCOLO PARA O MANEJO DE CASOS DE PALUDISMO.* S. TOME E PRÍNCIPE: MS (2018).
4. World Health Organization [WHO]. *Terminology of Malaria and of Malaria Eradication*. Geneva: WHO (1963).
5. World Health Organization [WHO]. *Guidelines on the Elimination of Residual Foci of Malaria Transmission*. Geneva: WHO (2007).
6. World Health Organization [WHO]. *Basic Malaria Microscopy - Part I: Learner's Guide, 2nd Edn*. Geneva: WHO (2010).
7. World Health Organization [WHO]. *A Framework for Malaria Elimination*. Geneva: WHO (2017).

8. Ministério da Saúde [MS]. *SÃO TOMÉ E PRÍNCIPE EM NÚMEROS 2017*. S. TOME E PRÍNCIPE: MS (2017).
9. China Foreign Ministry. *Overview of Sao Tome and Principe* (2019). Available online at: https://www.fmprc.gov.cn/web/gjhdq_676201/gj_676203/fz_677316/1206_678452/1206x0_678454/ (accessed July 19, 2020).
10. World Health Organization [WHO]. *Mass Drug Administration for Falciparum Malaria: A Practical Field Manual*. Geneva: WHO (2017).
11. Hung T-Y, Davis TME, Ilett KF, Karunajeewa H, Hewitt S, Denis MB, et al. Population pharmacokinetics of piperaquine in adults and children with uncomplicated falciparum or vivax malaria. *Br J Clin Pharmacol*. (2004) 57:253–62. doi: 10.1046/j.1365-2125.2003.02004.x
12. Tarning J, Lindegårdh N, Annerberg A, Singtoroj T, Day NPJ, Ashton M, et al. Pitfalls in estimating piperaquine elimination. *Antimicrobial Agents Chemother*. (2005) 49:5127–8. doi: 10.1128/AAC.49.12.5127-5128.2005
13. Chinh NT, Quang NN, Thanh NX, Dai B, Geue JP, Addison RS, et a Pharmacokinetics and bioequivalence evaluation of two fixed-dose tablet formulations of dihydroartemisinin and piperaquine in vietnamese subjects. *Antimicrob Agents Chemother*. (2009) 53:828–31. doi: 10.1128/AAC.00927-08
14. Maude RJ, Socheat D, Nguon C, Saroth P, Dara P, Li G, et al. Optimising strategies for Plasmodium falciparum malaria elimination in Cambodia: primaquine, mass drug administration and artemisinin resistance. *PLoS One*. (2012) 7:e37166. doi: 10.1371/journal.pone.0037166
15. Deng C, Wang Q, Zheng S, Zhou C, Gao Y, Guo J, et al. Mass drug administration of artemisinin-piperaquine on high malaria epidemic area *Trop Med Health*. (2014) 42:33–41. doi: 10.2149/tmh.2014-S05
16. Deng C, Huang B, Wang Q, Wu W, Zheng S, Zhang H, et al. (2018). Large-scale Artemisinin-piperaquine mass drug administration with or witho ut primaquine dramatically reduces malaria in a highly endemic region of Africa *Clin Infect Dis*. (2018) 67:1670–6. doi: 10.1093/cid/ciy364
17. Kagaya W, Gitaka J, Chan CW, Kongere J, Md Idris Z, Deng C, et al. Malaria resurgence after significant reduction by mass drug administration on Ngodhe Island, Kenya. *Sci Rep*. (2019) 9:19060. doi: 10.1038/s41598-019-55437-8

11

Management of Malaria in Children Younger than 5 Years Old During Coronavirus Disease 2019 Pandemic in Sierra Leone

Danilo Buonsenso[1,2,3], Francesco Iodice[4], Bianca Cinicola[5], Francesca Raffaelli[6], Solia Sowa[7] and Walter Ricciardi[1,8]*

[1] Department of Woman and Child Health and Public Health, Fondazione Policlinico Universitario A. Gemelli IRCCS, Rome, Italy, [2] Dipartimento di Scienze Biotecnologiche di Base, Cliniche Intensivologiche e Perioperatorie, Università Cattolica del Sacro Cuore, Rome, Italy, [3] Center for Global Health Research and Studies, Università Cattolica del Sacro Cuore, Rome, Italy, [4] Institute of Neurology, Fondazione Policlinico Universitario A. Gemelli IRCCS, Rome, Italy, [5] Department of Pediatrics, Sapienza University of Rome, Policliclinico Umberto I, Rome, Italy, [6] Dipartimento Scienze di Laboratorio e Infettivologiche, Fondazione Policlinico Universitario Agostino Gemelli IRCCS, Rome, Italy, [7] Konta Wallah Community Health Center, Port Loko, Sierra Leone, [8] Sezione di Igiene, Istituto di Sanità Pubblica, Università Cattolica del Sacro Cuore, Rome, Italy

Edited by:
Kuldeep Dhama,
Indian Veterinary Research Institute (IVRI), India

Reviewed by:
Vikrant Sudan,
U.P. Pandit Deen Dayal Upadhyaya Veterinary University, India
Abhilash Perisetti,
University of Arkansas for Medical Sciences, United States

***Correspondence:**
Danilo Buonsenso
danilobuonsenso@gmail.com

Growing evidences are showing the potential indirect effects of the Coronavirus Disease 2019 (COVID-19) on the health systems of low-resource settings, where diseases such as Tuberculosis, Human Immunodeficiency Virus (HIV) and Malaria represent major killers. Therefore, we performed a retrospective study aimed to evaluate the impact of COVID-19 on Malaria programs in a peripheral region of Sierra Leone, previously involved by the Ebola outbreak in 2015, when malaria care have been impaired since local health systems were overwhelmed by Ebola cases. During COVID-19 in Sierra Leone, we did not notice a significant drop in malaria diagnosis in children, suggesting that a proactive approach in the management of malaria in endemic countries during COVID-19 may have had a positive impact. A comprehensive approach that include also educational activities to sensitize the local population, was useful to guarantee successful malaria diagnosis and treatment, and prevents excess of malaria deaths due to potential disruption of the local health systems related to the SARS-CoV-2 pandemic.

Keywords: malaria, COVID-19, SARS-CoV-2, children, Africa

INTRODUCTION

After the first description in China, severe acute respiratory syndrome coronavirus 2 (SARS-CoV-2) spread worldwide and reached Sub-Saharan Africa. In particular, the first cases in Africa have been described around March 2020 (1). In this part of the world, the number of coronavirus disease 2019 (COVID-19) cases and deaths is rising day by day, although not significantly compared with Europe, Asia, and North and South America (2). The reasons for such a difference are still unexplained, but multiple factors can be involved, including race, sex, socioeconomic status, genetic differences (3), and lack of testing points in most areas, particularly in the peripheries.

The arrival and continuous spread of SARS-CoV-2 in Africa are worrying major organizations (including the World Health Organization and major medical journals) because of the direct impact of the viral spread on a weak health system and the indirect effects of lockdown in a weak economic system (4). Preliminary data arrived from Sierra Leone, where we previously highlighted the social consequences of SARS-CoV-2 lockdown, with most people experiencing economic difficulties and losing their jobs (5). However, it was immediately clear that the health system should be paid special attention to the possible effects of the COVID-19 pandemic on other major killers in Africa. During the last decade, African countries greatly improved the care of patients with these conditions, thanks to a coordinated approach including government acts and the support of major international agencies (such as the World Health Organization and non-governmental organizations). The impact on tuberculosis and HIV care has been widely claimed (6), and there is evidence of the negative impact of the pandemic on immunizations (7) and TB services worldwide (8, 9).

Conversely, the impact of COVID-19 on malaria services in low-to-middle income countries (LMICs) is less established. Considering that malaria mainly kills children under 5 years of age, whereas COVID-19 is relatively mild in this group (10), the potential effects of disrupted malaria programs on children's health could be massive. Using spatiotemporal Bayesian geostatistical models, Weiss et al. estimated that, under pessimistic scenarios, COVID-19-related disruption to malaria control in Africa could almost double malaria mortality in 2020 and the following years. However, real-world data from LMICs are still missing (11). Therefore, we performed this retrospective study aimed to evaluate the impact of COVID-19 on malaria programs in a peripheral region of Sierra Leone.

METHODS

To understand the impact of COVID-19 on malaria care, we retrospectively evaluated the gross numbers of children aged 0–60 months diagnosed with confirmed *Plasmodium falciparum* malaria in the Konta Wallah Community Health Center of Port Loko District, Kamasondo Chiefdom, a peripheral government-recognized malaria inpatient and outpatient unit, referral for an area of ~8,000 people. In this setting, malaria is diagnosed either on a clinical basis or confirmed with a rapid antigen test able to detect *P. falciparum* antigen, with no further diagnostic resources available.

We collected the number of patients tested with confirmed *P. falciparum* malaria during the first 5 months of the year 2020 (January, February, March, April, and May) and compared it with the cases reported in 2018 and 2019 during the same months. In Sierra Leone, the first COVID-19 presumptive cases have been documented at the end of March 2020 and lockdown declared in April 2020. In May 2020, the lockdown has been removed, but people were not allowed to move between districts. Because data have been collected during the very first local peak and the lockdown, we did not calculate the sample size and collected all malaria diagnoses made during the three study periods.

The data were collected, as absolute numbers, by the center's health workers in accordance with the usual rules held in Sierra Leone. Cases were retrospectively obtained using the health facility routine activity reporting forms. In many peripheral Sub-Saharan Africa health centers, data are collected by the health facility on a register by crossing off with a pen the type of disease diagnosed, without registering personal data nor more detailed epidemiological data. Peripheral health centers have a registry book with dedicated pages for the registration of diagnoses, where operators include age groups and final diagnosis (7). Eventually, data were transferred on an Excel file.

The study was approved by a local committee composed of those responsible of the malaria unit of the local health center (S.S.), the research team of the Bureh Town Community Hospital of Sierra Leone, the headman of the community, and the older adults of the village, in a similar way to what happens for all the important political and economic decisions in the examined area (n25_may-2020).

Descriptive and statistical analyses have been performed with STATA v16: χ^2 or Fisher's exact tests to compare categorical variables. *P*-value was considered significant if <0.05. Dataset available upon reasonable request contacting the corresponding author.

RESULTS

During the period analyzed, a total of 785 children younger than 5 years old diagnosed with malaria have been evaluated. Details are reported in **Table 1**.

In March 2020, when the first cases of SARS-CoV-2 were reported in neighboring countries (Guinea and Liberia) but not in Sierra Leone, the number of cases was similar to those reported during the same month of the years 2018 and 2019.

A significant reduction of malaria diagnosis was noted on April 2020 (15 males, 18 females) compared with April 2019 (15 males, 15 females) (*p* 0.01; confidence interval 13–5; 95% confidence interval 7.05–19.95) but not compared with April 2018 (16 males, 20 females) ($P > 0.05$).

In May 2020, a new rise in malaria diagnoses was found (32 males, 40 females), compared with April 2020 (15 males, 18 females), but similar to May 2019 (28 males, 26 females) and 2018 (25 males, 31 females) ($P > 0.05$).

The number of malaria deaths in children younger than 5 years of age has been calculated from January 2018 to May 2020. The total numbers were similar: 9 deaths in 2018 (7 males, 2 females), 8 deaths in 2019 (3 males, 5 females), and 2 deaths (one male) detected from January to May 2020 (possibly a similar rate/year considering the short timeframe evaluated in 2020).

DISCUSSION

Our study allowed us to provide first data about the trends of malaria diagnoses in children younger than 5 years of age in three different years, showing that the number of diagnoses did not significantly change during COVID-19. Although an initial drop of malaria cases has been documented in April 2020, when Sierra

TABLE 1 | Malaria diagnoses in children younger than 5 years of age.

	2018		2019		2020		2018 vs. 2020	2019 vs. 2020
	Males	**Females**	**Males**	**Females**	**Males**	**Females**		
Jan	18	17	25	21	27	24	No COVID-19 In Sierra Leone	No COVID-19 In Sierra Leone
Feb	15	15	31	24	35	40	No COVID-19 In Sierra Leone	No COVID-19 In Sierra Leone
Mar	28	30	20	36	34	34	$p > 0.05$	$p > 0.05$
April	16	20	30	30	15	18	$p > 0.05$	p 0.01 (CI 13.5; 95% CI 7.05–19.95)
May	25	31	28	26	32	40	$p > 0.05$	$p > 0.05$

Leone started the lockdown due to the first cases of COVID-19, we cannot exclude that it is a casual fluctuation in malaria diagnoses. Interestingly, when the lockdown was removed at the beginning of May 2020, a sudden increase in malaria diagnoses has been registered. Again, a causal relationship with the reduction of restrictive measures related to COVID-19 cannot be demonstrated but not even excluded.

According to local doctors and community health workers, in Sierra Leone, health authorities and health-care workers worked hard to ensure that people would not miss malaria care like what happened during the 2014–2016 Ebola virus disease (EVD) outbreak, when the number of malaria diagnoses, the number of patients with malaria seeking appropriate health care, and the volume of malaria treatments being dispensed dropped significantly compared with previous years (12, 13)[1]. It was estimated that ~7,000 additional malaria-associated deaths among children younger than 5 years in Guinea, Liberia, and Sierra Leone due to the Ebola outbreak [(12, 14) vecchie]. In the case of Ebola, the clinical similarity of EVD with malaria, fear of contracting Ebola in the health-care facilities, and interruption of distribution of insecticide-treated bed-nets were all contributing factors leading to disruption of malaria care (15).

Despite the beginning of April 2020, local health workers reported an initial reduction in malaria diagnosis, mainly due to fear of contracting COVID-19 in the health centers; after several health education activities, people came back to the health facilities when needed. In particular, during World Malaria Day on April 25th, an active campaign has been established by the government with the active involvement of community health workers, aiming to prevent interruption of malaria control programs due to COVID-19 (12). In particular, the campaign focused on:

- Education and information strategies aimed to eliminate the perception that health staff is infecting people with COVID-19
- Continuous health education on the use of insecticide-treated net, which has helped greatly in the reduction of positive malaria cases
- Implementation of malaria intermittent preventive treatment in infants given during the routine immunization activities to infants aged 10 weeks–9 months
- Nationwide free distribution of insecticide-treated bed-nets given to every household in May 2020, whereas this campaign has been interrupted during the previous Ebola outbreak
- Systematic malaria diagnostics as part of fever management and measures for early detection and treatment of malaria, including presumptive malaria treatment
- Implementation of community-based health workers for social engagement and monitoring of peripheries
- Continuation of the malaria drug and test supply.

In fact, on May 2020, when COVID-19 cases were still increasing in the country, the number of malaria diagnoses in our center in children younger than 5 years of age rose as well. To achieve this result, the Sierra Leone Government took preventive strategies after the lessons learned during the EVD outbreak.

This experience in a local health center previously involved by the EVD shows how a proactive approach may help to keep appropriate care for major killers in Africa, performing proactive screening to diagnose not only COVID-19 but also malaria. This is a necessary step in Sub-Saharan Africa because a missed diagnosis of malaria bears significant public health consequences for the community allowing the further spread of malaria, similarly to a missed diagnosis of COVID-19 (16). The clinical presentation of malaria is similar to COVID-19; moreover, both can be asymptomatic or paucisymptomatic or even present with a critical systemic disease (16). This further emphasizes the need to actively look for both diagnoses in malaria-endemic countries.

We are aware that our report has several limitations to address. The retrospective nature is a limitation itself. Moreover, we have been able to collect absolute numbers, and no comprehensive epidemiological/demographic data from the health center are currently available because the pandemic and the related restrictions are creating a higher workload for local workers and, at the same time, limits their possibility of interacting with other offices. Moreover, the restrictive measures lead to local organizational changes, including a reduction of the number of health workers concomitantly working at each health post, to reduce the risk of contagion of local workers, already extremely low in the area. Therefore, there were insufficient human resources and time to allow us a timely and more detailed data collection. Also, ecological

[1] Available online at: http://blogs.biomedcentral.com/bugbitten/2020/04/17/malaria-during-the-covid-19-pandemic/ (accessed June 4, 2020).

changes during the three study periods may have potentially influenced the trend of local malaria diagnoses, although currently, there are no published pieces of evidence of unusually different rainy or dry seasons in the study period. Last, our data reflect the results of a national campaign in a single health center in Sierra Leone; therefore, these data cannot be generalized to the whole country or, in general, to Sub-Saharan Africa.

In conclusion, our preliminary data seem to suggest that a proactive approach in the management of malaria in endemic countries during COVID-19, including educational activities to sensitize the local population, is important and may be potentially useful to guarantee successful malaria diagnosis and treatment. However, long-term observational studies, including more centers, and particularly the peripheral health centers of LMICs, are needed to understand if a proactive and educational approach will be sufficient to prevent an excess of malaria deaths due to disruption of the local health systems related to the SARS-CoV-2 pandemic.

informed consent to participate in this study was provided by th participants' legal guardian/next of kine

AUTHOR CONTRIBUTIONS

DB, SS, and FI conceptualized the study. BC and FR collected data and performed the analyses. WR supervised the study team. epted All authors contributed to manuscript writing, read, and acc the last version of the manuscript.

ACKNOWLEDGMENTS

We are grateful to all our colleagues that supported the development of local health services and training of community health workers in the Western Rural Area of Sierra Leone and, in particular, Ismail Jaber, Matilda Yamba, Prince Williams, Memunatu N. Kallon, Nee Turay, Pietro Sollena, Alessia De Nisco, Stefano Rocchi, Irene Sollena, Francesca Vassallo, Vittorio Sabatino, Mara Caramia, Gregory Leeb, Valeria Pansini, Filippo Bruno, Andrea Deidda, Arianna Cafarotti, Davide Guglielmi, Maria Giulia Conti, Jessica Balerna, Francesco Madeddu, Mattia Belardinelli, Daniele Barbuto, Luigi Torricelli, Rachel Mannings, and Surf4Children Onlus. We are grateful to the Research Center of Global Health of the Istituto di Sanità Pubblica, Università Cattolica del Sacro Cuore, Roma, Italia, for the scientific and cultural support in this research project. We are also grateful to Cassa Galeno, which granted DB a project aimed at the development of an Italian-Sierra Leone research network in pediatrics.

REFERENCES

1. Perisetti A, Gajendran M, Boregowda U, Bansal P, Goyal H. COVID-19 and gastrointestinal endoscopies: current insights and emergent strategies. *Dig Endosc.* (2020) 32:715–22. doi: 10.1111/den.13693
2. Perisetti A, Gajendran M, Mann R, Elhanafi S, Goyal H. COVID-19 extrapulmonary illness - special gastrointestinal and hepatic considerations. *Dis Mon.* (2020) 66:101064. doi: 10.1016/j.disamonth.2020.101064
3. Kopel J, Perisetti A, Roghani A, Aziz M, Gajendran M, Goyal H. Racial and gender-based differences in COVID-19. *Front Public Health.* (2020) 8:418. doi: 10.3389/fpubh.2020.00418
4. El-Sadr WM, Justman J. Africa in the path of Covid-19. *N Engl J Med.* (2020) 383:e11. doi: 10.1056/NEJMp2008193
5. Buonsenso D, Cinicola B, Raffaelli F, Sollena P, Iodice F. Social consequences of COVID-19 in a low resource setting in Sierra Leone, West Africa. *Int J Infect Dis.* (2020) 97:23–6. doi: 10.1016/j.ijid.2020.05.104. [Epub ahead of print].
6. Adepoju P. Tuberculosis and HIV responses threatened by COVID-19. *Lancet HIV.* (2020) 7:e319–20. doi: 10.1016/S2352-3018(20)30109-0
7. Buonsenso D, Cinicola B, Kallon MN, Iodice F. Child healthcare an immunizations in sub-saharan africa during the COVID-19 pandemic. *Front Pediatr.* (2020) 8:517. doi: 10.3389/fped.2020.00517
8. Buonsenso D, Iodice F, Sorba Biala J, Goletti D. COVID-19 effects on tuberculosis care in Sierra Leone. *Pulmonology.* (2020). doi: 10.1016/j.pulmoe.2020.05.013
9. Migliori GB, Thong PM, Akkerman O, Alffenaar JW, Álvarez-Navascués F, Assao-Neino MM, et al. Worldwide effects of coronavirus disease pandemic on tuberculosis services, January-April 2020. *Emerg Infect Dis.* (2020) 26:2709–12. doi: 10.3201/eid2611.203163
10. Parri N, Lenge M, Cantoni B, Arrighini A, Romanengo M, Urbino A, et al. COVID-19 in 17 Italian pediatric emergency departments. *Pediatrics.* (2020) 146:e20201235. doi: 10.1542/peds.2020-1235
11. Weiss DJ, Bertozzi-Villa A, Rumisha SF, Amratia P, Arambepola R, Battle KE, et al. Indirect effects of the COVID-19 pandemic on malaria intervention coverage, morbidity, and mortality in Africa: a geospatial modelling analysis. *Lancet Infect Dis.* (2020). doi: 10.1016/S1473-3099(20)30700-3. [Epub ahead of print].
12. Wang J, Xu C, Wong YK, He Y, Adegnika AA, Kremsner PG, et al. Preparedness is essential for malaria-endemic regions during the COVID-19 pandemic. *Lancet.* (2020) 395:1094–6. doi: 10.1016/S0140-6736(20)30561-4
13. Plucinski MM, Guilavogui T, Sidikiba S, Diakité N, Diakité S, Dioubaté M, et al. Effect of the Ebola-virus-disease epidemic on malaria case management in Guinea, 2014: a cross-sectional survey of health facilities. *Lancet Infect Dis.* (2014) 15:1017–23. doi: 10.1016/S1473-3099(15)00061-4
14. Parpia AS, Ndeffo-Mbah ML, Wenzel NS, Galvani AP. Effects of response to 2014–2015 Ebola outbreak on deaths from malaria, HIV/AIDS, and tuberculosis, west Africa. *Emerg Infect Dis.* (2016) 22:433–41. doi: 10.3201/eid2203.150977
15. Walker PGT, White MT, Griffin JT, Reynolds A, Ferguson NM, Ghani AC. Malaria morbidity and mortality in Ebola-affected countries caused by decreased health-care capacity, and the potential effect of mitigation strategies: a modelling analysis. *Lancet Infect Dis.* (2015) 15:825–32. doi: 10.1016/S1473-3099(15)70124-6
16. Chanda-Kapata P, Kapata N, Zumla A. COVID-19 and malaria: a symptom screening challenge for malaria endemic countries. *Int J Infect Dis.* (2020) 94:151–3. doi: 10.1016/j.ijid.2020.04.007

12

Cytotoxic T Cell-Derived Granzyme B is Increased in Severe *Plasmodium Falciparum* Malaria

Lea-Christina Kaminski [1†], ***Mathias Riehn*** [1†], ***Annemieke Abel*** [1], ***Christiane Steeg*** [1], ***Denis Dekugmen Yar*** [2‡], ***Otchere Addai-Mensah*** [3], ***Francis Aminkiah*** [2], ***Ellis Owusu Dabo*** [2‡], ***Thomas Jacobs*** [1†] ***and Maria Sophia Mackroth*** [1,4*†]

Protozoa Immunology, Bernhard Nocht Institute for Tropical Medicine, Hamburg, Germany, [2] *Kumasi Centre for Collaborative Research in Tropical Medicine, Kumasi, Ghana,* [3] *Department of Medical Laboratory Technology, Faculty of Allied Health Sciences, Kwame Nkrumah University of Science and Technology, Kumasi, Ghana,* [4] *Divisions of Tropical Medicine and Infectious Diseases, I. Medical Department, University Medical Centre Hamburg Eppendorf, Hamburg, Germany*

Edited by:
Wanderley De Souza,
Federal University of Rio de Janeiro, Brazil

Reviewed by:
Beatrix Schumak,
University of Bonn, Germany
Sunil Joshi,
Miller School of Medicine, University of Miami, United States

***Correspondence:**
Maria Sophia Mackroth
m.mackroth@uke.de

† *These authors have contributed equally to this work*

Present address:
Denis Dekugmen Yar,
Department of Science Education, Faculty of Science and Environment Education, College of Agriculture Education, University of Education, Winneba, Ghana
Ellis Owusu Dabo,
Department of Global Health School of Public Health, College of Health Sciences, Kwame Nkrumah University of Science and Technology, Kumasi, Ghana

In *Plasmodium falciparum* malaria, $CD8^+$ T cells play a double-edged role. Liver-stage specific $CD8^+$ T cells can confer protection, as has been shown in several vaccine studies. Blood-stage specific $CD8^+$ T cells, on the other hand, contribute to the development of cerebral malaria in murine models of malaria. The role of $CD8^+$ T cells in humans during the blood-stage of *P. falciparum* remains unclear. As part of a cross-sectional malaria study in Ghana, granzyme B levels and $CD8^+$ T cells phenotypes were compared in the peripheral blood of children with complicated malaria, uncomplicated malaria, afebrile but asymptomatically infected children and non-infected children. Granzyme B levels in the plasma were significantly higher in children with febrile malaria than in afebrile children. $CD8^+$ T cells were the main T cell subset expressing granzyme B. The proportion of granzyme B^+ $CD8^+$ T cells was significantly higher in children with complicated malaria than in uncomplicated malaria, whereas the activation marker CD38 on $CD8^+$ T cells showed similar expression levels. This suggests a pathogenic role of cytotoxic $CD8^+$ T cells in the development of malaria complications in humans.

Keywords: granzyme B, $CD8^+$ T cells, malaria, severe malaria, *Plasmodium falciparum*

INTRODUCTION

Plasmodium falciparum (*P. falciparum*) malaria leads to the activation of $CD8^+$ T cells during the liver- as well as the blood-stage of the disease. Hepatocytes, the host cells for *plasmodia* in the liver-stage, express MHC-class-I and can be recognized by $CD8^+$ T cells having a potential protective capacity. Several vaccine strategies, based on the circumsporozoite protein (CSP), a protein expressed on sporozoites in the early liver-stage or whole sporozoite-based vaccines, have employed the induction of $CD8^+$ T cells against liver-stage antigens in murine models (1–4) as well as human vaccine studies (5, 6).

The role of $CD8^+$ T cells during the blood-stage of *P. falciparum* remains yet ill-defined, although an increased activation of $CD8^+$ T cells has been documented in humans (7). Most data on $CD8^+$ T cells in blood-stage malaria are derived from murine models addressing their function in experimental cerebral malaria (ECM) using *P. berghei* ANKA infection of C57BL/6 mice (8). In murine malaria it was clearly shown that $CD8^+$ T cells sequester in the brain and mediate endothelial leakage in a granzyme B (GrzB) and perforin-dependent cytolytic reaction (9–12).

In contrast to the pathogenic role of $CD8^+$ T cells in ECM, their contribution to human blood stage malaria remains controversial. At least indirect evidence exist that they may play a role in severe malaria by contributing to the induction of anemia (13). Moreover, soluble T-cell activation marker, as well as neutrophil and monocyte activation marker in the blood of malaria patients, could be linked to disease severity (14).

In *P. falciparum* malaria, numerous attempts were undertaken to correlate the T cell phenotype and or cytokine production with the clinical outcome of the disease. Several studies indicate that the ratio of pro-inflammatory TNFα and anti-inflammatory IL-10 may influence disease outcome (15). Although this might represent a reasonable explanation for disease manifestation this dichotomy is not present in every cohort studied.

In our study we aimed to further investigate a potential contribution of $CD8^+$ T cells in the development of malaria complications. By analyzing soluble T cell-derived mediators in plasma from Ghanaian children suffering either from uncomplicated malaria or severe malaria symptoms, we found an increase in GrzB levels when compared to healthy or asymptomatic children. We employed Hierarchical Stochastic Neighbor Embedding (HSNE) (16) to use an unbiased approach for identifying the main source of GrzB. $CD8^+$ T cells were confirmed as the main T cell subset expressing GrzB. Children suffering from severe malaria showed an increased population of $CD8^+GrzB^+$ T cells in peripheral blood when compared to children with uncomplicated malaria, indicating a potential pathogenic role of GrzB-producing $CD8^+$ T cells in malaria.

MATERIALS AND METHODS

Study Population

Blood samples were collected as part of a cross-sectional study between June and August 2015 in the Bosomtwi District, Ashanti Region, Ghana. A detailed description of the study participants, further inclusion and exclusion criteria, and study procedures have previously been published (17). In summary, samples were collected from children belonging to four different groups: (1) Healthy children, (2) asymptomatically infected children, (3) children with uncomplicated malaria, and (4) children with severe malaria.

Samples of healthy ($n = 41$) and asymptomatic ($n = 41$) children between the ages of 5–13 years of age were collected at Jachie D/A Primary school. Healthy children (healthy donor = HD) were defined as afebrile and negative for Malaria as detected by a HRP2-based rapid diagnostic test. Asymptomatic children (AS) were afebrile but positive for *P. falciparum* by HRP2. Blood samples from children with malaria (1–12 years of age) were collected at the St. Michael's Hospital, Pramso, Ghana. Children with uncomplicated malaria ($n = 32$) were treated with oral artemisinin combination drug as outpatients (OP). Children with clinically diagnosed severe malaria ($n = 34$) were treated with intravenous Artesunate as inpatients (IP).

The children in the HD group were 8.5 years of age, children in the AS group were on average 9.1 years of age. The children in the two groups with acute malaria were on average younger. Children in the OP group were on average 5.7 years of age, children in the IP group were 4.7 years of age.

All children with acute, symptomatic malaria and 15 of 41 of the asymptomatically infected children were microscopically positive for *P. falciparum* infection by thin blood smear. The children treated as inpatients for severe malaria showed the highest parasitemia with a mean parasitemia of 4.5% (range 0.3–17.3%) whereas children with uncomplicated malaria had a mean parasitemia of 1.4% (range 0.1–5.7%). Asymptomatically infected children showed only low parasitemia <1% ($n = 15$) or no microscopically detectable parasitemia by thin blood smear ($n = 26$). Individual parasitemia levels as well as additional information on the study participants have been described before (17).

Blood was drawn into heparinized tubes (1–2 mL) before initiation of treatment or directly at the school and processed within 5 h after collection for *ex vivo* flow cytometry staining.

Detection of *Plasmodium falciparum* Infection

Present *P. falciparum* infections were determined using CareStart™ Malaria HRP2 (PF) rapid diagnostic test. Implementation was carried out according to the manufacturer's protocol. Parasitemia was determined with thin blood smears stained with 4% Giemsa and examined under oil immersion (original magnification × 100).

T Cell Analysis by Flow Cytometric Assay

All antibodies were purchased from BioLegend. The surface immunostaining was performed by adding anti-PD-1 (PerCP/Cy5.5, clone EH12.2H7), anti-CD8 (AF700, clone RPA-T8), anti-CD4 (BV510, clone OKT4), anti-CD69 (FITC, clone FN50), anti-CD38 (PE, clone HB-7) and anti-CD39 antibodies (BV421, clone A1) to 100 μl of whole blood. After incubation for 30 min at 4°C samples were lysed and fixed with RBC lysis/fixation solution (BioLegend) for 15 min at room temperature and washed with cold PBS. Afterwards samples were stained intracellularly by adding anti-CD3 (APC/Cy7, clone HIT3a), anti-FoxP3 (AF647, clone 259D), and anti-Granzyme B antibodies (AF647, clone GB11) using the Foxp3 transcription factor staining buffer (eBioscience) according to the manufacturer's protocol. The samples were analyzed using a BD LSR II flow cytometer. If possible, at least 100,000 cells were acquired in the lymphocyte gate. The flow cytometry data analysis was conducted with FlowJo for Mac, version 10.5.0 (FlowJo LLC, Ashland, OR, USA). All acquired cells were gated based on FSC/SSC for lymphocytes. Lymphocytes were further gated for single cells and subsequently for $CD3^+$ and $CD3^-$ cells. $CD3^+$ cells were then gated for $CD8^+$, $CD4^+$, and $CD4^-CD8^-$ T cells. Fluorescence minus one (FMO) controls were used to set gates for granzyme B, CD38, and PD-1. The gating strategy and exemplary flow cytometry staining can be seen in **Supplementary Figure 1**.

Data Processing and HSNE by Cytosplore

Data were cleaned of doublets in FlowJo. $CD3^+$ lymphocytes of all patients were concatenated group wise (HD $n = 41$; AS $n = 41$; OP $n = 36$; IP $n = 32$) and exported as FCS-file. For further analysis, FCS-files were imported to Cytosplore version 2.2.0 and arcsin transformation with the factor of *150* were applied. The cell number of all concatenated groups were downsampled to 10^6 cells/group. Hierarchical stochastic neighbor embedding (HSNE) analysis of all groups based on the expression of CD8, CD4, Granzyme B, CD38, CD69, and PD-1 were computed. The algorithm for HSNE and the processing in the Cytosplore software was described before (16, 18). Advanced parameters of Cytosplore were used as suggested (*RNG Seed* of *-1*; *#Checks in AKNN* of *512*; *#RW for influence* of *100*; *#RW for Monte Carlo* of *15; Random walks threshold* of *1,5*; *Random walks length* of *15*; *Pruning threshold* of *0*; *Mean Shift Gridsize* of *256*.) The number of Scales were set to 3. Landmark development and clustering were complete data-driven. Cluster Scale was set to *27* with the *#Iters* of *1000*; *Exag* of *125*; *ExpDec* of *50* and *Cluster Res* of *256*. Landmark-based clusters were used for heat map generation.

Detection of GrzB in Plasma

Levels of GrzB in plasma were determined using LEGEND MAX™ Human Granzyme B ELISA Kit (BioLegend) with the application of 50 μl of plasma per well, according to the manufacturer's protocol.

Statistics

The statistical analysis was performed using Kruskal–Wallis tests with Dunn's post-testing in Graph Pad Prism 7.

Study Approval

Ethical approval was obtained from the Committee on Human Research, Publication and Ethics, School of Medical Sciences/Komfo Anokye Teaching Hospital, Kwame Nkrumah University of Sciences and Technology, Kumasi, Ghana on the 27th of November 2014 under the reference number CHRPE/AP/377/4. Written informed consent was given from legal guardians/parents of all participants prior to inclusion in the study.

RESULTS

Increased GrzB Plasma Levels in Severe Malaria

GrzB levels in plasma are reflecting a soluble marker for a recent activation of cytotoxic cells. Whereas, in plasma of healthy, non-infected children (HD) and asymptomatically infected children (AS) similar levels of GrzB were measured, children with uncomplicated malaria, treated as outpatients (OP) displayed a moderate increase, which did not reach statistical significance. In contrast, samples from children with severe malaria, treated as inpatients (IP), showed significantly increased levels compared to the afebrile children and healthy donors (**Figure 1**).

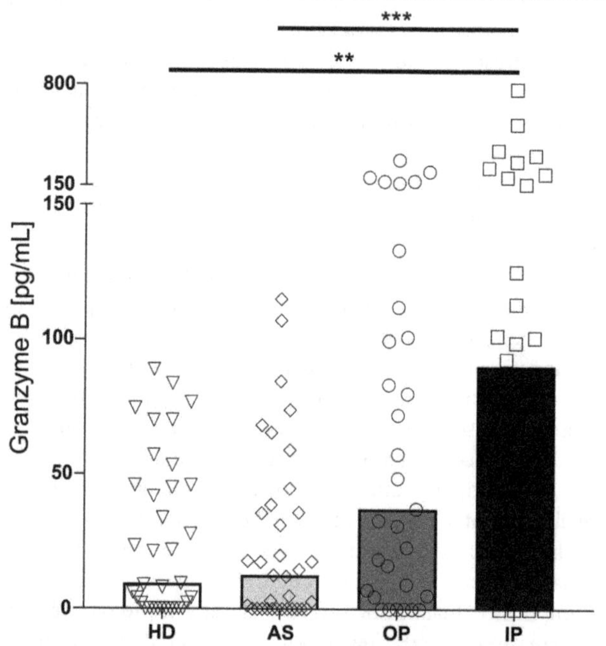

FIGURE 1 | Granzyme B level in the plasma of *P. falciparum* infected children is associated with disease severity. Blood samples were taken from healthy, non-infected children (healthy donors, HD; $n = 41$) and asymptomatically infected children (AS, asymptomatically infected; $n = 41$) as well as from children with uncomplicated malaria (outpatients, OP; $n = 35$) and severe malaria (inpatients, IP; $n = 32$). Granzyme B levels in the plasma were measured by ELISA. Statistical significance was determined using Kruskal–Wallis Test with *post-hoc* Dunn's test: $^{****}p < 0.0001$; $^{***}p < 0.001$; $^{**}p < 0.01$; $^{*}p < 0.05$.

Increased GrzB Production by $CD8^+$ T Cells in Severe Malaria

With hierarchical stochastic neighbor embedding (HSNE), we chose an unbiased approach to identify the source of the GrzB in the $CD3^+$ T cell subsets. HSNE calculates the similarity of cells and forms cluster, reflecting distinct cell subsets. Besides a moderate fraction of $CD4^-CD8^-$ T cells and a minor fraction of $CD4^+$ T cells producing GrzB, we could identify $CD8^+$ T cells as being the main GrzB producing T cell subset in malaria (**Figure 2**). The number of GrzB positive $CD3^+$ T cell subsets increased with more severe symptoms of malaria (**Figure 2**). One GrzB producing $CD4^+$ T cell subset was detectable in OP and IP groups, but none in healthy and asymptomatic individuals (blue boxes in **Figure 2**). Two $CD3^+CD4^-CD8^-$ T cell subsets were producing GrzB in the inpatient group, but only one in the healthy and asymptomatically infected groups (orange boxes in the heatmaps of **Figure 2**). However, already three T cell subsets, positive for CD8, produced GrzB in healthy controls. This increased to five distinct $GrzB^+CD8^+$ T cell subsets in the OP group and six in the IP group (red boxes in the heatmaps of **Figure 2**), indicating an increase of number and diversity of $CD8^+$ T cells positive for GrzB.

To directly compare the frequency of specific cell subsets and the expression levels of GrzB, we used a classical gating strategy

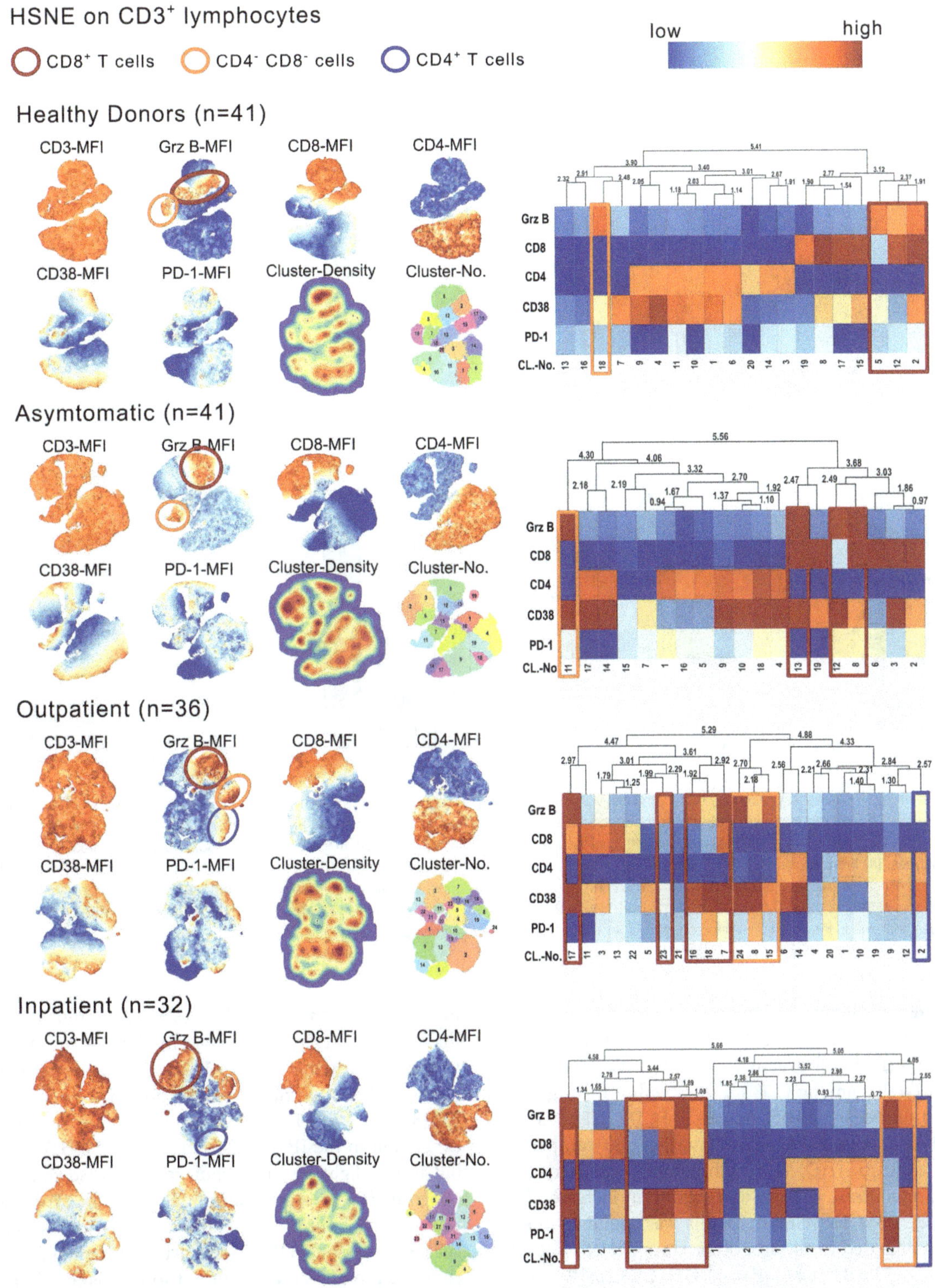

FIGURE 2 | $CD3^+CD8^+$ T cells express high amounts of GrzB in *P. falciparum* infected children. $CD3^+$ lymphocytes of all study participants were concatenated group wise (HD $n = 41$; AS $n = 41$; OP $n = 36$; IP $n = 32$). The cell number of all concatenated groups were downsampled to 10^6 cells/group. Hierarchical stochastic neighbor embedding (HSNE) analysis of all groups based on the expression of CD3, CD8, CD4, Granzyme B, CD38, and PD-1 were computed. Landmark development and clustering were complete data-driven. Landmark-based clusters were used for heat map generation. Color code represents mean fluorescence intensity (red = high; blue = low). Blue boxes indicate GrzB-producing $CD4^+$ T cell subsets, red boxes indicate GrzB-producing $CD8^+$ T cells. Orange boxes highlight $CD3^+CD4^-CD8^-$ T cell subsets, producing GrzB.

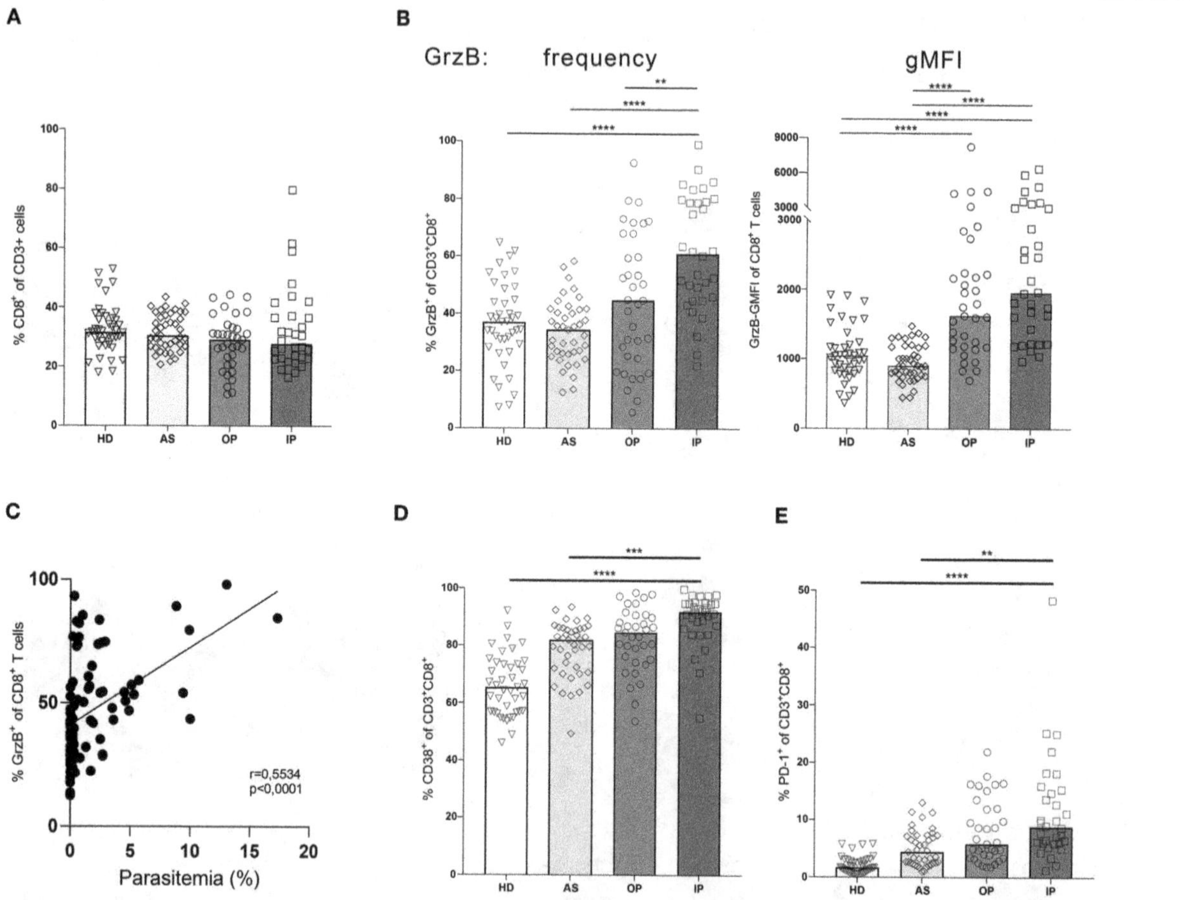

FIGURE 3 | Granzyme B expression in CD8+ T cells correlates with disease progression. Blood samples from children infected with *P. falciparum* but lacking symptoms (AS, $n = 41$), children treated as outpatients for uncomplicated malaria (OP, $n = 35$), children treated as inpatients for severe malaria (IP, $n = 32$), as well healthy, non-infected children (HD, $n = 41$) were stained with fluorescent labeled αCD3, αCD8, αCD4, αGranzyme B, αCD38, and αPD-1 antibodies for flow cytometric analyses. **(A)** Frequencies of CD8+ T cells among CD3+ cells were assessed in all 4 groups. **(B)** The $CD8^+CD3^+$ T cells were further analyzed for the expression of the effector molecule granzyme B, **(D)** CD38 and **(E)** PD-1 in all four groups. Statistical significance was determined using Kruskal–Wallis Test with *post-hoc* Dunn's test: $^{****}p < 0.0001$; $^{***}p < 0.001$; $^{**}p < 0.01$; $^{*}p < 0.05$. **(C)** The correlation between the frequency of GrzB expression by $CD3^+CD8^+$ T cells and parasitemia was analyzed in the blood of all infected children ($n = 89$), using Spearman rank correlation.

(see **Supplementary Figure 1**). Importantly, we could not detect differences in the frequency of $CD8^+$ T cells contributing to the total $CD3^+$ T cells in all groups (**Figure 3A**). Comparing the frequency of $GrzB^+$ among $CD8^+$ T cells within the 4 groups, the OP group showed a moderate increase of $CD3^+CD8^+GrzB^+$ T cells without reaching statistical significance in comparison to healthy controls (HD) or asymptomatic children (AS) (**Figure 3B**). In contrast, a strong and significant increase of the frequency of $CD3^+CD8^+GrzB^+$ T cells was found in the IP group when compared to all three other groups (HD = 36.48% ± 14.4; AS = 33.79% ± 10.90; OP = 44.47% ± 23.25; IP = 61.58 % ± 20.35). The HD and the AS group displayed similar fractions of $CD3^+CD8^+GrzB^+$ T cells. Similarly, the overall GrzB content of the $CD8^+$ T cell subset increased with disease severity, with OP and IP groups showing higher geometric mean fluorescent intensities of granzyme B (gMFI) (**Figure 3B**), compared to healthy and asymptomatically infected children. These results indicate that the $CD8^+$ T cell subset of IP children produced more GrzB than those of HD, AS and OP groups. Interestingly, the frequency of GrzB expression by $CD8^+$ T cells also correlated with the parasitemia (**Figure 3C**, $r = 0.5534$, $p < 0.0001$).

By further analyzing the induction of the activation marker CD38 on $CD8^+$ T cells we could show a significant higher expression in the IP group compared to the HD and AS group but just a slight and not significant increase compared to the OP group (**Figure 3D**). Interestingly, a similar expression pattern was observed for the exhaustion marker PD-1 on $CD8^+$ T cells. $CD3^+CD8^+PD1^+$ T cells were increased in the IP group compared to HD and AS but not to OP (**Figure 3E**), indicating that PD1 expression might reflect the activation status of $CD8^+$ T cells, rather than exhaustion in malaria.

Additionally, we compared the frequencies of $GrzB^+CD3^-$ cells and $GrzB^+CD3^+CD4^-CD8^-$ T cells between healthy controls, asymptomatically infected children as well as children with uncomplicated (OP) and severe malaria (IP) (**Supplementary Figure 2**). Of note, specific markers for unconventional T cell subsets or NK cells had not been included in our flow cytometry analyses. The frequencies of $GrzB^+CD3^-$ cells did not differ between all 4 groups (**Supplementary Figure 2A**). $CD3^+CD4^-CD8^-$ T cells showed a higher percentage of $GrzB^+$ cells in IP children compared to healthy and asymptomatically infected children but no significant difference was detected between the frequency of $GrzB^+CD3^+CD4^-CD8^-$ T cells in OP and IP children (**Supplementary Figure 2B**). Of note, the induction and role of GrzB producing $CD4^+$ T cells in malaria has already been analyzed and discussed before (17).

DISCUSSION

In the present study we found increased plasma levels of GrzB in children with acute malaria in comparison with healthy children and children with asymptomatic malaria.

GrzB is produced by cytotoxic cells like NK cells (19) and $CD8^+$ T cells (20). In various inflammatory diseases GrzB spills over from direct contact between cytotoxic cells and target cells and can be measured in the circulation, which might represent a surrogate marker of immune activation during infections (21) or autoimmune disease (22).

However, soluble GrzB failed to discriminate between children with uncomplicated and severe malaria in our study. Several factors might influence GrzB concentration in the circulation like half-life in plasma and binding to various matrix proteins. In addition, no data on the onset of disease is available in the present study and soluble GrzB might change over time. Therefore, the cellular source of GrzB was further investigated.

Using an unbiased approach based on flow cytometry data, we identified $CD8^+$ T cells as the major T cell producers of GrzB in our patients and showed a strong expansion of $GrzB^+CD8^+$ T cells in children with acute malaria compared to afebrile children. Importantly, the proportion of $GrzB^+CD3^+CD8^+$ T cells allowed a discrimination between uncomplicated and severe malaria in our patients, suggesting a role of $GrzB^+CD8^+$ T cells in the pathogenesis of malaria complications.

So far, data from human studies on $CD8^+$ T cells in blood stage malaria are limited. However, there is strong evidence that $CD8^+$ T cells play a protective role in the immune response to several other parasitic infections in humans such as *Toxoplasma gondi* or *Trypanosoma cruzi*, in which $CD8^+$ T cells are essential for controlling the infection in the chronic disease state (23, 24). $CD8^+$ T cells directed against pre-erythrocytic antigens of plasmodia can prevent the progression from liver stage to blood stage malaria and provide sterile immunity in human and murine malaria vaccine studies (25–28).

Yet in the blood stage of *P. falciparum*, $CD8^+$ T cells were thought to play a minor role as the activation of $CD8^+$ T cells depends on the expression of antigens via MHC I and red blood cells lack MHC I expression. In murine malaria models, however, it could be demonstrated that parasite-specific $CD8^+$ T cells are induced during blood-stage malaria, probably through cross presentation of parasite antigens by $CD8\alpha^+$ dendritic cells or stroma cells (29) or even endothelial cells (30) and contribute to the development of experimental cerebral malaria (9, 29, 31). In humans, at least indirect evidence of a pathologic role of $CD8^+$ T cells was given before by a study from Nigeria, in which high plasma sCD8 levels as surrogate marker for activated $CD8^+$ T cells were associated with the development of severe malaria anemia (13). Our study now shows for the first time a potential link between the expansion of cytotoxic $CD8^+$ T cells and severe malaria in pediatric patients. Interestingly, the expression of the activation marker CD38 and the immune checkpoint regulator PD-1 was not different between children with uncomplicated or severe malaria in our study. This supports the idea that not only the mere number of activated $CD8^+$ T cells but a difference in their function, namely GrzB production, might be causally linked to severe symptoms. Several studies using experimental cerebral malaria models already demonstrated that $CD8^+$ T cells contribute to endothelial dysfunction in a perforin (32) and GrzB-dependent mechanism (9). One could envisage a scenario in which endothelial cells present plasmodial antigens on MHC-I and are subsequently lysed by $CD8^+$ T cells (8). Apart from a direct cytolysis GrzB was shown to modify cell function by its proteolytic activity (33).

Importantly, we found a positive correlation between $CD3^+CD8^+GrzB^+$ T cells and parasitemia. This suggests that an increased antigen density influences the proportion of activated T cells producing GrzB. The strong GrzB production by $CD8^+$ T cells, however fails to control or lower the parasitaemia in *P. falciparum* malaria in our patients. This is in contrast to *P. vivax*, where a direct and protective interaction between infected erythrocytes and $CD8^+$ T cells has been demonstrated. This effect is attributed to the MHC-I expression of reticulocytes as host cells of *P. vivax*, which makes them susceptible for a granulysin-mediated permeabilization and subsequent GrzB-mediated killing (15).

Besides $CD8^+$ T cells, other cell subsets such as NK cells and γ/δ T cells are important producers of granzyme B. However, our study focused on the role of $CD8^+$ T cells in malaria and no specific markers for the analysis of NK cells or unconventional T cells or other cell groups such as monocytes or neutrophils were included, which is a limitation of the study. As surrogate markers, $CD3^+CD4^-CD8^-$ T cells as well as $CD3^-$ cells were analyzed for the proportion of $GrzB^+$ cells but no significant difference could be detected between children with uncomplicated and severe malaria. Future studies are needed to further dissect a potential role of NK cells and unconventional T cell subsets to the development of malaria complications.

In summary, our data show that the expansion of $GrzB^+CD8^+$ T cells correlates with parasitemia and is associated with the development of complications in children with *P. falciparum* malaria, supporting prior observations from murine malaria models.

Further studies are needed to examine how GrzB contributes to the pathophysiology of severe malaria in humans.

AUTHOR CONTRIBUTIONS

TJ, EO, and MM designed the study. AA, CS, FA, and MM conducted the experiments. OA-M, DY, and EO recruited the patients and supervised the study in Ghana. LK and MR analyzed the data and prepared the figures. L-CK, MR, MM, and TJ wrote the manuscript. All authors reviewed the manuscript.

ACKNOWLEDGMENTS

We thank Eric Fomevor, Isaac Yaw Asamoah, and Evans Gawu for their technical and logistical help during the study. We especially thank the children and their parents at St. Michael's Hospital and Jachie Primary School for participating in the study.

REFERENCES

1. Weiss WR, Sedegah M, Beaudoin RL, Miller LH, Good MF. CD8+ T cells (cytotoxic/suppressors) are required for protection in mice immunized with malaria sporozoites. *Proc Natl Acad Sci USA.* (1988) 85:573–6. doi: 10.1073/pnas.85.2.573
2. Chakravarty S, Cockburn IA, Kuk S, Overstreet MG, Sacci JB, Zavala F. CD8+ T lymphocytes protective against malaria liver stages are primed in skin-draining lymph nodes. *Nat Med.* (2007) 13:1035–41. doi: 10.1038/nm1628
3. Cockburn IA, Amino R, Kelemen RK, Kuo SC, Tse SW, Radtke A, et al. *In vivo* imaging of CD8 T cell-mediated elimination of malaria liver stages. *Proc Natl Acad Sci USA.* (2013) 110:9090–5. doi: 10.1073/pnas.1303858110.
4. Fernandez-Ruiz D, Ng WY, Holz LE, Ma JZ, Zaid A, Wong YC, et al. Liver-resident memory CD8+ T cells form a front-line defense against malaria liver-stage infection. *Immunity.* (2016) 45:889–902. doi: 10.1016/j.immuni.2016.08.011
5. Epstein JE, Tewari K, Lyke KE, Sim BKL, Billingsley PF, Laurens MB, et al. Live attenuated malaria vaccine designed to protect through hepatic CD8+ T cell immunity. *Science.* (2011) 334:475–80. doi: 10.1126/science.1211548
6. Sun P, Schwenk R, White K, Stoute JA, Cohen J, Ballou WR, et al. Protective immunity induced with malaria vaccine, RTS,S, is linked to *Plasmodium falciparum* circumsporozoite protein-specific CD4 + and CD8 + T cells producing IFN-gamma. *J Immunol.* (2003) 171:6961–67. doi: 10.4049/jimmunol.171.12.6961
7. Frimpong A, Kusi KA, Tornyigah B, Ofori MF, Ndifon W. Characterization of T cell activation and regulation in children with asymptomatic *Plasmodium falciparum* infection. *Malar J.* (2018) 17:263. doi: 10.1186/s12936-018-2410-6
8. Howland SW, Poh CM, Rénia L. Activated brain endothelial cells cross-present malaria antigen. *PLoS Pathog.* (2015) 11:e1004963. doi: 10.1371/journal.ppat.1004963
9. Haque A, Best SE, Unosson K, Amante FH, de Labastida F, Anstey NM, et al. Granzyme B expression by CD8+ T cells is required for the development of experimental cerebral malaria. *J Immunol.* (2011) 186:6148–56. doi: 10.4049/jimmunol.1003955
10. Nitcheu J, Bonduelle O, Combadiere C, Tefit M, Seilhean D, Mazier D, et al. Perforin-dependent brain-infiltrating cytotoxic CD8 + T lymphocytes mediate experimental cerebral malaria pathogenesis. *J Immunol.* (2003) 170:2221–8. doi: 10.4049/jimmunol.170.4.2221
11. Claser C, Malleret B, Gun SY, Wong AYW, Chang ZW, Teo P, et al. CD8+ T cells and IFN-γ mediate the time-dependent accumulation of infected red blood cells in deep organs during experimental cerebral malaria. *PLoS ONE.* (2011) 6:e18720. doi: 10.1371/journal.pone.0018720
12. Belnoue E, Kayibanda M, Vigario AM, Deschemin JC, Rooijen N van, Viguier M, et al. On the pathogenic role of brain-sequestered alphabeta CD8 + T cells in experimental cerebral malaria. *J Immunol.* (2002) 169:6369–75. doi: 10.4049/jimmunol.169.11.6369
13. Safeukui I, Gomez ND, Adelani AA, Burte F, Afolabi NK, Akondy R, et al. Malaria induces anemia through CD8+ T cell-dependent parasite clearance and erythrocyte removal in the spleen. *MBio.* (2015) 6:e02493–14. doi: 10.1128/mBio.02493-14
14. Otterdal K, Berg A, Michelsen AE, Patel S, Tellevik MG, Haanshuus CG, et al. Soluble markers of neutrophil, T-cell and monocyte activation are associated with disease severity and parasitemia in falciparum malaria. *BMC Infect Dis.* (2018) 18:670. doi: 10.1186/s12879-018-3593-8
15. Nyangoto EO. Cell-mediated effector molecules and complicated malaria. *Int Arch Allergy Immunol.* (2005) 137:326–42. doi: 10.1159/000086490
16. van Unen V, Höllt T, Pezzotti N, Li N, Reinders MJT, Eisemann E, et al. Visual analysis of mass cytometry data by hierarchical stochastic neighbour embedding reveals rare cell types. *Nat Commun.* (2017) 8:1740. doi: 10.1038/s41467-017-01689-9
17. Abel A, Steeg C, Aminkiah F, Addai-Mensah O, Addo M, Gagliani N, et al. Differential expression pattern of co-inhibitory molecules on CD4+ T cells in uncomplicated versus complicated malaria. *Sci Rep.* (2018) 8:4789. doi: 10.1038/s41598-018-22659-1
18. Höllt T, Pezzotti N, van Unen V, Koning F, Eisemann E, Lelieveldt B, et al. Cytosplore: interactive immune cell phenotyping for large single-cell datasets. *Comput Graph Forum.* (2016) 35:171–80. doi: 10.1111/cgf.12893
19. Böttger E, Multhoff G, Kun JFJ, Esen M. *Plasmodium falciparum*-infected erythrocytes induce granzyme B by NK cells through expression of host-Hsp70. *PLoS ONE.* (2012) 7:e33774. doi: 10.1371/journal.pone.0033774
20. Bijker EM, Teirlinck AC, Schats R, van Gemert GJ, van de Vegte-Bolmer M, van Lieshout L, et al. Cytotoxic markers associate with protection against malaria in human volunteers immunized with *Plasmodium falciparum* sporozoites. *J Infect Dis.* (2014) 210:1605–15. doi: 10.1093/infdis/jiu293
21. Dotiwala F, Sen Santara S, Binker-Cosen AA, Li B, Chandrasekaran S, Lieberman J. Granzyme B disrupts central metabolism and protein synthesis in bacteria to promote an immune cell death program. *Cell.* (2017) 171:1125–37.e11. doi: 10.1016/j.cell.2017.10.004
22. Russo V, Klein T, Lim DJ, Solis N, Machado Y, Hiroyasu S, et al. Granzyme B is elevated in autoimmune blistering diseases and cleaves key anchoring proteins of the dermal-epidermal junction. *Sci Rep.* (2018) 8:9690. doi: 10.1038/s41598-018-28070-0
23. Padilla AM, Bustamante JM, Tarleton RL. CD8+ T cells in *Trypanosoma cruzi* infection. *Curr Opin Immunol.* (2009) 21:385–90. doi: 10.1016/j.coi.2009.07.006
24. Tarleton RL. CD8+ T cells in *Trypanosoma cruzi* infection. *Semin Immunopathol.* (2015) 37:233–8. doi: 10.1007/s00281-015-0481-9
25. Ishizuka AS, Lyke KE, DeZure A, Berry AA, Richie TL, Mendoza FH, et al. Protection against malaria at 1 year and immune correlates following PfSPZ vaccination. *Nat Med.* (2016) 22:614–23. doi: 10.1038/nm.4110
26. Schofield L, Villaquiran J, Ferreira A, Schellekens H, Nussenzweig R, Nussenzweig V. Gamma Interferon, CD8+ T cells and antibodies required for immunity to malaria sporozoites. *Nature.* (1987) 330:664–6. doi: 10.1038/330664a0

27. Schmidt NW, Butler NS, Harty JT. *Plasmodium*-host interactions directly influence the threshold of memory CD8 T cells required for protective immunity. *J Immunol.* (2011) 186:5873–84. doi: 10.4049/jimmunol.1100194

28. Reyes-Sandoval A, Wyllie DH, Bauza K, Milicic A, Forbes EK, Rollier CS, et al. CD8+ T effector memory cells protect against liver-stage malaria. *J Immunol.* (2011) 187:1347–57. doi: 10.4049/jimmunol.1100302

29. Lundie RJ, de Koning-Ward TF, Davey GM, Nie CQ, Hansen DS, Lau LS, et al. Blood-stage *Plasmodium* infection induces CD8+ T lymphocytes to parasite-expressed antigens, largely regulated by CD8alpha+ dendritic cells. *Proc Natl Acad Sci USA.* (2008) 105:14509–14. doi: 10.1073/pnas.0806727105

30. Turner L, Lavstsen T, Berger SS, Wang CW, Petersen JE, Avril M, et al. Severe malaria is associated with parasite binding to endothelial protein C receptor. *Nature.* (2013) 498:502–5. doi: 10.1038/nature12216

31. Swanson PA II, Hart GT, Russo MV, Nayak D, Yazew T, Peña M, et al. CD8+ T cells induce fatal brainstem pathology during cerebral malaria via luminal antigen-specific engagement of brain vasculature. *PLoS Pathog.* (2016) 12:e1006022. doi: 10.1371/journal.ppat.1006022

32. Potter S, Chan-Ling T, Ball HJ, Mansour H, Mitchell A, Maluish L, et al. Perforin mediated apoptosis of cerebral microvascular endothelial cells during experimental cerebral malaria. *Int J Parasitol.* (2006) 36:485–96. doi: 10.1016/j.ijpara.2005.12.005

33. Afonina IS, Cullen SP, Martin SJ. Cytotoxic and non-cytotoxic roles of the CTL/NK protease granzyme B. *Immunol Rev.* (2010) 235:105–16. doi: 10.1111/j.0105-2896.2010.00908.x

13

Understanding *P. falciparum* Asymptomatic Infections: A Proposition for a Transcriptomic Approach

*Kelvin M. Kimenyi[1,2], Kevin Wamae[1] and Lynette Isabella Ochola-Oyier[1,3]**

[1] KEMRI-Wellcome Trust Research Programme, CGMRC, Kilifi, Kenya, [2] Centre for Biotechnology and Bioinformatics, University of Nairobi, Nairobi, Kenya, [3] Pwani University Bioscience Research Centre, Pwani University, Kilifi, Kenya

Edited by:
Jude Ezeh Uzonna,
University of Manitoba, Canada

Reviewed by:
Rajiv Kumar,
Banaras Hindu University, India
Giampietro Corradin,
Université de Lausanne, Switzerland

***Correspondence:**
Lynette Isabella Ochola-Oyier
liochola@kemri-wellcome.org

Malaria is still a significant public health burden in the tropics. Infection with malaria causing parasites results in a wide range of clinical disease presentations, from severe to uncomplicated or mild, and in the poorly understood asymptomatic infections. The complexity of asymptomatic infections is due to the intricate interplay between factors derived from the human host, parasite, and environment. Asymptomatic infections often go undetected and provide a silent natural reservoir that sustains malaria transmission. This creates a major obstacle for malaria control and elimination efforts. Numerous studies have tried to characterize asymptomatic infections, unanimously revealing that host immunity is the underlying factor in the maintenance of these infections and in the risk of developing febrile malaria infections. An in-depth understanding of how host immunity and parasite factors interact to cause malaria disease tolerance is thus required. This review primarily focuses on understanding anti-inflammatory and pro-inflammatory responses to asymptomatic infections in malaria endemic areas, to present the view that it is potentially the shift in host immunity toward an anti-inflammatory profile that maintains asymptomatic infections after multiple exposures to malaria. Conversely, symptomatic infections are skewed toward a pro-inflammatory immune profile. Moreover, we propose that these infections can be better interrogated using next generation sequencing technologies, in particular RNA sequencing (RNA-seq), to investigate the immune system using the transcriptome sampled during a clearly defined asymptomatic infection.

Keywords: asymptomatic infection, malaria, immunity, cytokines, RNA-seq

INTRODUCTION

Malaria is a significant public health burden with an estimated 219 million new cases and 435,000 deaths reported in 2017 (1). Nearly half of the world's population is at risk of contracting malaria, with tropical and subtropical areas showing the highest prevalence (2). Malaria infection is caused by protozoan parasites of the genus *Plasmodium* that affect humans. *P. falciparum* is globally the most deadly and is the most prevalent parasite in Africa (3). *P. falciparum* malaria ranges from severe to uncomplicated or mild and to the poorly understood asymptomatic infections. Such diverse outcomes are due to the intricate interplay between factors derived from the human host, parasite, and environment (4). At the genomic level, differences in gene expression by the host during host-parasite interactions may account for the various clinical manifestations (5).

Specifically, gene pathways that regulate cytokine signaling and complement regulation as well as the production of immunoglobulins have been implicated (6). A strong pro-inflammatory response has been associated with an increased risk of febrile malaria, severe malaria anemia (7) or cerebral malaria (8), while a weak response has been associated with asymptomatic infection (9). Hence, the balance between pro-inflammatory and anti-inflammatory cytokine production appears to be important in influencing the outcome of malaria infections. Identification of markers that can diagnose the clinical manifestations of *P. falciparum* infections, in addition to symptoms, is important in predicting prognosis and directing treatment strategies.

Malaria infections are mainly characterized by a recurrent cycle of fever and chills. Other symptoms include vomiting, shivering, convulsions, and anemia caused by hemolysis (10). In some cases, these symptoms are not observed, and the infection is described as asymptomatic in individuals without a recent history of antimalarial treatment (11). Once an individual is infected with the parasite, immune factors are tasked with reducing parasite numbers, i.e., anti-parasite immunity, and preventing manifestation of clinical symptoms, anti-disease immunity. In asymptomatic individuals, immunity is skewed toward anti-disease rather than anti-parasite immunity. The mechanisms behind this phenomena are still unclear and more studies are required to understand how anti-disease immunity is induced and its potential for application in vaccine development (12).

DEFINING ASYMPTOMATIC *Plasmodium falciparum* INFECTIONS

The study of asymptomatic infections is still hampered by the lack of standard criteria for defining these infections (4, 11). This is due to the wide range of definitions that complicates the comparison of results across studies (**Table 1**). The most basic definition seems to be the presence of parasitemia and the absence of malaria symptoms, mainly fever (axillary temperature $< 37.5°C$) (14, 19, 20). This definition is ambiguous and most studies have modified it by incorporating strict inclusion criteria. Laishram et al. (4) summarized the diagnostic criteria used to define asymptomatic individuals in different studies and made several recommendations. They suggested the use of longitudinal follow ups, quantifying parasitemia rather than reporting its presence or absence and the use of PCR to identify asymptomatic infections in a population (4). Since then, the criteria have improved by incorporating the latest advancement in PCR, the loop-mediated isothermal amplification (LAMP), biomarkers to detect the parasite and use of cohorts that ensure reliable information about clinical history and follow ups. This allows for the exclusion of those who experienced symptoms in the recent past and then sought treatment. However, there is no consensus on the duration of history and it ranges from 2 weeks to 1 month (5, 14, 20). The longitudinal follow-ups after diagnosis reduces the chances of "false" asymptomatic parasitemia that are defined during *P. falciparum* incubation toward a clinical outcome. The duration of follow-up varies depending on whether the study is interested in asymptomatic parasitemia or the eventual symptomatic outcome (5, 14). The method for asymptomatic parasitemia diagnosis is also important. Microscopy, with a detection threshold of $\sim$50 parasites μl^{-1}, may miss subpatent infections, while others use PCR whose sensitivity can extend to below one parasite μl^{-1} (21, 22). Studies in Kenya, Uganda and Brazil have reported a significantly high prevalence of asymptomatic parasitemia, as much as 6–7 times higher, using PCR when compared to microscopy (13, 23, 24). PCR has also helped to identify individuals with low-density parasitemia in low-transmission settings that were previously missed by microscopy (25). Although the use of PCR is technical and expensive, making it unrealistic in most field studies, it is important in improving the accuracy of diagnosing asymptomatic parasitemia (26). Interestingly, LAMP has been shown to accurately detect sub-microscopic asymptomatic *Plasmodium* infections (27). LAMP is cheap and easy to implement in a field setting as it does not require a thermocycler machine like PCR. In addition, several biomarkers such as lactate dehydrogenase, hemozoin and, in particular, Histidine-Rich Protein 2 that is utilized in rapid diagnostic tests (RDTs), have been used to diagnose malaria (28, 29). Hemozoin is an important metabolite of hemoglobin digestion by the malaria parasite and is associated with pathogenesis as well as inducing immunity to malaria (30–32). A hemozoin sensing assay has recently been shown to be 20 times more sensitive than RDTs in diagnosing *Plasmodium* species (33). It could be applied as a point of care test and more importantly in screening populations for asymptomatic individuals with submicroscopic parasitemia (33). More efficient diagnostic techniques are needed to effectively detect asymptomatic infections in various settings to improve the quality and reliability of data used in studying asymptomatic infections. **Table 1** outlines the different criteria used in transcriptomics studies to define asymptomatic *P. falciparum* infections.

UNDERSTANDING THE RISK OF DEVELOPING FEBRILE INFECTIONS

Asymptomatic infections can act as precursors to malaria illness (34). Mass drug administration (MDA) has been suggested as an effective way of treating chronic asymptomatic infections (35, 36). However, this may interfere with the immunity maintained by these infections, thus increasing the risk of developing clinical malaria in asymptomatic individuals (37). A study in Mali treated chronic asymptomatic individuals at the end of the dry season, followed them up during the subsequent rainy season and reported that treatment of asymptomatic infections is unlikely to influence the subsequent risk of developing clinical malaria (17). Similar findings were also reported in Burkina Faso (38). A risk-benefit analysis is required to determine the tradeoffs to inform the public health impact of MDA on asymptomatic infections. The possibility of developing febrile malaria among asymptomatic carriers has been shown to vary due to transmission intensity and age (**Figure 1**) (20, 39). A study in Kenya compared the risk of developing febrile malaria among

TABLE 1 | Examples of inclusion criteria used to define asymptomatic individuals in transcriptomic studies.

Country, year	Criteria for identifying asymptomatic cases	Study subjects (sample size)	Follow-up protocol, duration	References
Cameroon, 2009	Positive thick blood smear and afebrile. No history of fever and antimalarial treatment in the previous 1 and 2 weeks, respectively, at the time of mass screening	Children <12 years (13)	No follow-up	(5)
Mali, 2011	PCR-detected *P. falciparum* and no fever. No history of antimalarial or immunosuppressive medication in the last 30 days and helminths	Individuals >13 (5)	Bi-weekly and weekly surveillance for *Plasmodium infection* and malaria episode, respectively	(14)
Gabon, 2005	Thin and thick blood smear and no clinical symptoms	Children 0.5–6 years (ND)	Follow up for 5 consecutive days	(6)
Uganda, 2007–2008	Blood smear and no fever	Children 4–5 years (15)	Follow up for 7 days	(16)
Mali, 2006	Not defined	5–13 years (17)	Healthy baseline before the malaria season, 7 or 14 days after treatment of their first malaria episode of the ensuing malaria season, and a subset of children followed up to the 6-month dry season	(18)

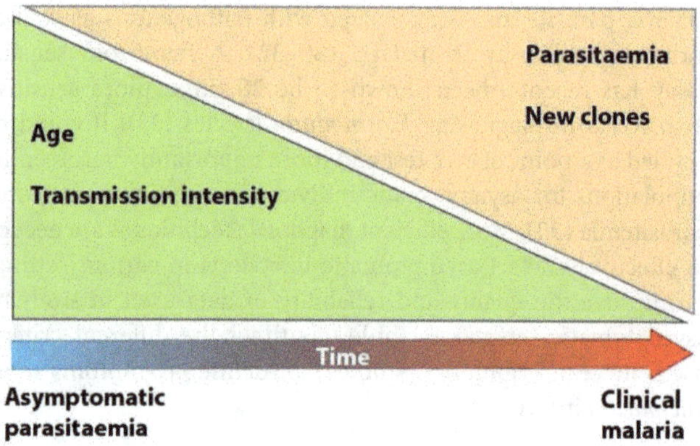

FIGURE 1 | Progression from asymptomatic to clinical malaria. Developing clinical malaria following an asymptomatic infection is influenced by host, parasite, and environmental factors. As individuals age and transmission intensity increases, the risk of developing clinical malaria decreases. This is primarily due to the development of acquired immunity in malaria endemic areas where exposure to repeated infection is common. An increase in parasitemia increases the risk of developing clinical malaria, while acquisition of new parasite clones increases the risk of developing symptoms due to lack of protective immunity against the new clones.

children (0–15 years) who were uninfected with *P. falciparum* and those with asymptomatic parasitemia. In lower transmission areas, asymptomatic parasitemia was linked to an increased risk of febrile malaria in children of all ages, while in moderate to high transmission areas, asymptomatic parasitemia was linked to a reduced risk of febrile malaria in children above 3 years (20). High asymptomatic parasitemia densities (≥2,500 parasites μL^{-1}) and every 10-fold increase in parasite density have been associated with an increased risk of developing febrile malaria, probably due to the underlying reduced host immunity (20, 39).

In addition, the transition from asymptomatic to symptomatic malaria may be influenced by the presence of new parasite genotypes to which an individual has not been previously exposed in the preceding asymptomatic infection, and hence they are likely to lack protective immune responses to the new genotype (40–42). *P. falciparum* infections in malaria endemic areas, primarily in sub-Saharan Africa, are characterized by the co-circulation of multiple *P. falciparum* clones in acute and persistent infections (43–47). This phenomenon is termed complexity of infection (COI). The presence of multiclonal infections has been associated with an increased range of anti-merozoite antibody responses. Together, COI and anti-merozoite antibody responses have been associated with a reduced risk of clinical malaria (48). Carriage of certain merozoite surface protein (*msp*) 1 genotypes have been associated with different clinical manifestations of malaria. In Nigerian children, *msp1* K1 and MAD20 alleles were associated with asymptomatic malaria and a minimal risk of becoming febrile (49). Similarly, using the *msp2* locus, the FC27 genotype was more prevalent in asymptomatic than in symptomatic Nigerian children (50). Other studies have shown that an increase in COI in children with asymptomatic infections is associated with an increased risk of febrile malaria in younger children, a lower risk in older children (51, 52) and in some cases, age had no influence (41, 53). Such conflicting findings on the role of COI in predicting febrile malaria could be due to methodology.

The traditional method for characterizing *P. falciparum* diversity uses nested-PCR with gel electrophoresis to detect polymorphisms in *msp1*, *msp2* and glutamine rich protein (GLuRP) (54) and recently by capillary electrophoresis (55). This technique has been shown to be limited in the number of variants detected within an individual infection (56, 57), is insensitive to less abundant variants and is not quantitative for relative proportions of circulating variants (57). Amplicon deep-sequencing overcomes these challenges as it is more sensitive than capillary electrophoresis in detecting minority clones and is able to quantify individual *P. falciparum* clones (58). This technique also uses less DNA since adequate amounts of amplicons are obtainable directly from dried blood spots used for screening large sample sizes (59). With increased sensitivity and number of samples that can be genotyped, deep-sequencing promises to increase our understanding of the dynamics of *P. falciparum* COI and how this relates to the outcomes of febrile malaria. An understanding of how host immunity mediates the development of febrile malaria in asymptomatic carriers is required to better understand these infections.

IMMUNITY TO MALARIA

Individuals residing in malaria endemic zones often harbor asymptomatic infections and are clinically immune due to exposure to multiple genetically complex *P. falciparum* infections over time (60). Children who have experienced repeated malaria episodes have a modified immune system (26, 61, 62) that is for instance characterized by an increased production of immunoregulatory cytokine IL-10 and activation of neutrophils, B cells and $CD8^+$ T cells (63). The immune system is involved in controlling disease outcome as exhibited by the fact that the parasitemia tolerated in high transmission settings is higher than that causing fever in low transmission settings (64). The chances of an infection being asymptomatic increases with age as repeated exposure to malaria leads to the development of partial anti-disease immunity (65). Unfortunately, the immunity developed is not sterile, only suppressing but not eliminating the infection leading to disease tolerance and asymptomatic infection (66, 67). This immunity may also be lost due to a lack of continuous exposure to the parasite, resulting in elevated pro-inflammatory responses and subsequently a high risk of illness (68).

IMMUNOMODULATION IN ASYMPTOMATIC MALARIA

Modulation of immune responses has been associated with different clinical malaria manifestations (66, 69). The immune responses are mediated by cytokines that regulate inflammation and are thus involved in protective immunity. These cytokines include interferon gamma (IFN-γ), tumor necrosis factor alpha (TNF-α) and IL-12 (70, 71). Overstimulation of the immune system leading to excessive production of these cytokines and activation of immune cells is detrimental to the host as they are likely to cause severe malaria symptoms through unknown mechanisms (72, 73). However, anti-inflammatory cytokines including IL-10, IL-27 and tissue growth factor beta (TGF-β) were shown to be involved in dampening pro-inflammatory cytokines, thereby minimizing disease severity (71, 74). The presence of anti-inflammatory cytokines, especially IL-10, suppresses parasite clearance, hindering the development of anti-parasite immunity, and clinical malaria (69), while promoting the development of asymptomatic infections (18). Elevated levels of IL-10 has also been linked to asymptomatic infections in pregnant women (75).

The production of anti-inflammatory cytokines has been shown to increase with repeated exposure to malaria, resulting in asymptomatic infection (18). Conversely, a lack of continuous exposure in historically exposed individuals can lead to the loss of anti-disease immunity (68, 76). This was exhibited by an increased production of pro-inflammatory cytokines and the proliferation of $CD4^+$ T cells (68). A study in Ugandan children revealed that the production of cytokines by $CD4^+$ T cells is influenced by prior exposure to malaria infections. $CD4^+$ T-cells in more exposed children were shown to produce higher levels of IL-10, while those in less exposed children produced higher levels of TNFα, hence promoting inflammation. The lack of TNFα production was associated with asymptomatic infections (9). A transcriptomic study in Mali described the activation of pro-inflammatory cytokine (IFN-γ, TNF, and IL-1β) production as being influenced by prior exposure to malaria, with asymptomatic infections having the least activation of these cytokines (14). Another study in Uganda revealed that frequent exposure to malaria infection causes decreased levels of pro-inflammatory cytokine (IFN-γ, TNF) producing $V\delta2^+$ $\gamma\delta$ T cells and increased expression of immunoregulatory genes potentially dampening symptom development upon subsequent infections (16). In addition to exposure, age differences have also been suggested to modulate the immune system, with older children having lower anti-inflammatory and pro-inflammatory responses as compared to younger children (15). Lower levels of regulatory T cells (T regs) has also been observed in asymptomatic compared to symptomatic individuals (77, 78). Additionally, high levels of T regs have been associated with increased parasitemia, TGF-β production and the development of clinical symptoms (77, 79, 80). Lower T reg levels, on the other hand, may result in a decreased risk of developing symptoms, which translates to anti-disease immunity (78).

Unlike in asymptomatic infections, the Fulani ethnic group, who have reduced susceptibility to *P. falciparum* infection compared to sympatric tribes, have a higher ratio of pro-inflammatory to anti-inflammatory cytokines (81). The higher levels of pro-inflammatory cytokines have been implicated in causing the reduced symptomatic cases and parasite densities. In a transcriptomic study of their monocytes, increased upregulation of gene pathways involved in the production of pro-inflammatory cytokines in uninfected Fulani was observed, potentially priming the immune system to respond more effectively to *P. falciparum* infections (82). Thus, it appears that a balance between inflammatory and regulatory cytokines is important in achieving anti-disease immunity.

Antibodies also play a significant role in malaria protection. Seminal studies in monkeys and humans reported a reduction in fever and parasitemia following the passive transfer of serum or IgG antibodies from immune to non-immune subjects with acute malaria (83, 84). However, antibody responses to malaria seem to be short lived as exposure to malaria may not lead to the production of sufficient antigen-specific memory B cells (85). In contrast, a study on Swedish travelers previously treated for malaria maintained long-lasting memory B cells for 16 years without subsequent exposure (86).

TABLE 2 | A list of selected cytokines and immune cells showing their levels as reported in studies from Africa comparing malaria clinical outcome.

	Levels	Study site	Clinical comparison	References
IL-10	High	Uganda	Asymptomatic/symptomatic	(9)
	High	Ghana	Asymptomatic/uninfected	(75)
	High	Mali	Asymptomatic/febrile	(18)
	High	Gabon	Asymptomatic/mild	(90)
IFN-γ	Low	Uganda	Asymptomatic/febrile	(9)
	High	Gabon	Asymptomatic/mild	(90)
TNFα	Low	Uganda	Asymptomatic/febrile	(16)
	Low	Uganda	Asymptomatic/symptomatic	(9)
Tregs	Low	Uganda	Asymptomatic/febrile	(77)
	Low	Ghana	Asymptomatic/symptomatic	(78)
$V\delta2^+$ γδ T cells	Low	Uganda	Asymptomatic/febrile	(16)
Natural killer cells	Low	Kenya	Asymptomatic/uninfected	(26)

Higher titers of antigen-specific IgG have been observed in asymptomatic individuals compared to individuals with other malaria outcomes (87–89). Furthermore, high antigen-specific antibody responses were associated with high levels of IL-10 and IFN-γ in Gabonese children with asymptomatic *P. falciparum* infection, suggesting that the antibody response may exert protective immune mechanisms (90). Further studies of immune cells and cytokines (**Table 2**) are necessary to understand the mechanisms underlying immunomodulation and how this can be applied to confer malaria protection. It is evident that there is a complex interplay of various components of the immune system (**Figure 2**), and one way of potentially interrogating this complexity is through an "omics" approach.

To add to this already complex immune process, co-endemicity of *P. falciparum* and helminths is very common in the tropics resulting in increased chances of co-infection (91). Interactions between the two parasites alter immune responses, thus influencing susceptibility to clinical malaria (92, 93). There are conflicting reports on the outcome of these interactions as some studies have reported enhanced severity (94, 95), others reduced severity (96, 97) yet others have revealed no association between helminth co-infection and malaria outcome (98, 99). These observations may be due to differences in the co-infecting helminth species (100), the host's level of immunity to *P. falciparum* (101) and differences in study design (91). Various helminths elicit different immune responses that have an impact on the immunopathology of malaria as a result of the imbalance between pro-inflammatory and anti-inflammatory cytokines (102). However, there are contradictory reports on cytokine profiles resulting from helminths and *P. falciparum* co-infection. Co-infection with *Schistosoma haematobium* in Senegal was shown to offset this balance in an age-dependent manner in children and adults when compared to *P. falciparum* mono-infections. Co-infected children had higher levels of pro-inflammatory cytokines, IFN-γ and TNF-α, and were more likely develop febrile malaria, while co-infected adults had higher levels of similar pro-inflammatory cytokines as well as anti-inflammatory cytokines IL-10 and TGF-β and were more protected from malaria morbidity (103). In Uganda, IL-10 and IL-6 levels were elevated during *P. falciparum* and soil-borne helminth co-infection, while the level of TGF-β was reduced (104). The level of IL-10 was also elevated in asymptomatic *P. falciparum* Malian patients with filaria co-infection while IFN-γ, TNF-α, and IL-17 levels were reduced (105). There is growing evidence that *P. falciparum* and helminth co-infections have a profound effect on the host immune system, preventing the immune clearance of either parasite over the other. Although modulation of pro-inflammatory and anti-inflammatory cytokines responses has been suggested as a possible mechanism, more studies are needed to understand the roles of these cytokines and how other aspects of the immune system are involved.

ASYMPTOMATIC *P. falciparum* TRANSCRIPTOMICS STUDIES

A number of studies have examined the transcriptomics of asymptomatic *P. falciparum* infections and revealed interesting findings that add to the current phenotypic knowledge of these infections. The first study compared parasite gene expression patterns between 18 cerebral and 18 asymptomatic malaria infections in Cameroonian children using microarrays. The major difference was observed in genes coding for exported proteins, transcriptional factor proteins, proteins involved in protein transport, variant surface antigen (VSA) proteins such as *P. falciparum* erythrocyte membrane proteins (PfEMP) and repetitive interspersed family (RIFIN) (5). A more recent study in Gabon compared the host transcriptomic profiles between children with uncomplicated, asymptomatic, severe and cerebral malaria and identified 36 genes, among 4,643 transcripts, which are specifically regulated during asymptomatic infections. These genes are involved in nucleotide binding and RNA processing alluding to gene regulation via chromatin remodeling as a potential mode of maintaining asymptomatic infections (6). Chromatin remodeling changes the chromatin architecture, making condensed genomic DNA accessible to the transcription proteins and thereby regulating gene expression. This was shown to influence activation of immune cells such as monocytes and macrophages (106). It is hypothesized that during asymptomatic infections, chromatin remodeling decreases the expression of immunoglobulin genes leading to reduced antibody mediated responses (6). An opposite effect of chromatin remodeling is observed in the Fulani ethnic group. Chromatin remodeling may have resulted in stronger transcriptional activity in the monocytes leading to a pro-inflammatory state and reduced susceptibility to malaria infections when compared to sympatric ethnic groups (82). Pre- and post-infection profiles of Malian adults who were either febrile, asymptomatic or naïve were compared. Interestingly, asymptomatic individuals had the least transcriptional changes in gene pathways that are regulated by pro-inflammatory cytokines,

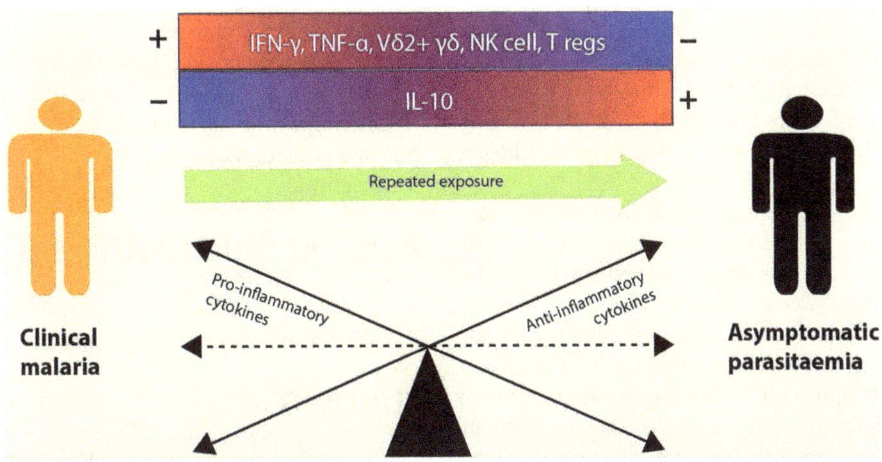

FIGURE 2 | Immune modulation during asymptomatic vs. symptomatic malaria infections. The outcome of a malaria infection is influenced by the balance between anti-inflammatory and pro-inflammatory cytokines. Clinical malaria is the result of elevated (+) production of pro-inflammatory cytokines (e.g., IFN-γ, TNF-α) and increased levels of immune cells (e.g., $V\delta2^+$ γδ, NK cells, and T regs) and the downregulation (–) of anti-inflammatory cytokines (e.g., IL-10). However, with repeated malaria exposure, the immune balance shifts toward an increased production of anti-inflammatory cytokines, leading to asymptomatic infection. The cytokines are encoded by immune genes, thus differential expression of these genes depicts that there is a balance between anti-inflammatory and pro-inflammatory cytokines.

IFN-γ, TNF, and IL-1β (14). This was probably caused by the downregulation of genes encoding pro-inflammatory cytokines, as observed in their lower levels in individuals with frequent exposure to *P. falciparum* in Mali (18). Chronic exposure to *P. falciparum* was shown to cause increased expression of immunoregulatory genes in $V\delta2^+$ T cells in Ugandan children (9). The results from the various transcriptomic studies in asymptomatic infections tend to agree that gene regulation mechanisms, either transcription factors or changes in the chromatin structure, may be involved in regulating inflammatory mechanisms that maintain malaria infections in the asymptomatic state. This can be confirmed by studying chromatin accessibility of gene regions that encode inflammatory regulators. Various techniques have been developed to assess genome-wide chromatin accessibility, with the Assay for Transposase-Accessible Chromatin using sequencing (ATAC-seq) proving to be the most effective (107). This technique has been applied in examining chromatin accessibility in *P. falciparum* and revealed insights into how the accessibility of specific transcriptome regulatory regions, i.e., promoter regions, are directly associated with an abundance of their corresponding transcripts (108, 109). The identification of regulatory regions that regulate expression of inflammatory genes in asymptomatic infections is important, as it would improve our understanding of how anti-disease immunity is maintained and reveal regions that can be targeted to achieve anti-parasite immunity and potentially, sterilizing immunity.

FUTURE PERSPECTIVES FOR ASYMPTOMATIC STUDIES

Asymptomatic malaria appears to be driven by host immunity, such that following multiple exposures to symptomatic infections an individual's immune system is potentially primed to control symptoms. Initially, at a young age, individuals in malaria endemic areas are likely to have high pro-inflammatory responses to control infection, which also results in the clinical manifestation of disease. With age, due to multiple exposure to infection, the immune system is perhaps trained and the balance shifts to a predominance of anti-inflammatory responses to control the infection with no clinical signs of disease, to a point that infection is tolerated and parasitemia is maintained. Since immunity to malaria is not sterile, there appears to be a trade-off between anti-parasite and anti-disease immunity, with the latter dominating in asymptomatic infections, where the focus is controlling disease rather than clearing parasites. This compromise in host immunity to control disease and not clear parasites is likely driven by the anti-inflammatory immune response. A transcriptomic approach to analyzing the cells and cytokines involved in the process would provide the necessary insight to unraveling the role of both anti- and pro-inflammatory responses to asymptomatic infections.

Though there is still a gap in our understanding of how the parasite remains in an asymptomatic state in individuals from malaria endemic areas, various studies have implicated genes responsible for gene regulation and chromatin remodeling and it is still unclear how host immunity is involved. High-throughput studies are needed to understand differential gene expression in immune cells that have shown differential activity in asymptomatic vs. symptomatic or uninfected states (5). Recently, single cell transcriptomics has emerged as a new approach in transcriptomic studies that characterizes individual cells, improving our ability to study cell to cell variability, unlike the conventional transcriptome method that assumes and treats cells from a certain tissue as homogenous (110). Reid et al. (111) used this technique to show transcription variation across all stages of the parasite life cycle and how genes involved in immune evasion aid the parasite in transiting from the asexual stage in humans to its sexual stage in the mosquito (111). Properly designed asymptomatic *P. falciparum* single cell RNA-seq studies of individual immune cells and parasites with good criteria for defining asymptomatic infections hold the key to understanding these chronic and debilitating infections as well as host pathogen interactions in general.

Furthermore, there is a need for a consensus on how asymptomatic infections are defined. Longitudinal cohorts or follow ups over a period of 6 weeks, 4 weeks prior to the asymptomatic case and 2 weeks following the case, with no history or evidence of the individual having taken antimalarials and no evidence of fever 48 h before and after the case, are likely to be the most feasible approach to defining an asymptomatic infection. More sensitive tools for defining the presence of parasitemia to minimize missing sub-patent infections requires methods such as PCR, LAMP, or the newly described hemozoin sensing assay (33). With a clear definition of asymptomatic infections, further downstream analyses become possible. Exploiting next generation sequencing platforms to conduct amplicon deep sequencing and RNA-Seq has the potential to allow for a comprehensive analysis of asymptomatic infections to a scale not previously explored. The scale to which COI can be defined using amplicon deep sequencing improves the accuracy of determining COI in asymptomatic infections, the impact of COI on the risk of developing febrile disease and immunity. RNA-seq promises to unravel the complexities of the host immune response to malaria infection, describing at the transcriptomic level which molecules are likely to be involved in particular processes of controlling infection or, in the case of asymptomatic infections, maintaining parasitemia with no clinical symptoms. Of interest in this review was the role of anti- and pro-inflammatory cytokines in determining the course of infection. A focused analysis of transcripts related to these pathways would provide a better understanding of the role cytokines play in regulating the immune system and influencing malaria outcome. Notably, a better understanding of chromatin remodeling pathways is required to determine whether they are associated with particular gene transcripts, and ATAC-Seq will allow further interrogation of these pathways.

AUTHOR CONTRIBUTIONS

KK and LO-O conceived, drafted, and reviewed the manuscript. KW drafted and reviewed the manuscript.

FUNDING

This work was supported through the DELTAS Africa Initiative (Grant No. DEL-15-003), an independent funding scheme of the African Academy of Sciences (AAS) Alliance for Accelerating Excellence in Science in Africa (AESA) and supported by the New Partnership for Africa's Development Planning and Coordinating Agency (NEPAD Agency) with funding from the Wellcome Trust and the UK government, DELGEME Grant 107740/Z/15/Z to support KK and IDeAL Grant No. 107769/Z/10/Z to support KW. The views expressed in this publication are those of the author(s) and not necessarily those of AAS, NEPAD Agency, Wellcome Trust or the UK government. There was also support from a Wellcome Trust Intermediate Fellowship (Grant No. 107568/Z/15/Z awarded to LO-O).

ACKNOWLEDGMENTS

We thank Dr. Eunice Nduati for her helpful comments on the manuscript and the Director of the Kenya Medical Research Institute, Dr. Yeri Kombe, for permission to publish this article.

REFERENCES

1. World Health Organization. *World Malaria Report 2018*. Global Malaria Programme; Geneva: World Health Organization (WHO) (2018).
2. World Health Organization. *World Malaria Report 2016*. Geneva: World Health Organization (WHO) (2016).
3. Snow RW, Guerra CA, Noor AM, Myint HY, Simon I. The global distribution of clinical episodes of *Plasmodium falciparum* malaria. *Nature.* (2005) 434:214–7. doi: 10.1038/nature03342
4. Laishram DD, Sutton PL, Nanda N, Sharma VL, Sobti RC, Carlton JM, et al. The complexities of malaria disease manifestations with a focus on asymptomatic malaria. *Malar J.* (2012) 11:29. doi: 10.1186/1475-2875-11-29
5. Almelli T, Nuel G, Bischoff E, Aubouy A, Elati M, Wang CW, et al. Differences in gene transcriptomic pattern of *Plasmodium falciparum* in children with cerebral malaria and asymptomatic carriers. *PLoS ONE.* (2014) 9:e114401. doi: 10.1371/journal.pone.0114401
6. Boldt ABW, van Tong H, Grobusch MP, Kalmbach Y, Dzeing Ella A, Kombila M, et al. The blood transcriptome of childhood malaria. *EBioMedicine.* (2019) 40:614–25. doi: 10.1016/j.ebiom.2018.12.055
7. Othoro C, Lal AA, Nahlen B, Koech D, Orago ASS, Udhayakumar V. A low interleukin-10 tumor necrosis factor-α ratio is associated with malaria anemia in children residing in a holoendemic malaria region in western Kenya. *J Infect Dis.* (1999) 179:279–82. doi: 10.1086/314548
8. Udomsangpetch R, Looareesuwan S, Viriyavejakul P, Pongponratn E, Riganti M, Chivapat S, et al. Involvement of cytokines in the histopathology of cerebral malaria. *Am J Trop Med Hyg.* (1997) 57:501–6. doi: 10.4269/ajtmh.1997.57.501
9. Jagannathan P, Eccles-James I, Bowen K, Nankya F, Auma A, Wamala S, et al. IFNγ/IL-10 co-producing cells dominate the CD4 response to malaria in highly exposed children. *PLoS Pathog.* (2014) 10:e1003864. doi: 10.1371/journal.ppat.1003864
10. Severe falciparum malaria. World Health Organization, communicable diseases cluster. *Trans R Soc Trop Med Hyg.* (2000) 94 (Suppl. 1):S1–90. doi: 10.1016/S0035-9203(00)90300-6
11. Lindblade KA, Steinhardt L, Samuels A, Kachur SP, Slutsker L. The silent threat: asymptomatic parasitemia and malaria transmission. *Expert Rev Anti Infect Ther.* (2013) 11:623–39. doi: 10.1586/eri.13.45
12. Ademolue TW, Awandare GA. Evaluating antidisease immunity to malaria and implications for vaccine design. *Immunology.* (2018) 153:423–34. doi: 10.1111/imm.12877
13. Idris ZM, Chan CW, Kongere J, Gitaka J, Logedi J, Omar A, et al. High and heterogeneous prevalence of asymptomatic and sub-microscopic malaria infections on islands in Lake Victoria, Kenya. *Sci Rep.* (2016) 6:36958. doi: 10.1038/srep36958
14. Tran TM, Jones MB, Ongoiba A, Bijker EM, Schats R, Venepally P, et al. Transcriptomic evidence for modulation of host inflammatory responses during febrile *Plasmodium falciparum* malaria. *Sci Rep.* (2016) 6:31291. doi: 10.1038/srep31291

15. Farrington L, Vance H, Rek J, Prahl M, Jagannathan P, Katureebe A, et al. Both inflammatory and regulatory cytokine responses to malaria are blunted with increasing age in highly exposed children. *Malar J.* (2017) 16:499. doi: 10.1186/s12936-017-2148-6
16. Jagannathan P, Kim CC, Greenhouse B, Nankya F, Bowen K, Eccles-James I, et al. Loss and dysfunction of Vδ2$^+$ $\gamma\delta$ T cells are associated with clinical tolerance to malaria. *Sci Transl Med.* (2014) 6:251ra117. doi: 10.1126/scitranslmed.3009793
17. Portugal S, Tran TM, Ongoiba A, Bathily A, Li S, Doumbo S, et al. Treatment of chronic asymptomatic *Plasmodium falciparum* infection does not increase the risk of clinical malaria upon reinfection. *Clin Infect Dis.* (2017) 64:645–53. doi: 10.1093/cid/ciw849
18. Portugal S, Moebius J, Skinner J, Doumbo S, Doumtabe D, Kone Y, et al. Exposure-dependent control of malaria-induced inflammation in children. *PLoS Pathog.* (2014) 10:e1004079. doi: 10.1371/journal.ppat.1004079
19. Botwe AK, Asante KP, Adjei G, Assafuah S, Dosoo D, Owusu-Agyei S. Dynamics in multiplicity of *Plasmodium falciparum* infection among children with asymptomatic malaria in central Ghana. *BMC Genet.* (2017) 18:67. doi: 10.1186/s12863-017-0536-0
20. Wamae K, Wambua J, Nyangweso G, Mwambingu G, Osier F, Ndung'u F, et al. Transmission and age impact the risk of developing febrile malaria in children with asymptomatic *Plasmodium falciparum* parasitemia. *J Infect Dis.* (2018) 219:936–44. doi: 10.1093/infdis/jiy591
21. Ashley EA, Pyae Phyo A, Woodrow CJ. Malaria. *Lancet.* (2018) 391:1608–21. doi: 10.1016/S0140-6736(18)30324-6
22. Vasoo S, Pritt BS. Molecular diagnostics and parasitic disease. *Clin Lab Med.* (2013) 33:461–503. doi: 10.1016/j.cll.2013.03.008
23. Alves FP, Durlacher RR, Menezes MJ, Krieger H, Silva LHP, Camargo EP. High prevalence of asymptomatic *Plasmodium vivax* and *Plasmodium falciparum* infections in native Amazonian populations. *Am J Trop Med Hyg.* (2002) 66:641–8. doi: 10.4269/ajtmh.2002.66.641
24. Nsobya SL, Parikh S, Kironde F, Lubega G, Kamya MR, Rosenthal PJ, et al. Molecular evaluation of the natural history of asymptomatic parasitemia in Ugandan children. *J Infect Dis.* (2004) 189:2220–6. doi: 10.1086/421281
25. Barbosa S, Gozze AB, Lima NF, Batista CL, Bastos MdS, Nicolete VC, et al. Epidemiology of disappearing *Plasmodium vivax* malaria: a case study in rural Amazonia. *PLoS Negl Trop Dis.* (2014) 8:e3109. doi: 10.1371/journal.pntd.0003109
26. Kijogi C, Kimura D, Bao LQ, Nakamura R, Chadeka EA, Cheruiyot NB, et al. Modulation of immune responses by *Plasmodium falciparum* infection in asymptomatic children living in the endemic region of Mbita, western Kenya. *Parasitol Int.* (2018) 67:284–93. doi: 10.1016/j.parint.2018.01.001
27. Sattabongkot J, Suansomjit C, Nguitragool W, Sirichaisinthop J, Warit S, Tiensuwan M, et al. Prevalence of asymptomatic Plasmodium infections with sub-microscopic parasite densities in the northwestern border of Thailand: a potential threat to malaria elimination. *Malar J.* (2018) 17:329. doi: 10.1186/s12936-018-2476-1
28. Krampa FD, Aniweh Y, Awandare GA, Kanyong P. Recent progress in the development of diagnostic tests for malaria. *Diagnostics.* (2017) 7:E54. doi: 10.3390/diagnostics7030054
29. Jain P, Chakma B, Patra S, Goswami P. Potential biomarkers and their applications for rapid and reliable detection of malaria. *Biomed Res Int.* (2014) 2014:852645. doi: 10.1155/2014/852645
30. Coronado LM, Nadovich CT, Spadafora C. Malarial hemozoin: from target to tool. *Biochim Biophys Acta.* (2014) 1840:2032–41. doi: 10.1016/j.bbagen.2014.02.009
31. Olivier M, Van Den Ham K, Shio MT, Kassa FA, Fougeray S. Malarial pigment hemozoin and the innate inflammatory response. *Front Immunol.* (2014) 5:25. doi: 10.3389/fimmu.2014.00025
32. Ihekwereme CP, Esimone CO, Nwanegbo EC. Hemozoin inhibition and control of clinical malaria. *Adv Pharmacol Sci.* (2014) 2014:984150. doi: 10.1155/2014/984150
33. Rifaie-Graham O, Pollard J, Raccio S, Balog S, Rusch S, Hernández-Castañeda MA, et al. Hemozoin-catalyzed precipitation polymerization as an assay for malaria diagnosis. *Nat Commun.* (2019) 10:1369. doi: 10.1038/s41467-019-09122-z
34. Galatas B, Bassat Q, Mayor A. Malaria parasites in the asymptomatic: looking for the hay in the haystack. *Trends Parasitol.* (2016) 32:296–308. doi: 10.1016/j.pt.2015.11.015
35. Newby G, Hwang J, Koita K, Chen I, Greenwood B, von Seidlein L, et al. Review of mass drug administration for malaria and its operational challenges. *Am J Trop Med Hyg.* (2015) 93:125–34. doi: 10.4269/ajtmh.14-0254
36. Sturrock HJW, Hsiang MS, Cohen JM, Smith DL, Greenhouse B, Bousema T, et al. Targeting asymptomatic malaria infections: active surveillance in control and elimination. *PLoS Med.* (2013) 10:e1001467. doi: 10.1371/journal.pmed.1001467
37. Smith T, Felger I, Tanner M, Beck HP. Premunition in *Plasmodium falciparum* infection: insights from the epidemiology of multiple infections. *Trans R Soc Trop Med Hyg.* (1999) 93 (Suppl. 1):59–64. doi: 10.1016/S0035-9203(99)90329-2
38. Tiono AB, Ouédraogo A, Ogutu B, Diarra A, Coulibaly S, Gansané A, et al. A controlled, parallel, cluster-randomized trial of community-wide screening and treatment of asymptomatic carriers of *Plasmodium falciparum* in Burkina Faso. *Malar J.* (2013) 12:79. doi: 10.1186/1475-2875-12-79
39. Njama-Meya D, Kamya MR, Dorsey G. Asymptomatic parasitemia as a risk factor for symptomatic malaria in a cohort of Ugandan children. *Trop Med Int Heal.* (2004) 9:862–8. doi: 10.1111/j.1365-3156.2004.01277.x
40. Roper C, Richardson W, Elhassan IM, Giha H, Hviid L, Satti GMH, et al. Seasonal changes in the *Plasmodium falciparum* population in individuals and their relationship to clinical malaria: a longitudinal study in a Sudanese village. *Parasitology.* (1998) 116:501–10. doi: 10.1017/S0031182098002650
41. Ofosu-Okyere A, Mackinnon MJ, Sowa MP, Koram KA, Nkrumah F, Osei YD, et al. Novel *Plasmodium falciparum* clones and rising clone multiplicities are associated with the increase in malaria morbidity in Ghanaian children during the transition into the high transmission season. *Parasitology.* (2001) 123:113–23. doi: 10.1017/S0031182001008162
42. Kun JFJ, Missinou MA, Lell B, Sovric M, Knoop H, Bojowald B, et al. New emerging *Plasmodium falciparum* genotypes in children during the transition phase from asymptomatic parasitemia to malaria. *Am J Trop Med Hyg.* (2002) 66:653–8. doi: 10.4269/ajtmh.2002.66.653
43. Babiker HA, Ranford-Cartwright LC, Currie D, Charlwood JD, Billingsley P, Teuscher T, et al. Random mating in a natural population of the malaria parasite *Plasmodium falciparum. Parasitology.* (1994) 109:413. doi: 10.1017/S0031182000080665
44. Babiker HA, Abdel-Muhsin AA, Hamad A, Mackinnon MJ, Hill WG, Walliker D. Population dynamics of *Plasmodium falciparum* in an unstable malaria area of eastern Sudan. *Parasitology.* (2000) 120 (Pt 2):105–11. doi: 10.1017/S0031182099005387
45. Magesa SM, Mdira KY, Babiker HA, Alifrangis M, Färnert A, Simonsen PE, et al. Diversity of *Plasmodium falciparum* clones infecting children living in a holoendemic area in north-eastern Tanzania. *Acta Trop.* (2002) 84:83–92. doi: 10.1016/S0001-706X(02)00179-1
46. Agyeman-Budu A, Brown C, Adjei G, Adams M, Dosoo D, Dery D, et al. Trends in multiplicity of *Plasmodium falciparum* infections among asymptomatic residents in the middle belt of Ghana. *Malar J.* (2013) 12:22. doi: 10.1186/1475-2875-12-22
47. Bereczky S, Liljander A, Rooth I, Faraja L, Granath F, Montgomery SM, et al. Multiclonal asymptomatic *Plasmodium falciparum* infections predict a reduced risk of malaria disease in a Tanzanian population. *Microbes Infect.* (2007) 9:103–10. doi: 10.1016/j.micinf.2006.10.014
48. Rono J, Osier FHA, Olsson D, Montgomery S, Mhoja L, Rooth I, et al. Breadth of anti-merozoite antibody responses is associated with the genetic diversity of asymptomatic *Plasmodium falciparum* infections and protection against clinical malaria. *Clin Infect Dis.* (2013) 57:1409–16. doi: 10.1093/cid/cit556
49. Amodu OK, Adeyemo AA, Ayoola OO, Gbadegesin RA, Orimadegun AE, Akinsola AK, et al. Genetic diversity of the msp-1 locus and symptomatic malaria in south-west Nigeria. *Acta Trop.* (2005) 95:226–32. doi: 10.1016/j.actatropica.2005.06.017
50. Amodu OK, Oyedeji SI, Ntoumi F, Orimadegun AE, Gbadegesin RA, Olumese PE, et al. Complexity of the *msp2* locus and the severity of childhood malaria, in south-western Nigeria. *Ann Trop Med Parasitol.* (2008) 102:95–102. doi: 10.1179/136485908X252340

51. Felger I, Smith T, Edoh D, Kitua A, Alonso P, Tanner M, et al. Multiple *Plasmodium falciparum* infections in Tanzanian infants. *Trans R Soc Trop Med Hyg.* (1999) 93:29–34. doi: 10.1016/S0035-9203(99)90324-3
52. Mayor A, Saute F, Aponte JJ, Almeda J, Gómez-Olivé FX, Dgedge M, et al. *Plasmodium falciparum* multiple infections in Mozambique, its relation to other malariological indices and to prospective risk of malaria morbidity. *Trop Med Int Heal.* (2003) 8:3–11. doi: 10.1046/j.1365-3156.2003.00968.x
53. Beck HP, Felger I, Huber W, Steiger S, Smith T, Weiss N, et al. Analysis of multiple *Plasmodium falciparum* infections in Tanzanian children during the phase III trial of the malaria vaccine SPf66. *J Infect Dis.* (1997) 175:921–6. doi: 10.1086/513991
54. Snounou G. Genotyping of *Plasmodium* spp.: nested PCR. In: Doolan DL, editor. *Malaria Methods and Protocols.* New Jersey, NY: Humana Press (2002). p. 103–16. doi: 10.1385/1-59259-271-6:103
55. Liljander A, Wiklund L, Falk N, Kweku M, Mrtensson A, Felger I, et al. Optimization and validation of multi-coloured capillary electrophoresis for genotyping of *Plasmodium falciparum* merozoite surface proteins (msp1 and 2). *Malar J.* (2009) 8:1–14. doi: 10.1186/1475-2875-8-78
56. Juliano JJ, Taylor SM, Meshnick SR. Polymerase chain reaction adjustment in antimalarial trials: molecular malarkey? *J Infect Dis.* (2009) 200:5–7. doi: 10.1086/599379
57. Juliano JJ, Porter K, Mwapasa V, Sem R, Rogers WO, Ariey F, et al. Exposing malaria in-host diversity and estimating population diversity by capture-recapture using massively parallel pyrosequencing. *Proc Natl Acad Sci USA.* (2010) 107:20138–43. doi: 10.1073/pnas.1007068107
58. Lerch A, Koepfli C, Hofmann NE, Kattenberg JH, Rosanas-Urgell A, Betuela I, et al. Longitudinal tracking and quantification of individual *Plasmodium falciparum* clones in complex infections. *Sci Rep.* (2019) 9:3333. doi: 10.1038/s41598-019-39656-7
59. Mideo N, Kennedy DA, Carlton JM, Bailey JA, Juliano JJ, Read AF. Ahead of the curve: next generation estimators of drug resistance in malaria infections. *Trends Parasitol.* (2013) 29:321–8. doi: 10.1016/j.pt.2013.05.004
60. Bull PC, Marsh K. The role of antibodies to *Plasmodium falciparum*-infected-erythrocyte surface antigens in naturally acquired immunity to malaria. *Trends Microbiol.* (2002) 10:55–8. doi: 10.1016/S0966-842X(01)02278-8
61. Day KP, Marsh K. Naturally acquired immunity to *Plasmodium falciparum*. *Immunol Today.* (1991) 12:A68–71. doi: 10.1016/S0167-5699(05)80020-9
62. Greenwood BM, Palit A, Bradley-Moore A, Bryceson ADM. Immunosuppression in children with malaria. *Lancet.* (1972) 299:169–72. doi: 10.1016/S0140-6736(72)90569-7
63. Bediako Y, Adams R, Reid AJ, Valletta JJ, Ndungu FM, Sodenkamp J, et al. Repeated clinical malaria episodes are associated with modification of the immune system in children. *BMC Med.* (2019) 17:60. doi: 10.1186/s12916-019-1292-y
64. Roucher C, Rogier C, Dieye-Ba F, Sokhna C, Tall A, Trape J-F. Changing malaria epidemiology and diagnostic criteria for *Plasmodium falciparum* clinical malaria. *PLoS ONE.* (2012) 7:e46188. doi: 10.1371/journal.pone.0046188
65. Ladeia-Andrade S, Ferreira MU, de Carvalho ME, Curado I, Coura JR. Age-dependent acquisition of protective immunity to malaria in riverine populations of the Amazon Basin of Brazil. *Am J Trop Med Hyg.* (2009) 80:452–9. doi: 10.4269/ajtmh.2009.80.452
66. Medzhitov R, Schneider DS, Soares MP. Disease tolerance as a defense strategy. *Science.* (2012) 335:936–41. doi: 10.1126/science.1214935
67. de Mendonça VR, Barral-Netto M. Immunoregulation in human malaria: the challenge of understanding asymptomatic infection. *Mem Inst Oswaldo Cruz.* (2015) 110:945–55. doi: 10.1590/0074-02760150241
68. Bediako Y, Ngoi JM, Nyangweso G, Wambua J, Opiyo M, Nduati EW, et al. The effect of declining exposure on T cell-mediated immunity to *Plasmodium falciparum* – an epidemiological "natural experiment." *BMC Med.* (2016) 14:143. doi: 10.1186/s12916-016-0683-6
69. Kumar R, Ng S, Engwerda C. The role of IL-10 in malaria: a double edged sword. *Front Immunol.* (2019) 10:229. doi: 10.3389/fimmu.2019.00229
70. Angulo I, Fresno M. Cytokines in the pathogenesis of and protection against malaria. *Clin Diagn Lab Immunol.* (2002) 9:1145–52. doi: 10.1128/CDLI.9.6.1145-1152.2002
71. Malaguarnera L, Musumeci S. The immune response to *Plasmodium falciparum* malaria. *Lancet Infect Dis.* (2002) 2:472–8. doi: 10.1016/S1473-3099(02)00344-4
72. Lyke KE, Burges R, Cissoko Y, Sangare L, Dao M, Diarra I, et al. Serum levels of the proinflammatory cytokines interleukin-1 beta (IL-1), IL-6, IL-8, IL-10, tumor necrosis factor alpha, and IL-12(p70) in malian children with severe *Plasmodium falciparum* malaria and matched uncomplicated malaria or healthy controls. *Infect Immun.* (2004) 72:5630–7. doi: 10.1128/IAI.72.10.5630-5637.2004
73. Butler NS, Harris TH, Blader IJ. Regulation of immunopathogenesis during *Plasmodium* and Toxoplasma infections: more parallels than distinctions? *Trends Parasitol.* (2013) 29:593–602. doi: 10.1016/j.pt.2013.10.002
74. Findlay EG, Greig R, Stumhofer JS, Hafalla JCR, de Souza JB, Saris CJ, et al. Essential role for IL-27 receptor signaling in prevention of Th1-mediated immunopathology during malaria infection. *J Immunol.* (2010) 185:2482–92. doi: 10.4049/jimmunol.0904019
75. Wilson NO, Bythwood T, Solomon W, Jolly P, Yatich N, Jiang Y, et al. Elevated levels of IL-10 and G-CSF associated with asymptomatic malaria in pregnant women. *Infect Dis Obstet Gynecol.* (2010) 2010:317430. doi: 10.1155/2010/317430
76. Deloron P, Chougnet C. Is immunity to malaria really short-lived? *Parasitol Today.* (1992) 8:375–8. doi: 10.1016/0169-4758(92)90174-Z
77. Boyle MJ, Jagannathan P, Farrington LA, Eccles-James I, Wamala S, McIntyre TI, et al. Decline of FoxP3+ regulatory CD4 T cells in peripheral blood of children heavily exposed to malaria. *PLoS Pathog.* (2015) 11:e1005041. doi: 10.1371/journal.ppat.1005041
78. Frimpong A, Kusi KA, Tornyigah B, Ofori MF, Ndifon W. Characterization of T cell activation and regulation in children with asymptomatic *Plasmodium falciparum* infection. *Malar J.* (2018) 17:263. doi: 10.1186/s12936-018-2410-6
79. Minigo G, Woodberry T, Piera KA, Salwati E, Tjitra E, Kenangalem E, et al. Parasite-dependent expansion of TNF receptor II–positive regulatory T cells with enhanced suppressive activity in adults with severe malaria. *PLoS Pathog.* (2009) 5:e1000402. doi: 10.1371/journal.ppat.1000402
80. Walther M, Tongren JE, Andrews L, Korbel D, King E, Fletcher H, et al. Upregulation of TGF-β, FOXP3, and $CD4^{+}CD25^{+}$ regulatory T cells correlates with more rapid parasite growth in human malaria infection. *Immunity.* (2005) 23:287–96. doi: 10.1016/j.immuni.2005.08.006
81. Boström S, Giusti P, Arama C, Persson J-O, Dara V, Traore B, et al. Changes in the levels of cytokines, chemokines and malaria-specific antibodies in response to *Plasmodium falciparum* infection in children living in sympatry in Mali. *Malar J.* (2012) 11:109. doi: 10.1186/1475-2875-11-109
82. Sanou GS, Qu Y, Quin JE, Bujila I, Che M, Homann MV, et al. Major transcriptional changes observed in the Fulani, an ethnic group less susceptible to malaria. (2017) 6:e29156. doi: 10.7554/eLife.29156
83. Cohen S, McGregor IA, Carrington S. Gamma-globulin and acquired immunity to human malaria. *Nature.* (1961) 192:733–7. doi: 10.1038/192733a0
84. Mshana RN, Boulandi J, Mshana NM, Mayombo J, Mendome G. Cytokines in the pathogenesis of malaria: levels of IL-I beta, IL-4, IL-6, TNF-alpha and IFN-gamma in plasma of healthy individuals and malaria patients in a holoendemic area. *J Clin Lab Immunol.* (1991) 34:131–9.
85. Dorfman JR, Bejon P, Ndungu FM, Langhorne J, Kortok MM, Lowe BS, et al. B cell memory to 3 *Plasmodium falciparum* blood-stage antigens in a malaria-endemic area. *J Infect Dis.* (2005) 191:1623–30. doi: 10.1086/429671
86. Ndungu FM, Lundblom K, Rono J, Illingworth J, Eriksson S, Färnert A. Long-lived *Plasmodium falciparum* specific memory B cells in naturally exposed Swedish travelers. *Eur J Immunol.* (2013) 43:2919. doi: 10.1002/eji.201343630
87. Kinyanjui SM, Mwangi T, Bull PC, Newbold CI, Marsh K. Protection against clinical malaria by heterologous immunoglobulin G antibodies against malaria-infected erythrocyte variant surface antigens requires interaction with asymptomatic infections. *J Infect Dis.* (2004) 190:1527–33. doi: 10.1086/424675
88. Moormann AM, Sumba PO, Chelimo K, Fang H, Tisch DJ, Dent AE, et al. Humoral and cellular immunity to *Plasmodium falciparum* merozoite surface protein 1 and protection from infection with blood-stage parasites. *J Infect Dis.* (2013) 208:149–58. doi: 10.1093/infdis/jit134

89. Braga EM, Barros RM, Reis TA, Fontes CJF, Morais CG, Martins MS, et al. Association of the IgG response to *Plasmodium falciparum* merozoite protein (C-terminal 19 kD) with clinical immunity to malaria in the Brazilian Amazon region. *Am J Trop Med Hyg.* (2002) 66:461–6. doi: 10.4269/ajtmh.2002.66.461
90. Guiyedi V, Bécavin C, Herbert F, Gray J, Cazenave P-A, Kombila M, et al. Asymptomatic *Plasmodium falciparum* infection in children is associated with increased auto-antibody production, high IL-10 plasma levels and antibodies to merozoite surface protein 3. *Malar J.* (2015) 14:162. doi: 10.1186/s12936-015-0658-7
91. Mwangi TW, Bethony JM, Brooker S. Malaria and helminth interactions in humans: an epidemiological viewpoint. *Ann Trop Med Parasitol.* (2006) 100:551–70. doi: 10.1179/136485906X118468
92. Druilhe P, Tall A, Sokhna C. Worms can worsen malaria: towards a new means to roll back malaria? *Trends Parasitol.* (2005) 21:359–62. doi: 10.1016/j.pt.2005.06.011
93. Vaumourin E, Vourc'h G, Gasqui P, Vayssier-Taussat M. The importance of multiparasitism: examining the consequences of co-infections for human and animal health. *Parasit Vectors.* (2015) 8:545. doi: 10.1186/s13071-015-1167-9
94. Midzi N, Mtapuri-Zinyowera S, Mapingure MP, Sangweme D, Chirehwa MT, Brouwer KC, et al. Consequences of polyparasitism on anaemia among primary school children in Zimbabwe. *Acta Trop.* (2010) 115:103–11. doi: 10.1016/j.actatropica.2010.02.010
95. Wilson S, Vennervald BJ, Kadzo H, Ireri E, Amaganga C, Booth M, et al. Hepatosplenomegaly in Kenyan schoolchildren: exacerbation by concurrent chronic exposure to malaria and *Schistosoma mansoni* infection. *Trop Med Int Heal.* (2007) 12:1442–9. doi: 10.1111/j.1365-3156.2007.01950.x
96. Hürlimann E, Houngbedji CA, Yapi RB, N'Dri PB, Silué KD, Ouattara M, et al. Antagonistic effects of *Plasmodium*-helminth co-infections on malaria pathology in different population groups in Côte d'Ivoire. *PLoS Negl Trop Dis.* (2019) 13:e0007086. doi: 10.1371/journal.pntd.0007086
97. Cot M, Garcia A, Le Hesran JY, Lemaitre M, Watier L, Briand V. Coinfection with *Plasmodium falciparum* and *Schistosoma haematobium*: additional evidence of the protective effect of schistosomiasis on malaria in Senegalese children. *Am J Trop Med Hyg.* (2014) 90:329–34. doi: 10.4269/ajtmh.12-0431
98. Lo AC, Faye B, Gyan BA, Amoah LE. Plasmodium and intestinal parasite perturbations of the infected host's inflammatory responses: a systematic review. *Parasit Vectors.* (2018) 11:387. doi: 10.1186/s13071-018-2948-8
99. Ojurongbe O, Adegbayi AM, Bolaji OS, Akindele AA, Adefioye OA, Adeyeba OA. Asymptomatic falciparum malaria and intestinal helminths co-infection among school children in Osogbo, Nigeria. *J Res Med Sci.* (2011) 16:680–6.
100. Shapiro AE, Tukahebwa EM, Kasten J, Clarke SE, Magnussen P, Olsen A, et al. Epidemiology of helminth infections and their relationship to clinical malaria in southwest Uganda. *Trans R Soc Trop Med Hyg.* (2005) 99:18–24. doi: 10.1016/j.trstmh.2004.02.006
101. Mboera LEG, Senkoro KP, Rumisha SF, Mayala BK, Shayo EH, Mlozi MRS. *Plasmodium falciparum* and helminth coinfections among schoolchildren in relation to agro-ecosystems in Mvomero District, Tanzania. *Acta Trop.* (2011) 120:95–102. doi: 10.1016/j.actatropica.2011.06.007
102. Maizels RM, Balic A, Gomez-Escobar N, Nair M, Taylor MD, Allen JE. Helminth parasites - masters of regulation. *Immunol Rev.* (2004) 201:89–116. doi: 10.1111/j.0105-2896.2004.00191.x
103. Diallo TO, Remoue F, Schacht AM, Charrier N, Dompnier J, Pillet S, et al. Schistosomiasis co-infection in humans influences inflammatory markers in uncomplicated *Plasmodium falciparum* malaria. (2005) 26:365–9. doi: 10.1111/j.0141-9838.2004.00719.x
104. Bwanika R, Kato CD, Welishe J, Mwandah DC. Cytokine profiles among patients co-infected with *Plasmodium falciparum* malaria and soil borne helminths attending Kampala International University Teaching Hospital, in Uganda. *Allergy Asthma Clin Immunol.* (2018) 14:10. doi: 10.1186/s13223-018-0235-z
105. Metenou S, Dembele B, Konate S, Dolo H, Coulibaly YI, Diallo AA, et al. Filarial infection suppresses malaria-specific multifunctional Th1 and Th17 responses in malaria and filarial coinfections. *J Immunol.* (2011) 186:4725–33. doi: 10.4049/jimmunol.1003778
106. Schultze JL. Chromatin remodeling in monocyte and macrophage activation. *Adv Protein Chem Struct Biol.* (2017) 106:1–15. doi: 10.1016/bs.apcsb.2016.09.001
107. Buenrostro JD, Giresi PG, Zaba LC, Chang HY, Greenleaf WJ. Transposition of native chromatin for fast and sensitive epigenomic profiling of open chromatin, DNA-binding proteins and nucleosome position. *Nat Methods.* (2013) 10:1213–8. doi: 10.1038/nmeth.2688
108. Ruiz JL, Tena JJ, Bancells C, Cortés A, Gómez-Skarmeta JL, Gómez-Díaz E. Characterization of the accessible genome in the human malaria parasite *Plasmodium falciparum*. *Nucleic Acids Res.* (2018) 46:9414–31. doi: 10.1093/nar/gky643
109. Toenhake CG, Fraschka SA-K, Vijayabaskar MS, Westhead DR, van Heeringen SJ, Bártfai R. Chromatin accessibility-based characterization of the gene regulatory network underlying *Plasmodium falciparum* blood-stage development. *Cell Host Microbe.* (2018) 23:557–69.e9. doi: 10.1016/j.chom.2018.03.007
110. Hwang B, Lee JH, Bang D. Single-cell RNA sequencing technologies and bioinformatics pipelines. *Exp Mol Med.* (2018) 50:96. doi: 10.1038/s12276-018-0071-8
111. Reid AJ, Talman AM, Bennett HM, Gomes AR, Sanders MJ, Illingworth CJR, et al. Single-cell RNA-seq reveals hidden transcriptional variation in malaria parasites. *Elife.* (2018) 7:e33105. doi: 10.7554/eLife.33105

14

Malaria Vaccines: Identifying *Plasmodium Falciparum* Liver-Stage Targets

*Rhea J. Longley**†, *Adrian V. S. Hill and Alexandra J. Spencer*

The Jenner Institute, Nuffield Department of Medicine, University of Oxford, Oxford, UK

Edited by:
Ute Frevert,
New York University School of Medicine, USA

Reviewed by:
Ann-Kristin Mueller,
University Hospital Heidelberg, Germany
Alberto Moreno,
Emory University, USA

***Correspondence:**
Rhea J. Longley,
The Jenner Institute, Nuffield Department of Medicine, University of Oxford, Oxford, UK
longley.r@wehi.edu.au

†Present address:
Rhea J. Longley,
The Walter and Eliza Hall Institute of Medical Research, Parkville, VIC, Australia;
Mahidol Vivax Research Unit, Faculty of Tropical Medicine, Mahidol University, Bangkok, Thailand;
Department of Medical Biology, University of Melbourne, Parkville, VIC, Australia

The development of a highly efficacious and durable vaccine for malaria remains a top priority for global health researchers. Despite the huge rise in recognition of malaria as a global health problem and the concurrent rise in funding over the past 10–15 years, malaria continues to remain a widespread burden. The evidence of increasing resistance to anti-malarial drugs and insecticides is a growing concern. Hence, an efficacious and durable preventative vaccine for malaria is urgently needed. Vaccines are one of the most cost-effective tools and have successfully been used in the prevention and control of many diseases, however, the development of a vaccine for the *Plasmodium* parasite has proved difficult. Given the early success of whole sporozoite mosquito-bite delivered vaccination strategies, we know that a vaccine for malaria is an achievable goal, with sub-unit vaccines holding great promise as they are simple and cheap to both manufacture and deploy. However a major difficulty in development of sub-unit vaccines lies within choosing the appropriate antigenic target from the 5000 or so genes expressed by the parasite. Given the liver-stage of malaria represents a bottle-neck in the parasite's life cycle, there is widespread agreement that a multi-component sub-unit malaria vaccine should preferably contain a liver-stage target. In this article we review progress in identifying and screening *Plasmodium falciparum* liver-stage targets for use in a malaria vaccine.

Keywords: malaria, vaccine, liver-stage, T cells, immunity

Introduction

Malaria is a disease caused by the parasite *Plasmodium*, of which five species are known to infect humans, and is transmitted by the bite of female *Anopheles* mosquitoes. In 2013, approximately 584 000 people died from malaria (WHO, 2014), the majority due to *Plasmodium falciparum*. There has been substantial success in reducing mortality rates by approximately 50% over the past 15 years (WHO, 2014), but there is still a considerable burden of disease and some worrying trends in resistance to anti-malarial drugs. There are increasing reports of resistance to artemisinin in several countries of South East Asia (Ashley et al., 2014), and in addition reports of insecticide resistance to pyrethroids, the only insecticide class licensed for use in impregnated bed-nets, have started to emerge (Ranson et al., 2011). Together, these issues highlight the importance, and potential reliance the global community may have, on developing a highly efficacious and durable vaccine for malaria.

An effective whole parasite vaccination approach for malaria was developed in the early 1970s (Clyde et al., 1973; Rieckmann et al., 1974), building on previous work in animal models

(Russell and Mohan, 1942; Nussenzweig et al., 1967). The parasite has a complex life cycle; within the human host, sporozoites injected by mosquitoes first travel to the liver. Here they develop for approximately 7 days, before entering into the bloodstream. The blood-stage is responsible for all symptoms associated with malaria, and gives rise to the sexual forms known as gametocytes. Researchers were able to demonstrate sterile protection - the complete absence of blood-stage parasites - after administration of irradiated sporozoites by mosquito bites. These irradiated sporozoites are able to invade the liver but development is arrested, providing a repertoire of antigens for the immune system to recognize without the host experiencing a blood-stage infection. Whilst this vaccination strategy was highly efficacious, it had numerous logistical issues, including the need to receive over 1000 bites from mosquitoes. Now, the biotechnology company Sanaria can cryopreserve sporozoites and vaccinate by needle-and-syringe, resulting in high levels of protection against subsequent challenge if 4–5 intravenous doses are administered (Seder et al., 2013), however, the durability of protection from this formulation has not yet been published. In addition, a number of manufacturing and logistical issues still remain, such as cost of manufacture, the route of administration, the need for storage in liquid nitrogen vapor phase and the requirement for large numbers of doses. An alternate, likely more practical, approach is sub-unit vaccination.

To-date, the most successful sub-unit vaccine is RTS,S Greenwood (2015), a particulate vaccine directed at the circumsporozoite protein (CSP). CSP is the major coat protein on the sporozoite surface (Yoshida et al., 1980; Nussenzweig and Nussenzweig, 1985) and is implicated in protection mediated by irradiated sporozoites (Gwadz et al., 1979; Nardin et al., 1982). The Phase III trial of RTS,S/AS01 conducted at eleven sites within seven African countries demonstrated 28% efficacy for 5–17 month-old children and 18% efficacy for 6–12 week-old infants with three doses, over the entire course of the study (~3–4 years of follow-up; Greenwood, 2015). Our group has also had some success with a virally vectored sub-unit vaccine directed at the pre-erythrocytic antigen thrombospondin-related adhesion protein (TRAP) fused to a multi-epitope (ME) string (Gilbert et al., 1997; McConkey et al., 2003). When delivered in the vectors chimpanzee adenovirus 63 (ChAd63) and modified vaccinia virus Ankara (MVA), ME-TRAP provided 21% sterile protection in malaria-naïve adults, associated with $CD8^+$ T cells inducing IFN-γ (Ewer et al., 2013). In the first field trial of this approach, significant efficacy (67%) in preventing PCR-detectable parasites was observed in Kenyan adults (Ogwang et al., 2015). Sub-unit vaccines with antigenic targets from the blood-stage of infection are also in clinical development (Drew and Beeson, 2015).

Given neither TRAP nor CSP alone (nor any blood-stage candidate) can match the protection induced by irradiated sporozoites, it is likely that a broad immune response to multiple target antigens will contribute to improved sub-unit vaccine efficacy. Only a minority of potential candidate antigens have been assessed as vaccine candidates, and CSP and TRAP may not be the best targets (Doolan et al., 2003; Kumar et al., 2006; Trieu et al., 2011). Furthermore, including multiple antigenic targets in one vaccine might overcome limitations in genetically restricted responses to certain epitopes (Doolan et al., 1996). The difficulty is choosing which antigenic targets from the 5000 or so genes expressed by the parasite (Gardner et al., 2002) should be incorporated. There is widespread agreement that a liver-stage target would be a desirable addition to a multi-component sub-unit malaria vaccine targeting another life-cycle stage, given that it represents a bottle-neck in the parasite's life-cycle and could also be transmission blocking, by preventing development to the blood-stage and hence the formation of gametocytes.

In this article we therefore review what has been learnt so far in terms of identification and screening of novel liver-stage vaccine targets.

Identifying Liver-Stage Targets

The discovery of the *Plasmodium* genome (Gardner et al., 2002) and proteome (Florens et al., 2002) has yielded a huge number of potential liver-stage targets, but has not necessarily provided information as to which should or could be included in a vaccine. In this section we will discuss a number of methods that could be used to prioritize antigens.

Transcriptomic Profiling

Transcriptomic profiling of the *P. falciparum* liver-stage would uncover genes that are actively being expressed. This has, however, not been a simple task to undertake, even in murine models, given the high proportion of uninfected hepatocytes (Lau et al., 2001). Nevertheless, using techniques such as laser capture microdissection, axenically cultured exo-erythrocytic forms and fluorescent parasites, the *P. yoelii* transcriptome has been described, with around 1000 proteins likely expressed at the liver-stage (Wang et al., 2004; Sacci et al., 2005; Tarun et al., 2008). The *P. yoelii* liver-stage lasts for only 2 days, compared to 7 days for *P. falciparum*, and hence there are likely important differences in the transcriptomic profiles of these species. For example, the *P. falciparum* liver-stage specific protein liver-stage antigen 1 (LSA1) does not have a murine ortholog but is critical for late-liver-stage development (Mikolajczak et al., 2011).

Only one published study to our knowledge has attempted to define the *P. falciparum* liver-stage specific transcriptome. Siau et al. (2008) found 532 genes up-regulated following co-culture of *P. falciparum* sporozoites and primary human hepatocytes *in vitro* when compared to genes expressed in sporozoites alone. We recently demonstrated sterile protection following vaccination with one candidate identified in this study, liver-stage associated protein 2 (LSAP2; Longley et al., 2015b). This transcriptomic study was designed to identify genes important in the invasive period of the liver-stage, and hence they co-cultured the sporozoites and hepatocytes for only 1 h. Further research is now needed to determine the complete transcriptome, including late liver-stage development.

Epitope Identification

To be immunogenic and targeted by T cells, the proteins need to be processed and epitopes presented on the hepatocyte cell surface in association with the major histocompatibility complex (MHC). Identifying which epitopes are presented at the liver-stage is hence also a rational method of choosing functionally important antigens. One method of epitope identification is prediction software (Trolle et al., 2015), used to predict the MHC binding capacity. This method has been applied to *P. falciparum* (Doolan et al., 2003) and reviewed in detail (Doolan, 2011) so will not be discussed further here, except to note that these predictions were made using the sporozoite proteome and that once the liver-stage specific *P. falciparum* proteome is known, they should be revisited. The risk with epitope prediction software is the rate of false positive identification (Zhong et al., 2003).

A direct method of epitope identification is the elution of peptides from *P. falciparum* infected hepatocytes. Generally, MHC-peptide complexes are isolated, the peptides eluted and separated by mass spectrometry, and subsequently sequenced (Hunt et al., 1992). This methodology has been used to identify epitopes for influenza (Testa et al., 2012), hepatitis C (Wolk et al., 2012), ovarian cancer (Ramakrishna et al., 2003), and tuberculosis (Flyer et al., 2002), but to our knowledge has not yet been used for *P. falciparum* due to the constraints on access to and infectability of hepatocytes.

Another method of epitope identification is a proprietary approach developed by Genocea Biosciences, Inc., known as ATLAS™. They created a 'high throughput, proteomic technology that facilitates unbiased and comprehensive identification of both $CD4^+$ and $CD8^+$ T cell antigens' (Long et al., 2014). The rationale is to use whole proteins, rather than peptides, to stimulate immune cells from large numbers of individuals from two groups, those naturally protected from the pathogen and those susceptible. By developing a high-throughput technology able to screen large numbers of individuals they reduce the effect of HLA-restrictions. Furthermore, utilizing whole proteins, which are then processed by each volunteer's own APCs, the resultant epitopes should be unbiased. This methodology is currently being explored for the identification of *P. falciparum* T cell targets.

Source of Hepatocytes

The major limitations for both transcriptomic profiling and epitope identification are the source of infected hepatocytes and an absence of a perfect model of *P. falciparum* liver-stage infection. Whilst both hepatoma cell lines and primary human hepatocytes can be infected with *P. falciparum in vitro*, the infectivity rates are very low (~0.1%; Mazier et al., 1985; Sattabongkot et al., 2006; March et al., 2013). In addition, *P. falciparum* sporozoites cannot naturally infect small rodents. Murine *Plasmodium* species are commonly used to study the liver-stage of infection in mice and *in vitro*, yet it is not clear how well these models reflect *P. falciparum* infections in humans. Whilst non-human primates can be infected with adapted human malaria parasites, they are not widely available and cost and ethical considerations of studies on higher order species are limiting factors.

An alternative model is the use of humanized mice; a number of laboratories now routinely infect various models of humanized mice with *P. falciparum* parasites (Morosan et al., 2006; Sacci et al., 2006; Vaughan et al., 2012b), after repopulation of 80–90% of the liver with human hepatocytes. The advantages over an *in vitro* model are that larger liver-stage parasites develop, up to 80 μm compared to 15–40 μm in culture (Mazier et al., 1985; Sattabongkot et al., 2006; Vaughan et al., 2012b). The larger size is more similar to results from studies of human infections (Shortt et al., 1951; Jeffery et al., 1952). Furthermore, liver-stage artifacts or abortive forms of parasites are often detected in cultures, yet this has not been observed in humanized mice. Whilst there are a number of disadvantages to this model (especially cost), it may be the most practical for obtaining large numbers of infected hepatocytes for antigen identification.

Human Whole Sporozoite Immmunization for Antigen Identification

Once potential antigens or epitopes have been prioritized, cells from irradiated sporozoite immunization studies can be utilized to confirm that down-selected target antigens are immunogenic in vaccinated volunteers and to try and identify protective antigens. This is possible as protection in irradiated sporozoite vaccination models is dependent on T cells targeting the liver-stage (Schofield et al., 1987; Weiss et al., 1988; Hoffman et al., 1989; Seguin et al., 1994; Weiss and Jiang, 2012). Doolan et al. (2003) adopted this method to attempt to validate their antigens identified using epitope prediction software.

Alternatively, immunity can now be induced in humans with cryopreserved sporozoites (Sanaria®PfSPZ-CVac) or mosquito bite delivered sporozoites under drug cover (Roestenberg et al., 2011; Bijker et al., 2013). A major difficulty with this general approach is that of statistical power. With whole sporozoite strategies only tens of subjects are generally immunized and challenged and it is difficult to quantify degrees of protection precisely in each individual. Because there are hundreds of possible liver-stage antigens to be assayed, and most people respond weakly to most antigens, it is likely to be difficult to pinpoint the best individual protective antigen(s) standing out above the level of efficacy provided by the cumulative effects of large numbers of other antigens.

Unfortunately, this is also a limitation for the ATLAS™ technology, as it relies on access to cells from humans whom are protected by whole pathogen exposure: for other pathogens they have used cells from exposed individuals (Long et al., 2014), whereas for malaria naturally exposed or challenged individuals generally have weak T cell responses (Offeddu et al., 2012; Sheehy et al., 2013). Hence, immunization models, such as described below, may be more useful.

Screening Targets

Once candidate antigens have been identified, a functional assay to assess pre-clinical efficacy needs to be employed. The challenges are twofold: *P. falciparum* does not infect small animals, and there is no standardized *in vitro* assay to measure T cell killing of liver-stage parasites.

Mouse Models

In the past, candidate antigens have been screened in mice using *P. berghei* or *P. yoelii* orthologs of the *P. falciparum* antigen of interest. It is still unclear how well these results translate to human trials, and importantly, not all *P. falciparum* antigens have murine orthologs. Alternate options are the use of transgenic parasites and humanized mice.

Transgenic parasites are a powerful tool that can enable functional screening of *P. falciparum* (or *P. vivax*) vaccine efficacy in mice (Persson et al., 2002; Mlambo et al., 2008; Cao et al., 2009; Espinosa et al., 2013; Porter et al., 2013; Bauza et al., 2014; Deal et al., 2014; Mizutani et al., 2014; Schwenk et al., 2014). Two methods are commonly used: (1) replacement of the endogenous *P. berghei* (or *P. yoelii*) gene with the *P. falciparum* ortholog under control of the relevant *P. berghei* promoter, or (2) addition of the *P. falciparum* copy of the gene inserted at a different and dispensable point in the genome (required when no murine ortholog exists). For example, the *230p* locus in both *P. berghei* and *P. yoelii* is considered "silent", and replacement of this gene has no adverse effect on expression of other genes and no impact on parasite viability or behavior (Janse et al., 2006; van Dijk et al., 2010; Lin et al., 2011). We have recently used this method of screening to identify PfLSA1 and PfLSAP2 as potential candidates for a liver-stage malaria vaccine (Longley et al., 2015b): we were able to screen ten antigens for homologous efficacy in mice, and both PfLSA1 and PfLSAP2 outperformed CSP and TRAP in this model. We were also able to utilize the transgenic parasites to demonstrate that efficacy was primarily dependent on $CD8^+$ T cells.

The main limitation of the addition rather than replacement technique is that the *P. falciparum* transgene is under control of a non-native promoter, potentially leading to differential patterns of gene expression. In addition, for both the replacement and addition strategies experiments are still undertaken in mice and the limited MHC system favors immunodominant responses, although this can be mitigated if outbred mice are studied. It is important to note that this is an artificial model system, and only once clinical trials of candidates selected in this manner have been undertaken successfully will we know its true value.

An alternative option is the use of humanized mice permissible to *P. falciparum* infection. As these mice are immunodeficient (Morosan et al., 2006; Sacci et al., 2006; Vaughan et al., 2012b) they would not be suitable for vaccination, but T cells from classical inbred mice could be adoptively transferred. To our knowledge this option has not yet been explored, but warrants some attention and preliminary experimentation to determine the feasibility.

In Vitro Assays

In vitro assays could also be used for screening liver-stage vaccine candidates. *P. falciparum*-infected primary human hepatocytes and hepatoma cell lines have been used to measure antibody inhibition of invasion and growth (Mazier et al., 1986; Hollingdale et al., 1987, 1990; Mellouk et al., 1990; Fidock et al., 1997; Brahimi et al., 2001; House et al., 2009; Zou et al., 2013; Finney et al., 2014). To-date, only murine *Plasmodium* infected hepatocytes have been used to measure T cell-mediated protection (Hoffman et al., 1989; Weiss et al., 1990; Renia et al., 1991, 1993; Trimnell et al., 2009). T-cell assays require MHC effector-target cell matching, complicating the assay, and perhaps explaining in part why it has received little attention for many years. We have since revisited this assay, incorporating a number of technological advances such as fluorescent parasites to simplify the assay design and interpretation (Longley et al., 2015a). We utilized *P. berghei* TRAP as a model antigen and demonstrated TRAP-specific $CD8^+$ T cell enriched splenocytes were able to inhibit *P. berghei* infected hepatoma cells in an effector-to-target ratio dependent manner.

However, the assessment of inhibition of *P. falciparum* infected human hepatocytes or hepatoma cell lines by human T cells is still an elusive goal. The difficulties are fourfold: (1) the rate of infectivity of *P. falciparum* sporozoites into human hepatocytes or hepatoma cells is inherently lower than that of murine *Plasmodium* species (Mazier et al., 1985; Sattabongkot et al., 2006); (2) *P. falciparum* sporozoites are more difficult to produce in the laboratory than murine species; (3) the lack of a *P. falciparum* parasite line with strong expression of a fluorescent or other visual marker throughout the entire lifecycle; and (4) the limited choice of human hepatoma cell lines with different HLA types (Karnasuta et al., 1995; Sattabongkot et al., 2006). Yet these barriers are constantly being reduced with improvements to liver-stage culture techniques (March et al., 2013; Zou et al., 2013; Ng et al., 2014) and the availability of cryopreserved *P. falciparum* parasites that could also reduce variability between assays (Sheehy et al., 2013). In addition, new *P. falciparum* parasites expressing fluorescent or luminescent markers are becoming available (Talman et al., 2010; Vaughan et al., 2012a), and flow cytometry detection of *P. falciparum* infected human hepatocytes and hepatoma cells has recently been demonstrated (Dumoulin et al., 2015). Finally the availability of cryopreserved primary human hepatocytes enriches the HLA-repertoire of target cells available (Li, 2014).

The remaining hurdle is the source of vaccine-induced human T cells. One option is through vaccination of human volunteers in clinical trials, however, this is not amenable to screening a large number of candidate antigens/vaccines. An alternate option is stimulation of naïve T cells *in vitro* (Gaucher et al., 2008), or alternatively (re-)stimulation of malaria-exposed T cells (for instance, sourced from whole sporozoite immunization studies, as described above).

The main advantage of using an *in vitro* system over *in vivo* murine models is the limited MHC repertoire of mice. Vaccination in mice often induces a response to only one immunodominant epitope; in humans, there are multiple epitopes that are often different between vaccinated individuals. However, as mentioned above, this can be overcome using outbred mice, although this still does not reflect the HLA-types of a human population. In turn, the *in vitro* model is still an artificial system, and likely does not recapitulate all immunological processes (such as signaling pathways) that would occur *in vivo*. Ultimately, screening liver-stage targets in both models (*in vivo* and *in vitro*) would be preferential.

Immune Correlates of Protection

Ideally, these methods would not only provide a useful model for screening liver-stage vaccine candidates, but also be used to define correlates of protection. If any of the functional assays of immunity described above (*in vivo* or *in vitro*) could accurately predict which vaccines provided protection in CHMI trials, the assay could then be used as a surrogate for protection. This could potentially alleviate the need for very large and expensive CHMI trials at the initial stages of vaccine assessment and would be extremely beneficial for the development of second-generation malaria vaccines.

Summary and Conclusion

In summary, in the current absence of a deployable and highly efficacious malaria vaccine, significant advances are enabling the identification of new *P. falciparum* liver-stage vaccine targets. Various antigen identification platforms are helping to reduce the number of potential candidates, and simultaneously, methods to screen such candidates are greatly improving. It will be of great interest to see whether any recently identified candidates, such as PfLSAP2, translate into protective efficacy in CHMI trials of non-immune adults. We believe these new identification and screening platforms will greatly enhance the development of second-generation malaria vaccines. In addition, it is also acknowledged that control and elimination of *P. vivax*, the most widespread of the *Plasmodium* sp. causing human disease, would be accelerated by the development of a *P. vivax* vaccine. Whilst this species has not been considered in this review, it is important to note that recent developments of novel tools to study *P. vivax* liver-stage biology, such as infection and generation of *P. vivax* dormant liver-stage forms both in humanized mice (Mikolajczak et al., 2015) and *in vitro* (Dembele et al., 2014), will be of great use in identifying *P. vivax* liver-stage targets in the future.

References

Ashley, E. A., Dhorda, M., Fairhurst, R. M., Amaratunga, C., Lim, P., Suon, S., et al. (2014). Spread of artemisinin resistance in *Plasmodium falciparum* malaria. *N. Engl. J. Med.* 371, 411–423. doi: 10.1056/NEJMoa1314981

Bauza, K., Malinauskas, T., Pfander, C., Anar, B., Jones, E. Y., Billker, O., et al. (2014). Efficacy of a *Plasmodium vivax* malaria vaccine using ChAd63 and modified vaccinia Ankara expressing thrombospondin-related anonymous protein as assessed with transgenic *Plasmodium berghei* parasites. *Infect. Immun.* 82, 1277–1286. doi: 10.1128/iai.01187-1113

Bijker, E. M., Bastiaens, G. J., Teirlinck, A. C., Van Gemert, G. J., Graumans, W., Van De Vegte-Bolmer, M., et al. (2013). Protection against malaria after immunization by chloroquine prophylaxis and sporozoites is mediated by preerythrocytic immunity. *Proc. Natl. Acad. Sci. U.S.A.* 110, 7862–7867. doi: 10.1073/pnas.1220360110

Brahimi, K., Badell, E., Sauzet, J. P., Benmohamed, L., Daubersies, P., Guerin-Marchand, C., et al. (2001). Human antibodies against *Plasmodium falciparum* liver-stage antigen 3 cross-react with *Plasmodium yoelii* preerythrocytic-stage epitopes and inhibit sporozoite invasion in vitro and in vivo. *Infect. Immun.* 69, 3845–3852. doi: 10.1128/iai.69.6.3845-3952.2001

Cao, Y., Zhang, D., and Pan, W. (2009). Construction of transgenic *Plasmodium berghei* as a model for evaluation of blood-stage vaccine candidate of *Plasmodium falciparum* chimeric protein 2.9. *PLoS ONE* 4:e6894. doi: 10.1371/journal.pone.0006894

Clyde, D. F., Most, H., Mccarthy, V. C., and Vanderberg, J. P. (1973). Immunization of man against sporozite-induced falciparum malaria. *Am. J. Med. Sci.* 266, 169–177. doi: 10.1097/00000441-197309000-00002

Deal, C., Balazs, A. B., Espinosa, D. A., Zavala, F., Baltimore, D., and Ketner, G. (2014). Vectored antibody gene delivery protects against *Plasmodium falciparum* sporozoite challenge in mice. *Proc. Natl. Acad. Sci. U.S.A.* 111, 12528–12532. doi: 10.1073/pnas.1407362111

Dembele, L., Franetich, J. F., Lorthiois, A., Gego, A., Zeeman, A. M., Kocken, C. H., et al. (2014). Persistence and activation of malaria hypnozoites in long-term primary hepatocyte cultures. *Nat. Med.* 20, 307–312. doi: 10.1038/nm.3461

Doolan, D. L. (2011). *Plasmodium immunomics. Int. J. Parasitol.* 41, 3–20. doi: 10.1016/j.ijpara.2010.08.002

Doolan, D. L., Sedegah, M., Hedstrom, R. C., Hobart, P., Charoenvit, Y., and Hoffman, S. L. (1996). Circumventing genetic restriction of protection against malaria with multigene DNA immunization: CD8+ cell-, interferon gamma-, and nitric oxide-dependent immunity. *J. Exp. Med.* 183, 1739–1746. doi: 10.1084/jem.183.4.1739

Doolan, D. L., Southwood, S., Freilich, D. A., Sidney, J., Graber, N. L., Shatney, L., et al. (2003). Identification of *Plasmodium falciparum* antigens by antigenic analysis of genomic and proteomic data. *Proc. Natl. Acad. Sci. U.S.A.* 100, 9952–9957. doi: 10.1073/pnas.1633254100

Drew, D. R., and Beeson, J. G. (2015). PfRH5 as a candidate vaccine for *Plasmodium falciparum* malaria. *Trends Parasitol.* 31, 87–88. doi: 10.1016/j.pt.2015.02.001

Dumoulin, P. C., Trop, S. A., Ma, J., Zhang, H., Sherman, M. A., and Levitskaya, J. (2015). Flow cytometry based detection and isolation of *Plasmodium falciparum* liver stages in vitro. *PLoS ONE* 10:e0129623. doi: 10.1371/journal.pone.0129623

Espinosa, D. A., Yadava, A., Angov, E., Maurizio, P. L., Ockenhouse, C. F., and Zavala, F. (2013). Development of a chimeric *Plasmodium berghei* strain expressing the repeat region of the *P. vivax* circumsporozoite protein for in vivo evaluation of vaccine efficacy. *Infect. Immun.* 81, 2882–2887. doi: 10.1128/iai.00461-413

Ewer, K. J., O'hara, G. A., Duncan, C. J., Collins, K. A., Sheehy, S. H., Reyes-Sandoval, A., et al. (2013). Protective $CD8^+$ T-cell immunity to human malaria induced by chimpanzee adenovirus-MVA immunisation. *Nat. Commun.* 4, 2836. doi: 10.1038/ncomms3836

Fidock, D. A., Pasquetto, V., Gras, H., Badell, E., Eling, W., Ballou, W. R., et al. (1997). *Plasmodium falciparum* sporozoite invasion is inhibited by naturally acquired or experimentally induced polyclonal antibodies to the STARP antigen. *Eur. J. Immunol.* 27, 2502–2513. doi: 10.1002/eji.1830271007

Finney, O. C., Keitany, G. J., Smithers, H., Kaushansky, A., Kappe, S., and Wang, R. (2014). Immunization with genetically attenuated *P. falciparum* parasites induces long-lived antibodies that efficiently block hepatocyte invasion by sporozoites. *Vaccine* 32, 2135–2138. doi: 10.1016/j.vaccine.2014.02.055

Florens, L., Washburn, M. P., Raine, J. D., Anthony, R. M., Grainger, M., Haynes, J. D., et al. (2002). A proteomic view of the *Plasmodium falciparum* life cycle. *Nature* 419, 520–526. doi: 10.1038/nature01107

Flyer, D. C., Ramakrishna, V., Miller, C., Myers, H., Mcdaniel, M., Root, K., et al. (2002). Identification by mass spectrometry of $CD8^+$-T-cell *Mycobacterium tuberculosis* epitopes within the Rv0341 gene product. *Infect. Immun.* 70, 2926–2932. doi: 10.1128/IAI.70.6.2926-2932.2002

Gardner, M. J., Hall, N., Fung, E., White, O., Berriman, M., Hyman, R. W., et al. (2002). Genome sequence of the human malaria parasite *Plasmodium falciparum*. *Nature* 419, 498–511. doi: 10.1038/nature01097

Gaucher, D., Therrien, R., Kettaf, N., Angermann, B. R., Boucher, G., Filali-Mouhim, A., et al. (2008). Yellow fever vaccine induces integrated multilineage and polyfunctional immune responses. *J. Exp. Med.* 205, 3119–3131. doi: 10.1084/jem.20082292

Gilbert, S. C., Plebanski, M., Harris, S. J., Allsopp, C. E., Thomas, R., Layton, G. T., et al. (1997). A protein particle vaccine containing multiple malaria epitopes. *Nat. Biotechnol.* 15, 1280–1284. doi: 10.1038/nbt1197-1280

Greenwood, B. M. (2015). Efficacy and safety of RTS,S/AS01 malaria vaccine with or without a booster dose in infants and children in Africa: final results of a phase 3, individually randomised, controlled trial. *Lancet* 386, 31–45. doi: 10.1016/s0140-6736(15)60721-60728

Gwadz, R. W., Cochrane, A. H., Nussenzweig, V., and Nussenzweig, R. S. (1979). Preliminary studies on vaccination of rhesus monkeys with irradiated sporozoites of *Plasmodium knowlesi* and characterization of surface antigens of these parasites. *Bull. World Health Organ.* 57(Suppl. 1), 165–173.

Hoffman, S. L., Isenbarger, D., Long, G. W., Sedegah, M., Szarfman, A., Waters, L., et al. (1989). Sporozoite vaccine induces genetically restricted T cell elimination of malaria from hepatocytes. *Science* 244, 1078–1081. doi: 10.1126/science.2524877

Hollingdale, M. R., Appiah, A., Leland, P., Do Rosario, V. E., Mazier, D., Pied, S., et al. (1990). Activity of human volunteer sera to candidate *Plasmodium falciparum* circumsporozoite protein vaccines in the inhibition of sporozoite invasion assay of human hepatoma cells and hepatocytes. *Trans. R. Soc. Trop. Med. Hyg.* 84, 325–329. doi: 10.1016/0035-9203(90)90303-V

Hollingdale, M. R., Ballou, W. R., Aley, S. B., Young, J. F., Pancake, S., Miller, L. H., et al. (1987). *Plasmodium falciparum*: elicitation by peptides and recombinant circumsporozoite proteins of circulating mouse antibodies inhibiting sporozoite invasion of hepatoma cells. *Exp. Parasitol.* 63, 345–351. doi: 10.1016/0014-4894(87)90182-2

House, B. L., Hollingdale, M. R., Sacci, J. B. Jr., and Richie, T. L. (2009). Functional immunoassays using an in-vitro malaria liver-stage infection model: where do we go from here? *Trends Parasitol.* 25, 525–533. doi: 10.1016/j.pt.2009.08.004

Hunt, D. F., Henderson, R. A., Shabanowitz, J., Sakaguchi, K., Michel, H., Sevilir, N., et al. (1992). Characterization of peptides bound to the class I MHC molecule HLA-A2.1 by mass spectrometry. *Science* 255, 1261–1263. doi: 10.1126/science.1546328

Janse, C. J., Franke-Fayard, B., Mair, G. R., Ramesar, J., Thiel, C., Engelmann, S., et al. (2006). High efficiency transfection of *Plasmodium berghei* facilitates novel selection procedures. *Mol. Biochem. Parasitol.* 145, 60–70. doi: 10.1016/j.molbiopara.2005.09.007

Jeffery, G. M., Wolcott, G. B., Young, M. D., and Williams, D. Jr. (1952). Exo-erythrocytic stages of *Plasmodium falciparum*. *Am. J. Trop. Med. Hyg.* 1, 917–925.

Karnasuta, C., Pavanand, K., Chantakulkij, S., Luttiwongsakorn, N., Rassamesoraj, M., Laohathai, K., et al. (1995). Complete development of the liver stage of *Plasmodium falciparum* in a human hepatoma cell line. *Am. J. Trop. Med. Hyg.* 53, 607–611.

Kumar, K. A., Sano, G., Boscardin, S., Nussenzweig, R. S., Nussenzweig, M. C., Zavala, F., et al. (2006). The circumsporozoite protein is an immunodominant protective antigen in irradiated sporozoites. *Nature* 444, 937–940. doi: 10.1038/nature05361

Lau, A. O., Sacci, J. B. Jr., and Azad, A. F. (2001). Detection of *Plasmodium yoelii* stage mRNA in BALB/c mice. *J. Parasitol.* 87, 19–23. doi: 10.1645/0022-3395(2001)087[0019:dopysm]2.0.co;2

Li, A. P. (2014). In vitro human hepatocyte-based experimental systems for the evaluation of human drug metabolism, drug-drug interactions, and drug toxicity in drug development. *Curr. Top. Med. Chem.* 14, 1325–1338. doi: 10.2174/1568026614666140506114411

Lin, J. W., Annoura, T., Sajid, M., Chevalley-Maurel, S., Ramesar, J., Klop, O., et al. (2011). A novel 'gene insertion/marker out' (GIMO) method for transgene expression and gene complementation in rodent malaria parasites. *PLoS ONE* 6:e29289. doi: 10.1371/journal.pone.0029289

Long, D., Skoberne, M., Gierahn, T. M., Larson, S., Price, J. A., Clemens, V., et al. (2014). Identification of novel virus-specific antigens by CD4^{+} and CD8^{+} T cells from asymptomatic HSV-2 seropositive and seronegative donors. *Virology* 464–465, 296–311. doi: 10.1016/j.virol.2014.07.018

Longley, R. J., Bauza, K., Ewer, K. J., Hill, A. V., and Spencer, A. J. (2015a). Development of an in vitro assay and demonstration of *Plasmodium berghei* liver-stage inhibition by TRAP-specific CD8^{+} T cells. *PLoS ONE* 10:e0119880. doi: 10.1371/journal.pone.0119880

Longley, R. J., Salman, A. M., Cottingham, M. G., Ewer, K., Janse, C. J., Khan, S. M., et al. (2015b). Comparative assessment of vaccine vectors encoding ten malaria antigens identifies two protective liver-stage candidates. *Sci. Rep.* 5, 11820. doi: 10.1038/srep11820

March, S., Ng, S., Velmurugan, S., Galstian, A., Shan, J., Logan, D. J., et al. (2013). A microscale human liver platform that supports the hepatic stages of *Plasmodium falciparum* and vivax. *Cell Host Microbe* 14, 104–115. doi: 10.1016/j.chom.2013.06.005

Mazier, D., Beaudoin, R. L., Mellouk, S., Druilhe, P., Texier, B., Trosper, J., et al. (1985). Complete development of hepatic stages of *Plasmodium falciparum* in vitro. *Science* 227, 440–442. doi: 10.1126/science.3880923

Mazier, D., Mellouk, S., Beaudoin, R. L., Texier, B., Druilhe, P., Hockmeyer, W., et al. (1986). Effect of antibodies to recombinant and synthetic peptides on *P. falciparum* sporozoites in vitro. *Science* 231, 156–159. doi: 10.1126/science.3510455

McConkey, S. J., Reece, W. H., Moorthy, V. S., Webster, D., Dunachie, S., Butcher, G., et al. (2003). Enhanced T-cell immunogenicity of plasmid DNA vaccines boosted by recombinant modified vaccinia virus Ankara in humans. *Nat. Med.* 9, 729–735. doi: 10.1038/nm881

Mellouk, S., Berbiguier, N., Druilhe, P., Sedegah, M., Galey, B., Yuan, L., et al. (1990). Evaluation of an in vitro assay aimed at measuring protective antibodies against sporozoites. *Bull. World Health Organ.* 68(Suppl.), 52–59.

Mikolajczak, S. A., Sacci, J. B. Jr., De La Vega, P., Camargo, N., Vanbuskirk, K., Krzych, U., et al. (2011). Disruption of the *Plasmodium falciparum* liver-stage antigen-1 locus causes a differentiation defect in late liver-stage parasites. *Cell Microbiol.* 13, 1250–1260. doi: 10.1111/j.1462-5822.2011.01617.x

Mikolajczak, S. A., Vaughan, A. M., Kangwanrangsan, N., Roobsoong, W., Fishbaugher, M., Yimamnuaychok, N., et al. (2015). *Plasmodium vivax* liver stage development and hypnozoite persistence in human liver-chimeric mice. *Cell Host Microbe* 17, 526–535. doi: 10.1016/j.chom.2015.02.011

Mizutani, M., Iyori, M., Blagborough, A. M., Fukumoto, S., Funatsu, T., Sinden, R. E., et al. (2014). Baculovirus-vectored multistage *Plasmodium vivax* vaccine induces both protective and transmission-blocking immunities against transgenic rodent malaria parasites. *Infect. Immun.* 82, 4348–4357. doi: 10.1128/iai.02040-2014

Mlambo, G., Maciel, J., and Kumar, N. (2008). Murine model for assessment of *Plasmodium falciparum* transmission-blocking vaccine using transgenic *Plasmodium berghei* parasites expressing the target antigen Pfs25. *Infect. Immun.* 76, 2018–2024. doi: 10.1128/iai.01409-1407

Morosan, S., Hez-Deroubaix, S., Lunel, F., Renia, L., Giannini, C., Van Rooijen, N., et al. (2006). Liver-stage development of *Plasmodium falciparum*, in a humanized mouse model. *J. Infect. Dis.* 193, 996–1004. doi: 10.1086/500840

Nardin, E. H., Nussenzweig, V., Nussenzweig, R. S., Collins, W. E., Harinasuta, K. T., Tapchaisri, P., et al. (1982). Circumsporozoite proteins of human malaria parasites *Plasmodium falciparum* and *Plasmodium vivax*. *J. Exp. Med.* 156, 20–30. doi: 10.1084/jem.156.1.20

Ng, S., March, S., Galstian, A., Hanson, K., Carvalho, T., Mota, M. M., et al. (2014). Hypoxia promotes liver-stage malaria infection in primary human hepatocytes in vitro. *Dis. Model. Mech.* 7, 215–224. doi: 10.1242/dmm.013490

Nussenzweig, R. S., Vanderberg, J., Most, H., and Orton, C. (1967). Protective immunity produced by the injection of x-irradiated sporozoites of *Plasmodium berghei*. *Nature* 216, 160–162. doi: 10.1038/216160a0

Nussenzweig, V., and Nussenzweig, R. S. (1985). Circumsporozoite proteins of malaria parasites. *Cell* 42, 401–403. doi: 10.1016/0092-8674(85)90093-5

Offeddu, V., Thathy, V., Marsh, K., and Matuschewski, K. (2012). Naturally acquired immune responses against *Plasmodium falciparum* sporozoites and liver infection. *Int. J. Parasitol.* 42, 535–548. doi: 10.1016/j.ijpara.2012.03.011

Ogwang, C., Kimani, D., Edwards, N. J., Roberts, R., Mwacharo, J., Bowyer, G., et al. (2015). Prime-boost vaccination with chimpanzee adenovirus and modified vaccinia Ankara encoding TRAP provides partial protection against *Plasmodium falciparum* infection in *Kenyan adults. Sci Trans. Med.* 7, 286re285. doi: 10.1126/scitranslmed.aaa2373

Persson, C., Oliveira, G. A., Sultan, A. A., Bhanot, P., Nussenzweig, V., and Nardin, E. (2002). Cutting edge: a new tool to evaluate human pre-erythrocytic malaria vaccines: rodent parasites bearing a hybrid *Plasmodium falciparum* circumsporozoite protein. *J. Immunol.* 169, 6681–6685. doi: 10.4049/jimmunol.169.12.6681

Porter, M. D., Nicki, J., Pool, C. D., Debot, M., Illam, R. M., Brando, C., et al. (2013). Transgenic parasites stably expressing full-length *Plasmodium falciparum* circumsporozoite protein as a model for vaccine down-selection in mice using sterile protection as an endpoint. *Clin. Vaccine Immunol.* 20, 803–810. doi: 10.1128/cvi.00066-13

Ramakrishna, V., Ross, M. M., Petersson, M., Gatlin, C. C., Lyons, C. E., Miller, C. L., et al. (2003). Naturally occurring peptides associated with HLA-A2 in ovarian cancer cell lines identified by mass spectrometry are targets of HLA-A2-restricted cytotoxic T cells. *Int. Immunol.* 15, 751–763. doi: 10.1093/intimm/dxg074

Ranson, H., N'guessan, R., Lines, J., Moiroux, N., Nkuni, Z., and Corbel, V. (2011). Pyrethroid resistance in African anopheline mosquitoes: what are the implications for malaria control? *Trends Parasitol.* 27, 91–98. doi: 10.1016/j.pt.2010.08.004

Renia, L., Grillot, D., Marussig, M., Corradin, G., Miltgen, F., Lambert, P. H., et al. (1993). Effector functions of circumsporozoite peptide-primed $CD4^+$ T cell clones against *Plasmodium yoelii* liver stages. *J. Immunol.* 150, 1471–1478.

Renia, L., Marussig, M. S., Grillot, D., Pied, S., Corradin, G., Miltgen, F., et al. (1991). In vitro activity of $CD4^+$ and $CD8^+$ T lymphocytes from mice immunized with a synthetic malaria peptide. *Proc. Natl. Acad. Sci. U.S.A.* 88, 7963–7967. doi: 10.1073/pnas.88.18.7963

Rieckmann, K. H., Carson, P. E., Beaudoin, R. L., Cassells, J. S., and Sell, K. W. (1974). Letter: sporozoite induced immunity in man against an Ethiopian strain of *Plasmodium falciparum*. *Trans. R. Soc. Trop Med. Hyg.* 68, 258–259. doi: 10.1016/0035-9203(74)90129-1

Roestenberg, M., Teirlinck, A. C., Mccall, M. B., Teelen, K., Makamdop, K. N., Wiersma, J., et al. (2011). Long-term protection against malaria after experimental sporozoite inoculation: an open-label follow-up study. *Lancet* 377, 1770–1776. doi: 10.1016/s0140-6736(11)60360-60367

Russell, P. F., and Mohan, B. N. (1942). The immunization of fowls against mosquito-borne *Plasmodium gallinaceum* by injections of serum and of inactivated homologous sporozoites. *J. Exp. Med.* 76, 477–495. doi: 10.1084/jem.76.5.477

Sacci, J. B. Jr., Alam, U., Douglas, D., Lewis, J., Tyrrell, D. L., Azad, A.F., et al. (2006). *Plasmodium falciparum* infection and exoerythrocytic development in mice with chimeric human livers. *Int. J. Parasitol.* 36, 353–360. doi: 10.1016/j.ijpara.2005.10.014

Sacci, J. B. Jr., Ribeiro, J. M., Huang, F., Alam, U., Russell, J. A., Blairet, P. L., et al. (2005). Transcriptional analysis of in vivo *Plasmodium yoelii* liver stage gene expression. *Mol. Biochem. Parasitol.* 142, 177–183. doi: 10.1016/j.molbiopara.2005.03.018

Sattabongkot, J., Yimamnuaychoke, N., Leelaudomlipi, S., Rasameesoraj, M., Jenwithisuk, R., Coleman, R. E., et al. (2006). Establishment of a human hepatocyte line that supports in vitro development of the exo-erythrocytic stages of the malaria parasites *Plasmodium falciparum* and *P. vivax*. *Am. J. Trop. Med. Hyg.* 74, 708–715.

Schofield, L., Villaquiran, J., Ferreira, A., Schellekens, H., Nussenzweig, R., and Nussenzweig, V. (1987). Gamma interferon, $CD8^+$ T cells and antibodies required for immunity to malaria sporozoites. *Nature* 330, 664–666. doi: 10.1038/330664a0

Schwenk, R., Debot, M., Porter, M., Nikki, J., Rein, L., Spaccapelo, R., et al. (2014). IgG2 antibodies against a clinical grade *Plasmodium falciparum* CSP vaccine antigen associate with protection against transgenic sporozoite challenge in mice. *PLoS ONE* 9:e111020. doi: 10.1371/journal.pone.0111020

Seder, R. A., Chang, L. J., Enama, M. E., Zephir, K. L., Sarwar, U. N., Gordon, I. J., et al. (2013). Protection against malaria by intravenous immunization with a nonreplicating sporozoite vaccine. *Science* 341, 1359–1365. doi: 10.1126/science.1241800

Seguin, M. C., Klotz, F. W., Schneider, I., Weir, J. P., Goodbary, M., Slayter, M., et al. (1994). Induction of nitric oxide synthase protects against malaria in mice exposed to irradiated *Plasmodium berghei* infected mosquitoes: involvement of interferon gamma and $CD8^+$ T cells. *J. Exp. Med.* 180, 353–358. doi: 10.1084/jem.180.1.353

Sheehy, S. H., Spencer, A. J., Douglas, A. D., Sim, B. K., Longley, R. J., Edwards, N. J., et al. (2013). Optimising controlled human malaria infection studies using cryopreserved parasites administered by needle and syringe. *PLoS ONE* 8:e65960. doi: 10.1371/journal.pone.0065960

Shortt, H. E., Fairley, N. H., Covell, G., Shute, P. G., and Garnham, P. C. (1951). The pre-erythrocytic stage of *Plasmodium falciparum*. *Trans. R. Soc. Trop. Med. Hyg.* 44, 405–419. doi: 10.1016/S0035-9203(51)80019-1

Siau, A., Silvie, O., Franetich, J. F., Yalaoui, S., Marinach, C., Hannoun, L., et al. (2008). Temperature shift and host cell contact up-regulate sporozoite expression of *Plasmodium falciparum* genes involved in hepatocyte infection. *PLoS Pathog.* 4:e1000121. doi: 10.1371/journal.ppat.1000121

Talman, A. M., Blagborough, A. M., and Sinden, R. E. (2010). A *Plasmodium falciparum* strain expressing GFP throughout the parasite's life-cycle. *PLoS ONE* 5:e9156. doi: 10.1371/journal.pone.0009156

Tarun, A. S., Peng, X., Dumpit, R. F., Ogata, Y., Silva-Rivera, H., Camargo, N., et al. (2008). A combined transcriptome and proteome survey of malaria parasite liver stages. *Proc. Natl. Acad. Sci. U.S.A.* 105, 305–310. doi: 10.1073/pnas.0710780104

Testa, J. S., Shetty, V., Hafner, J., Nickens, Z., Kamal, S., Sinnathamby, G., et al. (2012). MHC class I-presented T cell epitopes identified by immunoproteomics analysis are targets for a cross reactive influenza-specific T cell response. *PLoS ONE* 7:e48484. doi: 10.1371/journal.pone.0048484

Trieu, A., Kayala, M. A., Burk, C., Molina, D. M., Freilich, D. A., Richie, T. L., et al. (2011). Sterile protective immunity to malaria is associated with a panel of novel P. *falciparum* antigens. *Mol. Cell Proteomics* 10, M111007948. doi: 10.1074/mcp.M111.007948

Trimnell, A., Takagi, A., Gupta, M., Richie, T. L., Kappe, S. H., and Wang, R. (2009). Genetically attenuated parasite vaccines induce contact-dependent $CD8^+$ T cell killing of *Plasmodium yoelii* liver stage-infected hepatocytes. *J. Immunol.* 183, 5870–5878. doi: 10.4049/jimmunol.0900302

Trolle, T., Metushi, I. G., Greenbaum, J. A., Kim, Y., Sidney, J., Lund, O., et al. (2015). Automated benchmarking of peptide-MHC class I binding predictions. *Bioinformatics* 31, 2174–2181. doi: 10.1093/bioinformatics/btv123

van Dijk, M. R., Van Schaijk, B. C., Khan, S. M., Van Dooren, M. W., Ramesar, J., Kaczanowski, S., et al. (2010). Three members of the 6-cys protein family of *Plasmodium* play a role in gamete fertility. *PLoS Pathog* 6:e1000853. doi: 10.1371/journal.ppat.1000853

Vaughan, A. M., Mikolajczak, S. A., Camargo, N., Lakshmanan, V., Kennedy, M., Lindner, S. E., et al. (2012a). A transgenic *Plasmodium falciparum* NF54 strain that expresses GFP-luciferase throughout the parasite life cycle. *Mol. Biochem. Parasitol.* 186, 143–147. doi: 10.1016/j.molbiopara.2012.10.004

Vaughan, A. M., Mikolajczak, S. A., Wilson, E. M., Grompe, M., Kaushansky, A., Camargo, N., et al. (2012b). Complete *Plasmodium falciparum* liver-stage development in liver-chimeric mice. *J. Clin. Invest.* 122, 3618–3628. doi: 10.1172/jci62684

Wang, Q., Brown, S., Roos, D. S., Nussenzweig, V., and Bhanot, P. (2004). Transcriptome of axenic liver stages of *Plasmodium yoelii*. *Mol. Biochem. Parasitol.* 137, 161–168. doi: 10.1016/j.molbiopara.2004.06.001

Weiss, W. R., and Jiang, C. G. (2012). Protective $CD8^+$ T lymphocytes in primates immunized with malaria sporozoites. *PLoS ONE* 7:e31247. doi: 10.1371/journal.pone.0031247

Weiss, W. R., Mellouk, S., Houghten, R. A., Sedegah, M., Kumar, S., Good, M. F., et al. (1990). Cytotoxic T cells recognize a peptide from the circumsporozoite protein on malaria-infected hepatocytes. *J. Exp. Med.* 171, 763–773. doi: 10.1084/jem.171.3.763

Weiss, W. R., Sedegah, M., Beaudoin, R. L., Miller, L. H., and Good, M. F. (1988). $CD8^+$ T cells (cytotoxic/suppressors) are required for protection in mice immunized with malaria sporozoites. *Proc. Natl. Acad. Sci. U.S.A.* 85, 573–576. doi: 10.1073/pnas.85.2.573

WHO. (2014). *World Malaria Report 2013*. (Geneva: World Health Organization).

Wolk, B., Trautwein, C., Buchele, B., Kersting, N., Blum, H. E., Rammensee, H. G., et al. (2012). Identification of naturally processed hepatitis C virus-derived major histocompatibility complex class I ligands. *PLoS ONE* 7:e29286. doi: 10.1371/journal.pone.0029286

Yoshida, N., Nussenzweig, R. S., Potocnjak, P., Nussenzweig, V., and Aikawa, M. (1980). Hybridoma produces protective antibodies directed against the sporozoite stage of malaria parasite. *Science* 207, 71–73. doi: 10.1126/science.6985745

Zhong, W., Reche, P. A., Lai, C. C., Reinhold, B., and Reinherz, E. L. (2003). Genome-wide characterization of a viral cytotoxic T lymphocyte epitope repertoire. *J. Biol. Chem.* 278, 45135–45144. doi: 10.1074/jbc.M307417200

Zou, X., House, B. L., Zyzak, M. D., Richie, T. L., and Gerbasi, V. R. (2013). Towards an optimized inhibition of liver stage development assay (ILSDA) for *Plasmodium falciparum*. *Malar. J.* 12, 394. doi: 10.1186/1475-2875-12-394

Heme on Pulmonary Malaria: Friend or Foe?

*Tatiana Almeida Pádua and Mariana Conceição Souza**

Laboratory of Applied Pharmacology, Institute of Drug Technology (Farmanguinhos), Oswaldo Cruz Foundation, Rio de Janeiro, Brazil

Edited by:
Nicola Conran, Campinas State University, Brazil

Reviewed by:
Padmanaban Govindarajan, Indian Institute of Science (IISc), India
Claudio Romero Farias Marinho, University of São Paulo, Brazil

***Correspondence:**
Mariana Conceição Souza
mariana.souza@fiocruz.br

Malaria is a hemolytic disease that, in severe cases, can compromise multiple organs. Pulmonary distress is a common symptom observed in severe malaria caused by *Plasmodium vivax* or *Plasmodium falciparum*. However, biological components involved in the development of lung malaria are poorly studied. In experimental models of pulmonary malaria, it was observed that parasitized red blood cell-congested pulmonary capillaries are related to intra-alveolar hemorrhages and inflammatory cell infiltration. Thus, it is very likely that hemolysis participates in malaria-induced acute lung injury. During malaria, heme assumes different biochemical structures such as hemin and hemozoin (biocrystallized structure of heme inside *Plasmodium* sp.). Each heme-derived structure triggers a different biological effect: on the one hand, hemozoin found in lung tissue is responsible for the infiltration of inflammatory cells and consequent tissue injury; on the other hand, heme stimulates heme oxygenase-1 (HO-1) expression and CO production, which protect mice from severe malaria. In this review, we discuss the biological mechanism involved in the dual role of heme response in experimental malaria-induced acute lung injury.

Keywords: hemolysis, MA-RD, *Plasmodium*, heme, severe malaria, HO-1

INTRODUCTION

Malaria remains one of the major public health problems. In 2018, 228 million cases and 405,000 deaths from malaria were estimated worldwide (1). Malaria is particularly prevalent in tropical and subtropical low-income regions of the world such as the African region, which accounts for 93% of the cases, followed by the Southeast Asia region with 3.4% and the Eastern Mediterranean region with 2.1% (1). The World Health Organization's (WHO) mission is to reduce global malaria mortality rates by 90% by 2030 (2). Malaria is caused by at least six known species of *Plasmodium* infecting humans: *Plasmodium falciparum*, *Plasmodium vivax*, *Plasmodium malariae*, *Plasmodium ovale*, *Plasmodium knowlesi* (3), and the more recently described *Plasmodium simium* (4). Its transmission occurs by female anopheles mosquito bites, transfusion of infected blood, or transplacentally, from infected mother to fetus [reviewed in (5)]. The vast majority of human malaria worldwide is uncomplicated resulting in fever, and factors involved in disease complications are unknown.

Severe malaria is a complication that affects multiple organs, including lungs (6). (7) reviewed the incidence of lung dysfunction in malaria patients and showed data ranging from 2 to 29%. The wide range is related to different methods to diagnose dysfunction severity. Considering the classification of pulmonary complications, it is worth mentioning that malaria is most prevalent in poor countries where methods of diagnoses, documentation, and reporting are weak. Furthermore, a large proportion of severe malaria illnesses and deaths occur in people's homes without coming to the attention of a formal health service. In accordance, although the Berlin definition is a robust and reproducible tool for identifying acute respiratory distress syndrome (ARDS), it could not be applied in low-income countries because of inaccessibility of mechanical ventilators, arterial blood gas diagnostics, and chest radiography. For instance, none of the patients with malaria in the studies of Leopold et al. (8) could be diagnosed with ARDS using the conventional Berlin definition because the requirements for positive end-expiratory pressure criteria were not known since patients were managed outside of the intensive care unit (ICU). This limitation could have the unintended consequence of underestimating and undertreating the burden of malaria-induced ARDS in many countries (9). Thus, available data concerning malaria induced-ARDS incidence worldwide may be underestimated. Herein, we use the term malaria-induced respiratory distress (MA-RD) to present studies in which ARDS has not been formally diagnosed.

Almost all *Plasmodium* species that infect humans can induce MA-RD [reviewed in (10)], including *P. malariae* (11), *P. ovale* (12), and *P. knowlesi* (13); however, this syndrome is more common in *P. falciparum* and *P. vivax* malaria (14–17). MA-RD can be observed at early time points after diagnosis or even when the parasitemia decreases or disappears [reviewed in (7)]. Besides, antimalarial treatment can also lead to lung dysfunction. For instance, during quinine therapy, it is possible to observe pulmonary exacerbated inflammatory response and reduced alveolar-capillary gas exchange (18). Primaquine treatment also leads to hemolysis and consequent ARDS in malaria patients that present G6PD deficiency (19).

The most common pathologies associated with MA-RD are pulmonary edema, dyspnea, reduction in the capacity of gas exchange, and increased levels of inflammatory mediators (7). Autopsies in patients who have died of severe malaria and ARDS symptoms showed pleural and pulmonary hemorrhages, sequestered parasitized red blood cells (PRBC), neutrophils, and monocytes containing malarial pigment in lung tissue (20). Nevertheless, the biological process that triggers MA-RD is not clear. In this way, animal models have been an indispensable tool to understand lung dysfunction during malaria. However, since most experimental studies did not evaluate all factors that characterize ARDS, it is more appropriate to use the term malaria-induced acute lung injury (MA-ALI) to depict experimental results. Unlike cerebral malaria, which is mainly studied in *P. berghei*-infected C57BL/6 mice (21), lung malaria can be observed in *P. berghei* ANKA-infected C57BL/6 (22, 23), *P. berghei* NK65-infected C57BL/6 (24, 25), *P. berghei* ANKA-infected DBA mice (26), *P. berghei* ANKA-infected CBA mice (27), among others (28). These models show that malaria-induced experimental lung dysfunction is characterized by vascular dysfunction induced by $CD8^+$ T cells, presence of PRBC, hemorrhages, neutrophils, and monocytes containing malarial pigment. On the other hand, it has been shown that, at 24 h after infection, a time point at which inflammatory mediators are not yet detected, it is possible to observe PRBC, neutrophils, and mononuclear cells in the lung tissue (29, 30). Thus, it is unclear whether inflammatory cells, PRBC, blood, and pigment from malaria are a consequence or trigger the pulmonary pathology seen during malaria.

THE ROLE OF HEME DERIVATIVES IN LUNG PATHOLOGY DURING MALARIA

The study of heme and its derivatives in MA-RD is not elementary. The complex named heme (protoporphyrin IX + Fe II) is an important cofactor in several biological processes such as oxygen transfer, storage and activation, and electron transfer (31). During the respiratory process, the hemoglobin (Hb) containing heme captures and releases the oxygen without modifying iron oxidative state (32). However, 1–3% of Hb undergoes auto-oxidation, and oxygen is reduced to superoxide anion ($O_2^{\bullet-}$) and generates methemoglobin [Hb plus hemin (Fe III)] (32).

Heme and its analogs localize differently on erythrocyte membranes and exhibit distinct roles in its partitioning, leakage, and fusion (33). Under physiological conditions, when intravascular hemolysis occurs during the destruction of senescent erythrocytes and/or enucleation of erythroblasts, some hemoglobin, free heme, or hemin can be released into the plasma where they bind to soluble haptoglobin (Hp) or hemopexin (Hx) (reviewed by 27; 28). In the liver, the complexes are recognized by specific receptors on Kupffer cells such as CD163 and CD91/LRP-1, respectively, and metabolized by heme oxygenase-1 (HO-1) to iron, carbon monoxide, and biliverdin that will be stored or act as antioxidant molecules (34–36) (**Figure 1A**).

However, in hemolytic diseases, intravascular hemolysis increases, becoming a serious pathological complication (37). During the intraerythrocytic stage, parasites lyse the erythrocyte to release merozoites that rapidly invade new host cells (38). This lytic process also releases the infected red blood cell contents into the host bloodstream, including undigested hemoglobin, free heme, and hemozoin. The augment of extracellular levels of hemoglobin may reduce levels of available free Hp, making this pathway ineffective (39), while the large content of heme and hemin circulating in plasma can exhaust the binding capacity of Hx and their metabolism by HO-1. These events result in the increase in oxidation from heme to hemin and consequently methemoglobin (hemoglobin plus hemin) formation (40). It is important to note that the binding affinity of globin to hemin is weak and can lead to free heme release (32). The free heme leads to oxidative damage by the generation of reactive oxygen species (ROS) [e.g., superoxide ($O_2^{\bullet-}$), hydrogen peroxide (H_2O_2), and hydroxyl radical ($HO\bullet$)], reactive nitrogen species (RNS) (e.g., nitric oxide ($\bullet NO$), nitrogen dioxide ($\bullet NO_2$)], and peroxynitrite ($ONOO^-$) (41). These reactive species mediate the activation of inflammatory pathways and tissue damage, in addition to the loss of erythrocyte deformation ability and the endothelial barrier integrity by inducing lipid peroxidation of the membrane (42–44). Therefore, the consequences of heme derivative release might depend on their concentration and the environment in which they are found (38, 40).

As mentioned above, malaria is a hemolytic disease; thus, free heme and hemin released during hemolysis due

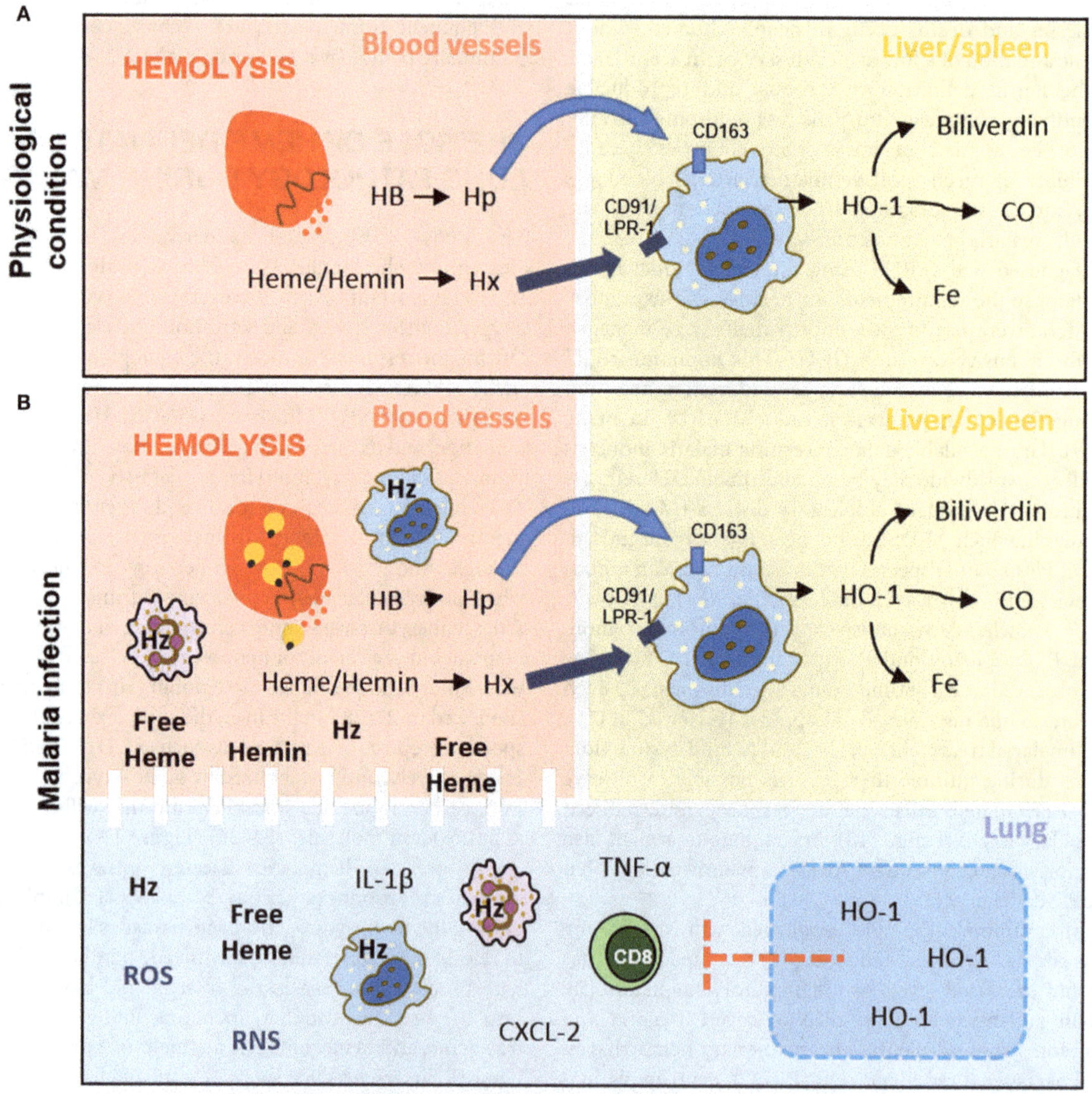

FIGURE 1 | Hemolysis under physiological conditions and malaria infection. **(A)** During hemolysis, hemoglobin (HB) and free heme/hemin are captured by haptoglobin (Hp) and hemopexin (Hx), respectively, in blood vessels. These complexes (HB-Hp and Heme-Hx) target macrophages CD163$^+$ and CD91/LRP-1$^+$ in the liver and spleen to be metabolized by heme oxygenase 1 (HO-1) to biliverdin, carbon monoxide (CO), and iron (Fe). **(B)** The hemolysis increases during the release of merozoites saturates the activity of haptoglobin (Hp) and hemopexin (Hx), leading to heme, hemin, and hemozoin (Hz) circulating in plasma. These heme derivatives increase ROS and RNS production and activate leukocytes to produce cytokines and chemokines that damage lung tissue and endothelial barriers. HO-1 induction would decrease leukocyte activation and migration, reduce inflammatory mediators production, and restore the integrity of the endothelial cell barrier in lung tissue.

to erythrocyte rupture during the plasmodium life cycle exert effects that contribute to malaria pathology. Beyond the free heme and hemin, heme can also be found in a biocrystallized structure named hemozoin in the *Plasmodium* sp. *Plasmodium* digest ~65% of total erythrocyte hemoglobin during intraerythrocytic development. Part of the hemoglobin's amino acids is incorporated in parasite proteins; however, since free heme released during hemoglobin digestion is a toxic by-product, *Plasmodium* biocrystallizes heme to hemozoin to store it as a nontoxic molecule in the digestive vacuole (45, 46).

The erythrocyte content (cytoplasm, parasite components, hemozoin, and free heme) released during hemolysis is engulfed by phagocytes such as macrophages, neutrophils, and dendritic cells (47). The accumulation of hemozoin in these immune phagocytic cells reflects the parasite burden and coincides with periodic fevers and high circulating levels of proinflammatory cytokines. In this way, this pigment is used to measure malaria severity and identify parasite developmental stages (6). Adult patients who died of severe *P. falciparum* malaria had significantly higher proportions of neutrophils and monocytes containing hemozoin than surviving patients (48). In addition, patients with MA-RD demonstrated high lung deposition of hemozoin and internal alveolar hemorrhage compared with those with non-MA-RD lungs (49). The same group also showed that hemozoin leads to loss of alveolar integrity by increasing the production of interleukin (IL)-1β by monocytes, which induces pneumocytes type II apoptosis (50). These observations are also seen in mouse lungs. The C57BL/6 mice infected with *P. berghei* NK65 showed a grayish-brown discoloration due to hemorrhages and hemozoin deposition, in addition to tissue edema and a marked inflammatory cells influx (24, 51).

The use of purified hemozoin has already been proposed to access its pathological role *in vitro* and *in vivo* (52). However, the method used to extract hemozoin is not effective in purifying it, since biological effects observed were attributed to a DNA contamination in hemozoin extract (53). In this context, some authors resort to the use of β-hematin, a compound produced *in vitro* using parasite lysate to provide necessary enzymes to biocrystallization. However, the artificial process to produce β-hematin results in substances different in shape and size from the natural ones, which could mask the results [reviewed in (46)]. Despite the immunological activity of synthetic hemozoin being controversial, several studies have demonstrated that both parasite-derived hemozoin and synthetically produced hemozoin, once phagocytized, activates both mouse and human leukocytes to produce proinflammatory cytokines such as tumor necrosis factor alpha (TNF-α) and IL-1β (54) and macrophage inflammatory protein (MIP)-1α/CCL3, MIP-1β/CCL4, MIP-2/C-X-C Motif Chemokine Ligand 2 (CXCL2), and MCP-1/CCL2 chemokines through oxidative stress-dependent and stress-independent mechanisms (55). Besides, Huy and coworkers showed that the treatment with β-hematin increased myeloperoxidase activity of peritoneal cells *in vivo* and neutrophil chemotaxis *in vitro* (56).

Despite the compelling data showing the deleterious effects of heme during malaria, in the last decade, several studies have shown that heme pathway could be beneficial to host outcomes. Balb/c mice, a resistant strain to multiorgan dysfunction (MOD) triggered by *P. berghei*-ANKA infection, expressed HO-1 in brain tissue during *P. berghei* infection. In addition, HO-1 knockout Balb/c mice succumb to *P. berghei* infection, through a mechanism that can be reversed by $CD8^+$ T cell depletion, which suggests that heme metabolism is involved in malaria resistance by modulating immunological response. Interestingly, studies with C57BL/6 mice, a susceptible strain to MOD triggered by *P. berghei*-ANKA infection, also produced HO-1 in brain tissue, however, correlated with parasite inoculum. It is well established that parasite inoculum modulates disease outcome (57). Additionally, the 10^5 *P. berghei* pRBC inoculum did not induce HO-1 expression in the brain tissue (58), while the 10^6 *P. berghei* pRBC inoculum induces HO-1 expression in the brain 4 days postinfection (59). It is noteworthy that parasite inoculum did not interfere in increased levels of free heme in plasma, which suggests that heme in malaria-susceptible hosts is not enough to induce HO-1; HO-1 is insufficiently produced/activated to induce free heme clearance, or the produced HO-1 is saturated. For instance, C57BL/6 *P. berghei*-infected mice treated with cobalt protoporphyrin, a pharmacological intervention that stimulates HO-1 production and activity, reduced brain edema and microvascular congestion (58). The authors also gave CO, a downstream metabolite in the heme clearance pathway, and further observed a reduction in $CD8^+$ T cells in the brain tissue, showing that the appropriate amounts of HO-1 are effective to protect susceptible mice from MOD. In accordance, the balance between free heme and HO-1 production is important to improve the outcome of *P. berghei*-infected mice that carry hemoglobin beta-chain mutation, named sickle Hb (HbS). The authors observed that mice with HbS phenotype did not develop cerebral malaria by two different mechanisms, and both pathways depend on low levels of free heme on the bloodstream. The first mechanism involves the stimulation of HO-1 production, and the second one involves heme-induced immunoregulatory roles. The authors suggest that there is a pathogenic and a protective concentration of circulating free heme during malaria (60).

In recent reviews by Frimat et al. (61) and Immenschuh et al. (40), the heme clearance pathway has been proposed as targets to treat hemolytic diseases. Frimat suggests that two different approaches should be considered to treat hemolytic disease: first, by modulating molecules from the heme clearance pathway as by administering hemopexin or inducing HO-1, and second, by treating oxidative stress and inflammation induced by heme (61). In addition, Immenschuh and colleagues state that heme exerts different effects depending on the target cell. Endothelial cells rapidly respond to heme by means of HO-1 production, which suggests that the lung, as a highly vascularized organ, is an important organ to study therapeutic interventions aiming at heme clearance. Compounds such as desoxyrhapontigenin, statins, curcumin, hemin, quercetin, and cobalt protoporphyrin have already been used to attenuate experimental lung dysfunction by inducing HO-1 expression (40). However, few studies have been dedicated to assessing whether HO-1 induction would attenuate malaria-induced ALI. Pereira et al. (62), using the *P. berghei*-infected DBA/2 mice model of MA-ALI, gave hemin to infected mice and observed an increase in HO-1 production correlated with attenuation of lung dysfunction and inflammatory response associated to alteration in lung histoarchitecture. As well, Liu et al. (59) showed that HO-1 expression in the lung tissue during experimental malaria depends on CXCL10 and signal transducer and activator of transcription 3 (STAT3). The authors further show that free heme is detectable in plasma since the second day of infection. At the same time point, they also observed HO-1 expression in the lung tissue but not in the brain tissue, supporting the idea that the lung is one of the most important organs for the heme clearance pathway (**Figure 1B**).

Thus, considering the biological mechanism by which HO-1 induction attenuates brain dysfunction during experimental cerebral malaria, we can speculate that during experimental MA-ALI, the induction of HO-1 downmodulates $CD8^+$ T cell activation and migration to lung tissue, reduces the production of inflammatory mediators, and restores endothelial cell barrier integrity.

CONCLUSION

Free heme and heme derivatives have been widely recognized as pathological molecules in several hemolytic conditions. The participation of heme in malaria is very peculiar because it exerts its effects through different molecular structures as free heme, hemin, and hemozoin. Several studies concerning malaria-induced lung dysfunction show that heme derivatives affect alveolar integrity, induce the production of inflammatory mediators, and accumulate the inflammatory cells in the lung tissue. On the other hand, more recent studies propose that heme exerts a beneficial role during malaria infection by inducing cytoprotective pathways such as HO-1 production. Indeed, more studies are necessary to define the role of heme during malaria-induced lung dysfunction. Overall, we can conclude that the imbalance between free concentration, production/saturation of HO-1, and the activation of coexisting anti-inflammatory pathways dictate if heme is a friend or foe to malaria patients.

AUTHOR CONTRIBUTIONS

TP and MS wrote the manuscript. All authors contributed to the article and approved the submitted version.

REFERENCES

1. World Health Organization (WHO). *World Malaria Report 2019*. Geneva (2019).
2. World Health Organization (WHO). *World Malaria Report 2018*. Guinea (2018).
3. Phillips MA, Burrows JN, Manyando C, van Huijsduijnen RH, Van Voorhis WC, Wells TNC. Malaria. *Nat Rev Dis Prim.* (2017) 3:17050. doi: 10.1038/nrdp.2017.50
4. Brasil P, Zalis MG, de Pina-Costa A, Siqueira AM, Júnior CB, Silva S, et al. Outbreak of human malaria caused by *Plasmodium simium* in the atlantic forest in rio de janeiro: a molecular epidemiological investigation. *Lancet Glob Health.* (2017) 5:e1038–e1046. doi: 10.1016/S2214-109X(17)30333-9
5. Basu S, Sahi PK. Malaria: an update. *Ind J Pedi.* (2017) 84:521–8. doi: 10.1007/s12098-017-2332-2
6. World Health Organization (WHO). WHO severe malaria 2014. *Trop Med Int Health.* (2014) 19 Suppl 1:7–131. doi: 10.1111/tmi.12313_2
7. Alladi M, Surendra MK, Srinivas B. Acute lung injury and acute respiratory distress syndrome in malaria. *J Vector Borne Dis.* (2008) 45:179–93.
8. Leopold SJ, Ghose A, Plewes KA, Mazumder S, Pisani L, Kingston HWF, et al. Point-of-care lung ultrasound for the detection of pulmonary manifestations of malaria and sepsis: an observational study. *PLoS ONE.* (2018) 13:e0204832. doi: 10.1371/journal.pone.0204832
9. Riviello ED, Kiviri W, Twagirumugabe T, Mueller A, Banner-Goodspeed VM, Officer L, et al. Hospital incidence and outcomes of the acute respiratory distress syndrome using the kigali modification of the berlin definition. *Am J Resp Crit Care Med.* (2016) 193:52–9. doi: 10.1164/rccm.201503-0584OC
10. Souza MC, Tatiana PA, Maria das Graças H. Multiple organ dysfunction during severe malaria: the role of the inflammatory response world's largest science, technology & medicine. In: *Current Topics in Malaria*. Rijeka: InTech. (2015). p. 85–104.
11. Hwang J, Cullen KA, Kachur SP, Arguin PM, Baird JK. Severe morbidity and mortality risk from malaria in the United States, 1985 – 2011. *Open Forum Infect Dis.* (2014) 1:ofu034. doi: 10.1093/ofid/ofu034
12. Haydoura S, Mazboudi O, Charafeddine K, Bouakl I, Baban TA, Taher AT. Transfusion-related plasmodium ovale malaria complicated by acute respiratory distress syndrome (ARDS) in a non-endemic country. *Parasitol Int.* (2011) 60:114–6. doi: 10.1016/j.parint.2010.10.005
13. Seilmaier M, Hartmann W, Beissner M, Fenzl T, Haller C, Guggemos W, et al. Severe *Plasmodium knowlesi* infection with multi-organ failure imported to Germany from Thailand/Myanmar. *Malaria J.* (2014) 13:422. doi: 10.1186/1475-2875-13-422
14. Mohapatra BN, Jangid SK, Mohanty R. GCRBS score: a new scoring system for predicting outcome in severe *Falciparum malaria. J Assoc Phys India.* (2014) 62:14–7.
15. Sulaiman H, Ismail MD, Jalalonmuhali M, Atiya N, Ponnampalavanar S. Severe *Plasmodium falciparum* infection mimicking acute myocardial infarction. *Malaria J.* (2014) 13:341. doi: 10.1186/1475-2875-13-341
16. Lacerda MV, Fragoso SC, Alecrim MG, Alexandre MA, Magalhães BM, Siqueira AM, et al. Postmortem characterization of patients with clinical diagnosis of plasmodium vivax malaria: to what extent does this parasite kill? *Clin Infect Dis.* (2012) 55:67–74. doi: 10.1093/cid/cis615
17. Londhe C, Ganeriwal A, deSouza R. Study of clinical profile of acute respiratory distress syndrome and acute lung injury in *Plasmodium vivax* malaria. *J Vector Borne Dis.* (2014) 51:339–42.
18. Maguire GP, Handojo T, Pain MC, Kenangalem E, Price RN, Tjitra E, et al. Lung injury in uncomplicated and severe falciparum malaria: a longitudinal study in Papua, Indonesia. *J Infect Dis.* (2005) 192:1966–74. doi: 10.1086/497697
19. Ramos Júnior WM, Sardinha JF, Costa MR, Santana MS, Alecrim MG, Lacerda MV. Clinical aspects of hemolysis in patients with *P. vivax* malaria treated with primaquine, in the Brazilian Amazon. *Brazil J Infect Dis.* (2010) 14:410–2. doi: 10.1016/S1413-8670(10)70084-2
20. Taylor WRJ, Hanson J, Turner GDH, White NJ, Dondorp AM. Respiratory manifestations of malaria. *Chest.* (2012) 142:492–505. doi: 10.1378/chest.11-2655
21. de Souza JB, Hafalla JC, Riley EM, Couper KN. Cerebral malaria: why experimental murine models are required to understand the pathogenesis of disease. *Parasitology.* (2009) 137:755–72. doi: 10.1017/S0031182009991715
22. Pádua TA, Torres ND, Candéa ALP, Costa MFS, Silva JD, Silva-Filho JL, et al. Therapeutic effect of lipoxin a4 in malaria-induced acute lung injury. *J Leukoc Biol.* (2018) 103:657–70. doi: 10.1002/JLB.3A1016-435RRR
23. Carla C, Samantha N, Teng Y, Akhila B, Howland W, Becht S, et al. Lung endothelial cell antigen cross-presentation to CD8+T cells drives malaria-associated lung injury. *Nat Commun.* (2019) 10:4241. doi: 10.1038/s41467-019-12017-8
24. Van den Steen PE, Geurts N, Deroost K, Van Aelst I, Verhenne S, Heremans H, et al. Immunopathology and dexamethasone therapy in a new model for malaria-associated acute respiratory distress syndrome. *Am J Resp Crit Care Med.* (2010) 181:957–68. doi: 10.1164/rccm.200905-0786OC
25. Pham TT, Verheijen M, Vandermosten L, Deroost K, Knoops S, Van den Eynde K, et al. Pathogenic CD8+ T cells cause increased levels of VEGF-A in experimental malaria-associated acute respiratory distress syndrome, but therapeutic VEGFR inhibition is not effective. *Front Cell Infect Microbiol.* (2017) 7:416. doi: 10.3389/fcimb.2017.00416
26. Epiphanio S, Campos MG, Pamplona A, Carapau D, Pena AC, Ataíde R, et al. VEGF promotes malaria-associated acute lung injury in mice. *PLoS Pathog.* (2010) 6:1–10. doi: 10.1371/journal.ppat.1000916
27. Carvalho LJM, Lenzi HL, Pelajo-Machado M, Oliveira DN, Daniel-Ribeiro CT, Ferreira-da-Cruz MF. *Plasmodium berghei*: cerebral malaria in CBA mice is not clearly related to plasma TNF levels or intensity of histopathological changes. *Exp Parasitol.* (2000) 95:1–7. doi: 10.1006/expr.2000.4508

28. Pereira MLM, Marinho CRF, Epiphanio S. Could heme oxygenase-1 be a new target for therapeutic intervention in malaria-associated acute lung injury/acute respiratory distress syndrome? *Front Cell Infect Microbiol.* (2018) 8:161. doi: 10.3389/fcimb.2018.00161
29. Souza MC, Silva JD, Pádua TA, Capelozzi VL, Rocco PR, da Henriques M. Early and late acute lung injury and their association with distal organ damage in murine malaria. *Resp Physiol Neurobiol.* (2013) 186:65–72. doi: 10.1016/j.resp.2012.12.008
30. Franke-Fayard B, Janse CJ, Cunha-Rodrigues M, Ramesar J, Büscher P, Que I, et al. Murine malaria parasite sequestration: CD36 is the major receptor, but cerebral pathology is unlinked to sequestration. *Proc Natl Acad Sci USA.* (2005) 102:11468–73. doi: 10.1073/pnas.0503386102
31. Tohru F, Hideo H. Biology of heme in mammalian erythroid cells and related disorders. *BioMed Research Int.* (2015) 2015:278536. doi: 10.1155/2015/278536
32. Quaye IK. Extracellular hemoglobin: the case of a friend turned foe. *Front Physiol.* (2015) 6:96. doi: 10.3389/fphys.2015.00096
33. Das D, Tarafdar PK, Chakrabarti A. Structure-activity relationship of heme and its analogues in membrane damage and inhibition of fusion. *FEBS Lett.* (2018) 592:2458–65. doi: 10.1002/1873-3468.13165
34. Umbreit J. Methemoglobin—it's not just blue: a concise review. *Am J Hematol.* (2007) 82:807–11. doi: 10.1002/ajh.20738
35. Gianrico F, Joseph SH. Carbon monoxide, hydrogen sulfide, and nitric oxide as signaling molecules in the gastrointestinal tract. *Gastroenterology.* (2014) 147:303–13. doi: 10.1053/j.gastro.2014.04.041
36. Schmidt HM, Kelley EE, Straub AC. The impact of xanthine oxidase (XO) on hemolytic diseases. *Redox Biol.* (2019) 21:101072. doi: 10.1016/j.redox.2018.101072
37. Ascenzi P, Bocedi A, Visca P, Altruda F, Tolosano E, Beringhelli T, et al. Hemoglobin and heme scavenging. *IUBMB Life.* (2005) 57:749–59. doi: 10.1080/15216540500380871
38. Sigala PA, Goldberg DE. The peculiarities and paradoxes of Plasmodium heme metabolism. *Ann Rev Microbiol.* (2014) 68:259–78. doi: 10.1146/annurev-micro-091313-103537
39. Schaer DJ, Vinchi F, Ingoglia G, Tolosano E, Buehler PW. Haptoglobin, hemopexin and related defense pathways-basic science, clinical perspectives and drug development. *Front Physiol.* (2014) 5:415. doi: 10.3389/fphys.2014.00415
40. Immenschuh S, Vijayan V, Janciauskiene S, Gueler F. Heme as a target for therapeutic interventions. *Front Pharmacol.* (2017) 8:146. doi: 10.3389/fphar.2017.00146
41. Man SS. Reactive oxygen and nitrogen species in pathogenesis of vascular complications of diabetes. *Diab Metab J.* (2012) 36:190–8. doi: 10.4093/dmj.2012.36.3.190
42. Aslan M, Ryan TM, Adler B, Townes TM, Parks DA, Thompson JA, et al. Oxygen radical inhibition of nitric oxide-dependent vascular function in sickle cell disease. *Proc Natl Acad Sci USA.* (2001) 98:15215–20. doi: 10.1073/pnas.221292098
43. Vinchi F, Costa da Silva M, Ingoglia G, Petrillo S, Brinkman N, Zuercher A, et al. Hemopexin therapy reverts heme-induced proinflammatory phenotypic switching of macrophages in a mouse model of sickle cell disease. *Blood.* (2016) 127:473–86. doi: 10.1182/blood-2015-08-663245
44. Matthews K, Duffy SP, Myrand-Lapierre ME, Ang RR, Li L, Scott MD, et al. Microfluidic analysis of red blood cell deformability as a means to assess hemin-induced oxidative stress resulting from *Plasmodium falciparum* intraerythrocytic parasitism. *Integr Biol.* (2017) 9:519–28. doi: 10.1039/c7ib00039a
45. Krugliak M, Zhang J, Ginsburg H. Intraerythrocytic *Plasmodium falciparum* utilizes only a fraction of the amino acids derived from the digestion of host cell cytosol for the biosynthesis of its proteins. *Mol Biochem Parasitol.* (2002) 119:249–56. doi: 10.1016/S0166-6851(01)00427-3
46. Timothy EJ. Haemozoin formation. *Mol Biochem Parasitol.* (2008) 157:127–36. doi: 10.1016/j.molbiopara.2007.11.005
47. Olivier M, Van Den Ham K, Shio MT, Kassa FA, Fougeray S. Malarial pigment hemozoin and the innate inflammatory response. *Front Immunol.* (2014) 5:25. doi: 10.3389/fimmu.2014.00025
48. Nguyen PH, Day N, Pram TD, Ferguson DJ, White NJ. Intraleucocytic malaria pigment and prognosis in severe malaria. *Trans R Soc Trop Med Hyg.* (1995) 89:200–4. doi: 10.1016/0035-9203(95)90496-4
49. Maknitikul S, Luplertlop N, Grau GER, Ampawong S. Dysregulation of pulmonary endothelial protein C receptor and thrombomodulin in severe falciparum malaria-associated ARDS relevant to hemozoin. *PLoS ONE.* (2017) 12:e0181674. doi: 10.1371/journal.pone.0181674
50. Maknitikul S, Luplertlop N, Chaisri U, Maneerat Y, Ampawong S. Featured article: immunomodulatory effect of hemozoin on pneumocyte apoptosis via CARD9 pathway, a possibly retarding pulmonary resolution. *Exp Biol Med.* (2018) 243:395–407. doi: 10.1177/1535370218757458
51. Deroost K, Tyberghein A, Lays N, Noppen S, Schwarzer E, Vanstreels E, et al. Hemozoin induces lung inflammation and correlates with malaria-associated acute respiratory distress syndrome. *Am J Resp Cell Mol Biol.* (2013) 48:589–600. doi: 10.1165/rcmb.2012-0450OC
52. Coban C, Ishii KJ, Kawai T, Hemmi H, Sato S, Uematsu S, et al. Toll-like receptor 9 mediates innate immune activation by the malaria pigment hemozoin. *J Exp Med.* (2005) 201:19–25. doi: 10.1084/jem.20041836
53. Parroche P, Lauw FN, Goutagny N, Latz E, Monks BG, Visintin A, et al. Malaria hemozoin is immunologically inert but radically enhances innate responses by presenting malaria DNA to toll-like receptor 9. *Proc Natl Acad Sci USA.* (2007) 104:1919–24. doi: 10.1073/pnas.0608745104
54. Giribaldi G, Prato M, Ulliers D, Gallo V, Schwarzer E, Akide-Ndunge OB, et al. Involvement of inflammatory chemokines in survival of human monocytes fed with malarial pigment. *Infect Immun.* (2010) 78:4912–21. doi: 10.1128/IAI.00455-10
55. Jaramillo M, Godbout M, Olivier M. Hemozoin induces macrophage chemokine expression through oxidative stress-dependent and -independent mechanisms. *J Immunol.* (2005) 174:475–84. doi: 10.4049/jimmunol.174.1.475
56. Nguyen Tien H, Xuan TDT, Tohru K, Motohiro S, Katsuya S, Shigeharu H, et al. Leukocyte activation by malarial pigment. *Parasitol Int.* (2006) 55:75–81. doi: 10.1016/j.parint.2005.10.003
57. Amani V, Boubou MI, Pied S, Marussig M, Walliker D, Mazier D, et al. Cloned lines of *Plasmodium berghei* ANKA differ in their abilities to induce experimental cerebral malaria. *Infect Immun.* (1998) 66:4093–9. doi: 10.1128/.66.9.4093-4099.1998
58. Pamplona A, Ferreira A, Balla J, Jeney V, Balla G, Epiphanio S. Heme oxygenase-1 and carbon monoxide suppress the pathogenesis of experimental cerebral malaria. *Nat Med.* (2007) 13:703–10. doi: 10.1038/nm1586
59. Liu M, Amodu AS, Pitts S, Patrickson J, Hibbert JM, Battle M, et al. Heme mediated STAT3 activation in severe malaria. *PLoS ONE.* (2012) 7:e34280. doi: 10.1371/journal.pone.0034280
60. Ferreira A, Marguti I, Bechmann I, Jeney V, Chora A, Palha NR. Sickle hemoglobin confers tolerance to plasmodium infection. *Cell.* (2011) 145:398–409. doi: 10.1016/j.cell.2011.03.049
61. Frimat M, Boudhabhay I, Roumenina LT. Hemolysis derived products toxicity and endothelium: model of the second hit. *Toxins.* (2019) 11:660. doi: 10.3390/toxins11110660
62. Pereira ML, Ortolan LS, Sercundes MK, Debone D, Murillo O, Lima FA. Association of heme oxygenase 1 with lung protection in malaria-associated ALI/ARDS. *Med Inflam.* (2016) 2016:4158698. doi: 10.1155/2016/4158698

16

NF-κB-Like Signaling Pathway REL2 in Immune Defenses of the Malaria Vector *Anopheles gambiae*

Suzana Zakovic and Elena A. Levashina *

Vector Biology, Max-Planck Institute for Infection Biology, Berlin, Germany

Edited by:
Susanne Hartmann,
Freie Universität Berlin, Germany

Reviewed by:
Tony Nolan,
Imperial College London,
United Kingdom
Antonio M. Mendes,
Instituto de Medicina Molecular (IMM),
Portugal

***Correspondence:**
Elena A. Levashina
levashina@mpiib-berlin.mpg.de

The blood feeding requirements of insects are often exploited by pathogens for their transmission. This is also the case of the protozoan parasites of genus *Plasmodium,* the causative agents of malaria. Every year malaria claims the lives of a half million people, making its vector, the *Anopheles* mosquito, the deadliest animal in the world. However, mosquitoes mount powerful immune responses that efficiently limit parasite proliferation. Among the immune signaling pathways identified in the main malaria vector *Anopheles gambiae*, the NF-κB-like signaling cascades REL2 and REL1 are essential for eliciting proper immune reactions, but only REL2 has been implicated in the responses against the human malaria parasite *Plasmodium falciparum.* Instead, constitutive activation of REL1 causes massive killing of rodent malaria parasites. In this review, we summarize our present knowledge on the REL2 pathway in *Anopheles* mosquitoes and its role in mosquito immune responses to diverse pathogens, with a focus on *Plasmodium*. Mosquito-parasite interactions are crucial for malaria transmission and, therefore, represent a potential target for malaria control strategies.

Keywords: ***Anopheles gambiae, Plasmodium*, NF-κB signaling, IMD, REL2 pathway, malaria, vector biology, innate immunity**

INTRODUCTION

Mosquitoes are vectors of human infectious diseases with immense importance for public health. Malaria, caused by the *Plasmodium* protozoa, is the deadliest disease transmitted by *Anopheles* mosquitoes. *Plasmodium* development in the mosquito takes about 3 weeks. A series of mosquito factors affect malaria transmission, among them female longevity, nutritional fitness and efficient immune responses. The ookinete is by far the most fragile parasite stage, attracting the majority of immune responses. It swiftly develops from the sexually created zygote, and its task is to escape the dangerous gut environment by traversing the unicellular epithelium and to hide beneath the basal lamina that lines the mosquito midgut. If successful, ookinetes transform within the second day into vegetative protective oocysts that in a fortnight give rise to thousands of sporozoites that migrate and invade the salivary glands to be ready for a new transmission. Vector-parasite molecular interactions have been studied mostly in the laboratory model of infections of *A. gambiae,* the major malaria vector in the sub-Saharan Africa, with the rodent malaria parasite *P. berghei.* Although rodent and human parasites have similar invasion strategies in the insect vector, their elimination is mediated by two distinct nuclear factor-κB (NF-κB) immune pathways, REL2/Imd and REL1/Toll. NF-κB, initially discovered for its DNA-binding activity to an immunoglobulin-κ light chain enhancer in B lymphocytes, emerged as the central regulator of immune responses in animal kingdom (Sen and Baltimore, 1986). In *Anopheles*, experimental activation of REL2 aborts development of *P. falciparum* ookinetes, while constitutive induction of REL1 kills rodent parasites (Frolet et al., 2006; Garver et al., 2009). However, in both cases the molecular mechanisms of parasite recognition and killing remain unknown. In this review, we discuss immune responses of *A. gambiae,* with a focus on the REL2 signaling pathway, which is believed to be the major regulator of mosquito immune responses against human malaria parasites.

IMMUNE SIGNALING AND PATHOGEN RECOGNITION

The Toll and Imd pathways in *Drosophila* regulate expression of hundreds of infection-inducible genes. While the Toll pathway, initially described in *Drosophila* embryonic development, is essential for defenses against Gram-positive bacteria and fungi (Lemaitre et al., 1996; Rutschmann et al., 2002), the Imd pathway orchestrates responses against Gram-negative bacteria and viruses (Kaneko et al., 2004; Costa et al., 2009).

Immune activation is mediated by recognition of pathogen derived molecules, such as metabolites, nucleic acids, or cell wall components that are released during pathogen growth and division (Vance et al., 2009). Among microbial and host factors that induce Imd signaling, the best characterized is the DAP-type peptidoglycan (DAP-PGN), a cell wall component of Gram-negative bacteria. DAP-PGN recognition at the cell surface is mediated by transmembrane peptidoglycan recognition proteins (PGRPs) (Choe et al., 2002; Gottar et al., 2002; **Figure 1**). In contrast, activation of the Toll pathway is initiated by binding of circulating recognition complexes to the lysine-type PGNs or glucans (Gobert et al., 2003; Leulier et al., 2003). This binding triggers downstream serine protease cascades, leading to processing and binding of the endogenous factor Spaetzle to the transmembrane receptor Toll (Morisato and Anderson, 1994; Schneider et al., 1994). Activation of both pathways culminates in the phosphorylation and release of the NF-κB-like transcription factors Dif, Dorsal and Relish from the inhibitors, and their translocation into the nucleus. The release of the Imd transcription factor Relish involves Caspar, which in its inactive state prevents cleavage of the Relish inhibitory domain (Kim et al., 2006; **Figure 1**). Phosphorylation of Cactus, the negative regulator of the Toll pathway, leads to its degradation and release of the transactivators Dif and Dorsal (Wu and Anderson, 1998).

The Imd role in *Drosophila* immunity has been recently extended to antiviral responses. Surprisingly, instead of protection, constitutive activation of the Imd pathway by depletion of a secreted cytokine-like molecule Diedel, enhances viral pathogenesis (Lamiable et al., 2016). Although the underlying mechanism is not entirely clear, in the absence of Diedel, viral infection triggers the pathway through an alternative, non-canonical cytoplasmic route by bypassing the function of the PGRP receptors (Lamiable et al., 2016). Similarly, non-canonical activation of this pathway was also reported in ticks that lack transmembrane PGRP-LC and death domain proteins, Imd and FADD, but feature a conserved ubiquitination module, Relish and Caspar (**Figure 1**). The tick pathway is induced by lipid components of membranes specific to PGN-deficient bacteria (Shaw et al., 2017). Importantly, the same lipids also induce the Imd pathway in Drosophila cell lines, suggesting that non-canonical activation of the Imd pathway may be evolutionarily conserved (Shaw et al., 2017).

REL2 PATHWAY IN *A. GAMBIAE*

The vast knowledge that accumulated on the immune signaling in Drosophila has served as a blueprint for studying *Anopheles* mosquitoes. Sequencing of the *A. gambiae* genome benefited identification of the conserved components of the pathway (Christophides et al., 2002; Holt et al., 2002). However, in spite of considerable interest and potential importance in antiparasitic responses, surprisingly little is known about the targets of the Imd/REL2 pathway in *Anopheles.*

Genomic searches in *A. gambiae* identified three potential receptors: PGRP-SD, PGRP-LB and PGRP-LC. PGRP-SD has not been characterized, whereas functional analysis of PGRP-LB did not reveal its role in mosquito survival upon bacterial infections (Meister et al., 2009). Instead, the structure and function of PGRP-LC were characterized in a great detail (Meister et al., 2009). PGRP-LC encodes three splice variants (LC1-3) that differ in the organization of their extracellular PGN-binding domains. Structural modeling uncovered the potential of all three isoforms to bind both types of PGNs, highlighting a striking difference between the mosquito PGRP-LC with broad sensing capacities and the *Drosophila* PGRP-LC, which binds exclusively DAP-PGNs. The broad specificity of PGN binding of the *Anopheles* PGRP-LC was further substantiated by functional analyses that demonstrated equally critical role of the receptor in mosquito survival to Gram-negative and Gram-positive bacteria (Meister et al., 2009). Although infections with both bacteria induced expression of genes encoding antimicrobial peptides (AMPs) Cecropin1 and Defensin1, their transcriptional induction was PGRP-LC independent (Meister et al., 2009), therefore, the mechanisms underlying the PGRP-LC-mediated resistance to bacteria remain to be elucidated.

PGRP-LC plays an important role in regulating proliferation of the mosquito microbiota after blood feeding (Meister et al., 2009) and may, in big part, explain the role of the pathway in modulating development of *Plasmodium* parasites. Indeed, similar to the phenotype of *PGRP-LC* silencing, clearing mosquito microbiota by antibiotics prior to infections increases *Plasmodium* loads, whereas feeding mosquitoes with bacteria boosts their resistance to *Plasmodium* in a *PGRP-LC*-dependent manner (Meister et al., 2009). Therefore, it is possible that the REL2 pathway is activated after blood feeding by massive bacterial proliferation, whereas *Plasmodium* parasites are simple bystanders in this process and do not directly induce mosquito immune responses. Further transcriptomics studies examined mosquito responses to infections with *P. falciparum* and *P. berghei* and identified species-specific patterns of gene expression

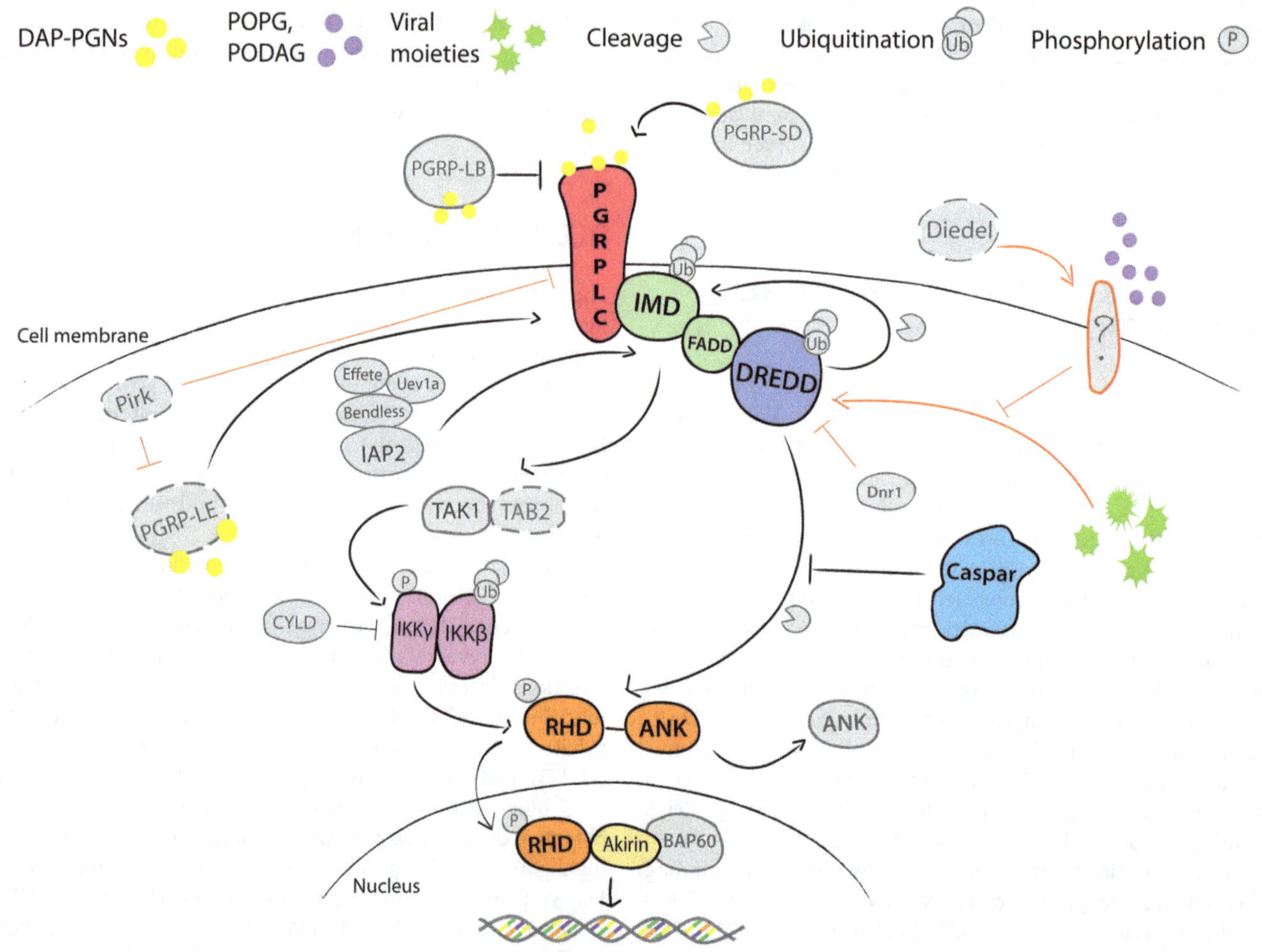

FIGURE 1 | Schematic overview of Imd pathway in *Drosophila melanogaster.* DAP-type PGNs trigger the activation of Imd signaling by direct interaction with the immune cell. Of Peptido-Glycan Recognition Proteins (PGRPs) that bind these pathogen-derived molecules, transmembrane PGRP-LC is the main receptor linked to activation of Imd pathway (Choe et al., 2002; Gottar et al., 2002). Its activity is enhanced in circulation by secreted PGRP-SD and intracellularly by the cytosolic PGRP-LE (Takehana et al., 2002; Iatsenko et al., 2016). Both proteins can directly bind DAP-PGNs and promote PGRP-LC activity. Another extracellular PGN-binding protein PGRP-LB antagonizes PGRP-LC activity by scavenging PGNs in circulation (Zaidman-Rémy et al., 2006). PGN binding induces conformational changes in PGRP-LC that promotes recruitment of the death domain-containing proteins Imd, FADD and DREDD caspase from the nucleus to the plasma membrane, and it is followed by subsequent polyubiquitination of DREDD by ubiquitin E3 ligase IAP2, cleavage of Imd by DREDD and exposure of K63 site for polyubiquitination by IAP2 and E2 conjugating enzymes Bendless, Effete and Uev1a (Paquette et al., 2010; Meinander et al., 2012). The K63-polyubiquitin chains, most likely, serve as activators of TAK1 kinase via the ubiquitin-binding domain of its regulatory protein TAB2 (Paquette et al., 2010). TAK1/TAB2 complex phosphorylates IKK complex, which consists of β and γ subunits. IKKβ further phosphorylates the NF-κB-like transcription factor Relish, while a regulatory IKKγ subunit regulates DREDD-mediated cleavage of Relish (Ertürk-Hasdemir et al., 2009). Relish consists of the Rel Homology Domain (RHD) and the inhibitory ankyrin-repeat rich domain (ANK) (Dushay et al., 1996). DREDD caspase cleaves the ANK domain from RHD. RHD translocates to the nucleus and initiates transcription of target genes. Caspar acts as a negative regulator of the pathway by inhibiting DREDD-dependent cleavage of Relish (Kim et al., 2006). Immunomodulatory cytokine Diedel restrains deleterious non-canonical activation of Imd in presence and absence of viral infection (Lamiable et al., 2016). Receptor that activates the pathway to viruses is not yet known However, epistasis analyses placed Diedel function between Imd and IKKγ, as mutants for both Diedel and Imd were more prone to spontaneous pathogenesis than Diedel/IKKγ double mutants (Lamiable et al., 2016). Additionally, activation of the pathway is held in check by other factors, including CYLD, Dnr1, and Pirk. Finally, transcriptional activity of Relish is regulated at the chromatin level through interactions with a nuclear co-factor Akirin and BAP60 component of Brahma chromatin remodeling complex. Akirin recruits BAP60 complex to promoters of a subset of Relish effector genes and hence regulates their transcription (Goto et al., 2008; Bonnay et al., 2014). Positive and inhibitory interactions are depicted with → and ⊣, respectfully; black—well established, and red—yet unknown interactions. Color coding highlights our current knowledge on the pathway in *Anopheles gambiae*. Confirmed pathway components are indicated in color. Components depicted in gray represent orthologs identified by genomic searches, but whose function was not experimentally validated. Components in gray with dashed lines are absent in *A. gambiae*.

(Dimopoulos et al., 2002; Dong et al., 2006). Nevertheless, a significant overlap observed in the responses to bacterial and *Plasmodium* infections provides further support to the hypothesis that REL2 modulation of *Plasmodium* development may be triggered by the PGRP-LC-mediated recognition of bacteria.

Regardless of the trigger, it is expected from the *Drosophila* model that conformational changes of PGRP-LC will recruit the death-domain containing receptor-adaptor complex (Imd, FADD and DREDD), which will, via the TAK1/TAB2 complex, activate the IKK signalosome and inhibit the negative regulator Caspar (**Figure 1**). Relish activation is achieved by phosphorylation by the IKK signalosome and by cleavage of the inhibitory ankirin domain by the DREDD caspase (**Figure 1**). Transcriptional activity of Relish at the promoters of some genes is further regulated by its nuclear co-factor Akirin. Using RNAi silencing and its effects on *P. falciparum* infections, most of the pathway components were functionally confirmed in *A. gambiae*, except for TAK1, whose depletion did not impact *Plasmodium* development (Meister et al., 2005; Garver et al., 2012; Ramphul et al., 2015).

Further studies of the REL2 pathway identified some mosquito-specific particularities. In contrast to *Drosophila, REL2* in mosquitoes encodes *three* alternatively-spliced isoforms that were first identified in another mosquito species, *Aedes aegypti* (Shin et al., 2002; Antonova et al., 2009). In *A. gambiae,* Meister et al. (2005) described two *REL2* forms: a long transcript (*REL2-F*) coding for the full-length protein consisting of Rel-homology domain (RHD) and ankyrin-rich repeat (ANK), and a short form (*REL2-S*) encoding only RHD. Although authors proposed that the isoforms regulate expression of distinct sets of genes, both isoforms regulate *Plasmodium* development (Garver et al., 2012). Currently, the molecular mechanisms underlying activation of REL2 in *Anopheles* remain unresolved. It is unknown whether REL2 requires proteolytic activation by CaspL1 (*Anopheles* ortholog of DREDD) and how Caspar inhibits its activation. Surprisingly, functional analyses by gene silencing suggested a genetic interaction between Caspar and REL2-S, whereas regulation of REL2-F was not investigated (Garver et al., 2012). These results are inconsistent with the proposed mechanism of Relish inhibition by Caspar in *Drosophila*, where Caspar binding to the inhibitory ankirin domain prevents its cleavage by DREDD. However, as REL2-S lacks the ANK domain, the inhibitory mechanism of Caspar in *Anopheles* remains unclear. Co-silencing of *Caspar* with *Imd, FADD, CaspL1* or *IKK2,* rescued the negative effect of the single *Caspar* knockdown on parasite development, confirming the role of these components in activation of REL2. Of particular interest is the role of Akirin, the nuclear co-factor of REL2, which regulates chromatin conformation and provides access to the promoter regions of a set of effector genes in *Drosophila* (Goto et al., 2008; Bonnay et al., 2014). As Akirin contributes to antiparasitic responses (Da Costa et al., 2014), better understanding of its function and of its target genes should shed light on regulation of *Plasmodium* killing.

So far, abortion of *Plasmodium* development was observed only upon experimentally-induced activation of the NF-κB pathways. Therefore, species-specific elimination of *Plasmodium* parasites by REL2 and REL1 seems to be independent of parasite recognition and may be explained by the activation of distinct sets of effectors. It is also plausible, that *Plasmodium* species differ in their susceptibility to the immune defenses triggered by these pathways. Therefore, understanding the molecular mechanisms underlying the pathway-specific parasite elimination may provide interesting insights into biology of *Plasmodium* species.

EFFECTORS

Antimicrobial peptides are powerful effectors of innate immunity (Jenssen et al., 2006). They bind and directly kill a broad spectrum of pathogens by disrupting cell membrane integrity (Yeaman and Yount, 2003). Insect AMPs are synthesized by the fat body with some contribution of hemocytes, and are secreted into the hemolymph shortly after infection. In addition, some AMPs are also produced by epithelial cells in a tissue-specific manner (Tzou et al., 2000). Expression of the AMP genes *Drosomycin* and *Diptericins* in the fat body is regulated by Toll and Imd, respectively, whereas both pathways contribute to expression of other AMP genes (e.g. *Defensin, Drosocin, Metchnikowin, Attacins,* and *Cecropins*) (Ferrandon et al., 2007).

Several AMP genes have been identified in *A. gambiae*: *Defensins* (*Def1-5*), *Cecropins* (*Cec1-4*), *Gambicin* (*Gamb*), and *Attacin* (Holt et al., 2002; Mongin et al., 2004). Antimicrobial and antifungal activities of the recombinant Cec1, Gamb, and Def1 peptides were demonstrated *in vitro* against filamentous fungi (Cec1, Gamb, Def1), Gram-negative (Cec1, Gamb) and Gram-positive bacteria (Def,1 Cec1, Gamb) (Vizioli et al., 2000, 2001a,b). *In vivo* silencing of *Def1* increases mosquito susceptibility to Gram-positive bacteria but does not affect development of *P. berghei* (Blandin et al., 2002). At the transcriptional level, however, expression of *Def1* was upregulated by infections with human and rodent parasites (Tahar et al., 2002). Gambicin, the only mosquito-specific AMP, exhibited some activity against *P. berghei* ookinetes *in vitro,* whereas depletion of *Gamb in vivo* increased mosquito susceptibility to Gram-positive bacteria, *P. berghei* and, to a lower extent, to *P. falciparum* (Vizioli et al., 2001a; Dong et al., 2006). Interestingly, transgenic over-expression of Cec1 fused to the Shiva toxin inhibited development of *P. berghei* oocysts in *A. gambiae* (Kim et al., 2004). In spite of these results, the exact role of antimicrobial peptides in the mosquito defenses against *Plasmodium* is still incompletely understood.

Identification of the effectors of REL2 and REL1 is crucial for understanding the specificity of malaria killing in the mosquito. However, only a handful of immune genes in *Anopheles* have been assigned to either pathway. Frolet et al. (2006) did not observe any changes in the expression of AMP genes upon constitutive activation of REL1, leaving an open possibility of their regulation by REL2. *In vitro* studies provided some support of *Cec1* and *Gamb* regulation by REL2 (Meister et al., 2005), but a more recent study *in vivo* suggested a dual regulation of AMP genes by both pathways (Garver et al., 2009).

The complement-like system emerged as a powerful arm of the mosquito immune responses to a broad spectrum of pathogens. The central component of this system, the thioester-containing protein 1 (TEP1), is a major determinant of malaria killing (Blandin et al., 2004; Garver et al., 2009; Molina-Cruz et al., 2012; Nsango et al., 2012). TEP1 binds to the surface of invading *Plasmodium* ookinetes and bacteria, and promotes their killing by lysis and phagocytosis, respectively (Blandin et al., 2004). TEP1 is a highly reactive protein and requires a complex of two leucine-rich repeat proteins [leucine-rich repeat immune protein 1 (LRIM1) and *Anopheles*

Plasmodium-responsive leucine-rich repeat 1C (APL1C)] to prevent its precocious activation and precipitation (Frolet et al., 2006; Fraiture et al., 2009). *TEP1* or *LRIM1* co-silencing with *Cactus* completely reverts the refractory phenotype of *Cactus* knockdown in *A. gambiae* infections with *P. berghei* (Frolet et al., 2006). Silencing of *TEP1* also results in higher intensities of *P. falciparum* infections (Garver et al., 2009), however, levels of TEP1 protection against *P. falciparum* vary with the genotype and genetic complexity of *Plasmodium* infections (Molina-Cruz et al., 2012; Nsango et al., 2012). Similar to AMPs, expression of the complement-like genes is regulated by both pathways (Frolet et al., 2006).

Another interesting multi-member protein family with potential roles in mosquito immune responses is the family of fibrinogen related proteins (FBNs or FREPs). It comprises 59 members in *A. gambiae*, 37 in *A. aegypti* and 14 in *D. melanogaster* (Christophides et al., 2002; Dong and Dimopoulos, 2009). Only few FBNs have been functionally characterized. Silencing of *FBN9*, *FBN22* and *FBN39* impairs mosquito survival upon bacterial infections; depletion of *FBN8*, *FBN9*, *FBN30*, and *FBN39* increases mosquito susceptibility to *Plasmodium* parasites, while silencing of *FBN1* decreases parasite loads (Dong and Dimopoulos, 2009; Li et al., 2013; Simões et al., 2017). Little is known about regulation of *FBN* expression, except for *FBN9*, whose expression is regulated by REL2 (Garver et al., 2009). FBN9 binds to malaria parasites and bacteria, thereby exposing them for killing by an as yet unknown mechanism (Dong and Dimopoulos, 2009). Surprisingly, transgenic expression of *FBN9* in the fat body driven by a blood feeding-inducible promoter did not enhance mosquito resistance to *P. falciparum* (Simões et al., 2017). This unexpected result highlights the importance of tissue-specific REL2 regulation, which has not been addressed yet.

CELLULAR IMMUNE RESPONSES

Several independent reports implicated REL2 pathway in the immune responses of hemocytes, the mosquito blood cells. Transcripts encoding the pathway components were identified in the hemocyte-enriched transcriptome and their expression levels were further upregulated by blood meal and by *P. berghei* ookinetes (Baton et al., 2009). Furthermore, hemocytes synthesize proteins whose expression is regulated by the REL2 pathway (e.g., AMPs, TEP1, LRIM1, and FBN9) (Levashina et al., 2001; Baton et al., 2009). Some of these proteins (TEP1, TEP3, PGRP-LC, and LRIM1) also contribute to the efficient phagocytosis of Gram-positive and Gram-negative bacteria (Moita et al., 2005). In *Drosophila*, hemocytes also serve as messengers in inter-organ communication. For example, an amplitude of systemic immune responses induced by localized infections is diminished in hemocyte-depleted fruit fly mutants, revealing hemocyte contribution to the amplification of the fat-body mediated immune responses (Charroux and Royet, 2009; Wu et al., 2012). The reactive oxygen species that act as local triggers of hemocyte activation, also efficiently activate the Imd pathway (Foley and O'Farrell, 2003; Wu et al., 2012), further supporting the potential role of this pathway in hemocyte activation.

MELANIZATION

The *Anopheles* REL2 pathway negatively regulates melanization, a process of melanin deposition in defense mechanisms (such as wound healing or pathogen killing), metamorphosis and tanning during development. Silencing of *PGRP-LC* and of both *REL2* isoforms not only renders mosquitoes more susceptible to *Plasmodium* but also induces melanization of *P. berghei* ookinetes (Meister et al., 2005, 2009; Frolet et al., 2006). The reverse is observed in *Drosophila,* where the intracellular receptor PGRP-LE is absolutely required for melanization (Takehana et al., 2004). REL1 pathway, on the other hand, promotes melanization in both insect species (Ligoxygakis et al., 2002; Frolet et al., 2006). Surprisingly, simultaneous activation of the REL1 pathway by *Cactus* knockdown and inhibition of the REL2 pathway by REL2 silencing abolishes *Plasmodium* melanization, revealing the complexity in the regulation of this immune reaction and a potential cross-talk between the two pathways (Frolet et al., 2006).

CONCLUSIONS

Although a significant progress has been achieved in identifying the components of the REL2 pathway in mosquitoes, many questions remain unanswered. Little is known about the role of post-translational modifications, such as ubiquitination and phosphorylation, which act as important pathway regulators in *Drosophila*. Moreover, completely unexplored areas are the contributions of the epigenetic modifications acting at the promoter level to fine tune immune responses. Understanding how chromatin conformations modulate expression patterns of effector genes may offer new insights into the complexity and specificity of REL2-mediated immune responses to a broad range of pathogens. However, even before considering the complexity of epigenetic modifications, it is pivotal to characterize the REL2-specific effectors, which are currently only vaguely known; and to address the questions of *Plasmodium* recognition and pathway activation upon infection in order to properly understand the parasite-host interaction and *Plasmodium* killing in the mosquito.

Recent studies in ticks and *Drosophila* discovered a non-canonical cytoplasmic route of pathway activation that bypasses the PGRP receptor-adaptor complex. These observations open new research avenues regarding receptor(s) and molecular mechanisms of pathway activation. The conservation of this non-canonical route in the evolutionarily distant organisms, such as ticks and *Drosophila*, may suggest that PGN recognition by PGRPs and further signal transduction by the death-domain module, appeared later in evolution, after separation of arachnids from insects. Instead, the core pathway from the ubiquitination module via Caspar to Relish seems to be broadly conserved across arthropods. Better understanding of the REL2 immune pathway in the malaria mosquitoes should advance our knowledge of conserved mechanisms of innate immunity and may identify new targets for vector-mediated malaria control.

AUTHOR CONTRIBUTIONS

All authors listed, have made substantial, direct and intellectual contribution to the work, and approved it for publication.

ACKNOWLEDGMENTS

The authors wish to thank Dr. Maiara Severo for critical reading of the manuscript. SZ is supported by a fellowship from German Research Foundation (DFG), GRK 2046.

REFERENCES

Antonova, Y., Alvarez, K. S., Kim, Y. J., Kokoza, V., and Raikhel, A. S. (2009). The role of NF-κB factor REL2 in the *Aedes aegypti* immune response. *Insect Biochem. Mol. Biol.* 39, 303–314. doi: 10.1016/j.ibmb.2009.01.007

Baton, L., Robertson, A., Warr, E., Strand, M. R., and Dimopoulos, G. (2009). Genome-wide transcriptomic profiling of *Anopheles gambiae* hemocytes reveals pathogen-specific signatures upon bacterial challenge and Plasmodium berghei infection. *BMC Genomics* 10:257. doi: 10.1186/1471-2164-10-257

Blandin, S., Moita, L. F., Köcher, T., Wilm, M., Kafatos, F. C., and Levashina, E. (2002). Reverse genetics in the mosquito *Anopheles gambiae*: targeted disruption of the Defensin gene. *EMBO Rep.* 3, 852–856. doi: 10.1093/embo-reports/kvf180

Blandin, S., Shiao, S. H., Moita, L. F., Janse, C. J., Waters, A. P., Kafatos, F. C., et al. (2004). Complement-like protein TEP1 is a determinant of vectorial capacity in the malaria vector *Anopheles gambiae*. *Cell* 116, 661–670. doi: 10.1016/S0092-8674(04)00173-4

Bonnay, F., Nguyen, X., Cohen-berros, E., Troxler, L., Batsche, E., Camonis, J., et al. (2014). Akirin specifies NF-κB selectivity of Drosophila innate immune response via chromatin remodeling. *EMBO J.* 33, 1–14. doi: 10.15252/embj.201488456

Charroux, B., and Royet, J. (2009). Elimination of plasmatocytes by targeted apoptosis reveals their role in multiple aspects of the Drosophila immune response. *Proc. Natl. Acad. Sci. U.S.A.* 106, 9797–9802. doi: 10.1073/pnas.0903971106

Choe, K. M., Werner, T., Stoven, S., Hultmark, D., and Anderson, K. V. (2002). Requirement for a Peptidoglycan Recognition Protein (PGRP) in Relish Activation and Antibacterial Immune Responses in Drosophila. *Science* 296, 359–362. doi: 10.1126/science.1070216

Christophides, G. K., Zdobnov, E., Barillas-Mury, C., Birney, E., Blandin, S., Blass, C., et al. (2002). Immunity-related genes and gene families in *Anopheles gambiae*. *Science* 298, 159–165. doi: 10.1126/science.1077136

Costa, A., Jan, E., Sarnow, P., and Schneider, D. (2009). The Imd pathway is involved in antiviral immune responses in Drosophila. *PLoS ONE* 4: e7436. doi: 10.1371/journal.pone.0007436

Da Costa, M., Pinheiro-Silva, R., Antunes, S., Moreno-Cid, J., Custódio, A., Villar, M., et al. (2014). Mosquito Akirin as a potential antigen for malaria control. *Malar. J.* 13, 470. doi: 10.1186/1475-2875-13-470

Dimopoulos, G., Christophides, G. K., Meister, S., Schultz, J., White, K. P., Barillas-Mury, C., et al. (2002). Genome expression analysis of *Anopheles gambiae*: responses to injury, bacterial challenge, and malaria infection. *Proc. Natl. Acad. Sci. U.S.A.* 99, 8814–8819. doi: 10.1073/pnas.092274999

Dong, Y., Aguilar, R., Xi, Z., Warr, E., Mongin, E., and Dimopoulos, G. (2006). *Anopheles gambiae* immune responses to human and rodent Plasmodium parasite species. *PLoS Pathog.* 2:e52. doi: 10.1371/journal.ppat.0020052

Dong, Y., and Dimopoulos, G. (2009). Anopheles fibrinogen-related proteins provide expanded pattern recognition capacity against bacteria and malaria parasites. *J. Biol. Chem.* 284, 9835–9844. doi: 10.1074/jbc.M807084200

Dushay, M. S., Asling, B., and Hultmark, D. (1996). Origins of immunity: Relish, a compound Rel-like gene in the antibacterial defense of Drosophila. *Proc. Natl. Acad. Sci. U.S.A.* 93, 10343–10347. doi: 10.1073/pnas.93.19.10343

Ertürk-Hasdemir, D., Broemer, M., Leulier, F., Lane, W. S., Paquette, N., Hwang, D., et al. (2009). Two roles for the Drosophila IKK complex in the activation of Relish and the induction of antimicrobial peptide genes. *Proc. Natl. Acad. Sci. U.S.A.* 106, 9779–9784. doi: 10.1073/pnas.0812022106

Ferrandon, D., Imler, J.-L., Hetru, C., and Hoffmann, J. A. (2007). The Drosophila systemic immune response: sensing and signalling during bacterial and fungal infections. *Nat. Rev. Immunol.* 7, 862–874. doi: 10.1038/nri2194

Foley, E., and O'Farrell, P. H. (2003). Nitric oxide contributes to induction of innate immune responses to gram-negative bacteria in Drosophila. *Genes Dev.* 17, 115–125. doi: 10.1101/gad.1018503

Fraiture, M., Baxter, R. H. G., Steinert, S., Chelliah, Y., Frolet, C., Quispe-Tintaya, W., et al. (2009). Two mosquito LRR proteins function as complement control factors in the TEP1-mediated killing of Plasmodium. *Cell Host Microbe* 5, 273–284. doi: 10.1016/j.chom.2009.01.005

Frolet, C., Thoma, M., Blandin, S., Hoffmann, J., and Levashina, E. (2006). Boosting NF-κB-dependent basal immunity of *Anopheles gambiae* aborts development of *Plasmodium berghei*. *Immunity* 25, 677–685. doi: 10.1016/j.immuni.2006.08.019

Garver, L. S., Bahia, A. C., Das, S., Souza-Neto, J., Shiao, J., Dong, Y., et al. (2012). Anopheles Imd pathway factors and effectors in infection intensity-dependent anti-plasmodium action. *PLoS Pathog.* 8:e1002737. doi: 10.1371/journal.ppat.1002737

Garver, L. S., Dong, Y., and Dimopoulos, G. (2009). Caspar controls resistance to *Plasmodium falciparum* in diverse anopheline species. *PLoS Pathog.* 5:e1000335. doi: 10.1371/journal.ppat.1000335

Gobert, V., Gottar, M., Matskevich, A. A., Rutschmann, S., Royet, J., Belvin, M., et al. (2003). Dual activation of the Drosophila Toll pathway by two pattern recognition receptors. *Science* 302, 2126–2130. doi: 10.1126/science.1085432

Goto, A., Matsushita, K., Gesellchen, V., El Chamy, L., Kuttenkeuler, D., Takeuchi, O., et al. (2008). Akirins are highly conserved nuclear proteins required for NF-κB-dependent gene expression in drosophila and mice. *Nat. Immunol.* 9, 97–104. doi: 10.1038/ni1543

Gottar, M., Gobert, V., Michel, T., Belvin, M., Duyk, G., Hoffmann, J., et al. (2002). The Drosophila immune response against Gram-negative bacteria is mediated by a peptidoglycan recognition protein. *Nature* 416, 640–644. doi: 10.1038/nature734

Holt, R., Subramanian, G., Halpern, A., Sutton, G., Charlab, R., Nusskern, D., et al. (2002). The genome sequence of the malaria mosquito *Anopheles gambiae*. *Science* 298, 129–149. doi: 10.1126/science.1076181

Iatsenko, I., Kondo, S., Mengin-Lecreulx, D., and Lemaitre, B. (2016). PGRP-SD, an extracellular pattern-recognition receptor, enhances peptidoglycan-mediated activation of the drosophila Imd pathway. *Immunity* 45, 1013–1023. doi: 10.1016/j.immuni.2016.10.029

Jenssen, H., Hamill, P., and Hancock, R. E. W. (2006). Peptide antimicrobial agents. *Clin. Microbiol. Rev.* 19, 491–511. doi: 10.1128/CMR.00056-05

Kaneko, T., Goldman, W. E., Mellroth, P., Steiner, H., Fukase, K., Kusumoto, S., et al. (2004). Monomeric and polymeric gram-negative peptidoglycan but not purified LPS stimulate the Drosophila IMD pathway. *Immunity* 20, 637–649. doi: 10.1016/S1074-7613(04)00104-9

Kim, M., Lee, J. H., Lee, S. Y., Kim, E., and Chung, J. (2006). Caspar, a suppressor of antibacterial immunity in Drosophila. *Proc. Natl. Acad. Sci. U.S.A.* 103, 16358–16363. doi: 10.1073/pnas.0603238103

Kim, W., Koo, H., Richman, A. M., Seeley, D., Vizioli, J., Klocko, A. D., et al. (2004). Ectopic expression of a Cecropin transgene in the human malaria vector Anopheles gambie (Diptera: Culicidae): Effects on susceptibility to Plasmodium. *Med. Entomol.* 41, 447–455. doi: 10.1603/0022-2585-4 1.3.447

Lamiable, O., Kellenberger, C., Kemp, C., Troxler, L., Pelte, N., Boutros, M., et al. (2016). Cytokine Diedel and a viral homologue suppress the IMD pathway in *Drosophila*. *Proc. Natl. Acad. Sci. U.S.A.* 113, 201516122. doi: 10.1073/pnas.1516122113

Lemaitre, B., Nicolas, E., Michaut, L., Reichhart, J. M., and Hoffmann, J. A. (1996). The dorsoventral regulatory gene cassette spatzle/Toll/Cactus controls the potent antifungal response in Drosophila adults. *Cell* 86, 973–983. doi: 10.1016/S0092-8674(00)80172-5

Leulier, F., Parquet, C., Pili-Floury, S., Ryu, J.-H., Caroff, M., Lee, W.-J., et al. (2003). The Drosophila immune system detects bacteria through specific peptidoglycan recognition. *Nat. Immunol.* 4, 478–484. doi: 10.1038/ni922

Levashina, E. A., Moita, L. F., Blandin, S., Vriend, G., Lagueux, M., and Kafatos, F. C. (2001). Conserved role of a complement-like protein in phagocytosis revealed by dsRNA knockout in cultured cells of the mosquito, *Anopheles gambiae*. *Cell* 104, 709–718. doi: 10.1016/S0092-8674(02)09026-8

Li, J., Wang, X., Zhang, G., Githure, J. I., Yan, G., and James, A. (2013). Genome-block expression-assisted association studies discover malaria resistance genes in *Anopheles gambiae*. *Proc. Natl. Acad. Sci. U.S.A.* 110, 20675–20680. doi: 10.1073/pnas.1321024110

Ligoxygakis, P., Pelte, N., Ji, C., Leclerc, V., Duvic, B., Belvin, M., et al. (2002). A serpin mutant links Toll activation to melanization in the host defence of Drosophila. *EMBO J.* 21, 6330–6337. doi: 10.1093/emboj/cdf661

Meinander, A., Runchel, C., Tenev, T., Chen, L., Kim, C.-H., Ribeiro, P. S., et al. (2012). Ubiquitylation of the initiator caspase DREDD is required for innate immune signalling. *EMBO J.* 31, 2770–2783. doi: 10.1038/emboj.2012.121

Meister, S., Agianian, B., Turlure, F., Relógio, A., Morlais, I., Kafatos, F. C., et al. (2009). *Anopheles gambiae* PGRPLC-Mediated Defense against Bacteria Modulates Infections with Malaria Parasites. *PLoS Pathog.* 5:e1000542. doi: 10.1371/journal.ppat.1000542

Meister, S., Kanzok, S. M., Zheng, X.-L., Luna, C., Li, T.-R., Hoa, N. T., et al. (2005). Immune signaling pathways regulating bacterial and malaria parasite infection of the mosquito *Anopheles gambiae*. *Proc. Natl. Acad. Sci. U.S.A.* 102, 11420–11425. doi: 10.1073/pnas.0504950102

Moita, L. F., Wang-Sattler, R., Michel, K., Zimmermann, T., Blandin, S., Levashina, E., et al. (2005). *In vivo* identification of novel regulators and conserved pathways of phagocytosis in *A. gambiae*. *Immunity* 23, 65–73. doi: 10.1016/j.immuni.2005.05.006

Molina-Cruz, A., DeJong, R. J., Ortega, C., Haile, A., Abban, E., Rodrigues, J., et al. (2012). PNAS Plus: Some strains of *Plasmodium falciparum*, a human malaria parasite, evade the complement-like system of *Anopheles gambiae* mosquitoes. *Proc. Natl. Acad. Sci. U.S.A.* 109, E1957–E1962. doi: 10.1073/pnas.1121183109

Mongin, E., Louis, C., Holt, R. A., Birney, E., and Collins, F. H. (2004). The *Anopheles gambiae* genome: an update. *Trends Parasitol.* 20, 49–52. doi: 10.1016/j.pt.2003.11.003

Morisato, D., and Anderson, K. V. (1994). The spätzle gene encodes a component of the extracellular signaling pathway establishing the dorsal-ventral pattern of the Drosophila embryo. *Cell* 76, 677–688. doi: 10.,1016/0092-8674(94)90507-X

Nsango, S. E., Abate, L., Thoma, M., Pompon, J., Fraiture, M., Rademacher, A., et al. (2012). Genetic clonality of *Plasmodium falciparum* affects the outcome of infection in *Anopheles gambiae*. *Int. J. Parasitol.* 42, 589–595. doi: 10.1016/j.ijpara.2012.03.008

Paquette, N., Broemer, M., Aggarwal, K., Chen, L., Husson, M., Reichhart, J., et al. (2010). Caspase mediated cleavage, IAP binding and ubiquitination: linking three mechanisms crucial for Drosophila NF-κB signaling. *Mol. Cell* 37, 172–182. doi: 10.1016/j.molcel.2009.12.036.Caspase

Ramphul, U. N., Garver, L. S., Molina-Cruz, A., Canepa, G. E., and Barillas-Mury, C. (2015). *Plasmodium falciparum* evades mosquito immunity by disrupting JNK-mediated apoptosis of invaded midgut cells. *Proc. Natl. Acad. Sci. U.S.A.* 112, 1273–1280. doi: 10.1073/pnas.1423586112

Rutschmann, S., Kilinc, A., and Ferrandon, D. (2002). Cutting edge: the toll pathway is required for resistance to gram-positive bacterial infections in Drosophila. *J. Immunol.* 168, 1542–1546. doi: 10.4049/jimmunol.168.4.1542

Schneider, D. S., Jin, Y., Morisato, D., and Anderson, K. V. (1994). A processed form of the Spätzle protein defines dorsal-ventral polarity in the Drosophila embryo. *Development* 120, 1243–1250.

Sen, R., and Baltimore, D. (1986). Inducibility of κ immunoglobulin enhancer-binding protein NF-κB by a posttranslational mechanism. *Cell* 47, 921–928. doi: 10.1016/0092-8674(86)90807-X

Shaw, D. K., Wang, X., Brown, L. J., Chávez, A. S. O., Reif, K. E., Smith, A. A., et al. (2017). Infection-derived lipids elicit an immune deficiency circuit in arthropods. *Nat. Commun.* 8:14401. doi: 10.1038/ncomms14401

Shin, S. W., Kokoza, V., Ahmed, A., and Raikhel, A. S. (2002). Characterization of three alternatively spliced isoforms of the Rel/NF-κB transcription factor Relish from the mosquito *Aedes aegypti*. *Proc. Natl. Acad. Sci. U.S.A.* 99, 9978–9983. doi: 10.1073/pnas.162345999

Simões, M. L., Dong, Y., Hammond, A., Hall, A., Crisanti, A., Nolan, T., et al. (2017). The Anopheles FBN9 immune factor mediates Plasmodium species-specific defense through transgenic fat body expression. *Dev. Comp. Immunol.* 67, 257–265. doi: 10.1016/j.dci.2016.09.012

Tahar, R., Boudin, C., Thiery, I., and Bourgouin, C. (2002). Immune response of *Anopheles gambiae* to the early sporogonic stages of the human malaria parasite *Plasmodium falciparum*. *Embo J.* 21, 6673–6680. doi: 10.1093/emboj/cdf664

Takehana, A., Katsuyama, T., Yano, T., Oshima, Y., Takada, H., Aigaki, T., et al. (2002). Overexpression of a pattern-recognition receptor, peptidoglycan-recognition protein-LE, activates imd/relish-mediated antibacterial defense and the prophenoloxidase cascade in Drosophila larvae. *Proc. Natl. Acad. Sci. U.S.A.* 99, 13705–13710. doi: 10.1073/pnas.212301199

Takehana, A., Yano, T., Mita, S., Kotani, A., Oshima, Y., and Kurata, S. (2004). Peptidoglycan recognition protein (PGRP)-LE and PGRP-LC act synergistically in Drosophila immunity. *EMBO J.* 23, 4690–4700. doi: 10.1038/sj.emboj.7600466

Tzou, P., Ohresser, S., Ferrandon, D., Capovilla, M., Reichhart, J. M., Lemaitre, B., et al. (2000). Tissue-specific inducible expression of antimicrobial peptide genes in Drosophila surface epithelia. *Immunity* 13, 737–748. doi: 10.1016/S1074-7613(00)00072-8

Vance, R. E., Isberg, R. R., and Portnoy, D. A. (2009). Patterns of pathogenesis: discrimination of pathogenic and nonpathogenic microbes by the innate immune system. *Cell Host Microbe* 6, 10–21. doi: 10.1016/j.chom.2009.06.007

Vizioli, J., Bulet, P., Charlet, M., Lowenberger, C., Blass, C., Muller, H. M., et al. (2000). Cloning and analysis of a cecropin gene from the malaria vector mosquito, *Anopheles gambiae*. *Insect. Mol. Biol.* 9, 75–84. doi: 10.1046/j.1365-2583.2000.00164.x

Vizioli, J., Bulet, P., Hoffmann, J. A., Kafatos, F. C., Müller, H.-M., and Dimopoulos, G. (2001a). Gambicin: a novel immune responsive antimicrobial peptide from the malaria vector *Anopheles gambiae*. *Proc. Natl. Acad. Sci. U.S.A.* 98, 12630–12635. doi: 10.1073/pnas.221466798

Vizioli, J., Richman, A. M., Uttenweiler-Joseph, S., Blass, C., and Bulet, P. (2001b). The defensin peptide of the malaria vector mosquito *Anopheles gambiae*: antimicrobial activities and expression in adult mosquitoes. *Insect Biochem. Mol. Biol.* 31, 241–248. doi: 10.1016/S0965-1748(00)00143-0

Wu, L. P., and Anderson, K. V. (1998). Regulated nuclear import of Rel proteins in the Drosophila immune response. *Nature* 392, 93–97. doi: 10.1038/32195

Wu, S. C., Liao, C. W., Pan, R. L., and Juang, J. L. (2012). Infection-induced intestinal oxidative stress triggers organ-to-organ immunological communication in Drosophila. *Cell Host Microbe* 11, 410–417. doi: 10.1016/j.chom.2012.03.004

Yeaman, M. R., and Yount, N. Y. (2003). Mechanisms of antimicrobial peptide action and resistance. *Pharmacol. Rev.* 55, 27–55. doi: 10.1124/pr.55.1.2.27

Zaidman-Rémy, A., Hervé, M., Poidevin, M., Pili-Floury, S., Kim, M. S., Blanot, D., et al. (2006). The Drosophila Amidase PGRP-LB Modulates the Immune Response to Bacterial Infection. *Immunity* 24, 463–473. doi: 10.1016/j.immuni.2006.02.012

17

Chloroquine neither Eliminates Liver Stage Parasites nor Delays their Development in a Murine Chemoprophylaxis Vaccination Model

Tejram Sahu*, Lynn Lambert, Jessica Herrod, Solomon Conteh, Sachy Orr-Gonzalez, Dariyen Carter and Patrick E. Duffy*

Laboratory of Malaria Immunology and Vaccinology, National Institute of Allergy and Infectious Diseases, National Institutes of Health, Rockville, MD, USA

Edited by:
Thomas Laurence Richie, Thomas L. Richie, Consulting, USA

Reviewed by:
Laurent Renia, Agency for Science, Research and Technology, Singapore
Else Bijker, Radboud University Medical Center, Netherlands

***Correspondence:**
Patrick E. Duffy, Laboratory of Malaria Immunology and Vaccinology, National Institute of Allergy and Infectious Diseases, National Institutes of Health, 5640 Fishers Lane, Room-1111, Rockville, MD 20852, USA duffype@niaid.nih.gov;
Tejram Sahu, Laboratory of Malaria Immunology and Vaccinology, National Institute of Allergy and Infectious Diseases, National Institutes of Health, 12735 Twinbrook Parkway, Room-3W15, Rockville, MD 20852, USA sahut@mail.nih.gov

Chemoprophylaxis Vaccination (CVac) confers long lasting sterile protection against homologous parasite strains in humans, and involves inoculation of infectious sporozoites (SPZ) under drug cover. CVac using the drug chloroquine (CQ) induces pre-erythrocytic immunity in humans that includes antibody to SPZ and T-cell responses to liver stage (LS) parasites. The mechanism by which CVac with CQ induces strong protective immunity is not understood as untreated infections do not confer protection. CQ kills blood stage parasites, but its effect on LS parasites is poorly studied. Here we hypothesized that CQ may prolong or perturb LS development of *Plasmodium*, as a potential explanation for enhanced pre-erythrocytic immune responses. Balb/c mice with or without CQ prophylaxis were infected with sporozoite forms of a luciferase-expressing rodent parasite, *Plasmodium yoelii*-Luc (*Py*-Luc). Mice that received primaquine, a drug that kills LS parasites, served as a positive control of drug effect. Parasite burden in liver was measured both by bioluminescence and by qRT-PCR quantification of parasite transcript. Time to appearance of parasites in the blood was monitored by microscopic analysis of Giemsa-stained thick and thin blood smears. The parasite load in livers of CQ-treated and untreated mice did not significantly differ at any of the time points studied. Parasites appeared in the blood smears of both CQ-treated and untreated mice 3 days after infection. Taken together, our findings confirm that CQ neither eliminates LS parasites nor delays their development. Further investigations into the mechanism of CQ-induced protection after CVac are required, and may give insights relevant to drug and vaccine development.

Keywords: *Plasmodium*, chloroquine, liver-stage, CVac, prepatent

Introduction

The most successful vaccination approach against malaria involves immunization with whole organism, generally by the liver-infective form called sporozoites (SPZ). SPZ attenuated by radiation (RAS; Nussenzweig et al., 1967; Clyde et al., 1973) or by genetic alterations (GAP;

Mikolajczak et al., 2010; Vaughan et al., 2010) infect hepatocytes but arrest during liver stage (LS) development and do not emerge in the blood stream. More recently, experimental infection and drug treatment has achieved impressive protection: in humans, inoculation of SPZ under drug cover, referred to here as Chemoprophylaxis Vaccination (CVac), required much lower SPZ doses than RAS to induce sterile immunity that persisted for >2 years in four of six individuals (Belnoue et al., 2004; Roestenberg et al., 2011). Chloroquine (CQ) prophylaxis has been studied most extensively as drug cover during CVac, and this regimen generates preerythrocytic immunity that includes anti-sporozoite antibody (Behet et al., 2014) and LS-specific T-cells in animals and humans (Belnoue et al., 2004; Renia, 2008; Bijker et al., 2013).

Chloroquine kills blood stage parasites as they reach the trophozoite stage of development (Yayon et al., 1983), but the effect of CQ on LS parasites has received less attention. It is widely believed that CQ does not affect LS development, allowing the immune system to encounter the full repertoire of LS antigens. However, the more durable protection achieved with CVac after ~16-fold fewer mosquito bites than required for RAS suggests that drug treatment effects might contribute independently to protection.

The effect of CQ on *Plasmodium* LS development is not completely settled. Based on an *in vivo* infection model, Belnoue et al. (2004) reported that CQ does not kill *Plasmodium* LS at 42 h post infection with SPZ. However, the effect of CQ on later time points including blood stage emergence has not been studied. Using an *in vitro* infection model, Fisk et al. (1989) reported a partial schizonticidal effect of CQ on late LS, but the CQ dose was relatively high, and had cytotoxic effects on hepatocytes as well. Here we report a systematic evaluation of the effects of therapeutic concentrations of CQ on late LS development, using a luciferase expressing *P. yoelii* parasite in Balb/c mice.

Materials and Methods

Mice

Female Balb/c mice, 4–6 week old were purchased from Taconic. Mice were housed in the NIH animal facility under pathogen free conditions and fed with autoclaved food *ad libitum*. All experiments were performed once mice reached 16 to 18 weeks of age. All experiments were approved and performed as per the guidelines by the Animal Care and Use Committee (ACUC) of NIAID/NIH.

Parasite and Mosquitoes

Plasmodium yoelii parasites (strain 17XNL), including the parental line and a transgenic line expressing firefly-luciferase and GFP (*Plasmodium yoelii*-Luc, *Py*-Luc), were maintained by cycling between Balb/c mice and *Anopheles stephensi* mosquitoes. Salivary gland SPZs were harvested on days 14–18 as described earlier (Ozaki et al., 1984; Guebre-Xabier et al., 1999).

Infection and Evaluation of LS Development by Bioluminescence Imaging

Female Balb/c mice (16–18 weeks old) were infected with 15,000 freshly dissected SPZ of *Py*-Luc in 100 μl of 1X PBS+2% normal mouse serum by IV injection. Development of LS was monitored by bioluminescence imaging (BLI) at different time points post-infection as described earlier (Mwakingwe et al., 2009; Miller et al., 2013). Briefly, mice were injected intradermally with 150 μl of Rediject D-Luciferin (Caliper Life Sciences, USA), then anesthetized with isoflurane-anesthesia system 8–10 min later to allow measurement of bioluminescence and image acquisition using IVIS-100 animal imager (Caliper Life Sciences, USA). Bioluminescence images were acquired at the following settings: 15 cm Field of View (FOV), medium binning, and exposure time of 30–60 s. Quantification of luminescence was performed using the ROI settings of the Living Image 4.4 software (Perkin Elmer, USA). ROI were drawn around the abdominal area locating the liver. ROI measurements were expressed as total flux photons per second (p/s).

Drug Treatment and LS Burden Estimation by Intravital Imaging

Infected mice comprised three groups that received different treatments in 100 μl of PBS by intraperitoneal (IP) route: one group received 0.8 mg/mouse of CQ diphosphate (SPZ+CQ; Sigma; Belnoue et al., 2004): one group received 1.5 mg/mouse of PQ bisphosphate (SPZ+PQ; Sigma; Putrianti et al., 2009); one group received PBS without drug (SPZ). Two drug control groups were also included, whereby mice received CQ or PQ but no SPZ infection. An additional control group received no drug and no SPZ. Drug was delivered at the time of infection (0 hours post infection, hpi) and at 24 hpi. Bioluminescence images were acquired *in vivo* with IVIS-100 (Perkin Elmer) at different time points after drug injection indicated in the figure legends. BLI was performed on whole livers that had been perfused (10 ml of RNAse free 1x PBS) and isolated at sequential time points from 40 hpi onward. Liver samples were also snap-frozen in liquid nitrogen for qRT-PCR.

Determination of LS Burden by qRT-PCR

Total RNA was extracted from the whole liver as described earlier (Schussek et al., 2013) using RNeasy mini kit (Qiagen Inc). cDNA was synthesized using High-Capacity cDNA Reverse Transcription Kit (Applied Biosystem, Foster City, CA, USA). Gene expression was measured with 1:40 dilutions of cDNA. Standard curve quantitative RT-PCR was performed (Bruna-Romero et al., 2001) in a 20 μl volume, which includes 1X ABI Power SYBR master mix (Applied Biosystems) and 0.25 μM of either *P. yoelii* 18S rRNA primer (forward- GGGGATTGGTTTTGACGTTTT, reverse- AAGCATTAAATAAAGCGAATA) or mouse β-actin primers (Forward- GGCTGTATTCCCCTCCAT; reverse-CCAGTTGGTAACAATGCAAT). PCR reactions were run on ABI 7500 machine (Applied Biosystems), using the following conditions: 50°C for 2 min; 95°C for 10 min; 40 cycles of 95°C for 15 s alternating with 60°C for 1 min.

cDNA standards for both 18S rRNA and β-actin were prepared as 10-fold dilutions (10^7–10^3 copies) from purified PCR product. Liver of naïve mouse was used as negative control. Parasite load was normalized to host β-actin as a ratio (absolute copy of *Py* 18S/ absolute copy of mouse β-actin).

Determination of Prepatent Period

Thick and thin blood smears were collected from the infected mice at different time points starting 42 hpi. Blood smears were Giemsa-stained and examined with a bright field microscope with 100× oil-immersion objective and by expert slide readers blinded to the study groups. Blood smears were considered positive if at least two infected RBCs were found in 100 adjacent fields.

Statistical Analysis

Mann–Whitney test was used to compare groups for LS burden measured by either BLI or qPCR. $P \leq 0.05$ was considered statistically significant. GraphPad Prism software (version 6) was used for statistical analysis.

Results

LS Parasites Persist 54 h after SPZ Inoculation into Untreated Mice

Plasmodium undergoes extensive multiplication during LS development, producing tens of thousands of merozoites from an individual sporozoite. Upon completion of LS development, merozoites are released into the blood stream as small merozoite-filled vesicles called merosomes. To quantify the multiplication and subsequent release of parasites in the liver, we infected mice with 1.5×10^4 luciferase expressing *Py*-Luc SPZ and performed BLI at 40, 44, 48, 54, and 62 hpi. Parasite biomass increased with time until 44 h and then gradually declined with the lowest LS parasite burden at 54 hpi (**Figures 1** and **2**; Supplementary Figure S2). We could detect measurable luciferase activity in the liver at 54 hpi with an average total flux of 5.0×10^6 photon/s (**Figure 1**). By 62 hpi, parasites are detected throughout the body, indicating a blood stage infection (Supplementary Figure S1E), and any residual parasites in the liver could not be distinguished from circulating blood stage parasites.

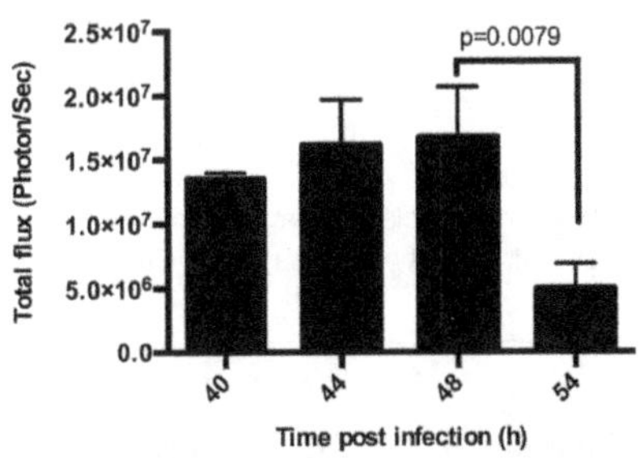

FIGURE 1 | Duration of *Plasmodium yoelii*-Luc (*Py*-Luc) liver stage (LS) growth. Graph representing quantification of total flux from infected and untreated mice imaged at 40, 44, 48, and 54 h after sporozoites (SPZ) injection. $n = 3$ for 40 h, 4 for 44 h, and 5 each for 48, and 54 h. Graph represents Mean ± SD. Mann–Whitney test was performed and $p < 0.05$ considered as significant.

CQ Neither Kills LS Parasites Nor Delays Their Development

To evaluate the effect of CQ on developing LS parasites, we infected mice with 1.5×10^4 *Py*-Luc SPZ, and then treated with either CQ (0.8 mg/mouse), PQ (1.5 mg/mouse), or an equal volume of PBS. Three groups of uninfected mice received same treatments (CQ, PQ, or PBS) but no SPZ. Imaging of whole bodies or of isolated livers was performed at 40, 44, 48, and 54 hpi. CQ-treated (SPZ+CQ) and untreated (SPZ) mice did not differ significantly at any time point (**Figures 2** and **3**; Supplementary Figure S2), whereas the SPZ+PQ group was completely devoid of any bioluminescence, as expected (**Figure 2**; Supplementary Figure S1). Parasite burden estimation with conventional qPCR gave similar results (**Figure 2D**). At 40 hpi, bioluminescence appeared lower in SPZ+CQ group than SPZ group but this trend was not statistically significant ($p = 0.06$; **Figure 2C**), and no such trend was observed in the corresponding qRT-PCR measurements at this time point ($P = 0.86$; **Figure 2D**).

To remove inter-subject variability in a second experiment, we followed individual mice over time, and acquired BLI at sequential time points. We infected each of 20 mice with SPZ of *Py*-Luc; half were treated with CQ while half received an equal volume of PBS. At 42, 44, 46, and 48 hpi, LS parasite burden was measured by whole body BLI. We did not observe significant differences in the parasite burden in the SPZ+CQ *versus* SPZ animals at any time point (Supplementary Figures S3 and S4). In a third experiment, using parental Py-17XNL infection, we confirmed by qPCR that the LS parasite burden at 48 hpi does not significantly differ between SPZ+CQ and SPZ animals ($p = 0.38$, Supplementary Figure S5). Both SPZ+CQ and SPZ mice became blood stage positive at 48 hpi by blood smear microscopy, further indicating that CQ does not delay LS development (**Figure 4**).

Discussion

The effect of CQ on *Plasmodium* blood stages is well characterized, with the inhibition of heme-polymerase enzyme leading to accumulation of toxic heme products, and parasite death (Slater and Cerami, 1992). CQ-CVac generates strong LS-specific immune responses and more durable protection at a log-fold lower SPZ dose as compared to RAS immunization (Clyde et al., 1973; Bijker et al., 2013). However, it is not clear how CQ treatment helps generate this strong and durable immune response. One school of thought holds that CQ-CVac allows the complete development of LS parasites that express a wide array of LS specific antigens, prior to killing the parasites in their first cycle of blood stage development; however, untreated *Plasmodium* infections also display the full antigen repertoire without inducing sterile preerythrocytic immunity. We hypothesized that

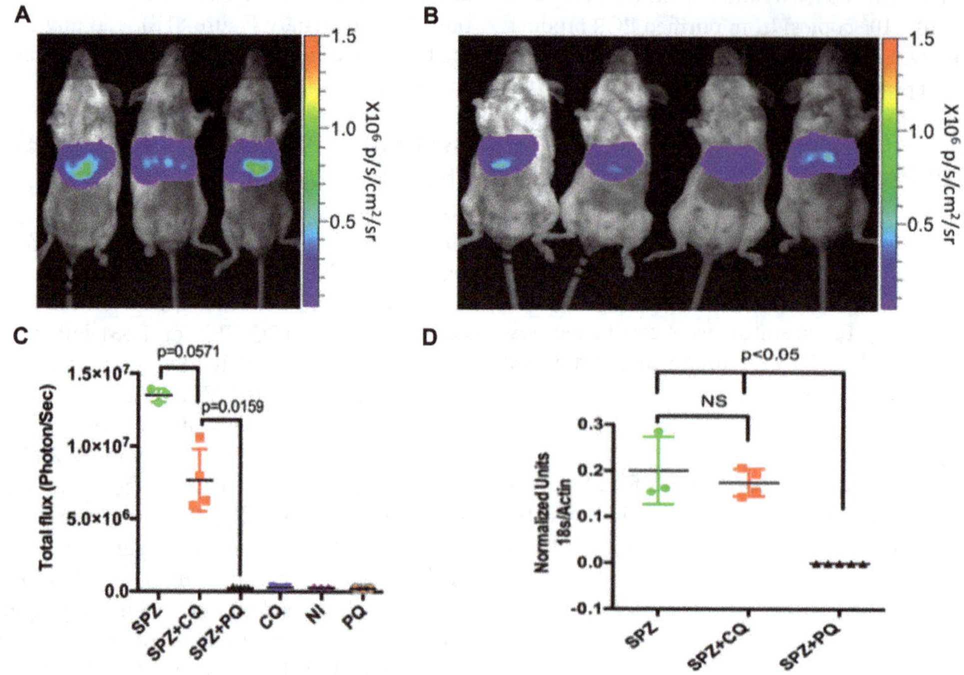

FIGURE 2 | Effect of CQ on LS parasite at 40 hours post infection (hpi). Rainbow images of mice infected and untreated **(A)** or CQ-treated **(B)** showing parasite load in liver 40 h after injection of 1.5 x 10^4 *Py*-Luc salivary gland SPZ. Rainbow scale represents radiance (p/s/cm^2/sr). **(C)** Quantification of total flux from whole body imaging of mice (shown in **A** and Supplementary Figure S1). $n = 3$ for SPZ (infected and untreated) and NI (neither infected nor treated) group, four for SPZ+CQ group and five each for SPZ+PQ and drug control (treated uninfected) groups. **(D)** Quantification of LS parasite burden 40 hpi in livers of SPZ ($n = 3$), SPZ+CQ ($n = 4$), and SPZ+PQ ($n = 5$) mice by qPCR. Graph represents Py-18S RNA normalized to murine β-actin RNA. Data in **(C,D)** represents Mean ± SD, Mann-Whitney test was performed and $p < 0.05$ considered as significant. CQ, Chloroquine; PQ, Primaquine; NI, non-infected and non-treated.

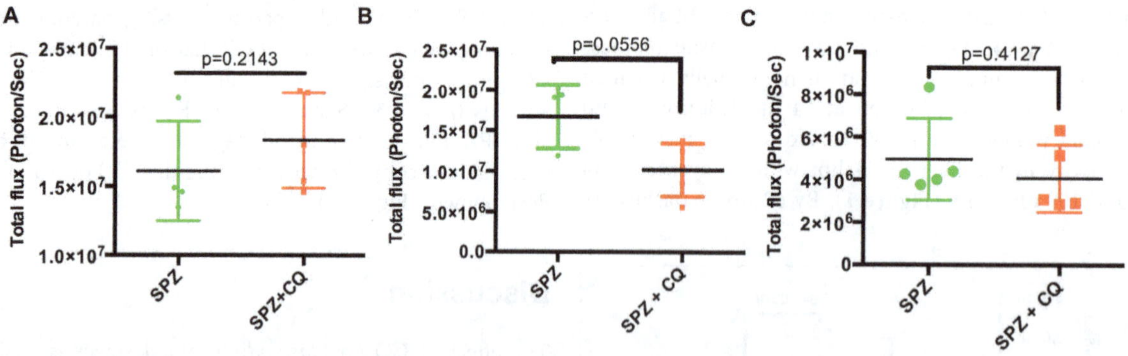

FIGURE 3 | Parasite load in liver at different time points after CQ treatment. Quantification of total flux from whole body imaging of mice (shown in Supplementary Figure S4). $n = 4$ for SPZ group at 44 hpi **(A)**, five each for both SPZ and SPZ+CQ at 48 h **(B)**, and 54 h **(C)** time points. Graph represents mean ± SD. Mann-Whitney test was performed and $p < 0.05$ considered as significant.

CQ may have partial or subtle effects on late LS development that contribute to enhanced immune responses, but we find no evidence that CQ decreases LS burden or delays LS development.

The effect of CQ on the LS of *Plasmodium* has previously been studied *in vivo* in a mouse model (Belnoue et al., 2004) and *in vitro* by infection of non-human primate hepatocytes (Fisk et al., 1989). Belnoue et al. (2004) reported that mice treated with 0.8 mg CQ and untreated mice had similar LS parasite burden 42 hpi, but did not examine effects beyond this time point; the CQ dose (~32 mg/kg) used by Belnoue et al. (2004, and also by us for this study) was based on earlier work (Orjih et al., 1982), and is in the dosing range (30–35 mg/kg) used for children of 10–20 kg body weight (Moore et al., 2011).

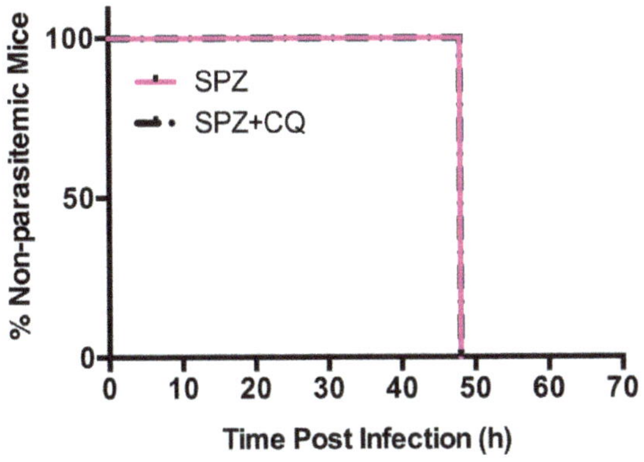

FIGURE 4 | Effect of CQ on prepatent period of *Py*-Luc. Mice ($n = 18$) were infected with 1.5 x 10^4 *Py*-Luc salivary gland SPZ and either CQ-treated (SPZ+CQ; $n = 9$) or not (SPZ; $n = 9$). Blood smears (both thick and thin smears) were collected starting from 48 hpi. Smears were stained and examined by expert smear reader blinded. Smears are considered positive if minimum two parasites were found in 100 adjacent fields.

Earlier, Fisk et al. (1989) reported that CQ at 1 μg/ml had a partial parasiticidal effect *in vitro* on late LS *P. cynomolgi* and *P. knowlesi* schizonts. However, these drug concentrations were ~2.5-fold higher than therapeutic concentrations (0.03–0.4 μg/ml) in humans (Tett et al., 1989; Carmichael et al., 2003), and had toxic effects on hepatocytes that may have contributed to parasiticidal activity.

We examined the effect of CQ on LS development *in vivo* by imaging luciferase expressing *P. yoelii* parasites in Balb/c mice, and followed parasite development in the liver, both by BLI and qPCR, at multiple time points from 40 h through 62 h. We observed no difference in the LS parasite load between CQ-treated (SPZ+CQ) and untreated (SPZ) groups at any time point during late LS development. Our observations at 42 hpi are consistent with those of Belnoue et al. (2004) and additionally showed no differences at 44, 46, 48, and 54 hpi.

We hypothesized that CQ might delay LS development, at least for a subset of parasites, thereby creating a condition of prolonged antigen exposure that might enhance LS specific immunity. All mice, both SPZ+CQ and SPZ, had parasites detectable by blood smear microscopy by 48 hpi, suggesting that there had been no delay in LS development with CQ treatment. This was further substantiated by similar LS parasite burdens in both groups of mice at 48 hpi (**Figure 3**; Supplementary Figures S3–S5). Our study cannot exclude the possibility that a small subset of parasite persist in liver of SPZ+CQ mice, because emerging blood stage parasites might mask the presence of LS forms in bioluminescence or qRT-PCR studies.

The potential effect of CQ to delay the prepatent period has also been examined in humans as part of CVac trials, using highly sensitive qPCR techniques to detect, and quantify blood stage parasites at densities below the sensitivity of microscopy (i.e, subpatent parasitemia; Roestenberg et al., 2009; Bijker et al., 2013). During CVac, blood stage parasites are detected by qPCR at the time expected of untreated individuals (Roestenberg et al., 2009; Bijker et al., 2013), although a direct comparison of blood stage parasite burden between CQ-treated and untreated individuals has not been reported. Similarly, we find that blood stage parasites are detected by microscopy at 48 hpi in both SPZ+CQ and SPZ mice. A previous study in mice reported that CQ suppressed blood stage growth during CVac (Peng et al., 2014), as is observed in human studies (Roestenberg et al., 2009; Bijker et al., 2013). Our results in mice confirm that CQ does not delay LS development nor kill LS parasites, and support the notion that the diminished first wave of parasitemia is likely to be solely due to its effects on blood stage growth, rather than the effect on the number of parasites released from liver.

Chloroquine was once widely used as an anti-malarial drug and was highly effective in clearing blood stage forms of sensitive *Plasmodium* parasites, but use of CQ has waned decisively with the global spread of CQ-resistant parasites. Recently, the impressive immunity observed after CVac has sparked renewed interest in CQ as a component of whole organism vaccines, whereby individuals are inoculated with infectious SPZ under CQ drug cover. However, the mechanisms by which drug treatment converts infectious SPZ into an effective vaccine remain unclear. Using a luciferase-expressing parasite and an *in vivo* mouse infection model, we have systematically evaluated the effect of CQ on *Plasmodium* late liver stages. We report that CQ given at a dose used for CVac studies neither kills nor delays LS parasite development. However, our study does not exclude other effects of CQ on *Plasmodium* LS biology that might impact immune responses, such as an altered repertoire of expressed antigens, and hence further investigation is warranted.

Author Contributions

Conceived and designed the experiments: TS and PD. Performed the experiments: TS, LL, JH, SC, SO-G, and DC. Analyzed the data: TS and PD. Wrote the manuscript: TS and PD.

Acknowledgments

We thank Prof. Jean Langhorne for her comments and suggestions on this work. We thank Dr. Stephan H. Kappe from Seattle Biomedical Research Institute, Seattle for providing the *Py*-Luc parasite line. Technical help by Yvette Robbins during experiments and Dr. Ankur Sharma during manuscript preparation is duly acknowledged. This work was funded by the Intramural Research Program, NIAID, NIH.

References

Behet, M. C., Foquet, L., Van Gemert, G. J., Bijker, E. M., Meuleman, P., Leroux-Roels, G., et al. (2014). Sporozoite immunization of human volunteers under chemoprophylaxis induces functional antibodies against pre-erythrocytic stages of *Plasmodium falciparum*. *Malar. J.* 13:136. doi: 10.1186/1475-2875-13-136

Belnoue, E., Costa, F. T., Frankenberg, T., Vigario, A. M., Voza, T., Leroy, N., et al. (2004). Protective T cell immunity against malaria liver stage after vaccination with live sporozoites under chloroquine treatment. *J. Immunol.* 172, 2487–2495. doi: 10.4049/jimmunol.172.4.2487

Bijker, E. M., Bastiaens, G. J., Teirlinck, A. C., Van Gemert, G. J., Graumans, W., Van De Vegte-Bolmer, M., et al. (2013). Protection against malaria after immunization by chloroquine prophylaxis and sporozoites is mediated by preerythrocytic immunity. *Proc. Natl. Acad. Sci. U.S.A.* 110, 7862–7867. doi: 10.1073/pnas.1220360110

Bruna-Romero, O., Hafalla, J. C., Gonzalez-Aseguinolaza, G., Sano, G., Tsuji, M., and Zavala, F. (2001). Detection of malaria liver-stages in mice infected through the bite of a single *Anopheles mosquito* using a highly sensitive real-time PCR. *Int. J. Parasitol.* 31, 1499–1502. doi: 10.1016/S0020-7519(01)00265-X

Carmichael, S. J., Charles, B., and Tett, S. E. (2003). Population pharmacokinetics of hydroxychloroquine in patients with rheumatoid arthritis. *Ther. Drug Monit.* 25, 671–681. doi: 10.1097/00007691-200312000-00005

Clyde, D. F., Most, H., Mccarthy, V. C., and Vanderberg, J. P. (1973). Immunization of man against sporozite-induced falciparum malaria. *Am. J. Med. Sci.* 266, 169–177. doi: 10.1097/00000441-197309000-00002

Fisk, T. L., Millet, P., Collins, W. E., and Nguyen-Dinh, P. (1989). In vitro activity of antimalarial compounds on the exoerythrocytic stages of *Plasmodium cynomolgi* and *P. knowlesi*. *Am. J. Trop. Med. Hyg.* 40, 235–239.

Guebre-Xabier, M., Schwenk, R., and Krzych, U. (1999). Memory phenotype CD8(+) T cells persist in livers of mice protected against malaria by immunization with attenuated *Plasmodium berghei* sporozoites. *Eur. J. Immunol.* 29, 3978–3986.

Mikolajczak, S. A., Vaughan, A. M., Soliman, J. M., and Kappe, S. H. (2010). A genetically attenuated parasite vaccine does not require liver stage persistence to elicit sterile protective immunity against sporozoite-induced malaria in mice. *J. Infect. Dis.* 201, 1270–1271. doi: 10.1086/651279

Miller, J. L., Murray, S., Vaughan, A. M., Harupa, A., Sack, B., Baldwin, M., et al. (2013). Quantitative bioluminescent imaging of pre-erythrocytic malaria parasite infection using luciferase-expressing *Plasmodium yoelii*. *PLoS ONE* 8:e60820. doi: 10.1371/journal.pone.0060820

Moore, B. R., Page-Sharp, M., Stoney, J. R., Ilett, K. F., Jago, J. D., and Batty, K. T. (2011). Pharmacokinetics, pharmacodynamics, and allometric scaling of chloroquine in a murine malaria model. *Antimicrob. Agents Chemother.* 55, 3899–3907. doi: 10.1128/AAC.00067-11

Mwakingwe, A., Ting, L. M., Hochman, S., Chen, J., Sinnis, P., and Kim, K. (2009). Noninvasive real-time monitoring of liver-stage development of bioluminescent *Plasmodium* parasites. *J. Infect. Dis.* 200, 1470–1478. doi: 10.1086/606115

Nussenzweig, R. S., Vanderberg, J., Most, H., and Orton, C. (1967). "Protective immunity produced by the injection of x-irradiated sporozoites of *Plasmodium berghei*." *Nature* 216, 160–162. doi: 10.1038/216160a0

Orjih, A. U., Cochrane, A. H., and Nussenzweig, R. S. (1982). Comparative studies on the immunogenicity of infective and attenuated sporozoites of *Plasmodium berghei*. *Trans. R. Soc. Trop. Med. Hyg.* 76, 57–61. doi: 10.1016/0035-9203(82)90019-0

Ozaki, L. S., Gwadz, R. W., and Godson, G. N. (1984). Simple centrifugation method for rapid separation of sporozoites from mosquitoes. *J. Parasitol.* 70, 831–833. doi: 10.2307/3281779

Peng, X., Keitany, G. J., Vignali, M., Chen, L., Gibson, C., Choi, K., et al. (2014). Artesunate versus chloroquine infection-treatment-vaccination defines stage-specific immune responses associated with prolonged sterile protection against both pre-erythrocytic and erythrocytic *Plasmodium yoelii* infection. *J. Immunol.* 193, 1268–1277. doi: 10.4049/jimmunol.1400296

Putrianti, E. D., Silvie, O., Kordes, M., Borrmann, S., and Matuschewski, K. (2009). Vaccine-like immunity against malaria by repeated causal-prophylactic treatment of liver-stage *Plasmodium* parasites. *J. Infect. Dis.* 199, 899–903. doi: 10.1086/597121

Renia, L. (2008). Protective immunity against malaria liver stage after vaccination with live parasites. *Parasite* 15, 379–383. doi: 10.1051/parasite/2008153379

Roestenberg, M., Mccall, M., Hopman, J., Wiersma, J., Luty, A. J., Van Gemert, G. J., et al. (2009). Protection against a malaria challenge by sporozoite inoculation. *N. Engl. J. Med.* 361, 468–477. doi: 10.1056/NEJMoa0805832

Roestenberg, M., Teirlinck, A. C., Mccall, M. B., Teelen, K., Makamdop, K. N., Wiersma, J., et al. (2011). Long-term protection against malaria after experimental sporozoite inoculation: an open-label follow-up study. *Lancet* 377, 1770–1776. doi: 10.1016/S0140-67361160360-7

Schussek, S., Groves, P. L., Apte, S. H., and Doolan, D. L. (2013). Highly sensitive quantitative real-time PCR for the detection of *Plasmodium* liver-stage parasite burden following low-dose sporozoite challenge. *PLoS ONE* 8:e77811. doi: 10.1371/journal.pone.0077811

Slater, A. F., and Cerami, A. (1992). Inhibition by chloroquine of a novel haem polymerase enzyme activity in malaria trophozoites. *Nature* 355, 167–169. doi: 10.1038/355167a0

Tett, S. E., Cutler, D. J., Day, R. O., and Brown, K. F. (1989). Bioavailability of hydroxychloroquine tablets in healthy volunteers. *Br. J. Clin. Pharmacol.* 27, 771–779. doi: 10.1111/j.1365-2125.1989.tb03439.x

Vaughan, A. M., Wang, R., and Kappe, S. H. (2010). Genetically engineered, attenuated whole-cell vaccine approaches for malaria. *Hum. Vaccin.* 6, 107–113. doi: 10.4161/hv.6.1.9654

Yayon, A., Vande Waa, J. A., Yayon, M., Geary, T. G., and Jensen, J. B. (1983). Stage-dependent effects of chloroquine on *Plasmodium falciparum* in vitro. *J. Protozool.* 30, 642–647. doi: 10.1111/j.1550-7408.1983.tb05336.x

18

Plasmodium Cellular Effector Mechanisms and the Hepatic Microenvironment

Ute Frevert[1*] *and Urszula Krzych*[2*]

[1] *Division of Medical Parasitology, Department of Microbiology, New York University School of Medicine, New York, NY, USA,* [2] *Division of Malaria Vaccine Development, Department of Cellular Immunology, Walter Reed Army Institute of Research, Silver Spring, MD, USA*

Edited by:
Abhay Satoskar, The Ohio State University, USA

Reviewed by:
Robin Stephens, University of Texas Medical Branch, USA
Andrew Taylor-Robinson, Central Queensland University, Australia

***Correspondence:**
Ute Frevert, Division of Medical Parasitology, Department of Microbiology, New York University School of Medicine, 341 E 25 Street, New York, NY 10010, USA ute.frevert@nyumc.org;
Urszula Krzych, Division of Malaria Vaccine Development, Department of Cellular Immunology, Walter Reed Army Institute of Research, 503 Robert Grant Avenue, Silver Spring, MD 20910, USA ukrzych@gmail.com

Plasmodium falciparum malaria remains one of the most serious health problems globally. Immunization with attenuated parasites elicits multiple cellular effector mechanisms capable of eliminating *Plasmodium* liver stages. However, malaria liver stage (LS) immunity is complex and the mechanisms effector T cells use to locate the few infected hepatocytes in the large liver in order to kill the intracellular LS parasites remain a mystery to date. Here, we review our current knowledge on the behavior of CD8 effector T cells in the hepatic microvasculature, in malaria and other hepatic infections. Taking into account the unique immunological and lymphogenic properties of the liver, we discuss whether classical granule-mediated cytotoxicity might eliminate infected hepatocytes via direct cell contact or whether cytokines might operate without cell–cell contact and kill *Plasmodium* LSs at a distance. A thorough understanding of the cellular effector mechanisms that lead to parasite death hence sterile protection is a prerequisite for the development of a successful malaria vaccine to protect the 40% of the world's population currently at risk of *Plasmodium* infection.

Keywords: *Plasmodium*, liver, antigen-presenting cells, CD8 T cells, liver lymphatics

Plasmodium falciparum malaria remains one of the most serious health problems globally and long-lasting protective malaria vaccine is desperately needed. The ability to interrupt the clinically silent liver phase of the malaria parasite would prevent an estimated 207 million clinical cases every year, leading to the death of one young African child almost every minute (WHO, 2013). Vaccination with attenuated parasites elicits multiple cellular effector mechanisms that lead to *Plasmodium* liver stage (LS) elimination. While granule-mediated cytotoxicity requires contact between CD8 effector T cells and infected hepatocytes, cytokine mediated parasite killing could occur without cell–cell contact. This review aims to put into context the biology of the pre-erythrocytic stages of *Plasmodium*, the unique immunological and lymphogenic properties of the liver, and recent insight into the dynamic behavior of CD8 effector T cells in the hepatic microvasculature to provide a better understanding of the cellular events involved in the blocking of *Plasmodium* LS development.

Abbreviations: APC, antigen-presenting cell; BM, bone marrow; BMT, bone marrow transfer; CSP, circumsporozoite protein; DC, dendritic cell; GAS, genetically attenuated sporozoites; KC, Kupffer cell; LSEC, liver sinusoidal endothelial cell; RAS, radiation-attenuated sporozoites; TCR-Tg, T cell receptor transgenic.

Immunity against Pre-Erythrocytic *Plasmodium* Antigens

While T cell priming against sporozoite antigens is thought to occur in the LNs draining the mosquito bite skin site (Chakravarty et al., 2007), the liver draining LNs are the most likely site of T cell activation against late-LS and early blood stage antigens. However, T cell priming may also occur in the liver itself, for example by direct recognition of infected hepatocytes and or via cross-presentation by the various non-parenchymal antigen-presenting cell (APCs) including hepatic dendritic cell (DCs; Jobe et al., 2009; Crispe, 2011; Bertolino and Bowen, 2015). For an overview on the induction phase of immunity against pre-erythrocytic *Plasmodium* antigens, the reader is referred to recent reviews (Crispe, 2014; Van Braeckel-Budimir and Harty, 2014; Radtke et al., 2015). Here, we focus on the effector phase of the disease and discuss how the various cellular effector mechanisms might operate in the liver, upon first infection of a naïve host leading to disease versus repeated exposure or vaccination resulting in immunity. We present this review in the context of the unique immunological and lymphogenic features of the liver.

The Liver, a Metabolic Organ with Unique Tolerogenic and Lymphogenic Properties

The liver is known as a lymphatic organ with unique immunological properties (Knolle and Limmer, 2001; Sheth and Bankey, 2001; Bertolino et al., 2002; Mackay, 2002; Racanelli and Rehermann, 2006; Crispe, 2009). Its tolerogenic properties, necessitated by continuous natural exposure to innocuous food antigens and commensal microbial products from the gastrointestinal tract, are now widely recognized (Racanelli and Rehermann, 2006; Crispe, 2009; Jenne and Kubes, 2013). It seems likely, therefore, that by choosing the liver as the initial site of multiplication, *Plasmodium* is able to exploit the tolerogenic properties of the liver (Frevert et al., 2006; Crispe, 2011; Bertolino and Bowen, 2015). Less appreciated is the generation of lymph in this large metabolic organ. Plasma flows continuously through the sinusoidal sieve plates and enters the space of Disse (**Figure 1**). Once in the perisinusoidal space, the lymph travels in a retrograde fashion around the sinusoids toward the periportal space of Mall (Reid et al., 1992). Despite more than half of the lymph of the entire body being of hepatic origin (Henriksen et al., 1984; Magari, 1990; Trutmann and Sasse, 1994; Ohtani and Ohtani, 2008), the contribution of lymph formation to liver immunology has been surprisingly underappreciated to date (reviewed in Frevert and Nacer, 2013). By influencing cytokine dissemination, the unique hepatic blood-lymph counterflow principle has important implications for the effector phase of immunity against *Plasmodium* LS.

Most non-parenchymal liver cells can function as APCs (Jobe et al., 2009; Crispe, 2011), inducing either tolerance or enhanced immune responses amongst liver T cells. The state of immune tolerance rather than immune activation is the more typical and frequent condition under the steady state. It prevents liver pathology arising from a constant inflow of bacterial and other microbes from the gastrointestinal tract and blood-borne antigens from the systemic circulation. The state of tolerance observed in the liver is maintained by the production of anti-inflammatory cytokines, in particular IL-10 (Knolle et al., 1995), and other modulators such as PGE2 produced by Kupffer cells (KCs) via ligation of TLR4. Together with nitric oxide, these mediators down-regulate antigen uptake by liver sinusoidal endothelial cells (LSECs) and DCs, which leads to a decreased T cell activation (Roland et al., 1994; Groux et al., 1996). However, KCs have also been shown to play a role in fighting infections by producing IL-12 and IL-18 and upregulating MHC I and II molecules as well as the co-stimulatory molecules CD40 and CD80 needed for activation of T cells to produce IFN-γ (Burgio et al., 1998). It appears therefore that signals received by KCs propel them either into poor and ineffective or efficient APC, promoting a reversal of immune tolerance. Tolerance induction or maintenance is also a particular property of the LSECs (Berg et al., 2006; Ebrahimkhani et al., 2011) with their typical fenestrations. Although LSECs express MHC I and II molecules as well as costimulatory molecules involved in T cell activation, they produce IL-10 upon TLR4 ligation; the ensuing down-regulation of IL-12 restricts the IFN-γ production by T cells thus reducing the size of the response (Berg et al., 2006; Ebrahimkhani et al., 2011). The anatomical location of the LSECs and KCs in the sinusoidal lumen makes them excellent scavengers of a plethora of exogenous antigens and enables them to present these efficiently in the context of MHC I and II molecules *in vivo* (Limmer et al., 2000) for the induction of tolerance. The tolerizing effects of anti-inflammatory responses of liver APCs is typically observed *in vivo* to low levels of LPS. Both human and rodent LSECs upregulate MHC I and express MHC II molecules in response, for example, to viral and bacterial infections or exposure of the liver to IFN-γ (Steinhoff et al., 1988; Steiniger et al., 1988; Steinhoff, 1990). Similar to KCs and classical splenic DCs, LSECs can cross-present hepatocyte-associated antigens to CD8 T cells (Berg et al., 2006; Ebrahimkhani et al., 2011). In contrast, several functional populations of DCs, the professional APCs, are located in the periportal connective tissue of the liver lobule (Sumpter et al., 2007), and they respond to virus infection by elaborating type I IFN, which ultimately leads to the induction of a pro-inflammatory environment in the liver. Apart from the most abundant plasmacytoid DCs, the mouse liver also harbors myeloid DCs and conventional CD8α^+DCs; thus far, the cCD8α^+DCs have no counterpart in the human liver. Amongst the three liver DC subsets, the cCD8α^+DCs have the highest APC capacity.

The Hepatic Cycle of *Plasmodium*—Implications for Antigen Presentation in the Liver

Following *Plasmodium* infection, mammalian hosts are exposed to *Plasmodium* antigens in multiple ways: (1) sporozoite surface antigens released from viable migrating parasites, (2) sporozoite antigens from parasites that degrade or are eliminated by phagocytosis before they reach their final destination in the liver, (3) early or late LS antigens from parasites that fail to complete the hepatic development cycle, and (4) early or late LS antigens, and potentially blood stage antigens, left behind in the remains of dead infected hepatocytes after successful merosome release.

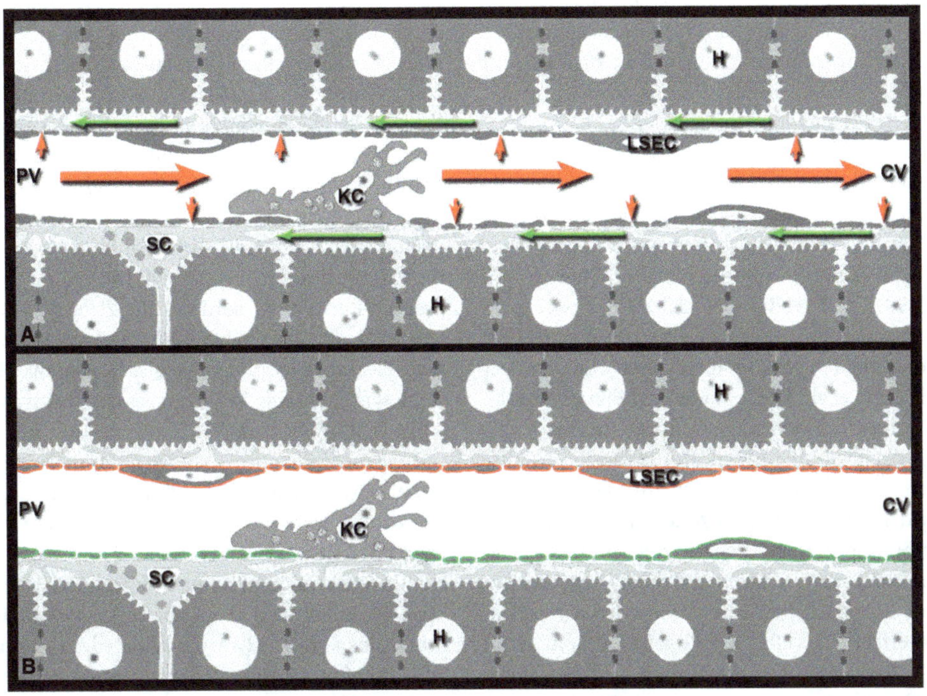

FIGURE 1 | Immunological implications of the hepatic blood-lymph countercurrent. (A) The liver generates lymph by filtering blood plasma (small red arrows) through the sieve plates of the sinusoidal endothelial cells (LSEC) into the perisinusoidal space of Disse formed by LSECs and hepatocytes. The lymph (green arrows) flows inside the space of Disse around the perisinusoidal stellate cells (SC) toward the portal field, while the blood (red arrows) continues its path in the opposite direction, from the portal venule (PV) to the central venule (CV). **(B)** LSECs represent the blood-lymph barrier of the liver: they express both the vascular marker PECAM-1 (red) and the lymphatic marker LYVE-1 (green). The two markers are depicted separately for clarity.

It has been widely accepted that responses to pre-erythrocytic stage antigens are rather low in persons residing in *P. falciparum* endemic areas (Doolan and Martinez-Alier, 2006). The current model suggests amongst others, that the few invading sporozoites leave inadequate antigen levels or that the sporozoites or the LS antigens that are invisible to the host undergo incomplete or faulty antigen processing for presentation to T cells. Consequently, induction of protective T cell and antibody responses by the erythrocytic stage antigens is rarely observed in naturally infected persons. It is also possible that the pre-erythrocytic antigens themselves induce some regulatory T cells or tolerance, both of which can dampen potential protective responses (Espinoza Mora Mdel et al., 2014; Wilson et al., 2015). Immunization with *P. falciparum* sporozoites, however, can induce high levels of sporozoite-neutralizing antibodies (Nardin, 2010) thus emphasizing the relevance of studying the presentation of sporozoite antigens such as circumsporozoite protein (CSP). Protective immunity requires CD8 memory T cells and CD4 helper T cell-derived cytokines such as IFN-γ that elicit sporozoite-neutralizing antibodies and inhibit LS development mainly through upregulation of iNOS and induction of NO in the infected hepatocytes (Doolan and Martinez-Alier, 2006; Nardin, 2010; Dups et al., 2014). Clinical trials conducted during the past decades revealed that synthetic CSP-derived peptide vaccines induce CD4 and CD8 T cells of similar fine specificity and function (Calvo-Calle et al., 2006; Oliveira et al., 2008; Othoro et al., 2009; Nardin, 2010). Another sporozoite surface antigen, the thrombospondin-related adhesive protein (TRAP), induces transient cytokine responses under natural exposure conditions (Moormann et al., 2009) and central memory T cell responses against TRAP are associated with a significantly reduced incidence of malaria (Todryk et al., 2008). These findings support recent vaccination strategies aimed at inducing durable protective T cell responses against TRAP (Ewer et al., 2013). Interestingly, it was shown that long-term residents of hyperendemic areas in Africa, who received protracted daily anti-malarial prophylactic chloroquine treatment to prevent the development of blood stage infection, developed a strong antibody response to sporozoites and LSs, but only a weak response to blood stages (Marchand and Druilhe, 1990; Gruner et al., 2003). In fact, sera from the individuals displaying responses to sporozoites and immunity against LS were used successfully to identify two LS-specific antigens in *P. falciparum* (Guerin-Marchand et al., 1987; Sangani et al., 1990). A similar example of T cell responses to pre-erythrocytic stage antigens comes from the *P. vivax* malaria. A recently published study shows that persons, who are negative for the Duffy antigen and hence are refractory to *P. vivax* blood-stage infection, do develop stronger T cell responses to sporozoite and LS antigens than Duffy antigen-positive subjects (Wang et al., 2005). These studies suggest that responses to the pre-erythrocytic stage antigens, be it those associated with sporozoites or with LS, are indeed inducible. As suggested by others, the presence of blood stage infection, which vastly exceeds the antigenic load of the sporozoites and the LS, may negatively influence the induction of T and B cell responses. Inhibition of antigen presentation by blood stage antigens has indeed been amply demonstrated in human (Urban et al., 2005) and animal (Ocana-Morgner et al., 2003) *Plasmodium* infections. In the following, we discuss how the main liver cell types could be involved in the acquisition and presentation of different *Plasmodium* antigens.

Sinusoidal Endothelia

In vitro studies revealed that during parasite invasion and traversal, *Plasmodium* sporozoites continuously release surface antigens such as CSP and TRAP as part of gliding motility (Stewart and Vanderberg, 1988, 1991, 1992; Hügel et al., 1996; Spaccapelo et al., 1997). In addition, sporozoites can also translocate CSP into the cytosol of mammalian cells by mere membrane contact (Hügel et al., 1996; Frevert et al., 1998; Pradel and Frevert, 2001). The implications for antigen processing and presentation of this phenomenon, which occurs in the absence of invasion, are discussed below. Various cell types of the liver are likely exposed to sporozoite-released antigens. As sporozoites glide extensively along the sinusoids before infecting hepatocytes (Frevert et al., 2005), a substantial number of LSECs are likely exposed to released CSP (**Figure 2**), which they can present for a recall of both CD8 and CD4 effector T cells (Knolle and Gerken, 2000; Crispe, 2011). LSECs have also been established as the primary cross-presenting APCs of the liver (Limmer et al., 2005). However, cross-presentation by LSECs can also lead to CD8 T cell tolerance (Berg et al., 2006). Thus, while LSECs are candidate APCs, their actual contribution to protective immunity against *Plasmodium* CSP or other sporozoite-associated antigens has not been fully investigated and remains rather difficult to predict.

Kupffer Cells

The vast majority of sporozoite entry events into the hepatic parenchyma involve KCs (Baer et al., 2007b; Tavares et al., 2013), resident macrophages and professional APCs of the liver (Crispe, 2011; **Figure 2**). Early evidence supporting this notion came from electron micrographs showing *P. berghei* sporozoites that stretch from the sinusoidal lumen through KCs all the way into hepatocytes (Meis and Verhave, 1988). Subsequently, *P. yoelii* sporozoites were shown to recognize KC-specific surface proteoglycans (Pradel et al., 2002, 2004) and to pass through KCs on their way into the hepatocytes (Frevert et al., 2005). The use of KC-deficient mouse models initially implied an obligatory role of these hepatic macrophages for liver infection (Baer et al., 2007b). A more recent *in vivo* study confirmed the involvement of KCs in the vast majority of all cell traversal events (Tavares et al., 2013), but also demonstrated that some intravenously injected sporozoites use a paracellular pathway for liver infection (Tavares et al., 2013). Thus, while there is no absolute requirement for KC passage, most sporozoite traversal events involve KCs, either directly or indirectly.

Based on the finding that the vast majority of SPECT$^{-/-}$ *P. berghei* sporozoites were trapped in lasting interactions with KCs, it was proposed that sporozoites must use cell traversal to avoid clearance by KC in the liver (Tavares et al., 2013). Of note, once intracellular, these mutant parasites cannot egress from the KC, and therefore die. This is in contrast to viable WT *Plasmodium* sporozoites, which are not killed by KCs, or other macrophages, from naïve mice (Pradel and Frevert, 2001; Frevert et al., 2006; Klotz and Frevert, 2008). Further, the infectious dose for naïve mice is often less than three intravenously injected *P. yoelii* sporozoites (Conteh et al., 2010). Thus, sporozoite infection of the liver is highly efficient, which renders the possibility unlikely that KCs from naïve mice kill sporozoites *in vivo*. On the other hand, 10% of intravenously injected WT *P. berghei* sporozoites were reported to be degraded during KC traversal (Tavares et al., 2013). This disparity could be due to the different parasite species used for the two studies. Alternatively, as the viability of isolated sporozoite preparations varies, some of the *P. berghei* parasites might have been already dead when they arrived in the liver resulting in their clearance by phagocytosis. In general, all available evidence suggests that viable WT sporozoites survive the interaction with naïve KCs unharmed.

In a separate study assessing the *in vivo* responses of KCs to radiation-attenuated *P. berghei* sporozoites (Pb-RAS), infectious sporozoites were shown to down-modulate MHC I and IL-12p40 expression (Steers et al., 2005). However, infectious sporozoite challenge of mice previously immunized with Pb-RAS has the opposite effect in that the expression of MHC I, co-stimulatory molecules, and IL-12 are upregulated. In addition, *in vitro* assessed APC function of these KCs was significantly enhanced in relation to KCs obtained from naïve mice, naïve mice exposed to infectious sporozoites or even mice immunized thrice with Pb-RAS (Steers et al., 2005). Thus, although the prevailing state of immune-tolerance in the liver might attract *Plasmodium* sporozoites to invade hepatocytes where they remain "incognito" as they expand in number, induction of an inflammatory milieu by Pb-RAS reverses the hospitality of the liver to a state of immunologic conflagration that is needed to eliminate the *Plasmodium* parasite. Exposure of mice to doses of IL-12 has a similar, albeit short-lived effect on *Plasmodium* LS (Sedegah et al., 1994; Hoffman et al., 1997). By contrast, Pb-RAS immunization induces lasting protection that becomes refractory to multiple challenges. The reason why KCs respond differentially to RAS versus viable sporozoites is unknown to date. Immunization with the similarly protective genetically attenuated sporozoites (GAS, Khan et al., 2012; Nganou-Makamdop and Sauerwein, 2013) or chemically attenuated sporozoites (CAS, Purcell et al., 2008) may provide insight into the response of KCs, or other hepatic APCs, to sporozoite encounters that are required for protection. Further, careful monitoring of location and fate of the various attenuated parasites may also provide valuable information.

Thus, the hepatic microenvironment from naïve and immune animals is functionally distinct. While KCs from naïve mice become deactivated upon contact with viable sporozoites and eventually succumb to apoptosis (Steers et al., 2005; Klotz and Frevert, 2008), activated KCs may phagocytose sporozoites, in particular if immunization has generated high antibody levels. As in other hepatic diseases (Nagy, 2003), the pro-inflammatory microenvironment created by activated KCs could further enhance the elimination of subsequent cohorts of sporozoites in a local fashion. Depending on the number of attenuated sporozoites used for immunization, challenge with viable sporozoites may allow a few parasites to enter the liver. The finding that challenge of immune mice with viable sporozoites resulted in a very low in

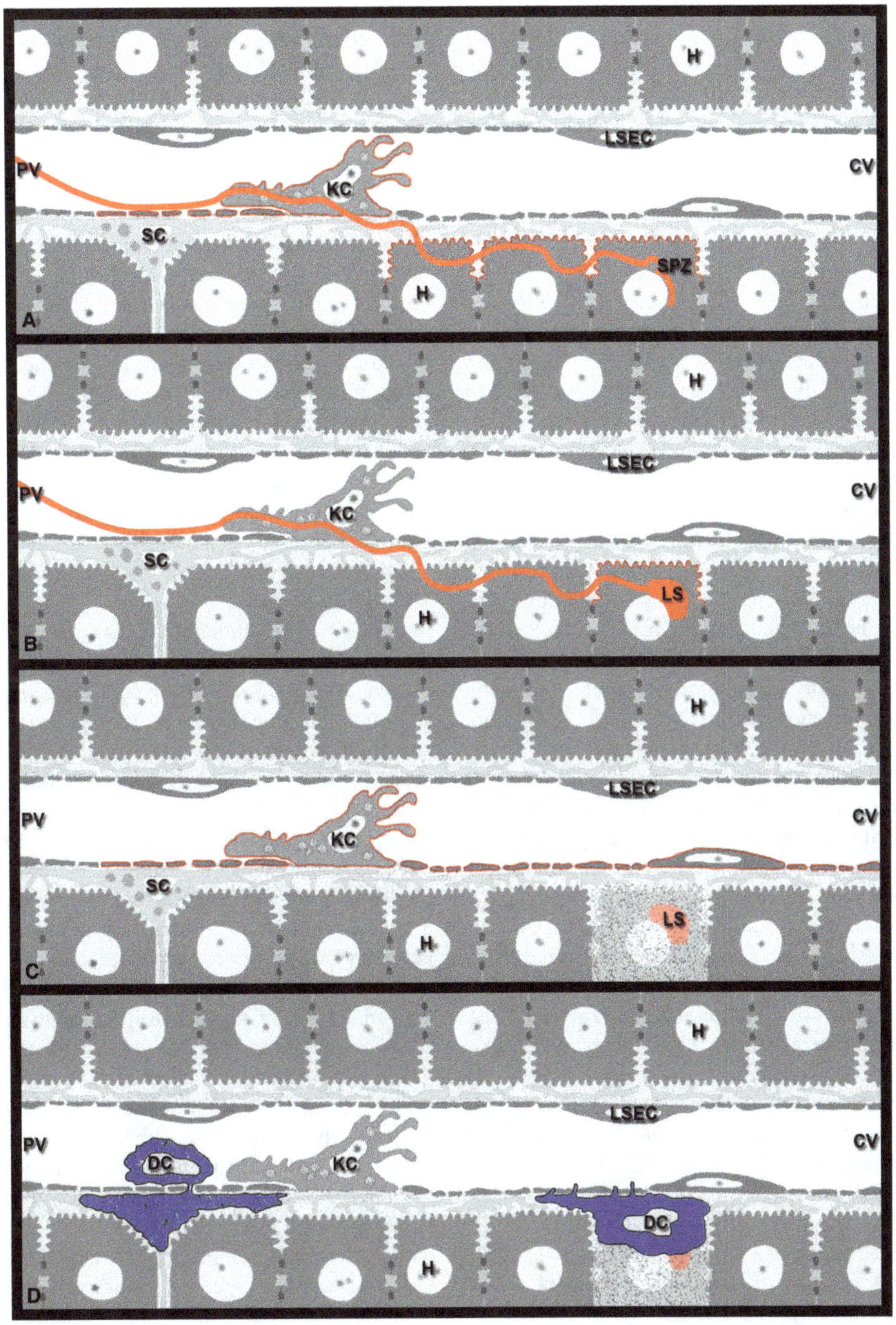

FIGURE 2 | Model for *Plasmodium* antigen presentation in the liver. **(A)** Sporozoites continuously release antigens such as CSP and TRAP from their surface. On their way from the sinusoidal lumen into the liver parenchyma, sporozoites glide along LSECs, traverse KCs, and migrate through several hepatocytes before infecting a final one (red line). In naïve mice, contact-mediated translocation of sporozoite antigens into the cytoplasm of these liver cells may result in antigen presentation by LSECs, KCs, as well as traversed and infected hepatocytes (red outline). **(B)** Sporozoite infection of naïve mice should allow late-LS antigen expression exclusively on infected hepatocytes, i.e., those cells in which the parasites develop (red outline). **(C)** During repeated exposure to viable sporozoites or multiple rounds of immunization with attenuated parasites, infected hepatocytes die after completion of LS development, resulting in the release of debris and leftover late-LS antigens into the environment. These late-LS antigens may then be internalized by nearby APCs such as LSECs and KCs and cross-presented to CD8 effector T cells monitoring the liver. **(D)** Of the various DC subsets that are involved in inflammatory processes of the liver, the conventional CD8α^+DCs are required for the CD8 T cell-mediated elimination of *Plasmodium* LS. While their exact location in the liver is unknown, *Plasmodium* infection likely attracts immature cCD8α^+DCs to the hepatic sinusoids, where they interact with KCs and acquire sporozoite antigens. Extravasation into the space of Disse would allow these DCs (blue) to communicate with CD8 effector T cells patrolling the sinusoids. DCs may also internalize cellular and parasite debris released from dead infected hepatocytes and subsequently cross-present these antigens to CD8 effector T cells, either from within the space of Disse or after traveling to the LNs that drain the liver.

number of very small LS supports this idea (Cabrera et al., 2013). In conclusion, the argument that sporozoites must avoid KC contact to successfully infect the liver (Tavares et al., 2013) could potentially be valid for the immune, but not for the naive host.

Whether KCs act as APCs to recall effector T cells in the *Plasmodium* infected liver is unknown to date (reviewed in Frevert, 2004; Frevert et al., 2006, 2008b, 2014; Frevert and Nardin, 2008). Owing to the unique immunological properties of the liver (Knolle and Limmer, 2001; Sheth and Bankey, 2001; Bertolino et al., 2002; Mackay, 2002; Racanelli and Rehermann, 2006; Crispe, 2009), KCs may respond to sporozoite contact with tolerance rather than inflammation and immunity (Frevert et al., 2006). *P. berghei* and *P. yoelii* sporozoites enter KCs actively by formation of a vacuole and release CSP into the cytosol of these APCs *in vitro* (Pradel and Frevert, 2001), suggesting that KCs can present sporozoite surface antigens to both CD8 and CD4 effector T cells (**Figure 2**). However, a number of reports support the notion that KCs and other macrophages do not survive sporozoite contact (Danforth et al., 1980; Smith and Alexander, 1986; Vanderberg et al., 1990; Klotz and Frevert, 2008). *In vitro* studies revealed that *P. yoelii* sporozoite CSP binds to the low density lipoprotein receptor-related protein (LRP) and proteoglycans on the surface of KCs, which leads to blockage of NADPH oxidase activation, suppression of the respiratory burst, and generation of an anti-inflammatory cytokine secretion profile (Usynin et al., 2007; Klotz and Frevert, 2008). Thus, traversed KCs may not be able to present sporozoite antigens, because they lose APC function and succumb to apoptosis (Klotz and Frevert, 2008). This notion is supported by data from other experimental systems, in which KCs generate tolerance by inducing apoptosis in naïve CD8 T cells in the absence of inflammation (Holz et al., 2012).

Another important finding was that sporozoites are able to introduce CSP into mammalian cells without invading them (Frevert et al., 1996; Hügel et al., 1996). CSP translocation across the cell membrane into the cytosol requires neither the metabolic nor the endocytic machinery of the affected cell (Hügel et al., 1996; Frevert et al., 1998; Pradel and Frevert, 2001) suggesting that it involves a PEXEL motif (Singh et al., 2007). Once in the cytosol, CSP binds to ribosomal RNA (Hügel et al., 1996), which interferes with initiation step of protein synthesis (Frevert, 1999). In contrast to the large number of enzymatically active cytotoxic plant, fungal, and bacterial proteins, which require only a few molecules in the cytosol to kill a cell (Stirpe et al., 1992; Barbieri et al., 1993; Lacadena et al., 2007), CSP has a stoichiometric mode of action (Frevert et al., 1998; Frevert, 1999). The effective concentration of CSP leading to complete inhibition of translation likely varies with the cell type, but complete blockage of the protein synthesis machinery renders uninfected mammalian cells moribund (Frevert et al., 1998). For example, large and metabolically highly active cells such as hepatocytes, which are filled with a huge amount of free and rough endoplasmic reticulum-associated ribosomes, are necessarily less sensitive to the stoichiometric ribotoxic effect of CSP than the much smaller LSECs and KC with a much less developed protein synthesis machinery. In agreement with this notion, macrophages appeared to be particularly sensitive to the ribotoxic action of CSP (Frevert et al., 1998). Nothing is known about the possibility that sporozoite-mediated CSP translocation induces apoptosis in LSECs and KCs. The resulting loss of these APCs from the normally continuous sinusoidal cell layer would expose the underlying parenchyma at the site of sporozoite gliding and KC traversal, similar to the gaps generated by clodronate-mediated KC removal from the sinusoidal cell layer (Baer et al., 2007b), albeit to a much larger extent. As a consequence, effector T cells might gain direct access to traversed and/or infected hepatocytes.

In conclusion, we are only beginning to understand the contribution of KC to sporozoite infection of the liver and the effector phase of immunity against *Plasmodium* LS. KC may be deactivated or even killed by contact with viable sporozoites or by the presence of cytosolic CSP. Alternatively, KC may be activated by exposure to opsonized sporozoites or immunization with attenuated parasites and turned into a source of pro-inflammatory cytokines. A better understanding of these very different scenarios will reveal whether KC (and LSEC) are able to process and present sporozoite antigens for priming of naïve CD8 and CD4 T cells and for induction of recall responses in effector memory T cells.

Dendritic Cells

Hepatic DCs are thought to play a major role in the cross-presentation of hepatocyte-derived antigens (Bertolino and Bowen, 2015). Under resting conditions, however, hepatic DCs are immature. Due to their location in the periportal interstitium and draining hepatic LNs, these professional APCs are not directly accessible to CD8 effector T cells patrolling the hepatic sinusoids (**Figure 2**). Pathological or inflammatory conditions trigger the recruitment of blood-borne DC precursors from the bone marrow to the liver sinusoids (Yoneyama and Ichida, 2005). In a murine model of *Propionibacterium acnes*-induced granuloma model, 6 h were required for a significant number of myeloid DCs and plasmacytoid DC precursors to accumulate in the liver of mice with preexisting granulomata (Yoneyama and Ichida, 2005). After antigen uptake, DCs enter the space of Disse, travel via the portal Glisson's capsule to the draining LNs for antigen presentation to T cells followed by their activation (Sato et al., 1998). Thus, unlike liver-resident APCs (LSECs and KCs), DCs must first travel to the liver, which takes time. Other immune cells also arrive in the liver with a considerable delay. For example, increased numbers of $Ly6C^{hi}$ monocytes, which enter sites of inflammation and get activated locally, were detectable 1 day after systemic infection with *Listeria monocytogenes* (Shi et al., 2010). Further, continuous intravital monitoring revealed that myelomonocytic cells begin to arrive in and extravasate out of hepatic sinusoids roughly an hour after surgical preparation of the liver for IVM (Frevert et al., 2005). Since leukocyte accumulation occurred independently of sporozoite infection, the recruitment of the cells is interpreted as a response to injury.

With respect to malaria, the relative contribution of liver resident versus recruited inflammatory DC is unknown to date (Mauduit et al., 2012). Several studies have demonstrated a critical role of $CD8\alpha^{+}$DCs in the activation of effector CD8 T cells responding to an epitope of CSP. Mice that are missing $CD8\alpha^{+}$DC succumbed to infection in the aftermath of exposure to infectious sporozoites (Layseca-Espinosa et al., 2013). In a murine model of protective immunity induced by *P. berghei* RAS, $CD8\alpha^{+}$DC accumulated in the liver coincident with the exposure to Pb-RAS sporozoites and induced CD8 T cells *in vitro* to produce IFN-γ, an activity that is IL-12 and MHC I dependent (Jobe et al., 2009). Several possible scenarios have been proposed for the cellular mechanisms by which CD8α^+DCs contribute to protective immunity (Jobe et al., 2009). CD8α^+DCs might activate effector CD8 T cells in the portal fields or in the draining hepatic LNs, similar to plasmacytoid DCs, which normally do not remain in the Disse spaces for extended periods of time (Yoneyama and Ichida, 2005). Alternatively, CD8α^+DCs might be recruited by KCs located in the vicinity of infected hepatocytes and extravasate into the spaces of Disse, similar to what has been observed for myeloid DCs in the *P. acnes* model (Yoneyama and Ichida, 2005). This would provide the advantage that *Plasmodium*-specific CTLs could be activated directly in the sinusoid and that the resulting release of cytokines and chemokines could kill LS at relatively close range. Quantitative aspects are worth considering as well. It could be argued that DC accumulation in the liver may not be necessary for CD8 T cell activation, because *in vitro* studies indicate that one CTL is sufficient to kill infected hepatocytes or *Plasmodium* peptide-primed target cells (Bongfen et al., 2007; Frevert et al., 2008a; Trimnell et al., 2009). However, sterile protection against *Plasmodium* infection requires extreme numbers of CD8 effector T cells in the mouse model (Schmidt et al., 2010) and the recruitment of large numbers of CD8 T cells to the vicinity of LS (Cockburn et al., 2013). Together with the apparent absence of direct CTL contact with the dying infected hepatocytes (Cockburn et al., 2013), these data suggest that parasite elimination is relatively inefficient *in vivo* (see below). Therefore, the recruitment of large numbers of DC to the liver may be required for optimal antigen uptake to assure efficient presentation to and activation of T cells in the draining LN. This unusual situation where antigens are loaded onto APCs (in this case DCs) in the liver for subsequent presentation in another organ, the draining LN, may cause a large fraction of the malaria antigens to undergo extensive proteolysis, resulting in a rather limited repertoire of antigenic peptides to activate T cells. Further, if effector memory CD8 T cells are activated in the draining LN they might return to the liver with a considerable delay to kill LS and prevent the erythrocytic phase of the infection.

In conclusion, a combination of DC recruitment to the liver, subsequent DC migration to the draining LN resulting in a limited peptide repertoire, delayed T cell migration back to the liver, and the impossibility to use direct contact-mediated cytotoxicity (see below) may indeed render the CTL response quite ineffective in conferring sterile protection to the host. Clearly, more work is required to elucidate the relative contribution of recruited versus resident hepatic DCs to the presentation of *Plasmodium* antigens to T cells. Dynamic *in vivo* studies should be particularly suitable to shed light onto the local cellular interactions involved in immunity.

Hepatocytes

After crossing the sinusoidal cell layer, sporozoites traverse several hepatocytes before selecting a final cell for multiplication and differentiation to thousands of merozoites (Mota et al., 2001; Frevert et al., 2005). As mentioned above, sporozoites continuously release surface antigens while migrating (Stewart and Vanderberg, 1988, 1991, 1992; Spaccapelo et al., 1997). The first microscopic evidence for the presence of sporozoite-released CSP in the cytosol of infected hepatoma cells came from the Frevert lab (Hügel et al., 1996; Frevert et al., 1998). Temporal analysis of infected HepG2 cells revealed that the amount of cytosolic CSP decreases with increasing maturity of the intracellular LS. Further, because only a few of the skin-deposited sporozoites get a chance to infect hepatocytes, the amount of CSP available in the liver for either direct presentation to CD8 T cells or for cross-presentation involving non-parenchymal cells is limited (Chakravarty et al., 2007). Nevertheless, as *Plasmodium* increases its chances for survival in the liver by preventing the death of its host cell (van de Sand et al., 2005; Sturm et al., 2006; Rennenberg et al., 2010; Graewe et al., 2012; Kaushansky et al., 2013), antigen presentation to CD8 T cells might continue until merozoite replication and merosome release are accomplished. Two groups proposed that *Plasmodium* LS antigen presentation to CD8 effector T cells is restricted to hepatocytes. First, by transplanting bone marrow from C57BL/6 donor mice into lethally irradiated BALB/c recipient mice, Chakravarty et al. (2007) created C57BL/6 $\rightarrow$ BALB/c (H-2K^b $\rightarrow$ H-2K^d) bone marrow chimera. Adoptive transfer of CS-TCR Tg CD8 T cells (H-2K^d) into these chimera inhibited LS development, but not in the reverse chimeric mice (Chakravarty et al., 2007). On the basis of these observations, the authors suggested that CD8 effector T cells must recognize CSP-derived antigen on hepatocytes to eliminate *Plasmodium* LS from the liver. However, a role of radio-resistant LSECs and stellate cells (SCs) cannot be excluded, because these cells do not originate from the bone marrow (Bertolino and Bowen, 2015). Further, sessile KCs are radiation-resistant (Klein et al., 2007) and kinetic studies revealed that 85% of the recipient KCs remain in the liver 2 months after standard bone marrow transfer (BMT); even after 1 year, less than half of the original KC population is replaced (Kennedy and Abkowitz, 1997; Seki et al., 2009; Inokuchi et al., 2011). Therefore, to fully reconstitute bone marrow derived cells in the liver, KCs must be depleted with clodronate liposomes prior to irradiation and BMT (Van Rooijen and Sanders, 1996). This strategy could be used to accurately address the question of the role of KCs as APCs for *Plasmodium*-specific effector T cells. In this scenario, KC may activate CD8 effector T cells to release inflammatory cytokines, such as IFN-γ, to eliminate *Plasmodium* parasites within infected hepatocytes. In a separate study involving OT-I cells, it was observed that these T cells significantly inhibited the parasite burden in C57BL/6 mice and bone marrow TAP$^{-/-}$ $\rightarrow$ C57BL/6 chimeras infected with *P. berghei*-OVA transgenic parasites, but not in C57BL/6 $\rightarrow$ TAP$^{-/-}$ chimeras and TAP$^{-/-}$ mice infected with the same parasites. Kimura et al. (2013) concluded that infected hepatocytes process and present the OVA epitope via the classical cytosolic MHC I pathway.

Two decades ago, immunoelectron microscopy demonstrated CSP in the cytosol of HepG2 cells harboring *P. berghei* sporozoites (Hügel et al., 1996). In retrospect, we know now that these sporozoites were traversing the hepatoma cells (Mota et al., 2001; Frevert et al., 2005), because they were not enclosed in a parasitophorous vacuole as required for productive infection (Mota et al., 2001). Based on these *in vitro* data, it seems likely that both traversed and infected hepatocytes contain sporozoite surface antigens in the liver (**Figure 2**). *In vivo* studies, on the other hand, suggest that hepatocytes do not survive sporozoite traversal, but undergo necrosis (Frevert et al., 2005). As a consequence, sporozoite antigens associated with the remains of these disintegrating hepatocytes are likely phagocytosed and could be cross-presented by liver APCs. In contrast, only infected hepatocytes would contain early-late-LS, and eventually merozoite antigens within the PV (Butler et al., 2011). Indeed, *in vitro* studies with primary hepatocytes indicate that both traversed and infected cells are able to process and present antigen to induce IFN-γ secretion in primed CD8 T cells (Bongfen et al., 2007). However, *in vitro* exposure of primary hepatocytes to either WT or cell traversal-deficient Pb-RAS revealed that only infected hepatocytes process and present CSP via the proteasome pathway (Bongfen et al., 2008), which led to the proposal that only infected hepatocytes could induce their own elimination (Balam et al., 2012). Results from *in vivo* experiments in a murine model revealed the capacity of hepatocytes to induce protection by priming naïve T cells and by presenting *Plasmodium* CSP to antigen-specific primed CD8 T cells (Balam et al., 2012). As mice immunized with WT and traversal-deficient sporozoites exhibited similar CD8 T cell responses to CSP, the authors suggested that infected hepatocytes play a dominant role in CD8 T cell priming *in vivo*. This interpretation appears to contrast with the observation that hepatic CD8α^+DCs play a critical role in the activation of CD8 effector T cells after immunization with Pb-RAS (Jobe et al., 2009). Although it is entirely possible that different cells act as APCs during CD8 T cell priming in response to infection with attenuated sporozoites, these APCs should express MHC-I:peptide complexes, co-stimulatory signals and produce inflammatory cytokines (Zarling et al., 2013). In addition, priming of CSP-specific responses may also depend on the source of peripheral DCs (Chakravarty et al., 2007; Cockburn et al., 2011). Together with the finding that apoptotic infected hepatocytes can provide antigens to hepatic DCs (Leiriao et al., 2005), and the notion that antigen presentation by hepatocytes tends to have a tolerizing effect (Crispe et al., 2006; Bertolino and Bowen, 2015), these data underscore the need for more work to elucidate the cellular events within the complex architecture of the intact liver with its large number of non-parenchymal cells (Racanelli and Rehermann, 2006; Frevert and Nardin, 2008; Crispe, 2011), some of which exhibit greater APC function than hepatocytes (Bertolino and Bowen, 2015).

Several different scenarios can be envisioned for cell-mediated immunity directed against late-LS antigens in the naïve versus the immunized host. For example, first-time infection of a naïve host with WT sporozoites leads to expression of late-LS antigens only in hepatocytes, the only liver cell type that supports parasite growth and differentiation. Consequently, under experimental conditions that involve adoptive transfer of late-LS antigen-specific CD8 CTLs into first-time infected recipient mice, these CTLs should be able to recognize late-LS antigens exclusively on infected hepatocytes (**Figure 2**). Although most merozoites are successfully released into the blood, some parasite debris and LS remnant bodies are left behind and inflammatory cells infiltrate the exhausted former host cell (Baer et al., 2007a). If some of these late-LS antigens are picked up by liver APC, then CTL responses could be activated that would take effect against subsequent generations of incoming parasites. For example, in mice immunized with parasites under drug cover (Belnoue et al., 2004, 2008; Renia et al., 2013), which have experienced several complete rounds of LS development, late-LS antigens left behind after merosome release are likely internalized and cross-presented by hepatic APCs, in particular LSECs and DCs (**Figure 2**). Similarly, repeated exposure of humans to infected mosquito bites in endemic areas may cause hepatic APCs to cross-present late-LS antigens. Thus, under natural infection conditions, CTLs patrolling the sinusoids might recognize late-LS antigens on LSECs, DCs, and/or KCs in addition to infected hepatocytes. Finally, hepatic APCs may also present late-LS antigens after vaccination with late-stage arrested GAS. We anticipate that advances in longitudinal imaging with sensitive molecular tools will reveal the time of parasite antigen persistence and the fate of GAS-infected host cells.

In conclusion, a few parasites engage with a minute number of hepatic APC in a highly local fashion within a huge organ. Consequently, the fate of the LSECs and KCs that have been touched or traversed by migrating sporozoites *in vivo* remains unknown to date. We are confident that tools can be developed and strategies designed to identify the few APCs at a time when the parasites have already left, be it by imaging or otherwise, for analysis of phenotypical changes in response to infection and immunization.

Contact-Dependent Mechanisms against *Plasmodium* Liver Stage Parasites

The mechanism by which effector cells eliminate *Plasmodium* LS from the liver has been a matter of contention for decades (Doolan and Hoffman, 2000). While *Plasmodium*-specific CTLs can induce apoptosis in target cells by formation of an immunological synapse (Frevert et al., 2008a; Trimnell et al., 2009), followed by contact-mediated cytotoxicity, the situation is more complex in the liver, where infected hepatocytes are hidden behind a layer of sinusoidal cells. Histological liver sections, although suggestive (Rodrigues et al., 1992), are inadequate to confirm CD8 T cell contact with infected hepatocytes and granule-mediated cytotoxicity. Electron microscopy offers the resolution to visualize CD8 T cell extravasation into the space of Disse, formation of an immunological synapse, and chromatin condensation indicating apoptotic target cell death (Frevert et al., 2008a). However, comprehensive analysis of the small number of LS developing in the large liver requires a more efficient method. For example, dynamic *in vivo* imaging has been used successfully to visualize subcellular details on the liver phase of *Plasmodium* including sporozoite invasion, merozoite maturation, and merosome release into the blood (Sturm et al., 2006; Baer et al., 2007a). However, identification of the exact position of effector T cells in the hepatic microenvironment by intravital imaging requires simultaneous labeling of several crucial structural elements: the vascular lumen, the sinusoidal endothelium, the space of Disse, hepatocytes, and the intracellular parasites. With the recent introduction of a novel imaging technique, intravital reflection recording, it is now possible to monitor the behavior of T cells in the hepatic microvasculature of non-fluorescent mice (Cabrera and Frevert, 2012). Combined with vascular tracers, cellular or molecular markers, and fluorescent reporter mice, intravital reflection recording represents a powerful technique to define the exact location of effector T cells with respect to infected hepatocytes and neighboring non-parenchymal cells, sinusoidal endothelia and KCs.

Three recent studies aimed to identify the mechanism by which CD8 effector T cells kill *Plasmodium* LS in the liver. Using a 70–90% pure preparation of PyCSP TCR-Tg CD8 T cells specific for the *P. yoelii* CSP epitope SYVPSAEQI, Cockburn et al. (2013) showed that CD8 effector T cells cluster around *Plasmodium* LS in the BALB/c mouse liver signaling via G protein-coupled receptors. Both antigen-specific and antigen-unrelated OT-I cells exhibited the same low velocity inside the cluster. Based on this report, PyCSP TCR-Tg cells were proposed to recruit antigen-unrelated OT-I cells to the site of *P. yoelii* LS development (Bayarsaikhan et al., 2015) supporting the argument that all patrolling CD8 T cells will slow down in an area where adhesion molecules are upregulated, because there is no mechanism for recruitment to be antigen specific, only engagement. Surprisingly, however, both the parasite-specific T cells and the OT-I cells moved at slow speed also outside the cluster (Cockburn et al., 2013). Other experimental systems showed that when non-lymphoid tissue resident memory CD8 T cells encounter cognate antigen, they recruit preformed circulating memory CD8 T cells of the same specificity to the site of infection (Schenkel et al., 2013). This specialized feature of tissue resident CD8 T cells allows for an accumulation of a large number of effector CD8 T cells prior to the protracted process re-activation and arrival of antigen-specific cells induced in the secondary lymphoid organs, e.g., the draining LN (Schenkel et al., 2013). Another example suggesting that recruitment of CD8 T cells is strictly antigen-dependent comes from studies of tumor killing by activated CTLs. The tumor antigen-specific CD8 T cells migrate at high velocity ($\sim$10 μm/min) in the periphery of tumors expressing cognate antigen, deeply infiltrate the tumors, and kill tumors in a contact-dependent fashion (Boissonnas et al., 2007). In contrast, the same CTLs do not infiltrate unrelated tumors and neither arrest nor kill tumor cells that fail to present cognate antigen.

One reason for the large size of the PyCSP TCR-Tg CD8 T cell clusters (80 μm diameter) may be that the CD8 T cells received MHCI:SYVPSAEQI signals from sporozoite-traversed cells in addition to sporozoite-infected hepatocytes. This possibility is difficult to evaluate, however, because the exact location of the PyCSP TCR-Tg cells with respect to the sinusoidal walls is not visible in that study (Cockburn et al., 2013). Whether these cells were intra- or extravascular in this experimental setting based on a single CSP-derived peptide remains to be shown. In addition, whether large numbers of effector T cells also accumulate around *Plasmodium* LS in natural infections or after immunization with attenuated sporozoites, in particular in the large human liver, also remains to be shown. Immunization with a viral prime boost regimen against multiple epitopes in the *P. falciparum* TRAP revealed that much lower levels of IFN-γ producing CD8 T cells were required for protection of humans (Ewer et al., 2013) compared to the high CD8 T cell frequencies necessary for protection in mice (Schmidt et al., 2010). According to the authors (Ewer et al., 2013), the significantly longer duration of *P. falciparum* LS development, which lasts about 7 days compared to the 2 days for rodent species, could be a plausible explanation for this difference.

In agreement with the concealed location of hepatocytes in the liver, CD8 T cells appear to use different mechanisms for *Plasmodium* LS elimination *in vitro* and *in vivo*. Similar to classical granule-mediated target cell killing, which is typically triggered within seconds of CTL conjugation (Berke, 1995; Keefe et al., 2005; Pipkin and Lieberman, 2007), *P. yoelii* specific CD8 T cells rapidly induce apoptosis in infected hepatocytes *in vitro* and kill the parasites efficiently using a contact- and perforin-dependent, but IFN-γ independent mechanism (Trimnell et al., 2009). In contrast, *P. yoelii* LS killing *in vivo* is a protracted process that is contact-independent and require multiple CD8 T cells per parasite (Cockburn et al., 2013). Together with the finding that CD8 T cells from *P. yoelii* GAS-immunized mice rely partly on IFN-γ for protection (Trimnell et al., 2009), these intravital observations suggest that cytokines are responsible for the PyCSP TCR-Tg cell-mediated LS killing (Cockburn et al., 2013). Compared to classical granule-mediated cytotoxicity, cytokine-mediated effector mechanisms operate slower and, depending on the local cytokine concentration, may range from mere growth stagnation to parasite death.

Another study showed that OT-I CD8 T cells accumulate in very large numbers around mature LS in the livers of naïve C57BL/6 mice 40–48 h after infection with *P. berghei*-gfpOVA (Kimura et al., 2013). Whether or not these T cell clusters formed around all LS was not reported, but as LS development is highly asynchronous, some LS had likely matured and released merosomes, which is typically followed by infiltration of the remains of the dead hepatocytes with inflammatory cells (Khan and Vanderberg, 1991a; Baer et al., 2007a). Alternatively, the clusters were formed by T cells specific for late-stage antigens that appear in the hepatocyte cytoplasm, in this case OVA (Bayarsaikhan et al., 2015). Depending on the host-parasite combination, mice can also mount inflammatory responses prior to LS maturation. For example, *P. berghei* sporozoites are 2000-fold less infectious to BALB/c mice than to C57BL/6 mice (Scheller et al., 1994). On the other hand, *P. yoelii* is 50–100 times more infectious to C57BL/6 mice than *P. berghei* (Briones et al., 1996). As a result, the *P. berghei* parasite biomass in the C57BL/6 mouse liver is significantly lower than that of *P. yoelii* suggesting that *P. berghei* induces an inflammatory response not only in BALB/c mice, but also in C57BL/6 mice. Granuloma formation in naïve *P. berghei*-infected mouse livers starts at 24 h after infection and is therefore clearly independent of adaptive immune mechanisms. The finding that *P. yoelii* LS develop basically undetected in the mouse until merosome release is accomplished (Khan and Vanderberg, 1991b; Liehl et al., 2014) supports this notion (see caveat below). Taken together, CD8 effector T cells appear to participate in granuloma formation around moribund *P. berghei*-infected hepatocytes (Kimura et al., 2013). The alternative hypothesis, namely that CD8 T cells cluster around healthy LS that successfully develop in the liver of naïve mice or humans, requires experimental confirmation.

A third study presents novel imaging techniques that proved essential for visualization of the exact location of CD8 effector memory T cells in the *Plasmodium*-infected liver (Cabrera and Frevert, 2012). Intravital reflection recording revealed that immunization of BALB/c mice with radiation-attenuated *P. yoelii* sporozoites (Py-RAS), early-stage genetically attenuated (Py-uis4$^{-/-}$), or late-stage genetically attenuated (Py-fabb/f$^{-/-}$) parasites significantly increased the velocity of CD8 T cells patrolling the hepatic microvasculature compared to naïve mice (Cabrera et al., 2013). After adoptive transfer, CD8 T cells from these immunized donor mice unexpectedly remained immobile in the hepatic microvasculature for at least 3 days, whether or not the recipient mice were infected (Cabrera et al., 2013). The same low velocity was observed after transfer of TCR-tg CD8 T cells specific for the *P. yoelii* $CSP_{280-288}$ epitope (Butler et al., 2010; Schmidt et al., 2011). Instead of migrating with a leading edge and a trailing uropod as in immunized mice, the transferred CD8 T cells were rounded (Cabrera et al., 2013) and met the definition of local confinement (Friedl and Weigelin, 2008). In fact, an 28% pure PyCSP TCR-tg CD8 effector memory T cells exhibited a similarly low average velocity after adoptive transfer as the 70–90% pure PyCSP TCR-Tg CD8 effector T cells mentioned above (Cockburn et al., 2013). Although recipient mice were infected with one million sporozoites, a parasite density that should have facilitated CTL encounters with LS, none of the transferred CD8 T cells, whether of hepatic or splenic origin, approached or made contact with infected hepatocytes under any of the experimental conditions used (Cabrera et al., 2013). Because neither immunized donor mice nor infected recipient mice provided any evidence for CD8 T cell extravasation into the space of Disse, the CD8 effector memory T cells from the immunized mice likely eliminated infected hepatocytes via release of soluble mediators, cytokines and/or chemokines (Frevert and Nacer, 2013; Miller et al., 2014). The finding that adoptive transfer of two million purified CD8 T cells from Pb-uis3$^{-/-}$ immunized mice conferred sterile protection to challenge with 50,000 viable sporozoites supports this notion (Mueller et al., 2007).

In conclusion, while conducted under very different conditions in terms of *Plasmodium* species, CD8 T cell specificity, and time of imaging, common denominators that emerge from these studies are (1) the low velocity of adoptively transferred CD8 T cells, whether antigen-specific or not and whether in proximity to the parasites or not, in the liver of recipient mice, (2) the lack of direct CD8 T cell contact with infected hepatocytes, and (3) the considerably slower LS killing *in vivo* compared to hepatocyte monocultures, where CTLs have direct access infected hepatocytes.

Adoptive Transfer-Associated Phenotypical CD8 T Cell Changes in Other Systems

Much of our current understanding of T cell functions comes from experiments using adoptive transfers of either enriched T cell subsets displaying a certain phenotype or T cells bearing a TCR-Tg for a given specificity. Recent advances in the use of intravital imaging have provided us with a much clearer understanding of T cell functions vis-à-vis the patterns of migratory behavior within the various lymphoid and non-lymphoid organs. The microarchitecture of each organ and the expression of MHC:peptide complexes, chemokines, adhesion molecules and cytokines provide signaling pathways that prompt specific movement and velocity patterns, as well as changes in T cell function. Collectively, these observations suggest a certain plasticity of most T cells is needed mainly to prevent tissue pathology, while simultaneously enhancing T cell effector function against invading pathogens. For example, liver CD8 T cells specific for HBV modulate their IFN-γ production and cytolytic function in an oscillatory and sequential fashion, which culminates in effective reduction of viral load (Isogawa et al., 2005). Th17 cells convert to IFN-γ producing Th1-like cells after adoptive transfer into NOD/SCID recipient mice (Bending et al., 2009; Martin-Orozco et al., 2009). Further, adoptively transferred resting memory CD8 T cells acquire an effector phenotype upon entry into non-lymphoid tissues as indicated by induction of lytic activity and granzyme B expression (Marzo et al., 2007). Some of these observed changes may simply reflect a programmed T cell differentiation, e.g., from resting memory to effector cells, upon reinfection. Changes in the profiles of cytokine production or lytic function may also indicate that anatomical location plays a role in local T cell differentiation.

Cytokine-Mediated Effector Mechanisms against *Plasmodium* Liver Stages

Nonspecific responses to microenvironmental changes could provide an alternative explanation for the finding that antibody-mediated blockage of IFN-γ abrogated protection against *Plasmodium* LS within 2 days (Schofield et al., 1987b; Rodrigues et al., 1991; Weiss et al., 1992), but neither 8 days after CD8 T cell transfer (Chakravarty et al., 2008) nor in immunized mice in the absence of adoptive transfer (Doolan and Hoffman, 2000). Whatever the cause of the immobility of adoptively transferred CD8 effector T cells, this phenomenon is useful to demonstrate that direct contact is not necessary for CTL-mediated protection against *Plasmodium* LS. Blockage of IFN-γ within 2 days after transfer abrogates protection (Schofield et al., 1987b; Rodrigues et al., 1991; Weiss et al., 1992), a result that supports the concept that soluble factors are obligatory for protection when CTLs are unable to approach infected hepatocytes. A role of cytokines, in particular IFN-γ and TNF-α, in parasite killing is clearly documented, both *in vivo* and *in vitro* (Ferreira et al., 1986; Mellouk et al., 1987, 1991; Schofield et al., 1987a; Rodrigues et al., 1991; Weiss et al., 1992; Seguin et al., 1994; Renggli et al., 1997; Doolan and Hoffman, 2000; Jobe et al., 2007; Mueller et al., 2007; Butler et al., 2010). For example, C57BL/6 mice deficient in both perforin and the CD95/CD95L pathway were protected after immunization with Pb-RAS suggesting that parasite-specific CD8 effector T cell-derived cytokines activate mechanisms responsible for the elimination of the intracellular LS (Renggli et al., 1997).

IFN-γ is now considered the central mediator of protection against LS (McCall and Sauerwein, 2010). However, the finding that (1) blockage of IFN-γ does not abolish protection in actively immunized mice (Doolan and Hoffman, 2000), (2) CD8 T cells from IFN-γ deficient mice protect mice challenge 8 days after transfer (Chakravarty et al., 2008), when the CTLs have likely regained motility, and (3) CD8 T cells protect IFN-γ KO mice against infection (Butler et al., 2010) all suggest that IFN-γ is not the only soluble factor involved. CD8 T cells monitor hepatocytes with small cytoplasmic projections that reach into the space of Disse (Warren et al., 2006), but they appear not to extravasate into the liver tissue or form immunological synapses with hepatocytes *in vivo* (Crispe, 2011). Interestingly, while perforin-dependent cytotoxicity plays an important role in the clearance of virus infections from extrahepatic organs, this mechanism was not involved in the elimination of hepatocytes infected with a non-cytopathic adenovirus from the liver (Kafrouni et al., 2001). Because hepatic CD8 T cells exhibited similar IFN-γ and TNF responses and were able to kill virus-infected cells *in vitro*, this finding was interpreted as a relative resistance of hepatocytes to perforin-mediated cytotoxicity (Kafrouni et al., 2001). Alternatively, however, CD8 T cells may be unable to use contact-dependent cytotoxicity because they cannot exit the hepatic sinusoid (Cabrera et al., 2013; Frevert and Nacer, 2013). Of note, CTLs can form two different types of immunological synapses (1) lytic synapses, used for target cell killing and (2) stimulatory synapses with APCs to induce cytokine secretion (Faroudi et al., 2003; Depoil et al., 2005; Wiedemann et al., 2006). It seems therefore possible that CTLs specific for *Plasmodium* sporozoite proteins recognize—from within the sinusoidal lumen—antigens at the site of parasite entry into the parenchyma, form stimulatory synapses with sinusoidal APC, in particular KCs, secrete IFN-γ in a multidirectional fashion (Kupfer et al., 1991; Huse et al., 2006; Sanderson et al., 2012), and trigger the secretion of additional cytokines such as IL-6 and IL-12 that then contribute to LS killing (Nüssler et al., 1991; Pied et al., 1991, 1992; Vreden et al., 1992; Belnoue et al., 2004). Synapse formation with sinusoidal APCs could involve cytotoxic granule proteins (Doolan and Hoffman, 2000; Butler et al., 2010), which might explain the requirement for perforin in protection of vaccinated humans (Seder et al., 2013) and mice (Butler et al., 2010). This scenario could also pertain to CTLs that recognize late-LS antigens on cross-presenting APCs.

How can CTL-derived cytokines reach infected hepatocytes (**Figure 1**)? Considering the high sinusoid-to-lymph filtration rate (Greenway and Lautt, 1970; Laine et al., 1979; Henriksen et al., 1984), the enhanced pressure gradients created by leukocytes moving through the sinusoidal lumen (Wisse et al., 1983), and the highly anastomosed sinusoidal microvasculature, CD8 T cells could conceivably exploit both the anterograde blood flow and the retrograde lymph flow to take control of a large portion of the liver lobule—without extravasation and granule-mediated cytotoxicity (Frevert and Nacer, 2013). This hypothesis is supported by the finding that intravenous IFN-γ inoculation reduced the *P. berghei* liver burden independently of the sporozoite challenge dose (Ferreira et al., 1986). Further, CD8 T cells protect against various viral liver infections and *in vivo* data indicate that virus replication is blocked without CD8 T cell extravasation and in the absence of hepatocyte death (Guidotti et al., 1999; Kafrouni et al., 2001; Guidotti, 2002; Crispe, 2011). Consistent with the notion that CTL-derived cytokines traverse the sieve plates of the sinusoidal endothelia and disseminate via the lymphatic conduits of the liver, adoptively transferred-specific CTLs acted against infected hepatocytes, but had no effect on not infected renal tubule or choroid plexus epithelia (Ando et al., 1994a), both of which are shielded from the bloodstream by a continuous layer of non-fenestrated endothelia.

While the crucial role of perforin expressing CD8 T cells in protection against *Plasmodium* LS is now well documented (Renggli et al., 1997; Doolan and Hoffman, 2000; Trimnell et al., 2009; Butler et al., 2010), the exact mechanism by which this cytotoxic granule protein contributes to the elimination of infected hepatocytes *in vivo* is unclear. CTLs typically release perforin into an immunological synapse (Lieberman, 2003; Pipkin and Lieberman, 2007; Lopez et al., 2013). Unlike Fas/FasL-mediated cytotoxicity, which requires only a few molecules on the target cell and which could therefore potentially be accomplished via small cytoplasmic projections such as TEHLI (Warren et al., 2006), immunological synapse formation involves a much larger area of contact between CTL and target cell (Dustin, 2005; Pipkin and Lieberman, 2007). For this reason, establishment of synapse with the basolateral hepatocyte membrane likely requires extravasation of the CTL. However, CTLs conjugating with hepatocytes from within the space of Disse have not been documented to date, neither in malaria nor in other liver infections. While CTLs specific for the were initially thought to exert a direct cytopathic effect on infected hepatocytes *in vivo* (Ando et al., 1994b), the use of a transgenic mouse model of hepatitis B infection revealed that adoptively transferred virus-specific CTLs abolish gene expression and replication of the virus in the liver in the absence of hepatocyte death (Guidotti and Chisari, 1996; Guidotti et al., 1999; Kafrouni et al., 2001; Wuensch et al., 2006; Giannandrea et al., 2009). Thus, rather than reflecting secretion of cytotoxic molecules and induction of apoptosis, which requires immunological synapse formation with the target cell, the requirement of perforin expression for protection may indicate CD8 T cell maturation in the liver. This model would also link perforin expression to IFN-γ secretion. It is now established that CTLs eliminate the virus by secretion of IFN-γ and TNF-α and that this cytokine-mediated, non-cytopathic mechanism represents a survival strategy of the host to control massive viral infections of vital organs such as the liver (Guidotti, 2002). Clearly, widespread takeover of the hepatocyte machinery by a hepatotropic virus differs from the very focal intracellular development of a large protozoan parasite such as *Plasmodium*. However, all available evidence suggests that both infectious agents can be eliminated via cytokines, i.e., in the absence of CTL extravasation and immunological synapse formation with antigen-presenting hepatocytes. Taken together, CTLs appear to be more likely to engage in stimulatory immunological synapse formation with sinusoidal APCs rather than establishing lytic synapses with infected hepatocytes. However, this aspect of effector CD8 T cell activity will need to be investigated further. Confocal or multi-photon microscopy, combined with cellular and molecular tools for intravital imaging of the hepatic microvasculature (Cabrera and Frevert, 2012), can provide the necessary spatio-temporal resolution to elucidate which liver cell types interact with which *Plasmodium* antigen-specific CD8 T cells and whether discrete epitopes of the still unknown liver-stage specific antigens require specific hepatocyte and/or APC contacts.

Much is known about the cytotoxic mechanisms associated with immunological synapse formation *in vitro* (Russell and Ley, 2002; Catalfamo and Henkart, 2003; Lieberman, 2003; Trambas and Griffiths, 2003). For example, upon *in vitro* conjugation of human-specific CD8 T cells with cognate target cells, perforin rapidly accumulates at the immunological synapse where it promotes cytotoxicity (Makedonas et al., 2009). Although cellular cytotoxicity against congenic hepatocytes has been studied extensively in various virus hepatitis models (Guidotti et al., 1999; Kafrouni et al., 2001; Wuensch et al., 2006; Giannandrea et al., 2009), CTL conjugation with target hepatocytes in the intact liver has not been documented to our knowledge, neither ultrastructurally nor with the combined use of modern fluorescent tools and state-of-the-art imaging techniques. Unlike the continuous endothelium of other organs, which prevents ready access of soluble mediators to the parenchyma, one of the essential functions of the fenestrated sinusoidal endothelium of the liver is to allow unrestricted passage of soluble and small corpuscular substances to hepatocytes for detoxification and a plethora of anabolic and catabolic processes. Further, the liver is unique in that every hepatocyte is in direct contact with sinusoidal endothelia thus allowing screening by patrolling immune cells and exposure to their secreted cytokines. This is in stark contrast to other organs, which require immune cell infiltration for elimination of infected, malignant, or otherwise abnormal target cells. This applies in particular to organs with a tight blood barrier such as brain or testes or tissues comprised of a dense parenchyma with a relatively low degree of vascularization such as joint or cartilage.

In conclusion, it appears that CD8 effector T cells recognize the site of sporozoite entry into the liver, either by detecting antigen presented on hepatic local APC or by screening hepatocytes via TEHLI. Being unable to extravasate and kill via classical granule-mediated cytotoxicity, CTLs appear to eliminate *Plasmodium* LS via secretion of cytokines, in particular IFN-γ.

Cytokine-Mediated Control of Parasite Growth

Cytokines alone can clearly confer protection against *Plasmodium* LS, further supporting the notion that CTL-mediated cytotoxicity does not require contact with infected hepatocytes. *In vitro* studies document that *P. yoelii* and *P. falciparum* infected hepatocytes can be eliminated by direct exposure to IFN-γ (Ferreira et al., 1986; Mellouk et al., 1991, 1994) and intravenous IFN-γ inoculation reduced liver burden in a *P. berghei* model (Ferreira et al., 1986). Antibodies against CD8 T cells or IFN-γ abrogated protection (Ferreira et al., 1986), suggesting that CD8 T cells either secrete sufficient IFN-γ or produce other cytokines that elicit IFN-γ secretion from other cellular sources (Schofield et al., 1987b). Clearly, IFN-γ mediated protection is dependent on iNOS-mediated production in infected hepatocytes (Mellouk et al., 1991, 1994; Nussler et al., 1993; Seguin et al., 1994; Klotz et al., 1995). However, despite the essential role of IFN-γ in iNOS upregulation in infected hepatocytes (Nussler et al., 1993; Seguin et al., 1994; Klotz et al., 1995), the exact mode of operation of this cytokine *in vivo* is not known (Doolan and Hoffman, 2000; Overstreet et al., 2008; Butler et al., 2010). Interestingly, IFN-γ induced iNOS activation was shown to regulate the replication of various obligatory intracellular microorganisms including *Toxoplasma* (Pfefferkorn, 1984, 1986; Pfefferkorn et al., 1986; Takacs et al., 2012), *Trypanosoma cruzi* (Silva et al., 2003), *Leishmania* (Bogdan et al., 2000), *Mycobacterium* (Herbst et al., 2011), and *Chlamydia* (Zhang et al., 2012). An IFN-γ based regulatory mechanism could explain why challenge of immunized mice results not only in a smaller number of *Plasmodium* LS (as expected for a direct killing mechanism), but also in a reduced LS size (Cabrera et al., 2013). In agreement with this finding, the effect of IFN-γ induced iNOS activation may range from a minor reduction in LS growth to complete cure of the host cell depending on the local CD8 T cell density, the level of IFN-γ secretion, the position of the T cells and the LS relative to the liver lobule, and the distance between them.

Thus, it appears that CTLs exert an IFN-γ mediated growth-regulatory effect on *Plasmodium* LS rather than acting in a parasitocidal fashion. To be efficient, this mechanism requires an organ with sinusoidal endothelia, a large *trans*-endothelial lymph filtration rate, and a high microvascular density that exposes every parenchymal cell to CTL-derived cytokines—properties uniquely combined in the liver. Considering that a similar mechanism of cellular immunity has been proposed to operate against viral infections of the liver (Guidotti, 2002; Guidotti and Iannacone, 2013), IFN-γ induced iNOS activation in hepatocytes (Chen et al., 2003) may have evolved as an efficient strategy to control hepatotropic microbes while promoting hepatocyte survival and preserving the function of this essential organ.

Contribution of Cellular Effector Mechanisms to Protection of Naïve Versus Immune Hosts

Plasmodium has developed multiple parallel strategies to evade detection in the liver: the choice of a tolerogenic environment for its initial round of replication, the limited infection of a minute number of hepatocytes in the huge liver, and the change of protein expression from sporozoite to late-LS antigens. For these reasons, it has been suggested that finding and killing all LS during the brief period of LS development represents the predominant challenge the CD8 T cell response is facing (Bertolino and Bowen, 2015). Indeed, this reasoning clearly applies to the most severe malaria cases, namely to first infections of naïve hosts that result in a fatal outcome after only one round of LS development. In these cases, effective CTL-mediated interruption of LS development would prevent the clinically symptomatic blood infection in young *P. falciparum*-infected children and also allow susceptible mice to survive experimental infection with large numbers of lethal *P. yoelii* XL or *P. berghei* ANKA sporozoites.

After repeated infections, for example with non-lethal parasite species/strains or with sub-lethal inoculation doses, protection increasingly relies on the humoral arm of immunity. Challenge of immunized mice by mosquito bite likely allows antibodies to immobilize most sporozoites in the skin (Vanderberg and Frevert, 2004). Should a few parasites manage to escape from the skin, they are likely opsonized in the bloodstream and phagocytosed by KCs. In contrast to liver infection of naïve mice, which is very fast and highly efficient (Shin et al., 1982; Conteh et al., 2010), studies with mice that had been vaccinated with *P. yoelii* RAS or GAS showed that the majority of intravenously inoculated sporozoites are unable to enter the liver (Cabrera et al., 2013). Thus, LS development in the immune host is impeded and extremely scarce, which drastically reduces the probability of parasite recognition by *Plasmodium*-specific CD8 T cells, in particular in the large human liver. These considerations emphasize the crucial role of antibodies in protection of the previously exposed host against recurring sporozoite infections (Vanderberg et al., 2007; Vanderberg, 2014).

Contribution of Innate Immune Responses to Protection against *Plasmodium* LS

Recent studies demonstrate a significant impact of the innate immune response on the survival of *Plasmodium* in the murine liver. Both *P. berghei* and *P. yoelii* infected hepatocytes were shown to sense *Plasmodium* LS and induce a type I IFN response that is propagated by hepatocytes in an interferon-a/b receptor dependent fashion and reduces the parasite burden in the liver (Liehl et al., 2014; Miller et al., 2014). In the *P. yoelii* model, primary infection with a late-stage GAP increased the number of IFN-γ secreting CD1d-restricted NKT cells in the liver thus implicating IFN-γ as a crucial innate factor in controlling secondary infection with WT XNL parasites (Miller et al., 2014). Although lymphocytes were required for the innate suppression of secondary liver infections, CD8 T cells, CD4 T cells, and NK cells, the latter of which constituted the largest subset of IFN-γ secreting cells, appeared to be dispensable as effector cells. Type I IFN signaling was responsible for the recruitment of both CD8 T cells and CD49b$^+$CD3$^+$ NKT cells to the liver, but only NKT cells reduced the LS burden significantly (Miller et al., 2014), which is in line with earlier work (Gonzalez-Aseguinolaza et al., 2000).

Certain differences between the two murine models are noteworthy. For example, the innate immune response to *P. berghei* infection involved the cytosolic pattern recognition receptor MDA5, the adaptor molecule for cytosolic RNA sensors, MAVS, suggesting parasite RNA sensing, and the transcription factors IRF3 and IRF7 (Liehl et al., 2014). In the *P. yoelii* model, IRF3, but not IRF7, was crucial for the induction of the type I IFN response and neither MDA5 nor MAVS contributed to a functional innate response against secondary infection (Miller et al., 2014). Further, *P. berghei* infection activated a considerably stronger innate immune response compared to *P. yoelii*, and interferon-stimulated gene expression was upregulated at 36 h after infection with WT *P. berghei*, but only at 42 h after infection with WT *P. yoelii* (Liehl et al., 2014). In agreement with earlier histological work (Khan and Vanderberg, 1991b), immune cell infiltration occurred midway through completion of LS development for *P. berghei*, but only at the time of merosome formation for *P. yoelii* (Miller et al., 2014). Finally, IFN-γ signaling pathways were upregulated as early as 24 h after infection with late-stage arrested *P. yoelii* parasites (Miller et al., 2014), while early stage-arrested *P. berghei* parasites (GAS or RAS) failed to induce such a response (Liehl et al., 2014).

Thus, many questions remain. For example, is the intense inflammation and early granuloma formation associated with *P. berghei* infection of the murine liver the cause or the consequence of the type I IFN response? Is parasite death required for RNA sensing and initiation of the innate response? Can LS sensing be improved by parasite attenuation? Addressing these issues may provide crucial clues as to which events in the life cycle reveal the presence of the parasite to the host. Perhaps most relevant for malaria endemic areas: does the human host indeed sense intracellular LS if infected with a well adapted *Plasmodium* species?

Outlook and Future Directions

We hope to have highlighted the vast number of open questions associated with the local cellular events leading to protection against *Plasmodium* LS. While much progress has been made on the biology and nutritional requirements of *Plasmodium* LS (Luder et al., 2009; Vaughan et al., 2009; Rankin et al., 2010; Labaied et al., 2011; Deschermeier et al., 2012; Graewe et al., 2012; Itoe et al., 2014), the liver is still a black box in terms of effector mechanisms mediating the detection and elimination of infected hepatocytes. Recent live attenuated malaria vaccination trials in humans and non-human primates as well as work in mice clearly demonstrate the requirement for protection of large quantities of IFN-γ producing CD8, CD4, and $\gamma\delta$ T cells as well as IFN-γ secreting NK and NKT cells in the liver (Epstein et al., 2011; Teirlinck et al., 2011; Seder et al., 2013). Neither location nor behavior in the liver of any of these cells nor their exact modes of action during adaptive and innate immunity has been determined, however. Elucidation of the protective cell-mediated mechanisms elicited by attenuated sporozoite vaccines will aid in the development of a cheap, safe, and easy-to-administer synthetic vaccine that matches this gold standard. As hundreds of millions of people living in endemic areas are in desperate need for protection against malaria, future vaccination protocols should be selected based on their capacity to boost the number of CD8 T cells. Indeed, a multi-epitope malaria vaccine that significantly increases the magnitude of T cell induction has already been developed (Ewer et al., 2013). This so-called ME-TRAP vaccine contains full-length *Plasmodium falciparum* TRAP fused to ME, a string of 20 malarial T and B cell epitopes (McConkey et al., 2003).

Acknowledgments

The authors would like to express their gratitude to all the past and the present members of the Frevert and Krzych Labs for many useful discussions about malaria and the liver. Work presented in this review was partly supported by a NIH grants RO1 AI070894 and S10 RR019288 (UF) and by NIH grant RO1 AI46438 and US Army Research and Materiel Command (UK). The opinions or assertions contained herein are the private views of the authors, and are not to be construed as official, or as reflecting true views of the Department of the Army or the Department of Defense.

References

Ando, K., Guidotti, L. G., Cerny, A., Ishikawa, T., and Chisari, F. V. (1994a). CTL access to tissue antigen is restricted in vivo. *J. Immunol.* 153, 482–488.

Ando, K., Guidotti, L. G., Wirth, S., Ishikawa, T., Missale, G., Moriyama, T., et al. (1994b). Class I-restricted cytotoxic T lymphocytes are directly cytopathic for their target cells in vivo. *J. Immunol.* 152, 3245–3253.

Baer, K., Klotz, C., Kappe, S. H., Schnieder, T., and Frevert, U. (2007a). Release of hepatic *Plasmodium yoelii* merozoites into the pulmonary microvasculature. *PLoS Pathog.* 3:e171. doi: 10.1371/journal.ppat.0030171

Baer, K., Roosevelt, M., Van Rooijen, N., Clarkson, A. B. Jr., Schnieder, T., et al. (2007b). Kupffer cells are obligatory for *Plasmodium yoelii* sporozoite infection of the liver. *Cell. Microbiol.* 9, 397–412. doi: 10.1111/j.1462-5822.2006.00798.x

Balam, S., Romero, J. F., Bongfen, S. E., Guillaume, P., and Corradin, G. (2012). CSP-A model for in vivo presentation of *Plasmodium berghei* sporozoite antigens by hepatocytes. *PLoS ONE* 7:e51875. doi: 10.1371/journal.pone.0051875

Barbieri, L., Battelli, M. G., and Stirpe, F. (1993). Ribosome-inactivating proteins from plants. *Biochim. Biophys. Acta* 1154, 237–282. doi: 10.1016/0304-4157(93)90002-6

Bayarsaikhan, G., Akbari, M., Yui, K., and Amino, K. (2015). Antigen-driven focal inflammatory death of malaria liver stages. *Front. Microbiol.* 6:47. doi: 10.3389/fmicb.2015.00047

Belnoue, E., Costa, F. T., Frankenberg, T., Vigario, A. M., Voza, T., Leroy, N., et al. (2004). Protective T cell immunity against malaria liver stage after vaccination with live sporozoites under chloroquine treatment. *J. Immunol.* 172, 2487–2495. doi: 10.4049/jimmunol.172.4.2487

Belnoue, E., Voza, T., Costa, F. T., Gruner, A. C., Mauduit, M., Rosa, D. S., et al. (2008). Vaccination with live *Plasmodium yoelii* blood stage parasites under chloroquine cover induces cross-stage immunity against malaria liver stage. *J. Immunol.* 181, 8552–8558. doi: 10.4049/jimmunol.181.12.8552

Bending, D., De La Pena, H., Veldhoen, M., Phillips, J. M., Uyttenhove, C., Stockinger, B., et al. (2009). Highly purified Th17 cells from BDC2.5NOD mice convert into Th1-like cells in NOD/SCID recipient mice. *J. Clin. Invest.* 119, 565–572. doi: 10.1172/JCI37865

Berg, M., Wingender, G., Djandji, D., Hegenbarth, S., Momburg, F., Hammerling, G., et al. (2006). Cross-presentation of antigens from apoptotic tumor cells by liver sinusoidal endothelial cells leads to tumor-specific $CD8^+$ T cell tolerance. *Eur. J. Immunol.* 36, 2960–2970. doi: 10.1002/eji.200636033

Berke, G. (1995). The CTL's kiss of death. *Cell* 81, 9–12. doi: 10.1016/0092-8674(95)90365-8

Bertolino, P., and Bowen, D. G. (2015). Malaria and the liver: immunological hide-and-seek or subversion of immunity from within? *Front. Microbiol.* 6:41. doi: 10.3389/fmicb.2015.00041

Bertolino, P., Mccaughan, G. W., and Bowen, D. G. (2002). Role of primary intrahepatic T-cell activation in the 'liver tolerance effect'. *Immunol. Cell Biol.* 80, 84–92. doi: 10.1046/j.0818-9641.2001.01048.x

Bogdan, C., Rollinghoff, M., and Diefenbach, A. (2000). The role of nitric oxide in innate immunity. *Immunol. Rev.* 173, 17–26. doi: 10.1034/j.1600-065X.2000.917307.x

Boissonnas, A., Fetler, L., Zeelenberg, I. S., Hugues, S., and Amigorena, S. (2007). In vivo imaging of cytotoxic T cell infiltration and elimination of a solid tumor. *J. Exp. Med.* 204, 345–356. doi: 10.1084/jem.20061890

Bongfen, S. E., Balam, S., Torgler, R., Romero, J. F., and Corradin, G. (2008). Processing of the circumsporozoite protein in infected hepatocytes is not dependent on aspartic proteases. *Parasite Immunol.* 30, 375–378. doi: 10.1111/j.1365-3024.2008.01032.x

Bongfen, S. E., Torgler, R., Romero, J. F., Renia, L., and Corradin, G. (2007). *Plasmodium berghei*-infected primary hepatocytes process and present the circumsporozoite protein to specific $CD8^+$ T cells in vitro. *J. Immunol.* 178, 7054–7063. doi: 10.4049/jimmunol.178.11.7054

Briones, M. R. S., Tsuji, M., and Nussenzweig, V. (1996). The large difference in infectivity for mice of *Plasmodium berghei* and *Plasmodium yoelii* sporozoites cannot be correlated with their ability to enter hepatocytes. *Mol. Biochem. Parasitol.* 77, 7–17. doi: 10.1016/0166-6851(96)02574-1

Burgio, V. L., Ballardini, G., Artini, M., Caratozzolo, M., Bianchi, F. B., and Levrero, M. (1998). Expression of co-stimulatory molecules by Kupffer cells in chronic hepatitis of hepatitis C virus etiology. *Hepatology* 27, 1600–1606. doi: 10.1002/hep.510270620

Butler, N. S., Schmidt, N. W., and Harty, J. T. (2010). Differential effector pathways regulate memory CD8 T cell immunity against *Plasmodium berghei* versus *P. yoelii* sporozoites. *J. Immunol.* 184, 2528–2538. doi: 10.4049/jimmunol.0903529

Butler, N. S., Schmidt, N. W., Vaughan, A. M., Aly, A. S., Kappe, S. H., and Harty, J. T. (2011). Superior antimalarial immunity after vaccination with late liver stage-arresting genetically attenuated parasites. *Cell Host Microbe* 9, 451–462. doi: 10.1016/j.chom.2011.05.008

Cabrera, M., and Frevert, U. (2012). Novel in vivo imaging techniques for the liver microvasculature. *Intravital* 1, 107–114. doi: 10.4161/intv.23423

Cabrera, M., Pewe, L. L., Harty, J. T., and Frevert, U. (2013). *In vivo* $CD8^+$ T cell dynamics in the liver of *Plasmodium yoelii* immunized and infected mice. *PLoS ONE* 8:e70842. doi: 10.1371/journal.pone.0070842

Calvo-Calle, J. M., Oliveira, G. A., Watta, C. O., Soverow, J., Parra-Lopez, C., and Nardin, E. H. (2006). A linear peptide containing minimal T- and B-cell epitopes of *Plasmodium falciparum* circumsporozoite protein elicits protection against transgenic sporozoite challenge. *Infect. Immun.* 74, 6929–6939. doi: 10.1128/IAI.01151-06

Catalfamo, M., and Henkart, P. A. (2003). Perforin and the granule exocytosis cytotoxicity pathway. *Curr. Opin. Immunol.* 15, 522–527. doi: 10.1016/S0952-7915(03)00114-6

Chakravarty, S., Baldeviano, G. C., Overstreet, M. G., and Zavala, F. (2008). Effector $CD8^+$ T lymphocytes against liver stages of *Plasmodium yoelii* do not require gamma interferon for antiparasite activity. *Infect. Immun.* 76, 3628–3631. doi: 10.1128/IAI.00471-08

Chakravarty, S., Cockburn, I. A., Kuk, S., Overstreet, M. G., Sacci, J. B., and Zavala, F. (2007). $CD8^+$ T lymphocytes protective against malaria liver stages are primed in skin-draining lymph nodes. *Nat. Med.* 13, 1035–1041. doi: 10.1038/nm1628

Chen, T., Zamora, R., Zuckerbraun, B., and Billiar, T. R. (2003). Role of nitric oxide in liver injury. *Curr. Mol. Med.* 3, 519–526. doi: 10.2174/1566524033479582

Cockburn, I. A., Amino, R., Kelemen, R. K., Kuo, S. C., Tse, S. W., Radtke, A., et al. (2013). In vivo imaging of $CD8^+$ T cell-mediated elimination of malaria liver stages. *Proc. Natl. Acad. Sci. U.S.A.* 110, 9090–9095. doi: 10.1073/pnas.1303858110

Cockburn, I. A., Tse, S. W., Radtke, A. J., Srinivasan, P., Chen, Y. C., Sinnis, P., et al. (2011). Dendritic cells and hepatocytes use distinct pathways to process protective antigen from *Plasmodium in vivo*. *PLoS Pathog.* 7:e1001318. doi: 10.1371/journal.ppat.1001318

Conteh, S., Chattopadhyay, R., Anderson, C., and Hoffman, S. L. (2010). *Plasmodium yoelii*-Infected *A. stephensi* inefficiently transmit malaria compared to intravenous route. *PLoS ONE* 5:e8947. doi: 10.1371/journal.pone.0008947

Crispe, I. N. (2009). The liver as a lymphoid organ. *Annu. Rev. Immunol.* 27, 147–163. doi: 10.1146/annurev.immunol.021908.132629

Crispe, I. N. (2011). Liver antigen-presenting cells. *J. Hepatol.* 54, 357–365. doi: 10.1016/j.jhep.2010.10.005

Crispe, I. N. (2014). APC licensing and CD4+T cell help in liver-stage malaria. *Front. Microbiol.* 5:617. doi: 10.3389/fmicb.2014.00617

Crispe, I. N., Giannandrea, M., Klein, I., John, B., Sampson, B., and Wuensch, S. (2006). Cellular and molecular mechanisms of liver tolerance. *Immunol. Rev.* 213, 101–118. doi: 10.1111/j.1600-065X.2006.00435.x

Danforth, H. D., Aikawa, M., Cochrane, A. H., and Nussenzweig, R. S. (1980). Sporozoites of mammalian malaria: attachment to, interiorization and fate within macrophages. *J. Protozool.* 27, 193–202. doi: 10.1111/j.1550-7408.1980.tb04680.x

Depoil, D., Zaru, R., Guiraud, M., Chauveau, A., Harriague, J., Bismuth, G., et al. (2005). Immunological synapses are versatile structures enabling selective T cell polarization. *Immunity* 22, 185–194. doi: 10.1016/j.immuni.2004.12.010

Deschermeier, C., Hecht, L. S., Bach, F., Rutzel, K., Stanway, R. R., Nagel, A., et al. (2012). Mitochondrial lipoic acid scavenging is essential for *Plasmodium berghei* liver stage development. *Cell. Microbiol.* 14, 416–430. doi: 10.1111/j.1462-5822.2011.01729.x

Doolan, D. L., and Hoffman, S. L. (2000). The complexity of protective immunity against liver-stage malaria. *J. Immunol.* 165, 1453–1462. doi: 10.4049/jimmunol.165.3.1453

Doolan, D. L., and Martinez-Alier, N. (2006). Immune response to pre-erythrocytic stages of malaria parasites. *Curr. Mol. Med.* 6, 169–185. doi: 10.2174/156652406776055249

Dups, J. N., Pepper, M., and Cockburn, I. A. (2014). Antibody and B cell responses to *Plasmodium* sporozoites. *Front. Microbiol.* 5:625. doi: 10.3389/fmicb.2014.00625

Dustin, M. L. (2005). A dynamic view of the immunological synapse. *Semin. Immunol.* 17, 400–410. doi: 10.1016/j.smim.2005.09.002

Ebrahimkhani, M. R., Mohar, I., and Crispe, I. N. (2011). Cross-presentation of antigen by diverse subsets of murine liver cells. *Hepatology* 54, 1379–1387. doi: 10.1002/hep.24508

Epstein, J. E., Tewari, K., Lyke, K. E., Sim, B. K., Billingsley, P. F., Laurens, M. B., et al. (2011). Live attenuated malaria vaccine designed to protect through hepatic CD8+ T cell immunity. *Science* 334, 475–480. doi: 10.1126/science.1211548

Espinoza Mora Mdel, R., Steeg, C., Tartz, S., Heussler, V., Sparwasser, T., Link, A., et al. (2014). Depletion of regulatory T cells augments a vaccine-induced T effector cell response against the liver-stage of malaria but fails to increase memory. *PLoS ONE* 9:e104627. doi: 10.1371/journal.pone.0104627

Ewer, K. J., O'Hara, G. A., Duncan, C. J., Collins, K. A., Sheehy, S. H., Reyes-Sandoval, A., et al. (2013). Protective CD8+ T-cell immunity to human malaria induced by chimpanzee adenovirus-MVA immunisation. *Nat. Commun.* 4, 2836. doi: 10.1038/ncomms3836

Faroudi, M., Utzny, C., Salio, M., Cerundolo, V., Guiraud, M., Muller, S., et al. (2003). Lytic versus stimulatory synapse in cytotoxic T lymphocyte/target cell interaction: manifestation of a dual activation threshold. *Proc. Natl. Acad. Sci. U.S.A.* 100, 14145–14150. doi: 10.1073/pnas.2334336100

Ferreira, A., Schofield, L., Enea, V., Schellekens, H., Van Der Meide, P., Collins, W. E., et al. (1986). Inhibition of development of exoerythrocytic forms of malaria parasites by gamma-interferon. *Science* 232, 881–884. doi: 10.1126/science.3085218

Frevert, U. (1999). Heparan sulphate and RNA-binding sites in the malaria circumsporozoite protein. *Biochem. Soc. Trans.* 27, 482–487.

Frevert, U. (2004). Sneaking in through the back entrance: the biology of malaria liver stages. *Trends Parasitol.* 20, 417–424. doi: 10.1016/j.pt.2004.07.007

Frevert, U., Engelmann, S., Zougbédé, S., Stange, J., Ng, B., Matuschewski, K., et al. (2005). Intravital observation of *Plasmodium berghei* sporozoite infection of the liver. *PLoS Biol.* 3:e192.

Frevert, U., Galinski, M. R., Hügel, F.-U., Allon, N., Schreier, H., Smulevitch, S., et al. (1998). Malaria circumsporozoite protein inhibits protein synthesis in mammalian cells. *EMBO J.* 17, 3816–3826. doi: 10.1093/emboj/17.14.3816

Frevert, U., Moreno, A., Calvo Calle, J. M., Klotz, C., and Nardin, E. (2008a). Imaging human cytotoxic CD4+ T cells specific for *Plasmodium falciparum* circumsporozoite protein. *Int. J. Parasitol.* 39, 119–132. doi: 10.1016/j.ijpara.2008.06.014

Frevert, U., Usynin, I., Baer, K., and Klotz, C. (2008b). *Plasmodium* sporozoite passage across the sinusoidal cell layer. *Subcell. Biochem.* 47, 182–197. doi: 10.1007/978-0-387-78267-6_15

Frevert, U., and Nacer, A. (2013). Immunobiology of *Plasmodium* in liver and brain. *Parasite Immunol.* 35, 267–282. doi: 10.1111/pim.12039

Frevert, U., Nacer, A., Cabrera, M., Movila, A., and Leberl, M. (2014). Imaging *Plasmodium* immunobiology in the liver, brain, and lung. *Parasitol. Int.* 63, 171–186. doi: 10.1016/j.parint.2013.09.013

Frevert, U., and Nardin, E. (2008). Cellular effector mechanisms against *Plasmodium* liver stages. *Cell. Microbiol.* 10, 1956–1967. doi: 10.1111/j.1462-5822.2008.01211.x

Frevert, U., Sinnis, P., Esko, J. D., and Nussenzweig, V. (1996). Cell surface glycosaminoglycans are not obligatory for *Plasmodium berghei* invasion in vitro. *Mol. Biochem. Parasitol.* 76, 257–266. doi: 10.1016/0166-6851(95)02563-4

Frevert, U., Usynin, I., Baer, K., and Klotz, C. (2006). Nomadic or sessile: can Kupffer cells function as portals for malaria sporozoites to the liver? *Cell. Microbiol.* 8, 1537–1546. doi: 10.1111/j.1462-5822.2006.00777.x

Friedl, P., and Weigelin, B. (2008). Interstitial leukocyte migration and immune function. *Nat. Immunol.* 9, 960–969. doi: 10.1038/ni.f.212

Giannandrea, M., Pierce, R. H., and Crispe, I. N. (2009). Indirect action of tumor necrosis factor-alpha in liver injury during the CD8+ T cell response to an adeno-associated virus vector in mice. *Hepatology* 49, 2010–2020. doi: 10.1002/hep.22869

Gonzalez-Aseguinolaza, G., De Oliveira, C., Tomaska, M., Hong, S., Bruna-Romero, O., Nakayama, T., et al. (2000). α-galactosylceramide-activated Vα14 natural killer T cells mediate protection against murine malaria. *Proc. Natl. Acad. Sci. U.S.A.* 97, 8461–8466. doi: 10.1073/pnas.97.15.8461

Graewe, S., Stanway, R. R., Rennenberg, A., and Heussler, V. T. (2012). Chronicle of a death foretold: *Plasmodium* liver stage parasites decide on the fate of the host cell. *FEMS Microbiol. Rev.* 36, 111–130. doi: 10.1111/j.1574-6976.2011.00297.x

Greenway, C. V., and Lautt, W. W. (1970). Effects of hepatic venous pressure on transsinusoidal fluid transfer in the liver of the anesthetized cat. *Circ. Res.* 26, 697–703. doi: 10.1161/01.RES.26.6.697

Groux, H., Bigler, M., De Vries, J. E., and Roncarolo, M. G. (1996). Interleukin-10 induces a long-term antigen-specific anergic state in human CD4+ T cells. *J. Exp. Med.* 184, 19–29. doi: 10.1084/jem.184.1.19

Gruner, A. C., Snounou, G., Brahimi, K., Letourneur, F., Renia, L., and Druilhe, P. (2003). Pre-erythrocytic antigens of *Plasmodium falciparum*: from rags to riches? *Trends Parasitol.* 19, 74–78. doi: 10.1016/S1471-4922(02)00067-3

Guerin-Marchand, C., Druilhe, P., Galey, B., Londono, A., Patarapotikul, J., Beaudoin, R. L., et al. (1987). A liver-stage-specific antigen of *Plasmodium falciparum* characterized by gene cloning. *Nature* 329, 164–167. doi: 10.1038/329164a0

Guidotti, L. G. (2002). The role of cytotoxic T cells and cytokines in the control of hepatitis B virus infection. *Vaccine* 20(Suppl. 4), A80–A82. doi: 10.1016/S0264-410X(02)00392-4

Guidotti, L. G., and Chisari, F. V. (1996). To kill or to cure: options in host defense against viral infection. *Curr. Opin. Immunol.* 8, 478–483. doi: 10.1016/S0952-7915(96)80034-3

Guidotti, L. G., and Iannacone, M. (2013). Effector CD8 T cell trafficking within the liver. *Mol. Immunol.* 55, 94–99. doi: 10.1016/j.molimm.2012.10.032

Guidotti, L. G., Rochford, R., Chung, J., Shapiro, M., Purcell, R., and Chisari, F. V. (1999). Viral clearance without destruction of infected cells during acute HBV infection. *Science* 284, 825–829. doi: 10.1126/science.284.5415.825

Henriksen, J. H., Horn, T., and Christoffersen, P. (1984). The blood-lymph barrier in the liver. A review based on morphological and functional concepts of normal and cirrhotic liver. *Liver* 4, 221–232. doi: 10.1111/j.1600-0676.1984.tb00932.x

Herbst, S., Schaible, U. E., and Schneider, B. E. (2011). Interferon gamma activated macrophages kill mycobacteria by nitric oxide induced apoptosis. *PLoS ONE* 6:e19105. doi: 10.1371/journal.pone.0019105

Hoffman, S. L., Crutcher, J. M., Puri, S. K., Ansari, A. A., Finkelman, F., Gately, M. K., et al. (1997). Sterile protection of monkeys against malaria after administration of interleukin-12. *Nat. Med.* 3, 80–83. doi: 10.1038/nm0197-80

Holz, L. E., Benseler, V., Vo, M., Mcguffog, C., Van Rooijen, N., Mccaughan, G. W., et al. (2012). Naive CD8 T cell activation by liver bone marrow-derived cells leads to a "neglected" IL-2^{low} Bim^{high} phenotype, poor CTL function and cell death. *J. Hepatol.* 57, 830–836. doi: 10.1016/j.jhep.2012.05.015

Hügel, F.-U., Pradel, G., and Frevert, U. (1996). Release of malaria circumsporozoite protein into the host cell cytoplasm and interaction with ribosomes. *Mol. Biochem. Parasitol.* 81, 151–170. doi: 10.1016/0166-6851(96)02701-6

Huse, M., Lillemeier, B. F., Kuhns, M. S., Chen, D. S., and Davis, M. M. (2006). T cells use two directionally distinct pathways for cytokine secretion. *Nat. Immunol.* 7, 247–255. doi: 10.1038/ni1304

Inokuchi, S., Tsukamoto, H., Park, E., Liu, Z. X., Brenner, D. A., and Seki, E. (2011). Toll-like receptor 4 mediates alcohol-induced steatohepatitis through bone marrow-derived and endogenous liver cells in mice. *Alcohol. Clin. Exp. Res.* 35, 1509–1518. doi: 10.1111/j.1530-0277.2011.01487.x

Isogawa, M., Furuichi, Y., and Chisari, F. V. (2005). Oscillating CD8+ T cell effector functions after antigen recognition in the liver. *Immunity* 23, 53–63. doi: 10.1016/j.immuni.2005.05.005

Itoe, M. A., Sampaio, J. L., Cabal, G. G., Real, E., Zuzarte-Luis, V., March, S., et al. (2014). Host cell phosphatidylcholine is a key mediator of malaria parasite survival during liver stage infection. *Cell Host Microbe* 16, 778–786. doi: 10.1016/j.chom.2014.11.006

Jenne, C. N., and Kubes, P. (2013). Immune surveillance by the liver. *Nat. Immunol.* 14, 996–1006. doi: 10.1038/ni.2691

Jobe, O., Donofrio, G., Sun, G., Liepinsh, D., Schwenk, R., and Krzych, U. (2009). Immunization with radiation-attenuated *Plasmodium berghei* sporozoites induces liver cCD8α+DC that activate CD8+T cells against liver-stage malaria. *PLoS ONE* 4:e5075. doi: 10.1371/journal.pone.0005075

Jobe, O., Lumsden, J., Mueller, A. K., Williams, J., Silva-Rivera, H., Kappe, S. H., et al. (2007). Genetically attenuated *Plasmodium berghei* liver stages induce sterile protracted protection that is mediated by major histocompatibility complex Class I-dependent interferon-γ-producing CD8+ T cells. *J. Infect. Dis.* 196, 599–607. doi: 10.1086/519743

Kafrouni, M. I., Brown, G. R., and Thiele, D. L. (2001). Virally infected hepatocytes are resistant to perforin-dependent CTL effector mechanisms. *J. Immunol.* 167, 1566–1574. doi: 10.4049/jimmunol.167.3.1566

Kaushansky, A., Ye, A. S., Austin, L. S., Mikolajczak, S. A., Vaughan, A. M., Camargo, N., et al. (2013). Suppression of host p53 is critical for *Plasmodium* liver-stage infection. *Cell Rep.* 3, 630–637. doi: 10.1016/j.celrep.2013.02.010

Keefe, D., Shi, L., Feske, S., Massol, R., Navarro, F., Kirchhausen, T., et al. (2005). Perforin triggers a plasma membrane-repair response that facilitates CTL induction of apoptosis. *Immunity* 23, 249–262. doi: 10.1016/j.immuni.2005.08.001

Kennedy, D. W., and Abkowitz, J. L. (1997). Kinetics of central nervous system microglial and macrophage engraftment: analysis using a transgenic bone marrow transplantation model. *Blood* 90, 986–993.

Khan, S. M., Janse, C. J., Kappe, S. H., and Mikolajczak, S. A. (2012). Genetic engineering of attenuated malaria parasites for vaccination. *Curr. Opin. Biotechnol.* 23, 1–9. doi: 10.1016/j.copbio.2012.04.003

Khan, Z. M., and Vanderberg, J. P. (1991a). Eosinophil-rich, granulomatous inflammatory response to *Plasmodium berghei* hepatic schizonts in non-immunized rats is age-related. *Am. J. Trop. Med. Hyg.* 45, 190–201.

Khan, Z. M., and Vanderberg, J. P. (1991b). Role of host cellular response in differential susceptibility of nonimmunized BALB/C mice to *Plasmodium berghei* and *Plasmodium yoelii* sporozoites. *Infect. Immun.* 59, 2529–2534.

Kimura, K., Kimura, D., Matsushima, Y., Miyakoda, M., Honma, K., Yuda, M., et al. (2013). $CD8^+$ T cells specific for a malaria cytoplasmic antigen form clusters around infected hepatocytes and are protective at the liver stage of infection. *Infect Immun.* 81, 3825–3834. doi: 10.1128/IAI.00570-13

Klein, I., Cornejo, J. C., Polakos, N. K., John, B., Wuensch, S. A., Topham, D. J., et al. (2007). Kupffer cell heterogeneity: functional properties of bone marrow derived and sessile hepatic macrophages. *Blood* 110, 4077–4085. doi: 10.1182/blood-2007-02-073841

Klotz, C., and Frevert, U. (2008). *Plasmodium yoelii* sporozoites modulate cytokine profile and induce apoptosis in murine Kupffer cells. *Int. J. Parasitol.* 38, 1639–1650. doi: 10.1016/j.ijpara.2008.05.018

Klotz, F. W., Scheller, L. F., Seguin, M. C., Kumar, N., Marletta, M. A., Green, S. J., et al. (1995). Co-localization of inducible-nitric oxide synthase and *Plasmodium berghei* in hepatocytes from rats immunized with irradiated sporozoites. *J. Immunol.* 154, 3391–3395.

Knolle, P. A., and Gerken, G. (2000). Local control of the immune response in the liver. *Immunol. Rev.* 174, 21–34. doi: 10.1034/j.1600-0528.2002.017408.x

Knolle, P. A., and Limmer, A. (2001). Neighborhood politics: the immunoregulatory function of organ-resident liver endothelial cells. *Trends Immunol.* 22, 432–437. doi: 10.1016/S1471-4906(01)01957-3

Knolle, P. A., Schlaak, J., Uhrig, A., Kempf, P., Meyer Zum Büschenfelde, K.-H., and Gerken, G. (1995). Human Kupffer cells secrete IL-10 in response to lipopolysaccharide (LPS) challenge. *J. Hepatol.* 22, 226–229. doi: 10.1016/0168-8278(95)80433-1

Kupfer, A., Mosmann, T. R., and Kupfer, H. (1991). Polarized expression of cytokines in cell conjugates of helper T cells and splenic B cells. *Proc. Natl. Acad. Sci. U.S.A.* 88, 775–779. doi: 10.1073/pnas.88.3.775

Labaied, M., Jayabalasingham, B., Bano, N., Cha, S. J., Sandoval, J., Guan, G., et al. (2011). *Plasmodium* salvages cholesterol internalized by LDL and synthesized *de novo* in the liver. *Cell. Microbiol.* 13, 569–586. doi: 10.1111/j.1462-5822.2010.01555.x

Lacadena, J., Alvarez-Garcia, E., Carreras-Sangra, N., Herrero-Galan, E., Alegre-Cebollada, J., Garcia-Ortega, L., et al. (2007). Fungal ribotoxins: molecular dissection of a family of natural killers. *FEMS Microbiol. Rev.* 31, 212–237. doi: 10.1111/j.1574-6976.2006.00063.x

Laine, G. A., Hall, J. T., Laine, S. H., and Granger, J. (1979). Transsinusoidal fluid dynamics in canine liver during venous hypertension. *Circ. Res.* 45, 317–323. doi: 10.1161/01.RES.45.3.317

Layseca-Espinosa, E., Korniotis, S., Montandon, R., Gras, C., Bouillie, M., Gonzalez-Amaro, R., et al. (2013). CCL22-producing $CD8\alpha^-$ myeloid dendritic cells mediate regulatory T cell recruitment in response to G-CSF treatment. *J. Immunol.* 191, 2266–2272. doi: 10.4049/jimmunol.1202307

Leiriao, P., Mota, M. M., and Rodriguez, A. (2005). Apoptotic *Plasmodium*-infected hepatocytes provide antigens to liver dendritic cells. *J. Infect. Dis.* 191, 1576–1581. doi: 10.1086/429635

Lieberman, J. (2003). The ABCs of granule-mediated cytotoxicity: new weapons in the arsenal. *Nat. Rev. Immunol.* 3, 361–370. doi: 10.1038/nri1083

Liehl, P., Zuzarte-Luis, V., Chan, J., Zillinger, T., Baptista, F., Carapau, D., et al. (2014). Host-cell sensors for *Plasmodium* activate innate immunity against liver-stage infection. *Nat. Med.* 20, 47–53. doi: 10.1038/nm.3424

Limmer, A., Ohl, J., Kurts, C., Ljunggren, H. G., Reiss, Y., Groettrup, M., et al. (2000). Efficient presentation of exogenous antigen by liver endothelial cells to CD8+ T cells results in antigen-specific T-cell tolerance. *Nat. Med.* 6, 1348–1354. doi: 10.1038/82161

Limmer, A., Ohl, J., Wingender, G., Berg, M., Jungerkes, F., Schumak, B., et al. (2005). Cross-presentation of oral antigens by liver sinusoidal endothelial cells leads to CD8 T cell tolerance. *Eur. J. Immunol.* 35, 2970–2981. doi: 10.1002/eji.200526034

Lopez, J. A., Susanto, O., Jenkins, M. R., Lukoyanova, N., Sutton, V. R., Law, R. H., et al. (2013). Perforin forms transient pores on the target cell plasma membrane to facilitate rapid access of granzymes during killer cell attack. *Blood* 121, 2659–2668. doi: 10.1182/blood-2012-07-446146

Luder, C. G., Stanway, R. R., Chaussepied, M., Langsley, G., and Heussler, V. T. (2009). Intracellular survival of apicomplexan parasites and host cell modification. *Int. J. Parasitol.* 39, 163–173. doi: 10.1016/j.ijpara.2008.09.013

Mackay, I. R. (2002). Hepatoimmunology: a perspective. *Immunol. Cell Biol.* 80, 36–44. doi: 10.1046/j.1440-1711.2002.01063.x

Magari, S. (1990). Hepatic lymphatic system: structure and function. *J. Gastroenterol. Hepatol.* 5, 82–93. doi: 10.1111/j.1440-1746.1990.tb01769.x

Makedonas, G., Banerjee, P. P., Pandey, R., Hersperger, A. R., Sanborn, K. B., Hardy, G. A., et al. (2009). Rapid up-regulation and granule-independent transport of perforin to the immunological synapse define a novel mechanism of antigen-specific $CD8^+$ T cell cytotoxic activity. *J. Immunol.* 182, 5560–5569. doi: 10.4049/jimmunol.0803945

Marchand, C., and Druilhe, P. (1990). How to select *Plasmodium falciparum* pre-erythrocytic antigens in an expression library without defined probe. *Bull. World Health Organ.* 68(Suppl.), 158–164.

Martin-Orozco, N., Chung, Y., Chang, S. H., Wang, Y. H., and Dong, C. (2009). Th17 cells promote pancreatic inflammation but only induce diabetes efficiently in lymphopenic hosts after conversion into Th1 cells. *Eur. J. Immunol.* 39, 216–224. doi: 10.1002/eji.200838475

Marzo, A. L., Yagita, H., and Lefrancois, L. (2007). Cutting edge: migration to nonlymphoid tissues results in functional conversion of central to effector memory CD8 T cells. *J. Immunol.* 179, 36–40. doi: 10.4049/jimmunol.179.1.36

Mauduit, M., See, P., Peng, K., Renia, L., and Ginhoux, F. (2012). Dendritic cells and the malaria pre-erythrocytic stage. *Immunol. Res.* 53, 115–126. doi: 10.1007/s12026-012-8269-7

McCall, M. B., and Sauerwein, R. W. (2010). Interferon-γ—central mediator of protective immune responses against the pre-erythrocytic and blood stage of malaria. *J. Leukoc. Biol.* 88, 1131–1143. doi: 10.1189/jlb.0310137

McConkey, S. J., Reece, W. H., Moorthy, V. S., Webster, D., Dunachie, S., Butcher, G., et al. (2003). Enhanced T-cell immunogenicity of plasmid DNA vaccines boosted by recombinant modified vaccinia virus Ankara in humans. *Nat. Med.* 9, 729–735. doi: 10.1038/nm881

Meis, J. F., and Verhave, J. P. (1988). Exoerythrocytic development of malarial parasites. *Adv. Parasitol.* 27, 1–61. doi: 10.1016/S0065-308X(08)60352-8

Mellouk, S., Green, S. J., Nacy, C. A., and Hoffman, S. L. (1991). IFN-γ inhibits development of *Plasmodium berghei* exoerythrocytic stages in hepatocytes by an L-arginine-dependent effector mechanism. *J. Immunol.* 146, 3971–3976.

Mellouk, S., Hoffman, S. L., Liu, Z. Z., De La Vega, P., Billiar, T. R., and Nussler, A. K. (1994). Nitric oxide-mediated antiplasmodial activity in human and murine hepatocytes induced by gamma interferon and the parasite itself: enhancement by exogenous tetrahydrobiopterin. *Infect. Immun.* 62, 4043–4046.

Mellouk, S., Maheshwari, R. K., Rhodes-Feuilette, A., Beaudoin, R. L., Berbibuier, N., Matile, H., et al. (1987). Inhibitory activity of interferons and interleukin 1 on the development of *Plasmodium falciparum* in human hepatocyte cultures. *J. Immunol.* 139, 4192–4195.

Miller, J. L., Sack, B. K., Baldwin, M., Vaughan, A. M., and Kappe, S. H. (2014). Interferon-mediated innate immune responses against malaria parasite liver stages. *Cell Rep.* 7, 436–447. doi: 10.1016/j.celrep.2014.03.018

Moormann, A. M., Sumba, P. O., Tisch, D. J., Embury, P., King, C. H., Kazura, J. W., et al. (2009). Stability of interferon-gamma and interleukin-10 responses to *Plasmodium falciparum* liver stage antigen 1 and thrombospondin-related adhesive protein immunodominant epitopes in a highland population from Western Kenya. *Am. J. Trop. Med. Hyg.* 81, 489–495.

Mota, M. M., Pradel, G., Vanderberg, J. P., Hafalla, J. C., Frevert, U., Nussenzweig, R. S., et al. (2001). Migration of *Plasmodium* sporozoites through cells before infection. *Science* 291, 141–144. doi: 10.1126/science.291.5501.141

Mueller, A. K., Deckert, M., Heiss, K., Goetz, K., Matuschewski, K., and Schluter, D. (2007). Genetically attenuated *Plasmodium berghei* liver stages persist and elicit sterile protection primarily via CD8 T cells. *Am. J. Pathol.* 171, 107–115. doi: 10.2353/ajpath.2007.060792

Nagy, L. E. (2003). Recent insights into the role of the innate immune system in the development of alcoholic liver disease. *Exp. Biol. Med. (Maywood)* 228, 882–890.

Nardin, E. (2010). The past decade in malaria synthetic peptide vaccine clinical trials. *Hum. Vaccin.* 6, 27–38.

Nganou-Makamdop, K., and Sauerwein, R. W. (2013). Liver or blood-stage arrest during malaria sporozoite immunization: the later the better? *Trends Parasitol.* doi: 10.1016/j.pt.2013.03.008 [Epub ahead of print].

Nüssler, A., Pied, S., Goma, J., Rénia, L., Miltgen, F., Grau, G. E., et al. (1991). TNF inhibits malaria hepatic stages in vitro via synthesis of IL-6. *Int. Immunol.* 3, 317–321. doi: 10.1093/intimm/3.4.317

Nussler, A. K., Renia, L., Pasquetto, V., Miltgen, F., Matile, H., and Mazier, D. (1993). In vivo induction of the nitric oxide pathway in hepatocytes after injection with irradiated malaria sporozoites, malaria blood parasites or adjuvants. *Eur. J. Immunol.* 23, 882–887. doi: 10.1002/eji.1830230417

Ocana-Morgner, C., Mota, M. M., and Rodriguez, A. (2003). Malaria blood stage suppression of liver stage immunity by dendritic cells. *J. Exp. Med.* 197, 143–151. doi: 10.1084/jem.20021072

Ohtani, O., and Ohtani, Y. (2008). Lymph circulation in the liver. *Anat. Rec. (Hoboken)* 291, 643–652. doi: 10.1002/ar.20681

Oliveira, G. A., Kumar, K. A., Calvo-Calle, J. M., Othoro, C., Altszuler, D., Nussenzweig, V., et al. (2008). Class II-restricted protective immunity induced by malaria sporozoites. *Infect. Immun.* 76, 1200–1206. doi: 10.1128/IAI.00566-07

Othoro, C., Johnston, D., Lee, R., Soverow, J., Bystryn, J.-C., and Nardin, E. (2009). Enhanced immunogenicity of *Plasmodium falciparum* peptide vaccines using a topical adjuvant containing a potent synthetic Toll-like receptor 7 agonist, imiquimod. *Infect. Immun.* 77, 739–748. doi: 10.1128/IAI.00974-08

Overstreet, M. G., Cockburn, I. A., Chen, Y. C., and Zavala, F. (2008). Protective CD8 T cells against *Plasmodium* liver stages: immunobiology of an 'unnatural' immune response. *Immunol. Rev.* 225, 272–283. doi: 10.1111/j.1600-065X.2008.00671.x

Pfefferkorn, E. R. (1984). Interferon gamma blocks the growth of *Toxoplasma gondii* in human fibroblasts by inducing the host cells to degrade tryptophan. *Proc. Natl. Acad. Sci. U.S.A.* 81, 908–912. doi: 10.1073/pnas.81.3.908

Pfefferkorn, E. R. (1986). Interferon gamma and the growth of *Toxoplasma gondii* in fibroblasts. *Ann. Inst. Pasteur. Microbiol.* 137A, 348–352. doi: 10.1016/S0769-2609(86)80047-3

Pfefferkorn, E. R., Eckel, M., and Rebhun, S. (1986). Interferon-gamma suppresses the growth of *Toxoplasma gondii* in human fibroblasts through starvation for tryptophan. *Mol. Biochem. Parasitol.* 20, 215–224. doi: 10.1016/0166-6851(86)90101-5

Pied, S., Civas, A., Berlot-Picard, F., Rénia, L., Miltgen, F., Gentilini, M., et al. (1992). IL-6 induced by IL-1 inhibits malaria pre-erythrocytic stages but its secretion is down-regulated by the parasite. *J. Immunol.* 146, 197–201.

Pied, S., Rénia, L., Nüssler, A., Miltgen, F., and Mazier, D. (1991). Inhibitory activity of IL-6 on malaria hepatic stages. *Parasite Immunol.* 13, 211–217. doi: 10.1111/j.1365-3024.1991.tb00276.x

Pipkin, M. E., and Lieberman, J. (2007). Delivering the kiss of death: progress on understanding how perforin works. *Curr. Opin. Immunol.* 19, 301–308. doi: 10.1016/j.coi.2007.04.011

Pradel, G., and Frevert, U. (2001). *Plasmodium* sporozoites actively enter and pass through Kupffer cells prior to hepatocyte invasion. *Hepatology* 33, 1154–1165. doi: 10.1053/jhep.2001.24237

Pradel, G., Garapaty, S., and Frevert, U. (2002). Proteoglycans mediate malaria sporozoite targeting to the liver. *Mol. Microbiol.* 45, 637–651. doi: 10.1046/j.1365-2958.2002.03057.x

Pradel, G., Garapaty, S., and Frevert, U. (2004). Kupffer and stellate cell proteoglycans mediate malaria sporozoite targeting to the liver. *Comp. Hepatol.* 3(Suppl. 1), S47. doi: 10.1046/j.1365-2958.2002.03057.x

Purcell, L. A., Wong, K. A., Yanow, S. K., Lee, M., Spithill, T. W., and Rodriguez, A. (2008). Chemically attenuated *Plasmodium* sporozoites induce specific immune responses, sterile immunity and cross-protection against heterologous challenge. *Vaccine* 26, 4880–4884. doi: 10.1016/j.vaccine.2008.07.017

Racanelli, V., and Rehermann, B. (2006). The liver as an immunological organ. *Hepatology* 43, S54–S62. doi: 10.1002/hep.21060

Radtke, A. J., Kastenmuller, W., Espinosa, D. A., Gerner, M. Y., Tse, S. W., Sinnis, P., et al. (2015). Lymph-node resident CD8α+ dendritic cells capture antigens from migratory malaria sporozoites and induce CD8$^+$ T cell responses. *PLoS Pathog.* 11:e1004637. doi: 10.1371/journal.ppat.1004637

Rankin, K. E., Graewe, S., Heussler, V. T., and Stanway, R. R. (2010). Imaging liver-stage malaria parasites. *Cell. Microbiol.* 12, 569–579. doi: 10.1111/j.1462-5822.2010.01454.x

Reid, L. M., Fiorino, A. S., Sigal, S. H., Brill, S., and Holst, P. A. (1992). Extracellular matrix gradients in the space of Disse: relevance to liver biology. *Hepatology* 15, 1198–1203. doi: 10.1002/hep.1840150635

Renggli, J., Hahne, M., Matile, H., Betschart, B., Tschopp, J., and Corradin, G. (1997). Elimination of *P. berghei* liver stages is independent of Fas (CD95/Apo-I) or perforin-mediated cytotoxicity. *Parasite Immunol.* 19, 145–148. doi: 10.1046/j.1365-3024.1997.d01-190.x

Renia, L., Gruner, A. C., Mauduit, M., and Snounou, G. (2013). Vaccination using normal live sporozoites under drug treatment. *Methods Mol. Biol.* 923, 567–576. doi: 10.1007/978-1-62703-026-7_39

Rennenberg, A., Lehmann, C., Heitmann, A., Witt, T., Hansen, G., Nagarajan, K., et al. (2010). Exoerythrocytic *Plasmodium* parasites secrete a cysteine protease inhibitor involved in sporozoite invasion and capable of blocking cell death of host hepatocytes. *PLoS Pathog.* 6:e1000825. doi: 10.1371/journal.ppat.1000825

Rodrigues, M., Nussenzweig, R. S., Romero, P., and Zavala, F. (1992). The in vivo cytotoxic activity of CD8$^+$ T cell clones correlates with their levels of expression of adhesion molecules. *J. Exp. Med.* 175, 895–905. doi: 10.1084/jem.175.4.895

Rodrigues, M. M., Cordey, A. S., Arreaza, G., Corradin, G., Romero, P., Maryanski, J. L., et al. (1991). CD8$^+$ cytolytic T cell clones derived against the *Plasmodium yoelii* circumsporozoite protein protect against malaria. *Int. Immunol.* 3, 579–585. doi: 10.1093/intimm/3.6.579

Roland, C. R., Walp, L., Stack, R. M., and Flye, M. W. (1994). Outcome of Kupffer cell antigen presentation to a cloned murine Th1 lymphocyte depends on the inducibility of nitric oxide synthase by IFN-gamma. *J. Immunol.* 153, 5453–5464.

Russell, J. H., and Ley, T. J. (2002). Lymphocyte-mediated cytotoxicity. *Annu. Rev. Immunol.* 20, 323–370. doi: 10.1146/annurev.immunol.20.100201.131730

Sanderson, N. S., Puntel, M., Kroeger, K. M., Bondale, N. S., Swerdlow, M., Iranmanesh, N., et al. (2012). Cytotoxic immunological synapses do not restrict the action of interferon-gamma to antigenic target cells. *Proc. Natl. Acad. Sci. U.S.A.* 109, 7835–7840. doi: 10.1073/pnas.1116058109

Sangani, B., Sukumaran, P. K., Mahadik, C., Yagnik, H., Telang, S., Vas, F., et al. (1990). Thalassemia in Bombay: the role of medical genetics in developing countries. *Bull. World Health Organ.* 68, 75–81.

Sato, T., Yamamoto, H., Sasaki, C., and Wake, K. (1998). Maturation of rat dendritic cells during intrahepatic translocation evaluated using monoclonal antibodies and electron microscopy. *Cell Tissue Res.* 294, 503–514. doi: 10.1007/s004410051201

Scheller, L. F., Wirtz, R. A., and Azad, A. F. (1994). Susceptibility of different strains of mice to hepatic infection with *Plasmodium berghei*. *Infect. Immun.* 62, 4844–4847.

Schenkel, J. M., Fraser, K. A., Vezys, V., and Masopust, D. (2013). Sensing and alarm function of resident memory CD8$^+$ T cells. *Nat. Immunol.* 14, 509–513. doi: 10.1038/ni.2568

Schmidt, N. W., Butler, N. S., Badovinac, V. P., and Harty, J. T. (2010). Extreme CD8 T cell requirements for anti-malarial liver-stage immunity following immunization with radiation attenuated sporozoites. *PLoS Pathog.* 6:e1000998. doi: 10.1371/journal.ppat.1000998

Schmidt, N. W., Butler, N. S., and Harty, J. T. (2011). *Plasmodium*-host interactions directly influence the threshold of memory CD8 T cells required for protective immunity. *J. Immunol.* 186, 5873–5884. doi: 10.4049/jimmunol.1100194

Schofield, L., Ferreira, A., Altszuler, R., Nussenzweig, V., and Nussenzweig, R. S. (1987a). Interferon-gamma inhibits the intrahepatocytic development of malaria parasites in vitro. *J. Immunol.* 139, 2020–2025.

Schofield, L., Villaquiran, J., Ferreira, A., Schellekens, H., Nussenzweig, R., and Nussenzweig, V. (1987b). Gamma interferon, CD8$^+$ T cells and antibodies required for immunity to malaria sporozoites. *Nature* 330, 664–666. doi: 10.1038/330664a0

Sedegah, M., Finkelman, F., and Hoffman, S. L. (1994). Interleukin 12 induction of interferon gamma-dependent protection against malaria. *Proc. Natl. Acad. Sci. U.S.A.* 91, 10700–10702. doi: 10.1073/pnas.91.22.10700

Seder, R. A., Chang, L. J., Enama, M. E., Zephir, K. L., Sarwar, U. N., Gordon, I. J., et al. (2013). Protection against malaria by intravenous immunization with a nonreplicating sporozoite vaccine. *Science* 341, 1359–1365. doi: 10.1126/science.1241800

Seguin, M. C., Klotz, F. W., Schneider, I., Weir, J. P., Goodbary, M., Slayter, M., et al. (1994). Induction of nitric oxide synthase protects against malaria in mice exposed to irradiated *Plasmodium berghei* infected mosquitoes: involvement of interferon γ and $CD8^+$ T cells. *J. Exp. Med.* 180, 353–358. doi: 10.1084/jem.180.1.353

Seki, E., De Minicis, S., Gwak, G. Y., Kluwe, J., Inokuchi, S., Bursill, C. A., et al. (2009). CCR1 and CCR5 promote hepatic fibrosis in mice. *J. Clin. Invest.* 119, 1858–1870. doi: 10.1172/JCI37444

Sheth, K., and Bankey, P. (2001). The liver as an immune organ. *Curr. Opin. Crit. Care* 7, 99–104. doi: 10.1097/00075198-200104000-00008

Shi, C., Velazquez, P., Hohl, T. M., Leiner, I., Dustin, M. L., and Pamer, E. G. (2010). Monocyte trafficking to hepatic sites of bacterial infection is chemokine independent and directed by focal intercellular adhesion molecule-1 expression. *J. Immunol.* 184, 6266–6274. doi: 10.4049/jimmunol.0904160

Shin, S. C. J., Vanderberg, J. P., and Terzakis, J. A. (1982). Direct infection of hepatocytes by sporozoites of *Plasmodium berghei*. *J. Protozool.* 29, 448–454. doi: 10.1111/j.1550-7408.1982.tb05431.x

Silva, J. S., Machado, F. S., and Martins, G. A. (2003). The role of nitric oxide in the pathogenesis of Chagas disease. *Front. Biosci.* 8, s314–s325. doi: 10.2741/1012

Singh, A. P., Buscaglia, C. A., Wang, Q., Levay, A., Nussenzweig, D. R., Walker, J. R., et al. (2007). *Plasmodium* circumsporozoite protein promotes the development of the liver stages of the parasite. *Cell* 131, 492–504. doi: 10.1016/j.cell.2007.09.013

Smith, J. E., and Alexander, J. (1986). Evasion of macrophage microbicidal mechanisms by mature sporozoites of *Plasmodium yoelii* yoelii. *Parasitology* 93, 33–38. doi: 10.1017/S0031182000049805

Spaccapelo, R., Naitza, S., Robson, K. J. H., and Crisanti, A. (1997). Thrombospondin-related adhesive protein (TRAP) of *Plasmodium berghei* and parasite motility. *Lancet* 350, 335. doi: 10.1016/S0140-6736(97)24031-6

Steers, N., Schwenk, R., Bacon, D. J., Berenzon, D., Williams, J., and Krzych, U. (2005). The immune status of Kupffer cells profoundly influences their responses to infectious *Plasmodium berghei* sporozoites. *Eur. J. Immunol.* 35, 2335–2346. doi: 10.1002/eji.200425680

Steinhoff, G. (1990). Major histocompatibility complex antigens in human liver transplants. *J. Hepatol.* 11, 9–15. doi: 10.1016/0168-8278(90)90264-R

Steinhoff, G., Wonigeit, K., and Pichlmayr, R. (1988). Analysis of sequential changes in major histocompatibility complex expression in human liver grafts after transplantation. *Transplantation* 45, 394–401. doi: 10.1097/00007890-198802000-00030

Steiniger, B., Falk, P., and Van Der Meide, P. H. (1988). Interferon-γ in vivo. Induction and loss of class II MHC antigens and immature myelomonocytic cells in rat organs. *Eur. J. Immunol.* 18, 661–669. doi: 10.1002/eji.1830180502

Stewart, M. J., and Vanderberg, J. P. (1988). Malaria sporozoites leave behind trails of circumsporozoite protein during gliding motility. *J. Protozool.* 35, 389–393. doi: 10.1111/j.1550-7408.1988.tb04115.x

Stewart, M. J., and Vanderberg, J. P. (1991). Malaria sporozoites release circumsporozoite protein from their apical end and translocate it along their surface. *J. Protozool.* 38, 411–421. doi: 10.1111/j.1550-7408.1991.tb01379.x

Stewart, M. J., and Vanderberg, J. P. (1992). Electron microscopic analysis of circumsporozoite protein trail formation by gliding malaria sporozoites. *J. Protozool.* 39, 663–671. doi: 10.1111/j.1550-7408.1992.tb04446.x

Stirpe, F., Barbieri, L., Battelli, M. G., Soria, M., and Lappi, D. A. (1992). Ribosome-inactivating proteins from plants: present status and future prospects. *Biotechnology* 10, 405–412. doi: 10.1038/nbt0492-405

Sturm, A., Amino, R., van de Sand, C., Regen, T., Retzlaff, S., Rennenberg, A., et al. (2006). Manipulation of host hepatocytes by the malaria parasite for delivery into liver sinusoids. *Science (New York, N.Y.)* 313, 1287–1290. doi: 10.1126/science.1129720

Sumpter, T. L., Abe, M., Tokita, D., and Thomson, A. W. (2007). Dendritic cells, the liver, and transplantation. *Hepatology* 46, 2021–2031. doi: 10.1002/hep.21974

Takacs, A. C., Swierzy, I. J., and Luder, C. G. (2012). Interferon-gamma restricts *Toxoplasma gondii* development in murine skeletal muscle cells via nitric oxide production and immunity-related GTPases. *PLoS ONE* 7:e45440. doi: 10.1371/journal.pone.0045440

Tavares, J., Formaglio, P., Thiberge, S., Mordelet, E., Van Rooijen, N., Medvinsky, A., et al. (2013). Role of host cell traversal by the malaria sporozoite during liver infection. *J. Exp. Med.* 210, 905–915. doi: 10.1084/jem.20121130

Teirlinck, A. C., McCall, M. B., Roestenberg, M., Scholzen, A., Woestenenk, R., De Mast, Q., et al. (2011). Longevity and composition of cellular immune responses following experimental *Plasmodium falciparum* malaria infection in humans. *PLoS Pathog.* 7:e1002389. doi: 10.1371/journal.ppat.1002389

Todryk, S. M., Bejon, P., Mwangi, T., Plebanski, M., Urban, B., Marsh, K., et al. (2008). Correlation of memory T cell responses against TRAP with protection from clinical malaria, and $CD4^+$ $CD25^{high}$ T cells with susceptibility in Kenyans. *PLoS ONE* 3:e2027. doi: 10.1371/journal.pone.0002027

Trambas, C. M., and Griffiths, G. M. (2003). Delivering the kiss of death. *Nat. Immunol.* 4, 399–403. doi: 10.1038/ni0503-399

Trimnell, A., Takagi, A., Gupta, M., Richie, T. L., Kappe, S. H., and Wang, R. (2009). Genetically attenuated parasite vaccines induce contact-dependent $CD8^+$ T cell killing of *Plasmodium yoelii* liver stage-infected hepatocytes. *J. Immunol.* 183, 5870–5878. doi: 10.4049/jimmunol.0900302

Trutmann, M., and Sasse, D. (1994). The lymphatics of the liver. *Anat. Embryol. (Berl.)* 190, 201–209. doi: 10.1007/BF00234299

Urban, B. C., Ing, R., and Stevenson, M. M. (2005). Early interactions between blood-stage *Plasmodium* parasites and the immune system. *Curr. Top. Microbiol. Immunol.* 297, 25–70. doi: 10.1007/3-540-29967-X_2

Usynin, I., Klotz, C., and Frevert, U. (2007). Malaria circumsporozoite protein inhibits the respiratory burst in Kupffer cells. *Cell. Microbiol.* 9, 2610–2628. doi: 10.1111/j.1462-5822.2007.00982.x

Van Braeckel-Budimir, N., and Harty, J. T. (2014). CD8 T-cell-mediated protection against liver-stage malaria: lessons from a mouse model. *Front. Microbiol.* 5:272. doi: 10.3389/fmicb.2014.00272

Vanderberg, J., Mueller, A.-K., Heiss, K., Goetz, K., Matuschewski, K., Deckert, M., et al. (2007). Assessment of antibody protection against malaria sporozoites must be done by mosquito injection of sporozoites. *Am. J. Pathol.* 171, 1405–1406; author reply 1406. doi: 10.2353/ajpath.2007.070661

Vanderberg, J. P. (2014). Imaging mosquito transmission of *Plasmodium* sporozoites into the mammalian host: immunological implications. *Parasitol. Int.* 63, 150–164. doi: 10.1016/j.parint.2013.09.010

Vanderberg, J. P., Chew, S., and Stewart, M. J. (1990). *Plasmodium* sporozoite interactions with macrophages in vitro: a videomicroscopic analysis. *J. Protozool.* 37, 528–536. doi: 10.1111/j.1550-7408.1990.tb01260.x

Vanderberg, J. P., and Frevert, U. (2004). Intravital microscopy demonstrating antibody-mediated immobilization of *Plasmodium berghei* sporozoites injected into skin by mosquitoes. *Int. J. Parasitol.* 34, 991–996. doi: 10.1016/j.ijpara.2004.05.005

van de Sand, C., Horstmann, S., Schmidt, A., Sturm, A., Bolte, S., Krueger, A., et al. (2005). The liver stage of *Plasmodium berghei* inhibits host cell apoptosis. *Mol. Microbiol.* 58, 731–742. doi: 10.1111/j.1365-2958.2005.04888.x

Van Rooijen, N., and Sanders, A. (1996). Kupffer cell depletion by liposome-delivered drugs: comparative activity of intracellular clodronate, propamidine, and ethylenediaminetetraacetic acid. *Hepatology* 23, 1239–1243. doi: 10.1002/hep.510230544

Vaughan, A. M., O'Neill, M. T., Tarun, A. S., Camargo, N., Phuong, T. M., Aly, A. S., et al. (2009). Type II fatty acid synthesis is essential only for malaria parasite late liver stage development. *Cell. Microbiol.* 11, 506–520. doi: 10.1111/j.1462-5822.2008.01270.x

Vreden, S. G. S., Broek, M. F., Oettinger, M. C., Verhave, J. P., Meuwissen, J. H. E. T., and Sauerwein, R. W. (1992). Cytokines inhibit the development of liver schizonts of the malaria parasite *Plasmodium berghei* in vivo. *Eur. J. Immunol.* 22, 2271–2275. doi: 10.1002/eji.1830220914

Wang, R., Arevalo-Herrera, M., Gardner, M. J., Bonelo, A., Carlton, J. M., Gomez, A., et al. (2005). Immune responses to *Plasmodium vivax* pre-erythrocytic stage antigens in naturally exposed Duffy-negative humans: a potential model for identification of liver-stage antigens. *Eur. J. Immunol.* 35, 1859–1868. doi: 10.1002/eji.200425807

Warren, A., Le Couteur, D. G., Fraser, R., Bowen, D. G., Mccaughan, G. W., and Bertolino, P. (2006). T lymphocytes interact with hepatocytes through fenestrations in murine liver sinusoidal endothelial cells. *Hepatology* 44, 1182–1190. doi: 10.1002/hep.21378

Weiss, W. R., Berzofsky, J. A., Houghten, R. A., Sedegah, M., Hollindale, M., and Hoffman, S. L. (1992). A T cell clone directed at the circumsporozoite protein which protects mice against both *Plasmodium yoelii* and *Plasmodium berghei*. *J. Immunol.* 149, 2103–2109.

WHO. (2013). "World malaria report: 2013," in *WHO Global Malaria Programme*. (Geneva: World Health Organization).

Wiedemann, A., Depoil, D., Faroudi, M., and Valitutti, S. (2006). Cytotoxic T lymphocytes kill multiple targets simultaneously via spatiotemporal uncoupling of lytic and stimulatory synapses. *Proc. Natl. Acad. Sci. U.S.A.* 103, 10985–10990. doi: 10.1073/pnas.0600651103

Wilson, K. L., Xiang, S. D., and Plebanski, M. (2015). Montanide, Poly I:C and nanoparticle based vaccines promote differential suppressor and effector cell expansion: a study of induction of CD8 T cells to a minimal *Plasmodium berghei* epitope. *Front. Microbiol.* 6:29. doi: 10.3389/fmicb.2015.00029

Wisse, E., De Zanger, R. B., Jacobs, R., and Mccuskey, R. S. (1983). Scanning electron microscope observations on the structure of portal veins, sinusoids and central veins in rat liver. *Scan. Electron Microsc.* 3, 1441–1452.

Wuensch, S. A., Pierce, R. H., and Crispe, I. N. (2006). Local intrahepatic $CD8^+$ T cell activation by a non-self-antigen results in full functional differentiation. *J. Immunol.* 177, 1689–1697. doi: 10.4049/jimmunol.177.3.1689

Yoneyama, H., and Ichida, T. (2005). Recruitment of dendritic cells to pathological niches in inflamed liver. *Med. Mol. Morphol.* 38, 136–141. doi: 10.1007/s00795-005-0289-0

Zarling, S., Berenzon, D., Dalai, S., Liepinsh, D., Steers, N., and Krzych, U. (2013). The survival of memory CD8 T cells that is mediated by IL-15 correlates with sustained protection against malaria. *J. Immunol.* 190, 5128–5141. doi: 10.4049/jimmunol.1203396

Zhang, Y., Wang, H., Ren, J., Tang, X., Jing, Y., Xing, D., et al. (2012). IL-17A synergizes with IFN-gamma to upregulate iNOS and NO production and inhibit chlamydial growth. *PLoS ONE* 7:e39214. doi: 10.1371/journal.pone.0039214

19

Autoantibodies and Malaria: Where We Stand? Insights into Pathogenesis and Protection

*Luiza Carvalho Mourão, Gustavo Pereira Cardoso-Oliveira and Érika Martins Braga**

Departamento de Parasitologia, Instituto de Ciências Biológicas, Universidade Federal de Minas Gerais, Belo Horizonte, Brazil

Edited by:
Patricia Sampaio Tavares Veras, Gonçalo Moniz Institute (IGM), Brazil

Reviewed by:
Kai Yang, Indiana University School of Medicine—Lafayette, United States
Surya Prakash Pandey, University of Pittsburgh, United States
Ann M. Moormann, University of Massachusetts Medical School, United States

***Correspondence:**
Érika Martins Braga
embraga@icb.ufmg.br

Autoantibodies are frequently reported in patients with malaria, but whether they contribute to protection or to pathology is an issue of debate. A large body of evidence indicates that antibodies against host-self components are associated to malaria clinical outcomes such as cerebral malaria, renal dysfunction and anemia. Nonetheless, self-reactive immunoglobulins induced during an infection can also mediate protection. In light of these controversies, we summarize here the latest findings in our understanding of autoimmune responses in malaria, focusing on *Plasmodium falciparum* and *Plasmodium vivax*. We review the main targets of self-antibody responses in malaria as well as the current, but still limited, knowledge of their role in disease pathogenesis or protection.

Keywords: malaria, autoantibodies, anemia, cerebral malaria, renal dysfunction

INTRODUCTION

Despite substantial progress in control efforts over the past decades, malaria still accounts for significant morbidity and mortality, mainly in underdeveloped countries. In 2018, an estimated 228 million cases of malaria occurred worldwide with 405,000 deaths, largely in Africa (WHO | World Malaria Report, 2019). Five species are known to cause malaria in humans, *Plasmodium falciparum*, *Plasmodium vivax*, *Plasmodium knowlesi*, *Plasmodium ovale*, and *Plasmodium malariae*. Since research emphasis has been placed on *P. falciparum* and *P. vivax*, parasites that are responsible for most of malaria cases, here we will focus in these two species.

Symptomatic disease occurs during the erythrocytic phase when the presence of asexual blood-stage parasites triggers a robust innate immune response. This response if properly regulated may clear infection, contributing to the development of a protective immunity. By the other hand, if not counterbalanced by anti-inflammatory responses, the exacerbated activation of the immune system may play a key role in the pathogenesis (reviewed by Antonelli et al., 2019), leading to complications such as cerebral malaria, anemia, acute kidney injury and respiratory distress syndrome (Moxon et al., 2019).

During infection, high levels of antibodies with a broad range of specificities are elicited. Although their functional activity is far from over, it is known that such molecules can have diverse effects. Antibodies are critical for the control of the disease by acting alone or in cooperation with host immune cells (For further details see Teo et al., 2016). But in some cases, antibodies that recognize host's own components may also promote pathology (Ludwig et al., 2017).

The presence of autoantibodies that recognize the host's own molecules has also been extensively reported in patients with malaria (Rosenberg et al., 1973; Berzins et al., 1983; Daniel-Ribeiro et al., 1983; Wozencraft et al., 1990; Jakobsen et al., 1993; Lacerda et al., 2011; Fernandez-Arias et al., 2016; Mourão et al., 2016, 2018; Rivera-Correa et al., 2019a). The mechanisms by which autoimmune responses could be triggered during an infection remains unclear but it is generally accepted that they may include: molecular mimicry (Damian, 1964; Greenwood, 1974), bystander activation (Fujinami et al., 2006; Münz et al., 2009), epitope spreading (Vanderlugt and Miller, 2002; Münz et al., 2009), persistent infection and B cells polyclonal activation (Freeman and Parish, 1978; Rosenberg, 1978; Daniel-Ribeiro et al., 1983; Minoprio, 2001).

Molecular mimicry is the sharing of structurally similar antigens between parasite and host components (Damian, 1964). In malaria, molecular mimicry occurs between *P. falciparum* translationally controlled tumor protein (PfTCTP) and human histamine-releasing factor (HRF) (MaCDonald et al., 2001). Another plasmodial protein that share motifs with host's components is *P. falciparum* erythrocyte membrane protein 1 (PfEMP1), which exhibits homology with human vitronectin (Ludin et al., 2011). An *in silico* analysis comparing *P. vivax* entire proteome and human RBC proteome also revealed that 23 *P. vivax* proteins shared similarity to human RBC proteins such as ankyrin, actin, and spectrin (Mourão et al., 2018). These structural similarities can activate cross-reactive autoreactive lymphocytes, consequently disordering the immune system. So, when T- or B- cells receptors recognize a parasite epitope that is similar enough to a self-protein, an autoimmune response is elicited, leading to cell or tissue destruction in addition to activation of other branches of the immune system (Fujinami et al., 2006; Münz et al., 2009).

Bystander activation is an antigen-independent phenomenon whereby parasitized cells, either through direct cell contact or paracrine signals, alert or instruct neighboring non-infected cells to produce inflammatory mediators (Holmgren et al., 2017). The inflammatory milieu evoked by the infection promotes the activation and expansion of autoreactive T or B cells, which can initiate an autoimmune response that damage host's cells or tissues, leading to the release of self-reactive antigens (Fujinami et al., 2006; Münz et al., 2009). Evidences of bystander activation in malaria came from *in vitro* studies investigating the pathways driving inflammation in infection. These studies have demonstrated that extracellular vesicles derived from plasma of mice infected with *Plasmodium berghei* or from *P. falciparum*-infected erythrocytes were able to activate naïve host cells (Couper et al., 2010; Mantel et al., 2013).

It is widely known that in early immune responses, epitopes of the initial antigens are recognized by the acquired immune system, but during infection, epitopes other than the dominant ones may also become immunogenic and be targets of T and B cells. This reactivity to newer endogenous epitopes is termed "epitope spreading" and may be induced against other epitopes in the same autoantigen (intramolecular epitope spreading) or against epitopes in other self-antigens (intermolecular epitope spreading) that are released after T- or B-cell-mediated bystander (Münz et al., 2009). Although epitope spreading is more commonly reported in autoimmune diseases, it may also occur in persistent infections, as it has been suggested by Flanagan et al. (2006) in a study conducted with adults naturally exposed to malaria in Kenya. These authors have investigated cellular immunity to the thrombospondin-related adhesive protein of *P. falciparum* (PfTRAP) and showed that the immunodominant response stimulated in the primary exposure to this protein has progressed to encompass lesser epitopes with repeated and prolonged exposure.

In vitro experiments with *P. falciparum*-infected RBCs revealed that culture supernatant containing parasite-derived products was able to induce polyclonal B-cell activation and non-specific immunoglobulin synthesis, suggesting that B-cell's proliferation and differentiation into antibody-secreting cells triggered by pathogen's molecules can also lead to autoimmune responses (Freeman and Parish, 1978; Minoprio, 2001). One of the molecules that has been incriminated as a potential activator of B-cells in malaria is the cysteine-rich interdomain region 1 (CIDR1) of *P. falciparum* erythrocyte membrane protein 1 (PfEMP-1). Evidence in this line has been provided by a study with B cells from non-immune donors stimulated with a recombinant version of CIDR1. The recombinant protein was able to promote *in vitro* proliferation, increase in B-cell size, and expression of immunoglobulins and cytokines in those cells (Donati et al., 2004). However, just a small proportion of antibodies secreted by them was specific for parasite antigens; the greater part was non-specific and could react with different host's components, leading to cell and tissue damage.

Self-reactive antibodies recognize different self-antigens such as erythrocyte proteins (Rosenberg et al., 1973; Fontaine et al., 2010; Mourão et al., 2016, 2018; Ventura et al., 2018), brain molecules (Bansal et al., 2009; Gitau et al., 2013), phospholipids (Adebajo et al., 1993; Jakobsen et al., 1993; Facer and Agiostratidou, 1994; Fernandez-Arias et al., 2016; Barber et al., 2019; Rivera-Correa et al., 2019a,b), and nucleic acids (Adu et al., 1982; Adebajo et al., 1993; Rivera-Correa et al., 2019b). Although the literature reporting the detection of autoantibodies in plasmodial infections is vast, the role of such molecules in malaria is still a controversial issue. Some authors have associated such autoimmune responses to pathology while others to protection. In this review, we summarize the latest breakthroughs regarding autoantibody responses in malaria, emphasizing what is new on the pathogenesis front, mainly with respect to cerebral malaria, kidney injury and anemia (**Figure 1**).

CEREBRAL MALARIA

Cerebral malaria (CM) is a clinical syndrome of severe falciparum malaria characterized by impaired consciousness assessed by Blantyre Coma Score ≤ 2 in children (Molyneux et al., 1989) or Glasgow Coma Score ≤ 11 in adults (Teasdale and Jennett, 1974), with no other cause of encephalitis (Taylor et al., 2004). Although this neurological syndrome only develops in a small percentage of *P. falciparum*-infected patients, it is responsible for more than 90% of malaria-related deaths. The treatment with anti-malarial drugs decreases mortality due to CM, but nearly 20% of treated patients still succumb and up to one-third of survivors frequently exhibit long-term neurological sequelae such as cognition and speech disorders, physical disability and cortical blindness (Birbeck et al., 2010).

Although the mechanisms leading to CM pathogenesis are not yet clearly defined, it is known that both parasite and host factors play a role in the clinical outcome of this syndrome (Idro

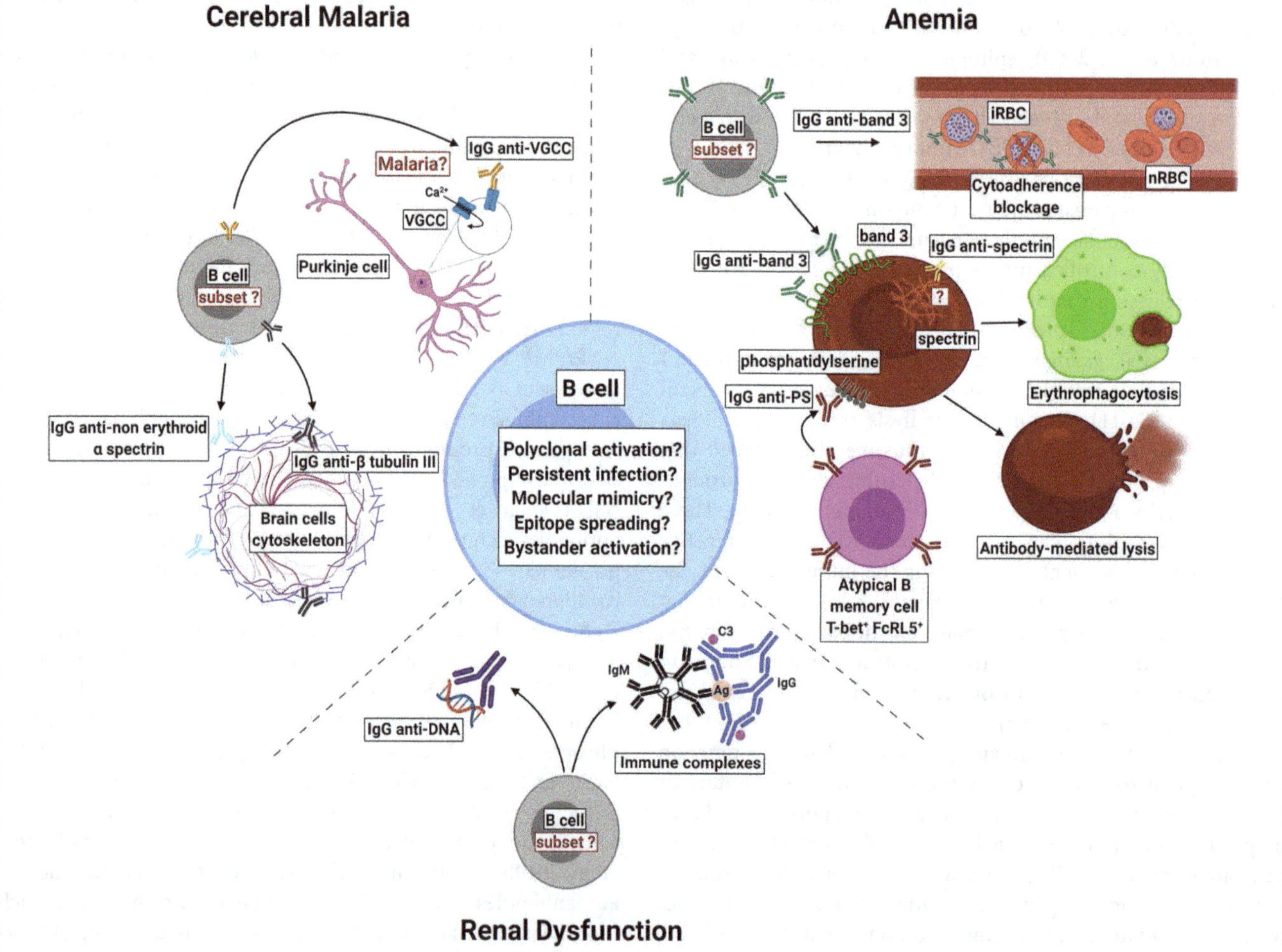

FIGURE 1 | Schematic representation of self-reactive antibodies and their proposed role in the pathogenesis or protection against malaria. Autoantibodies that recognize host's own molecules have been reported in patients with malaria but the mechanisms by which such autoimmune response is induced are still to be completely elucidated. In infections due to *P. falciparum*, self-reactive immunoglobulins against voltage-gated calcium channel (VGCC), non-erythroid alpha spectrin, and beta tubulin III have been associated to cerebral malaria. In *P. falciparum* and *P. vivax* infections, anti-phosphatidylserine antibodies (IgG anti-PS) have been shown to recognize non-infected red blood cells (nRBCs) exposing phosphatidylserine, mediating their clearance and contributing to malaria-associated anemia. During *P. vivax* malaria, autoimmune responses to anion exchanger 1 (band 3 protein) have been implicated in the removal of nRBCs by decreasing their deformability and enhancing their uptake by THP-1 cells. On the other hand, in *P. falciparum* malaria, anti-band 3 self-reactive antibodies have been associated to protection through the blockage of cytoadherence. Antibodies to erythrocytic spectrin are elicited during *P. vivax* malaria but it remains unclear how they bind to cytoplasmic proteins. It has been hypothesized that the inflammation triggered by infection may damage brain cells, leading to the exposure of spectrin, which may activate the complement, amplifying neuronal damage. Finally, anti-DNA autoantibodies and immune complexes containing self-immunoglobulins have been suggested to play a role in renal dysfunction by depositing in renal tissues. iRBC: infected red blood cell. Ag: antigen. C3: complement component 3. Figure created with BioRender.

et al., 2010). Among host components, B cells and antibodies are critical for the immune response against malaria. Large amounts of antibodies are produced in response to plasmodial infection, including those that recognize self-components such as host brain antigens (Guiyedi et al., 2007; Bansal et al., 2009; Duarte et al., 2012). However, whether such self-reactive immunoglobulins are a consequence of cerebral malaria or a factor that aggravates the disease is little explored. This could be, in part, due to the difficult in accessing human brain tissues because of the small proportion of *P. falciparum*-infected patients that develop CM. Moreover, the existence of ethical issues limits the study of CM to peripheral blood and *post-mortem* samples.

Although understudied, some research groups have associated a marked increase in specific anti-brain autoantibodies levels with disease severity in *P. falciparum* malaria. This is the case of self-reactive antibodies against the voltage-gated calcium channels (VGCCs), whose levels were shown to be higher in Kenyan children with CM than in those with uncomplicated disease or uninfected (Lang et al., 2005). Autoantibodies to VGCCs have been shown to downregulate calcium flow in Purkinje neurons and granule cells through a complement-independent process in autoimmune diseases such as limbic encephalitis and cerebellar ataxia (Pinto et al., 1998; Irani and Lang, 2008), thereby providing insight into the pathogenic role of such self-reactive molecules in malaria.

Furthermore, it has been reported that serum from Gabonese children with severe *P. falciparum* infection recognize a higher diversity of brain antigens in comparison to non-infected ones. Some of those autoantibodies display reactivity to the non-erythroid alpha spectrin (Guiyedi et al., 2007), a structural protein that is found in the cytoplasm of a variety of brain cells and is responsible for membrane structure and integrity. Since inflammation induced by malaria can damage brain cells exposing non-erythroid alpha spectrin, it is possible that this protein activates the complement system, amplifying the neuronal damage. In primary Sjögren's syndrome, an important autoimmune disease, non-erythroid spectrin undergoes proteolysis by caspase 3 and calpain, producing a fragment that acts as autoantigen (Nath et al., 1996; Haneji et al., 1997).

Other cytoskeletal protein that has also been described as a target of autoimmune responses in CM and which is considered as a disease-specific marker is beta tubulin III (TBB3) (Bansal et al., 2009), a protein that is abundant in cells from nervous system and in neoplastic cells of neural tumors (Katsetos et al., 2003). TBB3 is involved in axon guidance, thus mutations in this protein are associated with different nervous system disorders (Tischfield et al., 2010). In living cells and *in vitro* models, polyclonal antibodies with high affinity for beta tubulin have been shown to disrupt cytoplasmic microtubules, leading to their fragmentation into smaller units (Füchtbauer et al., 1985).

In addition to the self-reactive proteins mentioned above, the dendritic tree of Purkinje cell is another host component that has been considered a target of autoimmune responses in CM. In a cohort of Thai individuals, it has been demonstrated that levels of autoantibodies against dendrites are higher in *P. falciparum*-infected patients with CM than in those with uncomplicated malaria (Gallien et al., 2011). The pathogenic role of such autoantibodies was attributed to their ability in inhibiting *in vitro* development of Purkinje cells (Calvet et al., 1993). However, it is important to emphasize that these results were obtained from studies conducted with cat brain biopsies and thus, should be interpreted with caution.

On the other hand, a possible role in protection against severe *P. falciparum* malaria has already been suggested for self-reactive antibodies induced during plasmodial infection. This is the case of IgE autoantibodies to 14-3-3 ε brain protein, which induce *in vitro* mastocyte degranulation (Duarte et al., 2012). The 14-3-3 ε brain protein belongs to a family of adaptor proteins that interact with a multitude of binding partners that contain PSer/PThr motifs. Through this interaction, 14-3-3 ε protein affects the activity and localization of various substrate proteins, regulating signal cascades of a wide range of biological activities, including cell cycle and apoptosis (Cornell and Toyo-Oka, 2017). Therefore, 14-3-3 ε protein has been implicated in different neurodegenerative and neuropsychiatric diseases by mechanisms that vary from apoptosis to protein stabilization and aggregation (For further details see Foote and Zhou, 2012 and Cornell and Toyo-Oka, 2017). In Parkinson's disease, for example, the interaction of 14-3-3 ε protein with Bad and Bax proteins prevents neurons apoptosis. Neurodegeneration is avoided by interaction between 14-3-3 ε protein and phosphorylated tyrosine hydroxylase in parallel with the binding between α-synuclein to unphosphorylated tyrosine hydroxylase. An imbalance in those interactions leads to neurodegeneration in this nervous system disorder (Shimada et al., 2013). Thus, it is not surprising that an antibody response against 14-3-3 ε brain protein exert neuroprotective properties, as it has already been demonstrated in glaucoma, using a neuro-retinal cell line of mouse origin. In this case, cell viability and reduced reactive oxygen species levels were considered predictors of protection (Bell et al., 2015).

As highlighted herein, the repertoire of brain antigens that are targets of autoimmune responses during CM is vast and depends on a complex interplay of host, parasite and environmental factors. However, whether such autoantibodies have a pathogenic relevance, can be considered biomarkers of neuropathology or are merely innocent by-standers remains a focus of debate. More studies are needed in order to elucidate this, as well as to determine the epitopes, function and origin of such self-reactive immunoglobulins. Even though it is known that a breach in the blood brain barrier's (BBB) integrity is necessary to allow antibody influx into the brain (Huerta et al., 2006), studies conducted with *post mortem* brain tissues from Malawian children with fatal cerebral malaria revealed that, although BBB breakdown occurs in vessels containing cytoadherent parasitized RBCs, no gross leakage of plasma proteins occurs (Brown et al., 2001). Thus, the mechanisms by which immunoglobulins gain access to brain tissue are another issue that is still to be elucidated. Do they cross the BBB independently or do plasma cells secrete them? Further studies are necessary to understand in more details how BBB breakdown occurs in malaria. Understanding how this happens may provide new opportunities to find agents that are able to open the BBB, allowing the delivery of different molecules and shedding light on the effects of antibodies in the brain tissue. This knowledge may pave the way for the development of future interventions for malaria and other neurological diseases.

RENAL DYSFUNCTION

Acute renal failure is most reported in *P. falciparum* infections (Frutakul et al., 1974; Burchard et al., 2003; von Seidlein et al., 2012; Conroy et al., 2016; Sypniewska et al., 2017; Rivera-Correa et al., 2019b), but this complication can occasionally occurs in infection due to *P. malariae* (Neri et al., 2008; Badiane et al., 2016). Renal failure is considered a clinical manifestation with high prognostic value to severe malaria (von Seidlein et al., 2012; Sypniewska et al., 2017). In *P. malariae* infection, renal failure affects most children and is presented as steroid-resistant nephrotic syndrome. The pathogenesis is possibly mediated through immune-complex deposition containing IgM, IgG, C3, and malarial antigens in mesangiocapillary, glomerular, proximal tubules and subendothelial kidney tissues, with rarely IgA deposition (Ward and Kibuka-Musoke, 1969; Houba et al., 1971; van Velthuysen and Florquin, 2000; Das, 2008). Chronic glomerular disease due to *P. malariae* infection is usually not reversible even after treatment, raising the hypothesis that genetic and environmental factors are also involved (Houba, 1979). Although it is well-known that *P. malariae*-associated renal impairment is caused mainly because of immune complex deposits, there are no studies investigating if autoantibodies are involved in this process.

In *P. falciparum* malaria, acute renal failure is a common and serious complication in non-immune adults and adolescents and is more frequent in patients from non-endemic regions (Barsoum, 2000; Elsheikha and Sheashaa, 2007; Nguansangiam et al., 2007), but it can also occur in pediatric severe malaria (Olowu and Adelusola, 2004; von Seidlein et al., 2012; Conroy et al., 2016; Sypniewska et al., 2017; Rivera-Correa et al., 2019b). Although it is an important clinical manifestation associated with mortality and morbidity, the pathogenesis of renal failure in *P. falciparum* malaria is not well understood. However, unlikely *P. malariae*-associated renal failure, acute kidney injury in *P. falciparum* infection is usually transient and disappears after treatment (van Velthuysen and Florquin, 2000), suggesting that the parasite does not have a great role in the pathogenesis that is most likely to be caused by host's immune response. Several hypothesis on the pathogenesis of malarial renal failure have been proposed, including mechanical obstruction of glomerular and tubulointerstitial capillaries by infected erythrocytes (Seydel et al., 2006; Nguansangiam et al., 2007), possibly leading to renal ischemia (Conroy et al., 2016); immune complex deposits leading to renal impairment (Frutakul et al., 1974); and autoantibodies against nucleic acids (Wozencraft et al., 1990; Rivera-Correa et al., 2019b).

In a children population from Uganda, Rivera-Correa et al. (2019b) demonstrated that infants with severe *P. falciparum* malaria manifesting acute kidney injury have autoantibodies against nucleic acid and lipids. Additionally, they found a correlation between those autoantibodies and creatinine and blood urea nitrogen levels, two indicators of kidney health, suggesting that such immunoglobulins may play a role in kidney injury. It was also shown that anti-DNA autoantibodies were elevated in children with acute kidney injury, a result that is in accordance with Wozencraft et al. (1990), who obtained similar data, however, in mouse malaria. It is important to mention that no difference was found in levels of antibodies against parasite antigen, indicating that systemic changes in IgG metabolism and immune-mediated pathways may contribute to malaria-associated renal failure. This result corroborates the findings from Frutakul et al. (1974), who reported an absence of antibodies against parasite antigens in immune complexes deposited in glomeruli capillary walls from a Thai child's kidney. All these data demonstrate that renal dysfunction due to autoantibodies may be relevant in severe *P. falciparum*-associated renal failure. Future investigations should be conducted to further understand the role of those autoantibodies, their involvement in renal pathogenesis, as well as their use as disease biomarkers.

ANEMIA

Anemia is the most common feature and a major concern in malaria, mainly in young children and pregnant women (Accrombessi et al., 2015; Kenangalem et al., 2016; White, 2018). Despite its relevance, the pathogenesis of malaria-associated anemia is complex, and still incompletely understood. Malaria-induced anemia is thought to arise from the rupture of infected and non-infected red blood cells (nRBCs), as well as inappropriate erythropoiesis in the erythroid germinal centers (Douglas et al., 2012; White, 2018). But the greater loss is due to the clearance of nRBCs, which persist long after infection has resolved (Looareesuwan et al., 1987; Ritter et al., 1993; Collins et al., 2003; Douglas et al., 2012). An autoimmune component has been suggested to explain this removal, although the mechanisms underlying autoimmunity in malarial anemia have not been thoroughly explored (White, 2018; Rivera-Correa and Rodriguez, 2019). Self-reactive antibodies that recognize RBCs have been documented in plasmodial infections since 1970s, when host-serum components associated with the surface of nRBCs were detected in patients with malaria using different methodologies (Rosenberg et al., 1973; Facer et al., 1979; Berzins et al., 1983; Fernandez-Arias et al., 2016; Mourão et al., 2016). However, their roles in the pathophysiology of anemia have not been thoroughly explored. Evidence in this line is given by studies that have shown a reduction in RBC life span following the clearance of *P. falciparum* (Looareesuwan et al., 1987). This reduction in RBC survival time has been observed mainly in anemic patients and is associated with the deposition of complement containing immune complexes on RBCs surface (Rosenberg et al., 1973). Furthermore, it has been demonstrated that autoantibodies against triosephosphate isomerase purified from patients with *P. falciparum* malaria can bind to RBCs, promoting their lysis and activating complement cascade thereby, contributing to anemia (Ritter et al., 1993).

Since these early findings, autoantibodies with other specificities have already been identified and associated to anemia in malaria. This is the case of anti-phosphatidylserine (PS) antibodies, which were found to tag nRBCs exposing phosphatidylserine (Fernandez-Arias et al., 2016; Barber et al., 2019; Rivera-Correa et al., 2019a). These self-reactive immunoglobulins have been shown to increase *in vitro* phagocytosis and *in vivo* clearance of nRBCs, contributing to malarial anemia in a murine model (Fernandez-Arias et al., 2016). Moreover, a negative correlation between the magnitude of anti-PS antibodies and hemoglobin levels has been reported for patients infected with *P. falciparum* and *P. vivax* (Barber et al., 2019; Rivera-Correa et al., 2019a,b). In addition, it has been demonstrated that a population of atypical B cells, which is characterized by the expression of CD11c and T-bet, secretes anti-PS antibodies. The activation of these cells has been shown to be dependent of parasite DNA and different receptors have been suggested to be involved such as interferon-γ receptor (IFN-γR), B-cell receptor (BCR) and Toll-like receptor 9 (TLR9) (Rivera-Correa et al., 2017). However, the role of such atypical cells in human malaria was still unknown until a recent evidence has emerged from a study conducted with *P. falciparum*-infected returned travelers (Rivera-Correa et al., 2019a). In this study, it has been shown that FcRL5^{+}T-bet^{+} B-cells are expanded in acute malaria. Additionally, it has been observed that naïve human peripheral blood mononuclear cells are able to produce anti-PS antibodies when stimulated with lysates of *P. falciparum*-infected

TABLE 1 | Autoantibodies against self-antigens and their implications in *P. falciparum* and *P. vivax* malaria.

Self antigen	Possible functional activity of self-reactive antibody	Clinical outcome	References
14-3-3 ε brain protein	Degranulation of mast cells, basophils, eosinophils and/or monocytes/macrophages	Protection against severe *Plasmodium falciparum* malaria	Duarte et al., 2012
Beta tubulin III (TBB3)	Cytoplasm microtubule disruption	Cerebral malaria associated to *P. falciparum*	Füchtbauer et al., 1985; Bansal et al., 2009
Dendritic tree of Purkinje cell	*In vitro* inhibition of Purkinje cells development	Cerebral malaria associated to *P. falciparum*	Calvet et al., 1993; Gallien et al., 2011
Erythrocyte band 3 protein	Rigidity increase and *in vitro* clearance of non-parasitized RBCs	Anemia associated to *Plasmodium vivax*	Mourão et al., 2016, 2018
	In vitro P. falciparum cythoadherence blockage and *in vivo* adherence of RBCs; parasite growth inhibition	Protection against *P. falciparum* malaria	Hogh et al., 1994 ; Brahimi et al., 2011
Lipids	Kidney injury through immune complex deposition	Renal failure associated to *P. falciparum* malaria	Frutakul et al., 1974; Rivera-Correa et al., 2019b
Non-erythroid alpha spectrin	Disruption of brain cells cytoskeleton; complement activation and amplification of neuronal damage	Cerebral malaria associated to *P. falciparum*	Guiyedi et al., 2007
Nucleic acids	Kidney injury through immune complex deposition	Renal failure associated to *P. falciparum* malaria	Frutakul et al., 1974; Rivera-Correa et al., 2019b
Phosphatidylserine	Phagocytosis (*in vitro*) and clearance of non-parasitized RBCs	Anemia associated to *P. falciparum* and *P. vivax*	Fernandez-Arias et al., 2016; Barber et al., 2019; Rivera-Correa et al., 2019a
Spectrin	Disruption of RBCs cytoskeleton; amplification of RBCs damage	Anemia associated to *P. vivax*	Mourão et al., 2018
Triose-phosphate isomerase	*In vitro* lysis of RBC and activation of complement	Anemia associated to *P. falciparum*	Ritter et al., 1993
Voltage-gated calcium channels (VGCC)	Complement-independent downregulation of calcium flow in Purkinge and granule cells	Cerebral malaria associated to *P. falciparum*	Lang et al., 2005

RBCs, highlighting such atypical subset of memory B cells as a major promoter of autoimmune anemia in malaria. Besides anti-PS antibodies, self-reactive immunoglobulins triggered by other host cell targets are also involved in RBCs lysis, as it has been evidenced in a complement lysis assay using annexin V to block the binding of anti-PS antibodies to phosphatidylserine. After the binding of annexin to PS, RBC lysis could be partially inhibited by plasma from *P. falciparum*-infected patients (Rivera-Correa et al., 2019a).

Autoantibodies against RBCs have also been described for *P. vivax* infections (Mourão et al., 2016, 2018; Ventura et al., 2018; Barber et al., 2019). However, since this parasite has unique biological features that restricts its invasion to reticulocytes, lower densities of peripheral parasitemia are generally expected for infections due to *P. vivax* in comparison to *P. falciparum*. But despite this, *P. vivax* causes a greater loss of nRBCs. Thus, it is possible that the mechanisms leading to nRBCs removal in *P. vivax* malaria are distinct from those observed from *P. falciparum*. More work is needed to elucidate this.

Different erythrocytic antigens have been shown to be recognized by self-reactive immunoglobullins from anemic *P. vivax*-infected patients such as band 3 (Mourão et al., 2018), an anion exchanger protein which mediates the change of intracellular bicarbonate (HCO_3^-) to extracellular chloride (Cl^-) (Cordat and Reithmeier, 2014). Since IgGs purified from the same patients can bind to the surface of non-parasitized RBCs, increasing their rigidity and enhancing their clearance by THP-1 phagocytes (Mourão et al., 2018), it is also possible that anti-RBCs antibodies mediate malarial anemia through erythrophagocytosis or through decreasing RBC deformability (Mourão et al., 2016). Other possibility is the withdrawn from circulation by mechanisms like those tagging senescent RBCs for clearance (Lutz and Bogdanova, 2013), a hypothesis that should be better investigated.

Other RBC protein that has also been considered a target for autoimmune responses during *P. vivax* malaria is spectrin, although it is still unclear how anti-spectrin antibodies bind to an inner component of RBC membrane. Since *in silico* analysis revealed that human spectrin primary structure shares homology with a *P. vivax* hypothetical protein, it is possible that molecular mimicry drives autoimmune response against human spectrin (Mourão et al., 2018), a hypothesis that needs to be experimentally validated.

On the other hand, no association between anti-RBCs antibodies and anemia has been observed in a study conducted with *P. vivax*-infected children and adolescents from Pará, a State located in Brazilian Amazon (Ventura et al., 2018). A similar result was also found by (Fernandes et al., 2008), who evaluated the frequency of malarial anemia, as well as cytokines and autoantibodies levels, in an area in which *P. vivax* and *P. falciparum* coexists. It is important to mention that despite no significant association has been found in both studies,

BOX 1 | Outstanding questions in autoimmunity-mediated pathology in malaria:

- Which mechanisms are behind the generation of self-reactive antibodies in malaria?
- What are the self-antigens that trigger auto-immune responses in *P. falciparum* and *P. vivax* malaria?
- How self-reactive antibodies penetrate the blood-brain barrier, a high selective barrier that protects the central nervous system from invaders? Do they cross independently or do plasma cells secrete them?
- Do self-reactive antibody responses change with anti-malarial therapy?
- Is there any association between autoantibodies that persist after parasite clearance and long-term complications?
- What is the prevalence and the magnitude of autoantibody responses in different epidemiological settings?
- Can anti-self-antibody blockage prevent pathology?

higher frequency of anti-RBCs antibodies has been reported in patients with malaria (Fernandes et al., 2008; Ventura et al., 2018).

In other reports, a beneficial role has been attributed to anti-RBCs antibodies. This is the case of a study carried out in an area of intense transmission of malaria in Liberia, where it has been shown that immune responses to band 3 neoantigens are correlated with lower *P. falciparum* parasitemia and can block *in vitro* and *in vivo* RBCs' cytoadherence (Hogh et al., 1994). Moreover, an anti-plasmodial activity has been proposed to autoantibodies from patients with autoimmune diseases, which were able to inhibit parasite growth, suggesting a protective role for those molecules, although the authors have not ruled out the involvement of other serum components (Brahimi et al., 2011). Since the pathways involved in autoantibody-induced pathology differ among infections due to different parasites, it is possible that self-reactive antibodies exert diverse effects in infections by *P. vivax* and *P. falciparum*, an issue that should be target of future investigation.

As can be noted by the findings mentioned above, the literature concerning self-reactive antibodies against RBCs suggest a dual role for these immunoglobulins in malaria-associated anemia. But crucial gaps remain to be addressed (**Box 1**).

These scientific breakthroughs will allow the use of autoantibodies as signatures to predict disease severity or protection, as well as provide insights toward the best vaccination strategies. Furthermore, they will open new therapeutic possibilities to treat malarial anemia.

CONCLUDING REMARKS

Studies regarding autoantibodies and plasmodial infections have indicated that those molecules may play a dual role in malaria (**Figure 1** and **Table 1**). However, it is not clear if self-reactive antibodies lead to pathogenesis or are just a consequence of plasmodial infection. Although different self-reactive antibodies have been identified in distinct populations and associated with clinical complications, their epitopes as well as their origin and functional role remains to be elucidated. This information will be essential to the search and identification of epitopes and other molecules that can hijacks pathogenic autoantibodies from circulation, minimizing or inhibiting their pathogenic effects in host cells. This is an interesting field of work that should be focus of future investigation using *in vitro* and *in vivo* models. Since few reports have associated autoantibodies to protection, this is an issue that should also be better investigated. Additionally, it would be of interest to determine the prevalence and the magnitude of self-reactive responses in cohorts from different epidemiological settings, an analysis that should be extended including prospective studies. The role of self-immunoglobulins isotypes and IgG subclasses is another gap that should also be addressed. A better knowledge of all these points (**Box 1**) may allow the use of autoantibodies as signatures to predict malaria clinical outcome. Furthermore it may open new therapeutic possibilities to treat malaria-associated complications besides have implications for other autoimmune diseases.

AUTHOR CONTRIBUTIONS

LM, GC-O, and EB conceptualized and wrote the manuscript.

REFERENCES

Accrombessi, M., Ouédraogo, S., Agbota, G. C., Gonzalez, R., Massougbodji, A., Menéndez, C., et al. (2015). Malaria in pregnancy is a predictor of infant haemoglobin concentrations during the first year of life in Benin, West Africa. *PLoS ONE* 10:e0129510. doi: 10.1371/journal.pone.0129510

Adebajo, A. O., Charles, P., Maini, R. N., and Hazleman, B. L. (1993). Autoantibodies in malaria, tuberculosis and hepatitis B in a west African population. *Clin. Exp. Immunol.* 92, 73–76. doi: 10.1111/j.1365-2249.1993.tb05950.x

Adu, D., Williams, D. G., Quakyi, I. A., Voller, A., Anim-Addo, Y., Bruce-Tagoe, A. A., et al. (1982). Anti-ssDNA and antinuclear antibodies in human malaria. *Clin. Exp. Immunol.* 49, 310–316

Antonelli, L. R., Junqueira, C., Vinetz, J. M., Golenbock, D. T., Ferreira, M. U., and Gazzinelli, R. T. (2019). The immunology of *Plasmodium vivax* malaria. *Immunol. Rev.* 293, 163–189. doi: 10.1111/imr.12816

Badiane, A. S., Diongue, K., Diallo, S., Ndongo, A. A., Diedhiou, C. K., Deme, A. B., et al. (2016). Acute kidney injury associated with *Plasmodium malariae* infection. *Malar. J.* 13:226. doi: 10.1186/1475-2875-13-226

Bansal, D., Herbert, F., Lim, P., Deshpande, P., Bécavin, C., Guiyedi, V., et al. (2009). IgG autoantibody to brain beta tubulin III associated with cytokine cluster-II driscriminate cerebral malaria in central India. *PLoS ONE* 4:e8245. doi: 10.1371/journal.pone.0008245

Barber, B. E., Grigg, M. J., Piera, K., Amante, F. H., William, T., Boyle, M. J., et al. (2019). Antiphosphatidylserine immunoglobulin M and immunoglobulin G antibodies are higher in vivax than falciparum malaria, and associated with early anemia in both species. *J. Infect. Dis.* 220, 1435–1443. doi: 10.1093/infdis/jiz334

Barsoum, R. S. (2000). Malarial acute renal failure. *J. Am. Soc. Nephrol.* 11, 2147–2154. doi: 10.46-6673/1111-2147

Bell, K., Wilding, C., Funke, S., Pfeiffer, N., and Grus, F. H. (2015). Protective effect of 14-3-3 antibodies on stressed neuroretinal cells via the mitochondrial apoptosis pathway. *BMC Ophthalmol.* 15:64. doi: 10.1186/s12886-015-0044-9

Berzins, K., Wahlgren, M., and Perlmann, P. (1983). Studies on the specificity on anti-erythrocyte antibodies in the serum of patients with malaria. *Clin. Exp. Immunol.* 54, 313–318.

Birbeck, G. L., Molyneux, M. E., Kaplan, P. W., Seydel, K. B., Chimalizeni, Y. F., Kawaza, K., et al. (2010). Blantyre malaria project epilepsy study (BMPES) of neurological outcomes in retinopathy-positive paediatric cerebral malaria survivors: a prospective cohort study. *Lancet* 9, 1173–1181. doi: 10.1016/S1474-4422(10)70270-2

Brahimi, K., Martins, Y. C., Zanini, G. M., Ferreira-da-Cruz, M. F., and Daniel-Ribeiro, C. T. (2011). Monoclonal auto-antibodies and sera of autoimmune patients react with *Plasmodium falciparum* and inhibit its *in vitro* growth. *Mem. Inst. Oswaldo Cruz* 106, 44–51. doi: 10.1590/s0074-02762011000900006

Brown, H., Rogerson, S., Taylor, T., Tembo, M., Mwenechanya, J., Molyneux, M., et al. (2001). Blood-brain barrier function in cerebral malaria in Malawian children. *Am. J. Trop. Med. Hyg.* 64, 207–213. doi: 10.4269/ajtmh.2001.64.207

Burchard, G. D., Ehrhardt, S., Mockenhaupt, F. P., Mathieu, A., Agana-Nsiire, P., Anemana, S. D., et al. (2003). Renal dysfunction in children with uncomplicated *Plasmodium falciparum* malaria in Tamale, Ghana. *Ann. Trop. Med. Parasit.* 97, 345–350. doi: 10.1179/000349803235002281

Calvet, M. C., Druilhe, P., Camacho-Garcia, R., and Calvet, J. (1993). Culture model for the study of cerebral malaria: antibodies from *Plasmodium falciparum*-infected comatose patients inhibit the dendritic development of Purkinje cells. *J. Neurosci. Res.* 36, 235–240. doi: 10.1002/jnr.490360214

Collins, W. E., Jeffery, G. M., and Roberts, J. M. (2003). A retrospective examination of anemia during infection of humans with *Plasmodium vivax*. *Am. J. Trop. Med.* 68, 410–412.

Conroy, A. L., Hawkes, M., Elphinstone, R. E., Morgan, C., Hermann, L., Barker, K. R., et al. (2016). Acute kidney injury is common in pediatric severe malaria and is associated with increased mortality. *Open Forum Infect. Dis.* 3:ofw046. doi: 10.1093/ofid/ofw046

Cordat, E., and Reithmeier, R. A. (2014). Structure, function, and trafficking of SLC4 and SLC26 anion transporters. *Curr. Top. Membr.* 73, 1–67. doi: 10.1016/B978-0-12-800223-0.00001-3

Cornell, B., and Toyo-Oka, K. (2017). 14-3-3 proteins in brain development: neurogenesis, neuronal migration and neuromorphogenesis. *Front. Mol. Neurosci.* 10:318. doi: 10.3389/fnmol.2017.00318

Couper, K. N., Barnes, T., Hafalla, J. C. R., Combes, V., Ryffel, B., Secher, T., et al. (2010). Parasite-derived plasma microparticles contribute significantly to malaria infection-induced inflammation through potent macrophage stimulation. *PLoS Pathog.* 6:e1000744. doi: 10.1371/journal.ppat.1000744

Damian, R. T. (1964). Molecular mimicry: antigen sharing by parasite and host and its consequences. *Am. Nat.* 98, 129–149.

Daniel-Ribeiro, C., Druilhe, P., Monjour, L., Homberg, J. C., and Gentilini, M. (1983). Specificity of auto-antibodies in malaria and the role of polyclonal activation. *Trans. R. Soc. Trop. Med. Hyg.* 77, 185–188. doi: 10.1016/0035-9203(83)90064-0

Das, B. S. (2008). Renal failure in malaria. *J. Vector Borne Dis.* 45, 83–97.

Donati, D., Zhang, L. P., Chêne, A., Chen, Q., Flick, K., Nyström, M., et al. (2004). Identification of a polyclonal B-cell activator in *Plasmodium falciparum*. *Infect. Immun.* 72, 5412–5418. doi: 10.1128/IAI.72.9.5412-5418.2004

Douglas, N. M., Anstey, N. M., Buffet, P. A., Poespoprodjo, J. R., Yeo, T. W., White, N. J., et al. (2012). The anaemia of *Plasmodium vivax* malaria. *Malar. J.* 11:135. doi: 10.1186/1475-2875-11-135

Duarte, J., Herbert, F., Guiyedi, V., Franetich, J. F., Roland, J., Cazenave, P. A., et al. (2012). High levels of immunoglobulin E autoantibody to 14-3-3 epsilon protein correlate with protection against severe *Plasmodium falciparum* malaria. *J. Infect. Dis.* 206, 1781–1789. doi: 10.1093/infdis/jis595

Elsheikha, H. M., and Sheashaa, H. A. (2007). Epidemiology, pathophysiology, management and outcome of renal dysfunction associated with plasmodia infection. *Parasitol. Res.* 101, 1183–1190. doi: 10.1007/s00436-007-0650-4

Facer, C. A., and Agiostratidou, G. (1994). High levels of anti-phospholipid antibodies in uncomplicated and severe *Plasmodium falciparum* and *P. vivax malaria*. *Clin. Exp. Immunol.* 95, 304–309. doi: 10.1111/j.1365-2249.1994.tb06528.x

Facer, C. A., Bray, R. S., and Brown, J. (1979). Direct Coombs antiglobulin reactions in Gambian children with *Plasmodium falciparum* malaria. I. incidence and class specificity. *Clin. Exp. Immunol.* 35, 119–127.

Fernandes, A. A., Carvalho, L. J., Zanini, G. M., Ventura, A. M., Souza, J. M., Cotias, P. M., et al. (2008). Similar cytokine responses and degress of anemia in patients with *Plasmodium falciparum* and *Plasmodium vivax* infections in the Brazilian Amazon region. *Clin. Vaccine Immunol.* 15, 650–658. doi: 10.1128/CVI.00475-07

Fernandez-Arias, C., Rivera-Correa, J., Gallego-Delgado, J., Rudlaff, R., Fernandez, C., Roussel, C., et al. (2016). Anti-self-phosphatidylserine antibodies recognize uninfected erythrocytes promoting malarial anemia. *Cell Host Microbe.* 19, 194–203: doi: 10.1016/j.chom.2016.01.009

Flanagan, K. L., Plebanski, M., Odhiambo, K., Sheu, E., Mwangi, T., Gelder, C., et al. (2006). Cellular reactivity to the *P. falciparum* protein TRAP in adult kenyans: novel epitopes, complex cytokine patterns, and yhe impact of natural antigenic variation. *Am. J. Trop. Med. Hyg.* 74, 367–375.

Fontaine, A., Pophillat, M., Bourdon, S., Villard, C., Belghazi, M., Fourget, P., et al. (2010). Specific antibody responses against membrane proteins of erythrocytes infected by *Plasmodium falciparum* of individuals briefly exposed to malaria. *Malar. J.* 9:276. doi: 10.1186/1475-2875-9-276

Foote, M., and Zhou, Y. (2012). 14-3-3 proteins in neurological disorders. *Int. J. Biochem. Mol. Biol.* 3, 152–164.

Freeman, R. R., and Parish, C. R. (1978). Polyclonal B-cell activation during rodent malarial infections. *Clin. Exp. Immunol.* 32, 41–45

Frutakul, P., Boonpucknavig, V., Boonpucknavig, S., Mitrakul, C., and Bhamarapravati, N. (1974). Acute glomerulonephritis complicating *Plasmodium falciparum* infection. *Clin. Pediatr.* 13, 281–283. doi: 10.1177/000992287401300315

Füchtbauer, A., Herrmann, M., Mandelkowl, E., and Jockusch, M. (1985). Disruption of microtubules in living cells and cell models by high affinity antibodies to beta-tubulin. *EMBO.* 4, 2807–2814.

Fujinami, R. S., von Herrath, M. G., Christen, U., and Whitton, J. L. (2006). Molecular mimicry, bystander activation, por viral persistence: infections and autoimmune disease. *Clin. Microbiol. Rev.* 19, 80–94. doi: 10.1128/CMR.19.1.80-94.2006

Gallien, S., Roussilhon, C., Blanc, C., Pérignon, J. L., and Druilhe, P. (2011). Autoantibody against dendrite in *Plasmodium falciparum* infection: a singular auto-immune phenomenon preferentially in cerebral malaria. *Acta Trop.* 118, 67–70. doi: 10.1016/j.actatropica.2011.01.005

Gitau, E. N., Kokwaro, G. O., Karanja, H., Newton, C. R., and Ward, S. A. (2013). Plasma and cerebrospinal proteomes from children with cerebral malaria differ from those of children with other encephalopathies. *J. Infect. Dis.* 208, 1494–1503. doi: 10.1093/infdis/jit334

Greenwood, B. M. (1974). Possible role of a B-cell mitogen in hypergammaglobulinaemia in malaria and trypanosomiasis. *Lancet* 1, 435–436. doi: 10.1016/s0140-6736(74)92386-1

Guiyedi, V., Chanseaud, Y., Fesel, C., Snounou, G., Rousselle, J. C., Lim, P., et al. (2007). Self-reactivities to the non-erythroid alpha spectrin correlate with cerebral malaria in Gabonese children. *PLoS ONE* 2:e389. doi: 10.1371/journal.pone.0000389

Haneji, N. T., Nakamura, K., Takio, K., Yanagi, H., and Higashiyama, I. (1997). Identification of alpha-fodrin as a candidate autoantigen in primary Sjogren's syndrome. *Science,* 276, 604–607. doi: 10.1126/Science.276.5312.604

Hogh, B., Petersen, E., Crandall, I., Gottschau, A., and Sherman, I. W. (1994). Immune responses to band 3 neoantigens on *Plasmodium falciparum*-infected erythrocytes in subjects living in an area of intense malaria transmission are associated with low parasite density and high hematocrit value. *Infect. Immunol.* 62, 4362–4366.

Holmgren, A. M., McConkey, C. A., and Shin, S. (2017). Outrunning the red queen: bystander activation as a means of outpacing innate immune subversion by intracellular pathogens. *Cell. Mol. Immmunol.* 14, 14–21.

Houba, V. (1979). Immunologic aspects of renal lesions associated with malaria. *Kidney Int.* 16, 3–8. doi: 10.1038/ki.1979.96

Houba, V., Allison, A. C., Adeniyi, A., and Houba, J. E. (1971). Immunoglobulin classes and complement biopsies of Nigerian children with the nephrotic syndrome. *Clin. Exp. Immunol.* 8, 761–774.

Huerta, P. T., Kowal, C., DeGiorgio, L. A., Volpe, B. T., Diamond, B. (2006). Immunity and behavior: antibodies alter emotion. *Proc. Natl. Acad. Sci. U.S.A.* 103, 678–683. doi: 10.1073/pnas.0510055103

Idro, R., Marsh, K., John, C. C., Newton, C. R. (2010). Cerebral malaria: mechanisms of brain injury and strategies for improved neurocognitive outcome. *Pediatr. Res.* 68, 267–274. doi: 10.1203/00006450-201011001-00524

Irani, S., and Lang, B. (2008). Autoantibody-mediated disorders of the central nervous system. *Autoimmunity* 41, 55–65. doi: 10.1080/08916930701619490

Jakobsen, P. H., Morris-Jones, S. D., Hviid, L., Theander, T. G., Høier-Madsen, M., Bayoumi, R. A., et al. (1993). Anti-phospholipid antibodies in patients with *Plasmodium falciparum* malaria. *Immunology* 79, 653–657.

Katsetos, G. D., Herman, M. M., and Mörk, S. J. (2003). Class III β-tubullin in human development and cancer. *Cell Motil. Cytoskeleton* 55, 77–96. doi: 10.1002/cm.10116

Kenangalem, E., Karyana, M., Burdarm, L., Yeung, S., Simpson, J. A., Tjitra, E., et al. (2016). *Plasmodium vivax* infection: a major determinant of severe anaema in infancy. *Malar. J.* 15:321. doi: 10.1186/s12936-016-1373-8

Lacerda, M. V., Mourão, M. P., Coelho, H. C., and Santos, J. B. (2011). Thrombocytopenia in malaria: who cares? *Mem. Inst. Oswaldo Cruz.* 106(Suppl. 1), 52–63. doi: 10.1590/s0074-02762011000900007

Lang, B., Newbold, C. I., Williams, G., Peshu, N., Marsh, K., and Newton, C. R. (2005). Antibodies to voltage-gated calcium channels in children with falciparum malaria. *J. Infect. Dis.* 191, 117–121. doi: 10.1086/426512

Looareesuwan, S., Merry, A. H., Phillips, R. E., Pleehachinda, R., Wattanagoon, Y., Ho, M., et al. (1987). Reduced erythrocyte survival following clearance of malarial parasitaemia in Thai patients. *Br. J. Haematol.* 67, 473–478. doi: 10.1111/j.1365-2141.1987.tb06171.x

Ludin, P., Nilsson, D., and Maser, P. (2011). Genome-wide identification of molecular mimicry candidates in parasites. *PLoS One* 6:e17546. doi: 10.1371/journal.pone.0017546

Ludwig, R. J., Vanhoorelbeke, K., Leypoldt, F., Kaya, Z., Bieber, K., McLachlan, S. M., et al. (2017). Mechanisms of autoantibody-induced pathology. *Front. Immunol.* 8:603. doi: 10.3389/fimmu.2017.00603

Lutz, H. U., and Bogdanova, A. (2013). Mechanisms tagging senescent red blood cells for clearance in healthy humans. *Front. Physiol.* 4:387. doi: 10.3389/fphys.2013.00387

MaCDonald, S. M., Bhisutthiban, J., Shapiro, T. A., Rogerson, S. J., Taylor, T. E., Tembo, M., et al. (2001). Immune mimicry in malaria: *Plasmodium falciparum* secretes a functional histamine-releasing factor honmolog *in vitro* and *in vivo*. *Proc. Natl. Acad. Sci. U.S.A.* 98, 10829–10832. doi: 10.1073/pnas.20 1191498

Mantel, P., Hoang, A.n., Goldowitz, I., Potashnikova, D., Hamza, B., Vorobjev, I., et al. (2013). Malaria-infected erythrocyte-derived microvesicles mediate cellular communication within the parasite population and with the host immune system. *Cell Host Microbe.* 13, 521–534. doi: 10.1016/j.chom.2013.04.009

Minoprio, P. (2001). Parasite polyclonal activators: new targets for vaccination approaches? *Int. J. Parasitol.* 31, 583–591. doi: 10.1016/S0020-7519(01)00171-0

Molyneux, M. E., Taylor, T. E., Wirima, J. J., and Borgstein, A. (1989). Clinical features and prognostic indicators in paediatric cerebral malaria: a study of 131 comatose Malawian children. *Q. J. Med.* 71, 441–459.

Mourão, L. C., Baptista, R. P., Almeida, Z. B., Grynberg, P., Pucci, M. M., Castro-Gomes, T., et al. (2018). Anti-band 3 and anti-spectrin antibodies are increased in *Plasmodium vivax* infection and are associated with anemia. *Sci. Rep.* 6:8762. doi: 10.1038/s41598-018-27109-6

Mourão, L. C., Roma, P. M., Sultane-Aboobacar, J. S., Medeiros, C. M., de Almeida, Z. B., Fontes, C. J., et al. (2016). Anti-erythrocyte antibodies may contribute to anaemia in *Plasmodium vivax* malaria by decreasing red blood cell deformability and increasing erythrophagocytosis. *Malar. J.* 15:397. doi: 10.1186/s12936-016-1449-5

Moxon, C. A., Gibbins, M. P., McGuinness, D., Milner, D. A., and Marti, M. (2019). New insights into malaria pathogenesis. *Annu. Rev. Pathol.* 15. doi: 10.1146/annurev-pathmechdis-012419-032640

Münz, C., Lünemann, J. D., Getts, M. T., and Miller, S. D. (2009). Antiviral immune responses: triggers of or triggered by autoimmunity? *Nat. Rev. Immunol.* 9, 246–258. doi: 10.1038/nri2527

Nath, R., Raser, K. J., Stafford, D. (1996). Non-erythroid alpha-spectrin breakdown by calpain and interleukin I beta-converting-enzyme-like protease(s) in apoptotic cells: contributory roles of both protease families in neuronal apoptosis. *Biochem. J.* 319, 683–690. doi: 10.1042/bj3190683

Neri, S., Pulvirenti, D., Patamia, I., Zoccolo, A., and Castellino, P. (2008). Acute renal failure in *Plasmodium malariae* infection. *Neth. J. Med.* 66, 166–168.

Nguansangiam, S., Day, N. P. J., Hien, T. T., Mai, N. T. H., Chaisri, U., Riganti, M., et al. (2007). A quantitative ultrastructural study of renal pathology in fatal *Plasmodium falciparum* malaria. *Trop. Med. Int. Health.* 12, 1037–1050. doi: 10.1111/j.1365-3156.2007.01881.x

Olowu, W. A., and Adelusola, K. A. (2004). Pediatric acute renal failure in southwestern Nigeria. *Kidney Int.* 66, 1541–1548. doi: 10.1111/j.1523-1755.2004.00918.x

Pinto, A., Gillard, S., Moss, F., Whyte, K., Brust, P., Williams, M., et al. (1998). Human autoantibodies specific for the alpha1A calcium channel subunit reduce both P-type and Q-type calcium currents in cerebellar neurons. *Proc. Natl. Acad. Sci. U.S.A.* 95, 8328–8333. doi: 10.1073/PNAS.95.14.8328

Ritter, K., Kuhlencord, A., Thomssen, R., and Bommer, W. (1993). Prolonged haemolytic anaemia in malaria and autoantibodies against triosephosphate isomerase. *Lancet* 342, 1333–1334. doi: 10.1016/0140-6736(93)92248-r

Rivera-Correa, J., Conroy, A. L., Opoka, R. O., Batte, A., Namazzi, R., Ouma, B., et al. (2019b). Autoantibody levels are associated with acute kidney injury, anemia and post-discharge morbidity and mortality in Ugandan children with severe malaria. *Sci. Rep.* 9:14840. doi: 10.1038/s41598-019-51426-z

Rivera-Correa, J., Guthmiller, J. J., Vijay, R., Fernandez-Arias, C., Pardo-Ruge, M. A., Gonzalez, S., et al. (2017). *Plasmodium* DNA-mediated TLR9 activation of T-bet^{+} B cells contributes to autoimmune anaemia during malaria. *Nat. Commun.* 8:1282. doi: 10.1038/s41467-017-01476-6

Rivera-Correa, J., Mackroth, M. S., Jacobs, T., Schulze Zur Wiesch, J., Rolling, T., and Rodriguez, A. (2019a). Atypical memory B-cells are associated with *Plasmodium falciparum* anemia through anti-phosphatidylserine antibodies. *Elife* 8:e48309. doi: 10.7554/eLife.48309

Rivera-Correa, J., and Rodriguez, A. (2019). Autoimmune anemia in malaria. *Trends Parasitol.* 36, 91–97. doi: 10.1016/j.pt.2019.12.002

Rosenberg, E. B., Strickland, G. T., Yang, S. L., and Whalen, G. E. (1973). IgM antibodies to red cells and autoimmune anemia in patients with malaria. *Am. J. Trop. Med. Hyg.* 22, 146–152. doi: 10.4269/ajtmh.1973.22.146

Rosenberg, Y. J. (1978). Autoimmune and polyclonal B cell responses during murine malaria. *Nature* 264, 170–172. doi: 10.1038/274 170a0

Seydel, K. B., Milner, D. A., Kamiza, S. B., Molyneux, M. E., and Taylor, T. E. (2006). The distribution and intensity of parasite sequestration in comatose Malawian children. *J. Infect. Dis.* 194, 208–205. doi: 10.1086/50 5078

Shimada, T., Fournier, A. E., and Yamagat, K. (2013). Neuroprotective function of 14-3-3 proteins in neurodegeneration. *Biomed. Res. Int.* 2013:564534. doi: 10.1155/2013/564534

Sypniewska, P., Duda, J. F., Locatelli, I., Althaus, C. R., Althaus, F., Genton, B. (2017). Clinical and laboratory predictors of death in African children with features of severe malaria: a systematic review and meta-analysis. *BMC Med.* 15:147. doi: 10.1186/s12916-017-0906-5

Taylor, T. E., Fu, W. J., Carr, R. A., Whitten, R. O., Mueller, J. S., Fosiko, N. G., et al. (2004). Differentiating the pathologies of cerebral malaria by postmortem parasite counts. *Nat. Med.* 10, 143–145. doi: 10.1038/nm986

Teasdale, G., and Jennett, B. (1974). Assessment of coma and impaired consciousness. *a practical scale. Lancet* 2, 81–84. doi: 10.1016/s0140-6736(74)91639-0

Teo, A., Feng, G., Brown, G. V., Beeson, J. G., and Rogerson, S. J. (2016). Functional antibodies and protection against blood-stage malaria. *Trends Parasitol.* 32, 867–898. doi: 10.1016/j.pt.2016.07.003

Tischfield, M. A., Baris, H. N., Wu, C., Rudolph, G., Van Maldergem, L., He, W., et al. (2010). Human TUBB3 mutations perturb microtubule dynamics, kinesin interactions, and axon guidance. *Cell* 140, 74–87. doi: 10.1016/j.cell.2009.12.011

van Velthuysen, M. L. F., and Florquin, S. (2000). Glomerulopathy associated with parasitic infections. *Clin. Microbiol. Rev.* 13, 55–66. doi: 10.1128/cmr.13.1.55-66.2000

Vanderlugt, C. L., and Miller, S. D. (2002). Epitope spreading in immune-mediated diseases: implications fior immunotherapy. *Nat. Rev. Immunol.* 2, 85–95. doi: 10.1038/nri724

Ventura, A. M. R. S., Fernandes, A. A. M., Zanini, G. M., Pratt-Riccio, L. R., Sequeira, C. G., do Monte, C. R. S., et al. (2018). Clinical and immunological profiles of anaemia in children and adolescentes with *Plasmodium vivax* malaria in the Pará state. Brazilian Amazon. *Acta Trop.* 181, 122–131. doi: 10.1016/j.actatropica.2018.01.022

von Seidlein, L., Olaosebikan, R., Hendriksen, I. C. E., Lee, S. J., Adedoyin, O. T., Agbenyega, T., et al. (2012). Predicting the clinical outcome of severe falciparum malaria in African children: findings from a large randomized trial. *Clin. Infect. Dis.* 54, 1080–1090. doi: 10.1093/cid/cis034

Ward, P. A., and Kibuka-Musoke, J. W. (1969). Evidence for soluble immune complexes in the pathogenesis of the glomerulonephritis of quartan malaria. *Lancet* 1, 283–285.

White, N. J. (2018). Anaemia and malaria. *Malar. J.* 17:371. doi: 10.1186/s12936-018-2509-9

WHO | World Malaria Report (2019). *WHO. Available online at: https://www.who.int/publications-detail/world-malaria-report-2019 (accessed on January* 02, 2020).

Wozencraft, A. O., Lloyd, C. M., Staines, N. A., and Griffiths, V. J. (1990). Role of DNA-binding antibodies in kidney pathology associated with murine malaria infections. *Infect Immun.* 58, 2156–2164.

20

Chloroquine and Sulfadoxine–Pyrimethamine Resistance in Sub-Saharan Africa

*Alexandra T. Roux[1], Leah Maharaj[1], Olukunle Oyegoke[1], Oluwasegun P. Akoniyon[1], Matthew Adekunle Adeleke[1], Rajendra Maharaj[2] and Moses Okpeku[1]**

[1] *Discipline of Genetics, School of Life Sciences, University of KwaZulu-Natal, Westville, South Africa,* [2] *Office of Malaria Research, South African Medical Research Council, Cape Town, South Africa*

Edited by:
Apichai Tuanyok,
University of Florida, United States

Reviewed by:
Rajeev Kumar Mehlotra,
Case Western Reserve University, United States
Chenqi Wang,
University of South Florida, United States

***Correspondence:**
Moses Okpeku
okpekum@ukzn.ac.za

Malaria is a great concern for global health and accounts for a large amount of morbidity and mortality, particularly in Africa, with sub-Saharan Africa carrying the greatest burden of the disease. Malaria control tools such as insecticide-treated bed nets, indoor residual spraying, and antimalarial drugs have been relatively successful in reducing the burden of malaria; however, sub-Saharan African countries encounter great challenges, the greatest being antimalarial drug resistance. Chloroquine (CQ) was the first-line drug in the 20th century until it was replaced by sulfadoxine–pyrimethamine (SP) as a consequence of resistance. The extensive use of these antimalarials intensified the spread of resistance throughout sub-Saharan Africa, thus resulting in a loss of efficacy for the treatment of malaria. SP was replaced by artemisinin-based combination therapy (ACT) after the emergence of resistance toward SP; however, the use of ACTs is now threatened by the emergence of resistant parasites. The decreased selective pressure on CQ and SP allowed for the reintroduction of sensitivity toward those antimalarials in regions of sub-Saharan Africa where they were not the primary drug for treatment. Therefore, the emergence and spread of antimalarial drug resistance should be tracked to prevent further spread of the resistant parasites, and the re-emergence of sensitivity should be monitored to detect the possible reappearance of sensitivity in sub-Saharan Africa.

Keywords: antimalarial drug resistance, chloroquine, malaria, malaria control, sulfadoxine–pyrimethamine

INTRODUCTION

Malaria is a global health concern regarding morbidity and mortality, with approximately 228 million worldwide cases and an estimated 405,000 deaths in 2018 (World Health Organisation (WHO), 2019). Underprivileged, rural populations consisting of young children and pregnant women are disproportionately affected by malaria. The cornerstone of malaria control efforts for the past decade has been to address the inequalities, including the availability of commodities (Taylor et al., 2017). Sub-Saharan Africa experiences the greatest burden of the malaria disease, accounting for approximately 90% of the world's *Plasmodium falciparum* infections and deaths with almost all malaria caused by *P. falciparum* in this area (Yeka et al., 2012; Maitland, 2016).

P. falciparum is the most virulent of the malaria parasites that infect humans (Recker et al., 2018). Therefore, the utilization of effective tools for malaria control has increased to lessen the burden of malaria (Greenwood et al., 2005). In spite of increased efforts, many countries in Africa are still confronted with challenges with malaria control, partially as a consequence of the identified limitations in public health structures as well as the infrastructure of primary health care (Xia et al., 2014). The development of resistance toward antimalarial drugs is one of the main challenges when dealing with malaria control and elimination, as such antimalarial drug resistance in a setting where access to health care is limited has severe consequences (Takala-Harrison and Laufer, 2015). Drug pressure, which refers to the extensive and/or misuse of antimalarial drugs, is an identified factor associated with the emergence of resistance; additionally, the misuse or sole use of a drug can encourage selection of resistant strains (Hanboonkunupakarn and White, 2016).

In Africa, malaria control programs rest majorly on vector control and the use of antimalarial drugs (Conrad and Rosenthal, 2019). There are different types of malaria, namely, asymptomatic, uncomplicated, and severe malaria. Asymptomatic malaria refers to malaria parasites being present in the blood, providing a reservoir for transmission, without the individual displaying symptoms (Chourasia et al., 2017). Uncomplicated malaria refers to malaria symptoms presented by a patient together with a positive parasitological test (Grobusch and Kremsner, 2005). Severe malaria is defined by positive parasitological test (microscopy or rapid diagnostic test) detecting *P. falciparum* and at least one condition for severe disease such as severe anemia or respiratory distress (Conroy et al., 2019).

Sub-Saharan African countries used chloroquine (CQ) as the first-line drug for malaria up to the start of this millennium. However, it was replaced with sulfadoxine–pyrimethamine (SP) after CQ was declared ineffective as a result of resistant parasites (Lusingu and Von Seidlein, 2008) but soon lost its efficacy when parasites began to develop resistance toward it. Mutations in the *P. falciparum* CQ-resistant transporter (*pfcrt*) gene and the *P. falciparum* multidrug-resistance gene 1 (*pfmdr-1*) have been implicated in CQ resistance (CQR) (Bin Dajem and Al-Qahtani, 2010). CQR was observed on the Thai-Cambodian border and concurrently in South America in the late 1950s (Young and Moore, 1961; Harinasuta et al., 1965). In Southeast Asia, specifically Thailand and Myanmar, drug resistance in local parasite populations is a serious concern, with *P. falciparum* in the region tending to develop resistance (Parker et al., 2015). Key factors associated with drug resistance in these regions is drug pressure, which results in selection of resistant parasites and their propagation by local transmission and reservoir migration (Wernsdorfer, 1994). In 1978, resistance spread to Africa, with confirmed treatment failures in both Kenya and Tanzania, later reaching West Africa in 1980. CQ continued to be the first-line treatment for uncomplicated *P. falciparum* malaria in the most sub-Saharan countries until after 2,000 despite its declining use (Flegg et al., 2013). However, some countries, including South Africa, Zambia, Tanzania, and Kenya (D'Alessandro and Buttiëns, 2001; Mwendera et al., 2016), were only forced to switch to SP as the new first-line treatment for malaria, as levels of CQR increased (Gatton et al., 2004). Shortly after its introduction as the new first-line treatment for malaria, polymorphisms in the parasite's genes—*pfdhps* [*P. falciparum* dihydropteroate synthase (DHFR)] and *pfdhfr* [*P. falciparum* dihydrofolate reductase (DHPS)]—became widespread throughout Africa (Winstanley et al., 2004). The association of the mutations with SP treatment failure in children made the antimalarial unsuitable for therapy (Desai et al., 2015). In Africa, the use of SP for clinical malaria was stopped as a consequence of its extensive resistance. However, in malaria endemic areas, it is still used for intermittent preventative treatment during pregnancy (Zhao et al., 2020). By 2007, 90% of sub-Saharan Africa had implemented policies of artemisinin-based combination therapy (ACT) for the treatment of uncomplicated malaria as a consequence of widespread CQ and SP resistance (Frosch et al., 2011). The efficacy of ACTs leads to substantial declines in morbidity and mortality in areas with high malaria endemicity. But the success of such therapies is threatened by the appearance of artemisinin-resistant strains of *P. falciparum* from Thai-Cambodian and Thai-Myanmar borders (Ajayi and Ukwaja, 2013). There have been isolated reports of artemisinin-resistant parasites in sub-Saharan Africa, but they have not become established on the continent yet (Lu et al., 2017a). The emergence and spread of artemisinin-resistant parasites would have an immense impact on Africa's control efforts (Raman et al., 2019), especially as the world is anticipating a global elimination strategy (World Health Organisation (WHO), 2020). *P. falciparum* contains Kelch13 (*K13*), which is needed in the asexual erythrocytic development stage. Although details of its function are not fully known (Siddiqui et al., 2020), they are highly conserved, and single-point mutations are associated with artemisinin resistance (Birnbaum et al., 2020). According to Meshnick (1998), the mechanism of action of artemisinin is in two steps: first, an initial activation that catalyzes the cleavage of endoperoxide produces free radicals. In the second step, these free radicals are responsible for killing the parasites. However, a single-nucleotide polymorphism (SNP) in the gene associated with up-regulated pathway antagonizes the artemisinin oxidation activity (Fairhurst and Dondorp, 2016). A recent study revealed that parasites with inactivated *K13* or its mutated form displayed reduced hemoglobin endocytosis (Birnbaum et al., 2020). *K13* is important in the uptake and degradation of hemoglobin, which is vital for parasite survival. The mutations and mislocalization of *K13* induce artemisinin resistance (Xie et al., 2020); therefore, a close observation of ACT resistance is necessary, as they are the current first-line treatment for *P. falciparum* malaria (Siddiqui et al., 2020).

A key challenge for malaria control is the emergence and spread of antimalarial drug resistance, particularly in the malaria endemic areas of sub-Saharan Africa where disastrous consequences are observed as a result of the spread of CQ- and SP-resistant *P. falciparum* strains (von Seidlein and Dondorp, 2015). Furthermore, the development of ACT resistance threatens the control efforts in malaria elimination. This review aims to track the spread of CQ and SP resistance in sub-Saharan Africa. It identifies malaria control strategies employed and ways to combat the challenges being faced to further prevent the emergence and spread of resistant parasites.

MALARIA CONTROL IN SUB-SAHARAN AFRICA

A global public health concern of this century includes controlling vector-borne diseases such as malaria; therefore, much effort has focused on the development of vector control approaches (Tizifa et al., 2018). These approaches encompass methods directed toward the malaria vector by restricting its ability to transmit malaria by shielding areas that are recognized as receptive areas for transmission. Receptivity of the disease is dependent on the vectorial capacity of local vector populations, besides the presence of the vector; this includes the vector population size, biting habits, and the longevity of the sporogony period. These parameters are greatly affected by local ecology, climate, and human and vector behaviors (Smith Gueye et al., 2016). Examples of vector control strategies include insecticide-treated nets (ITNs) and indoor residual spraying (IRS).

In Africa, ITNs are the most extensively used intervention for malaria control, signifying the main tool for vector control in almost all malaria endemic African countries (World Health Organisation (WHO), 2017). ITNs act as a direct barrier to mosquito biting, hence proving effective in the reduction of malaria-related morbidity and mortality. Additionally, they reduce vector density and the average life span by providing community-wide protection through the killing of mosquitoes (Scates et al., 2020). They exploit the indoor feeding and resting behavioral patterns displayed by some *Anopheles* mosquitoes (Steinhardt et al., 2017). The universal coverage of ITN distribution, with mass distribution campaigns conducted in intervals, is implemented by most national malaria control programs (World Health Organisation (WHO), 2017). More than 800 million ITNs have been distributed in sub-Saharan Africa between 2011 and 2016, to ultimately achieve universal coverage (Olapeju et al., 2018). Through this initiative, a greater proportion (30% in 2010 to 54% in 2016) of Africans in malaria endemic areas slept under ITNs (Olapeju et al., 2018). In sub-Saharan Africa, 67–73% of the total 663 million prevented malaria cases in the past 15 years have been credited to the widespread distribution and use of ITNs (World Health Organisation (WHO), 2017). Another main method used for malaria control on a large scale includes the spraying of houses with insecticides, referred to as IRS. This method has aided the elimination of malaria from large parts of Latin America, Europe, Russia, and Asia. There are also successful IRS programs implemented in parts of Africa (Pluess et al., 2010). It is believed to function by repelling mosquitoes from entering houses as well as through killing female mosquitoes that rest inside houses after taking up a blood meal, thus suggesting that IRS is largely effective against endophilic mosquitoes (those species resting indoors). Additionally, this method is reliant on the vectorial mass effect, which refers to the reduction in transmission as a result of increased mortality of adult vectors typically after feeding (Najera and Zaim, 2001). Considering the slow development and implementation of alternative interventions, ITNs and IRS continue to be the foundation of the malaria control agenda. Consequently, a great challenge is the optimization of the continued use and sustained success of existing ITNs and IRS, while new vector control tools are being studied (Okumu and Moore, 2011).

Antimalarial drugs are used as a malaria control strategy to essentially reduce transmission. During the 20th century, CQ, a safe and inexpensive antimalarial, was a pillar of malaria control and eradication; however, it has lost its effectiveness. Of late, SP was the only alternative extensively available, but the increase and spread of drug resistance have compromised its effectiveness. Resistance to CQ and SP appeared in Southeast Asia, thereafter, spread to Africa (Naidoo and Roper, 2010). Therefore, the World Health Organization (WHO) recommended the implementation of policies approving ACTs as the primary treatment strategy for uncomplicated malaria in the majority of malaria endemic countries (Frosch et al., 2011). In spite of this, according to the 2008 World Malaria Report, ACTs were used to treat only 3% of children with suspected malaria (World Health Organisation (WHO), 2008), implying that CQ and SP were still used to treat malaria in children. Although ACTs are the recommended first-line treatment for malaria in both Asia and Africa, artemisinin-resistant *P. falciparum* strains have appeared and spread within Southeast Asia, subsequently leading to a reduction in treatment efficacy (Dondorp and Ringwald, 2013). Since Africa holds the greatest burden of malaria, there is a concern regarding the impact of artemisinin resistance on malaria morbidity and mortality (Slater et al., 2016).

THE MECHANISMS AND CONTRIBUTING FACTORS ASSOCIATED WITH ANTIMALARIAL DRUG RESISTANCE IN *Plasmodium falciparum*

Drug resistance is a growing problem in the fight to control malaria, as pathogens regularly develop mechanisms that allow them to survive the use of drugs. These mechanisms are generally the result of mutations that affect the drug's target site, thereby hindering or completely preventing binding between the drug and its target (**Table 1**). Another way that drug resistance may occur is by the increased levels of the target—this means that more drug is needed to reach inhibition of the parasite.

Chloroquine functions by accumulating in the parasite's acidic food vacuole (Lehane et al., 2012; Lawrenson et al., 2018). The xenobiotic inhibits heme catabolism (i.e., the mechanism by which the malaria parasite "feeds"). Upon infection, host hemoglobin is degraded by the parasite; this releases heme and leads to the ultimate development of an acidic lysosome-like digestive vacuole (Coban, 2020). Downstream, there is accumulation of heme–CQ complexes, which negatively impact parasite survival (Loria et al., 1999; Lehane et al., 2012).

CQ is able to move through biological membranes and accumulate in the acidic digestive vacuole (Ehlgen et al., 2012). This digestive vacuole functions to conduct

TABLE 1 | Summary of chloroquine- and sulfadoxine–pyrimethamine-resistant genes, their mutation sites, site, and mode of action.

Antimalarial and the stage it targets	Resistance gene(s)	Mutation site	Site of action	Mode of action
Chloroquine Stage of lifecycle—erythrocytic asexual stages (Lehane et al., 2012)	*Pfcrt* [located on chromosome 7 (Ikegbunam et al., 2019)]	Polymorphism at position 76 (K76T) in the first transmembrane domain (Pulcini et al., 2015)	Digestive vacuole (Shafik et al., 2020)	Mutant *Pfcrt*-mediated CQ efflux lessens access of CQ to its heme target (Ecker et al., 2012)
	pfmdr-1 [located on chromosome 5 (Ikegbunam et al., 2019)]	The amino-terminal mutations N86Y and F184Y—common to Asian and African parasites (Veiga et al., 2016). The 3 carboxy-terminal mutations S1034C, N1042D, and D1246Y—common to South American isolates (Veiga et al., 2016).	Digestive vacuole (Reiling et al., 2018)	Acts as an auxiliary mechanism alongside diffusion for drug entry into the digestive vacuole (Ibraheem et al., 2014)
Sulfadoxine–pyrimethamine **Stage of life cycle—liver and blood stages** (Raphemot et al., 2016)	*Pfdhfr* [located on chromosome 4 (Fortes et al., 2011)]	Amino acid point mutations at codons N51I, C59R, S108N, and I164L (Jiang et al., 2019)	Folate metabolic pathway (Sharma et al., 2015)	*Pfdhfr*—associated with pyrimethamine resistance (Sharma et al., 2015) *Pfdhps*—associated with sulfadoxine resistance (Sharma et al., 2015). These mutations reduce the binding affinity of SP to the targeted enzymes (Kümpornsin et al., 2014)
	Pfdhps [located on chromosome 8 (Fortes et al., 2011)]	Amino acid point mutations at codons S436A, A437G, K540E, A581G, and A613S (Jiang et al., 2019)	Folate metabolic pathway (Sharma et al., 2015)	

CQ, chloroquine; SP, sulfadoxine–pyrimethamine.

proteolysis of hemoglobin, which produces dipeptides and ferriprotoporphyrin IX (a substance that is toxic to the parasite at high concentrations). The parasite biocrystallizes ferriprotoporphyrin IX to hemozoin—this is inhibited by use of CQ (Reiling et al., 2018). CQR arises when CQ cannot accumulate at this active site to break the parasite's hemoglobin degradation cycle that *Plasmodium* needs (Loria et al., 1999).

CQR is often associated with genes *pfcrt* and/or *pfmdr-1*. The *P. pfcrt* gene is 424-amino acid long and is made up of 10 predicted transmembrane domains (Griffin et al., 2012). It is expressed at all infected erythrocyte stages with maximal expression at the trophozoite stage (Roepe, 2011). In its natural state, CQ is able to permeate the membrane of the food vacuole but becomes protonated in the vacuole and cannot pass the membrane to exit the vacuole (Homewood et al., 1972; Chinappi et al., 2010). As a result, there is a collection of CQ in the vacuole that binds to heme.

However, mutation on the gene increases export of CQ molecules. It has been reported that mutations in *pfcrt* lead to CQ and hydrogen ions being transported out of the food vacuole, which is where CQ exerts its effects from (Lehane and Kirk, 2008; Ecker et al., 2012). As a result, CQ is not activated and does not perform as it should. This is seen phenotypically as CQR.

Gene *pfmdr-1* has also been implicated in CQR. It mediates the production of P-glycoprotein homolog 1. The protein is localized to the food vacuole membrane (Cowman et al., 1991; Njokah et al., 2016). It is a member of a family of proteins that couple ATP hydrolysis to translocation of solutes across cell membranes (Cowman et al., 1991). Structural modeling of *pfmdr-1* assesses biophysical mechanisms of this gene and its protein in conferring resistance with respect to aminoquinoline (Ferreira et al., 2011). It has been established that *pfmdr-1* is involved in transporting xenobiotics (such as CQ) to the food vacuole. To do this, it is located along the food vacuole membrane and pushes CQ away off the cytosol (Dorsey et al., 2001; Ibraheem et al., 2014). The binding domain is on the cytosol-facing side of the food vacuole, allowing it to first encounter antimalarials—this side is where most resistance-causing mutations occur (Ibraheem et al., 2014). Mutations in *pfmdr-1* prevent movement of antimalarials from cytosol into the food vacuole—this reduces potency of some drugs such as CQ, which act in the food vacuole, but drugs that inhibit targets outside the food vacuole can become more potent (Wicht et al., 2020).

SP is an antifolate that is routinely used to treat uncomplicated malaria (Terlouw et al., 2003). Sulfadoxine (SDX) inhibits the activity of DHFR, and pyrimethamine (PYR) inhibits DHPS; these constituents are active against asexual erythrocytic stages of *P. falciparum* (Sandefur et al., 2007). Both DHFR and DHPS are central in parasite metabolism. Specifically, these enzymes are in the folate metabolic pathway. At the end of the pathway, reduced folate cofactors are produced, which are needed for DNA synthesis and metabolism of particular amino acids (Hyde, 2009).

Dihydrofolate reductase is the third enzyme involved in the folate-synthesis pathway in which it combines pteridine with *para*-amino benzoic acid to form dihydropteroate (Heinberg and Kirkman, 2015). SDX is a structural analog of *para*-amino benzoic acid, allowing it to inhibit the DHPS enzyme through competitive inhibition (Nzila, 2006). PYR is a competitive inhibitor of DHFR (Sandefur et al., 2007); thus, in its presence, the folate-metabolism pathway is halted or made less effective. Both SDX and PYR function through competitive inhibition of different targets. In combination, two different enzymes of the same pathway are disrupted and present as resistance to SP.

THE SPREAD OF CHLOROQUINE RESISTANCE IN SUB-SAHARAN AFRICA

Introduced in the mid-1940s, CQ became the most extensively utilized therapeutic antimalarial drug by 1950. Quinine was essentially swapped out for CQ in areas such as tropical Africa, which lacked systematic malaria eradication programs, therefore making it a pillar of presumptive and mass treatment in eradication campaigns (Nuwaha, 2001). CQ was used as the main malaria treatment therapy up to 1990, owing to its safety, efficacy, and low cost. However, CQR emerged in various parts of the world and quickly spread to West Africa in the 1980s and 1990s (Dagnogo et al., 2018) (**Figure 1**). Treatment failure, particularly in children who are too young to have acquired immunity, in malaria endemic regions is attributed to the presence of CQR (Trape et al., 1998). CQR is primarily related to an SNP in *pfcrt*, thus leading to an amino acid mutation from threonine to lysine at codon 76 (wild-type K to the mutant T-K76T) (Fidock et al., 2000); additionally, SNPs in exons 2, 3, 4, 6, 9, 10, and 11 of the *pfcrt* gene display possible association with CQR (Awasthi and Das, 2013). Three main haplotypes occur in codons 72–76 of *pfcrt*, thus resulting in the wild-type CVMNK and CQR haplotypes CVIET and SVMNT. In Africa, the most dominant mutant haplotype is CVIET (Thomsen et al., 2013). Another mutation conferring resistance to CQ is the N86Y allele of *pfmdr-1* (Ebel et al., 2020). The role of *pfmdr-1* mutations (N86Y, Y184F, S1034C, and D1246Y) in facilitating *in vitro* and *in vivo* CQR has received a lot of interest in research (Oladipo et al., 2015). CQR advances in three particular ways in each newly affected country, including its increasing spread over a number of locations and regions, the increased prevalence of resistant strains in each area, and the increase in the intensity of resistance (Trape, 2001).

The first reported cases of CQ-resistant infections were confirmed in non-immune tourists in Kenya and Tanzania in 1978, followed by semi–immune Kenyans in 1982 (Shretta et al., 2000). According to Annual Report: Diagnosis, Treatment and Prevention of Malaria: Nairobi, Kenyan Ministry of Health, 61–80% of isolated parasites were resistant to CQ, and 30% of cases treated with CQ experienced clinical treatment failure (Shretta et al., 2000). According to a study, 92% (22 of 24) of isolates assessed for CQR carried the point mutation, Asn to Tyr in *pfmdr-1* codon 86, which was the most frequently reported sequence variation related to CQR in Africa. Furthermore, 83% (20 of 24) had an Asp to Tyr mutation, and both mutations were observed in 82% (18 of 24) of the isolates. Both alleles have reported association with CQR. In addition, 75% (18 of 24) of samples each had polymorphisms on both *cg2* and *pfmdr-l* (Omar et al., 2001). Polymorphisms in the *cg2* gene, located in the 36-kb region on chromosome 7, are also related to CQR. This gene is characterized by 12 point mutations and three length polymorphisms, namely, kappa, gamma, and omega, and are associated with clones encompassing CQR phenotypes (Viana et al., 2006). Durand et al. (1999) used DNA sequencing to confirm the association of *cg2* with CQR. It was found that the *cg2* genotype including identical κ14 repeats and particular ω16 repeats displayed a strong association with CQR in all *P. falciparum* isolates from the African countries included in the study. CQR was heightened during the 1980s but continued to be the first-line treatment for uncomplicated malaria. In 1998, revised guideline for malaria treatment officially replaced CQ with a combination of SDX and PYR (Shretta et al., 2000).

In Tanzania, CQR was first demonstrated in semi-immune citizens in 1982 and in 1983 resistance spread and was reported at 34% among a Zanzibar school population. Furthermore, studies between 1982 and 1985 in various Tanzanian revealed a 20% average *in vivo*-resistant rate in schoolchildren (Trape, 2001). Consequently, CQ was the official first-line antimalarial drug for uncomplicated malaria until the end of July 2001. The parliament of Tanzania was notified by the Minister of Health, during the 2002–2003 budgetary session, that a decision was made to suspend CQ as the first-line antimalarial drug. The grounds for that decision were based on researched evidence of high cure-rate failure observed for CQ, of approximately 60% (Mubyazi and Gonzalez-Block, 2005).

By 1983, CQR had been reported in several sub-Saharan countries such as Madagascar, Burundi, Sudan, Uganda, Zambia, Comoros, Burkina Faso, Malawi, and Mozambique (Nuwaha, 2001).

The prevalence of CQR in Malawi by 1992 was an estimated 85% (Kublin et al., 2003), therefore prompting Malawi to be the first country in sub-Saharan Africa to terminate the routine use of CQ in 1993. This was supported by the increased failure of CQ treatment and its inability to produce sufficient clinical and hematological recovery. In 1990, more than 80% of Malawian children treated with CQ presented high-level parasitological resistance (Bloland et al., 1993). The removal for CQ in Malawi was supplemented by reduced prevalence of the CQR molecular marker, *pfcrt* T76, from 85% to 13% between 1992 and 2000 (Kublin et al., 2003). Widespread sensitivity to CQ was observed in Malawi after the removal of CQ as the first-line drug for malaria treatment. In 2005, a clinical trial estimated CQ efficacy at 99%, 12 years after removal. Furthermore, CQ susceptibility was maintained when used for recurring malaria episodes (Takala-Harrison and Laufer, 2015).

In 1999, a 90% prevalence of the *pfcrt* K76T mutation was identified in infected Mozambican children. A trial in southern Mozambique estimated an average of 47% for CQ's clinical efficacy between 2001 and 2002. Furthermore, another study revealed more than 90% occurrence of the mutant CVIET haplotype in the same area (Thomsen et al., 2013). This led to the abandonment of CQ treatment for malaria in 2003 (Galatas et al., 2017).

By 1984, CQR was observed in countries including Gabon, Angola, Namibia, Senegal, Zimbabwe, and South Africa (Nuwaha, 2001). A study in Senegal examined the prevalence of *pfcrt* to determine the molecular level of CQR. A high prevalence of single *pfcrt* CVMNK wild-type haplotype was observed in the study, and the data suggested that increased prevalence of *pfcrt* wild types is occurring country-wide (Ndiaye et al., 2012). The use of CQ was abandoned by health authorities in 2003

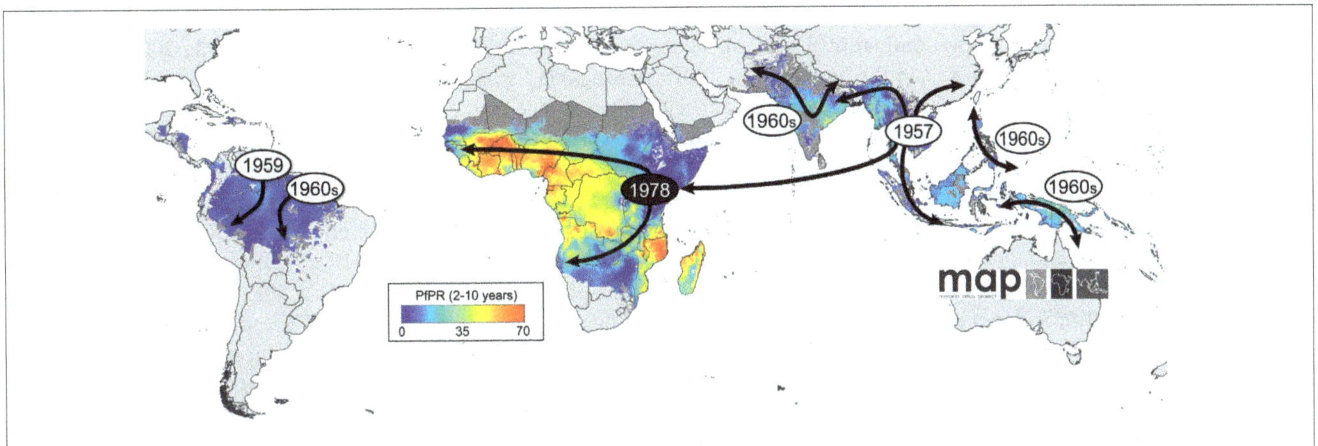

FIGURE 1 | The appearance and global spread of chloroquine resistance (CQR) in *P. falciparum*. Resistance is thought to have arisen in at least six independent origin (gray circles) and moved progressively as a CQ-driven selective sweep, including from Asia to Africa, where it established itself on the East coast in the late 1970s (black circle). The geographic spread of CQR is overlaid onto a current map of *P. falciparum* endemicity modeled for 2010. This map was derived from *P. falciparum* parasite rate (PfPR) surveys, age standardized to the 2- to 10-year age range, using model-based geostatistics (Ecker et al., 2012).

(Trape et al., 1998). In Zimbabwe, 50% of the population reside in malaria-risk areas, and malaria transmission occurs in 51 out of 59 administrative regions (Mlambo et al., 2007). Until 1983, there were no cases of CQR in Zimbabwe; however, in 1984, the first seven cases were reported in Zambezi Valley. CQR was initially confined to the Zambezi Valley, but by 1990, it was clear that the problem had spread throughout the country (Makono and Sibanda, 1999). According to a study facilitated in the Njelele area of Gokwe following a malaria outbreak, 83% of infections were CQ resistant, with only 3% of cases responding to CQ treatment (Mharakurwa and Mugochi, 1994). The establishment of maintainable national surveillance approaches was necessary to counteract the increasing CQR and monitor its spread throughout the country (Makono and Sibanda, 1999). The clinical failure of CQ was exceptionally high and, thus, only remained the drug of choice until 2000 (Mlambo et al., 2007).

Since 1932, South Africa had faced sporadic malaria epidemics, with KwaZulu Natal, Mpumalanga, and Limpopo bearing the greatest burden within the country (Knight et al., 2009). In 1985, KwaZulu Natal had its first report of *in vitro* CQR, which spread under persistent CQ pressure, thereby leading to an escalation in cases and treatment failures. In spite of being treated with CQ four times, 3% of malaria-treated patients remained positive (Ukpe et al., 2013). CQ was replaced and no longer used as the first-line drug for malaria treatment by February 1988 (Knight et al., 2009). Malaria parasites stayed susceptible to CQ in Mpumalanga and Limpopo until the mid-to-late 1990s. The number of CQ-resistant parasites escalated, thus prompting the replacement of CQ as the drug of choice in Mpumalanga and Limpopo in 1997 and 1998, respectively (Maharaj et al., 2013).

THE SPREAD OF SULFADOXINE–PYRIMETHAMINE RESISTANCE IN SUB-SAHARAN AFRICA

Africa, most predominantly, sub-Saharan Africa, still remains a home to malaria, bearing high morbidity, mortality, and risk of transmission, in spite of significant reduction in malaria incidence in the region, with children and pregnant women being the most vulnerable (Zareen et al., 2016). Malaria in pregnancy is estimated to cause hundreds of thousand infant deaths every year (Kajubi et al., 2019). Therefore, in 2012, WHO recommended SP as an intermittent preventive treatment (IPT) for fetal malaria prevention in pregnant women across malarious regions (Capan et al., 2010). However, efficacy of chemoprophylaxis with SP was halted by poor compliance of patients, which has led to emergence of drug-resistant strains of *P. falciparum* (Oyibo and Agomo, 2011).

The SP is a combination comprising SDX, which inhibits DHPS, a bifunctional protein that interacts with hydroxymethylpterin pyrophosphokinase, and PYR, which inhibits DHFR bifunctional protein (Nzila et al., 2000); it, therefore, synergistically inhibits the folate biosynthesis pathway of *P. falciparum* (Ahmed et al., 2006).

The molecular basis of *Plasmodium* resistance to SP is shown to be point mutations (Gatton et al., 2004) at seven sites in the DHPS gene (*dhfr*) that confer resistance to PYR and five sites in the DHFR (*dhps*) gene that confer resistance to SDX. Different combinations of mutations in each gene lead to varied resistance levels of SP (Pearce et al., 2003). For *pfdhps*, several point mutations—Ser → Ala at codon 436, Ala → Gly at codon 437, Lys → Glu at codon 540, Ala → Gly at codon 581, and Ser → Phe at codon 436—coupled with either Ala → Thr or Ala → Ser at codon 613 confer resistance to SDX. For *pfdhfr*, a point mutation of Ser → Asn changes at position 108 (S108N); resistance mutations Asn → Ile at codon 51 and/or Cys → Arg at codon 59 (C59R) and a Ser → Thr mutation at position 108 (S108N) with an Ala → Val change at position 16, synergistically confering PYR resistance in *Plasmodium* species (Kublin et al., 2003). The DHPS domain of the bifunctional 7,8-dihydro-6-hydroxymethylpterin pyrophosphokinase (PPPK)-dhps enzyme for SDX and the DHFR domain of the bifunctional DHFR-thymidylate synthase (DHFRTS) enzyme for PYR are key targets of SP drug, as these enzymes are responsible for the folic acid biosynthetic pathway (Basco et al., 1998). After approximately

50 years of SP's introduction, kinetics in children is still poorly understood; therefore, dosing is predominantly based on age for practical reasons, which may result in the administration of inaccurate quantities (De Kock et al., 2018). Increasing resistance to SP is linked to the stepwise acquisition of specific point mutations at specific codons in the *dhfrdhps* genes, which alter the drug-binding sites of SP (Oyibo and Agomo, 2011). However, the prophylaxis treatment of malaria was selected for double and triple mutations in *dhps* and *dhfr* genotypes, respectively, which are implicated in *Plasmodium* resistance to SP across sub-Saharan Africa (Capan et al., 2010; Sridaran et al., 2010). Accumulation of mutations within the genes (N51I, C59R, and S108N) in *pfdhfr* and mutations in codons A437G, K540E, and A581G within *pfdhps*, which confer resistance of *Plasmodium* to SP (Takala-Harrison and Laufer, 2015), has spread across sub-Saharan Africa (**Figure 2**).

In Benin, *pfdhps*, which confers resistance to SDX, contained a mixture of wild-type and mutant alleles (A437 and G437). High mutated alleles of *pfdhfr* were reported for codons N51I, C59R, and codon S108N. The *pfdhfr* (N51I, C59R, and S108N) proportion of single, triple, and quadruple mutations was very high in the study population (Ogouyèmi-Hounto et al., 2013). In Nigeria, parasite clearance was observed in pregnant women using SP (Kalanda et al., 2006), with mutations, N51I, C59R, S108N, and the triple mutation conferring a high level of *Plasmodium* resistance to SP (Iriemenam et al., 2012). A study conducted in Mali between August 2004 and January 2006 and in Ghana in 2003 supported the use of SP + AS (SP and amodiaquine) to treat young children with uncomplicated *P. falciparum* malaria and IPT in pregnant women (Tagbor et al., 2006; Tekete et al., 2011; Maiga et al., 2015). Additionally, in Mali, prevalence of each of the three *pfdhfr* mutations at codons N51I, C59R, and S108N was observed in 2007. Notably, *pfdhps* mutations at codons A437G and K540E as well as *pfdhfr* triple and *pfdhps* A437G quadruple mutations were present (Dicko et al., 2010). SP resistance was still quite low (Figueiredo et al., 2008; Dicko et al., 2012) in 2008 but rapidly increased in Mali in 2010 and Burkina Faso in 2012 (Coulibaly et al., 2014). The triple mutant *pfdhfr* in Africa evolved from the southeast Asian lineage (Coulibaly et al., 2014), while the N51I + S108N double-mutant *pfdhfr* alleles are a local origin. Both the *pfdhps* double mutants (Gly-437 and Glu-540) and the *pfdhfr* triple mutants were individually associated with SP treatment failure in children aged less than 5 years, with *pfdhps* and *pfdhfr* quintuple mutations being highly associated with SP treatment failure in Ibadan, Nigeria (Happi et al., 2005). The *pfdhfr* N51I, C59R, S108N triple mutation had a prevalence close to 100% in Cameroon, western Africa. The most frequent *pfdhps* mutation there was A437G, with a prevalence of 76.5% and had a higher significant prevalence in pregnant women with SP uptake (Chauvin et al., 2015).

Ghana, a western African country, in 2003 also recorded the quadruple mutation in *pfdhps* A437G and *pfdhfr*—N51I, C59R, and S108N (Marks et al., 2005)—but SP was still effective in 2001 for treating uncomplicated *P. falciparum* malaria whether as monotherapy or combined therapy in Cameroon (Basco et al., 2002). Meanwhile, emergence of SP combination resistance was sustained for many years before introduction of ACTs as a frontline antimalarial in Africa (Marks et al., 2005). There is a strong relationship between protective efficacy and the frequency of resistance mutations, as negative correlation exists between SP prophylaxis efficacy and parasite mutations, indicating that as resistance increases, protective efficacy decreases. This decreased efficacy of SP on IPTi was reported across Ghana and Gabon where decreased efficacy was linked to *pfdhfr* triple mutation (Griffin et al., 2010). A study in Niger showed a high proportion of *pfdhfr* N51I, C59R, and S108N haplotypes associated with resistance to PYR and *pfdhps* S436AFH and A437G mutations associated with reduced susceptibility to SDX (Grais et al., 2018). In 2004, a molecular genotyping study conducted in Laine, Guinea, found three *pfdhfr* mutations in 85.6% patients and quintuple *pfdhfr*/*pfdhps* mutations in 9.6% showing a progressive increase in resistance to SP (Bonnet et al., 2007). No *pfdhfr* I164L or *pfdhps* A581G mutations were found, but *pfdhps* K540E mutation was found in Mali, with a very low prevalence in Mali and Burkina-Faso (Coulibaly et al., 2014).

In Central Africa, between 2002 and 2003, there was adequate clearance of parasitemia in children treated with SP with low presence of *pfdhfr* S108N, *pfdhfr* triple, and *pfdhfr*/*pfdhps* quadruple mutation genotypes. This shows that studies conducted a decade ago still showed some SP efficacy despite accompanying resistance genotypes. The parasite population of Uige, Angola, revealed high frequency mutations in *pfcrt*, *pfdhps*, and *pfdhfr*, conferring resistance to CQ and SP (Coulibaly et al., 2014).

The frequency of the double A437G, K540E mutant *pfdhps* allele (conferring SDX resistance) increased from 200% to 300%, and the triple mutant *pfdhfr* (N51I, C59R, and S108N) allele (conferring PYR resistance) increased by 37–63% in Tanzanian population when SP was used as a first-line antimalarial (Malisa et al., 2010). A study conducted in 2002 in Tanzania confirmed the presence of *pfdhfr*/*pfdhps* mutations even when SP was efficient (Mbugi et al., 2006). SP resistance was reported across regions of Tanzania where the triple mutations (N51I, C59R, and S108N) were constantly predominant across all the regions, implying a high level of SP resistance (Schönfeld et al., 2007; Bertin et al., 2011; Baraka et al., 2015), which was corroborated by same result in Benin, a western African country (Bertin et al., 2011). No relationship exists between the number of mutations and the degree of parasitological resistance (Eriksen et al., 2004). Additionally, Tanzania not only reported SP failure, but its prophylaxis was of no significant effect in northern Tanzania in 2006, as triple mutations previously reported in other parts of Africa were also detected (Gesase et al., 2009). The highest mutations of *pfdhfr* and *pfdhps* genes were predominantly distributed across eastern and southern Africa where SP use has been the highest (Enosse et al., 2008; Griffin et al., 2010). In 2005, northwest Ethiopia displayed a gradual reduction of individual *pfdhps*/*pfdhfr* mutations; triple, quadruple, and quintuple mutations were observed after 5 years of SP withdrawal as a frontline antimalarial (Hailemeskel et al., 2013), but quintupled in western Kenya between 2008 and 2009 (Iriemenam et al., 2012). Moreover, by 2000, the East African Network for Monitoring Antimalarial Treatment (EANMAT)

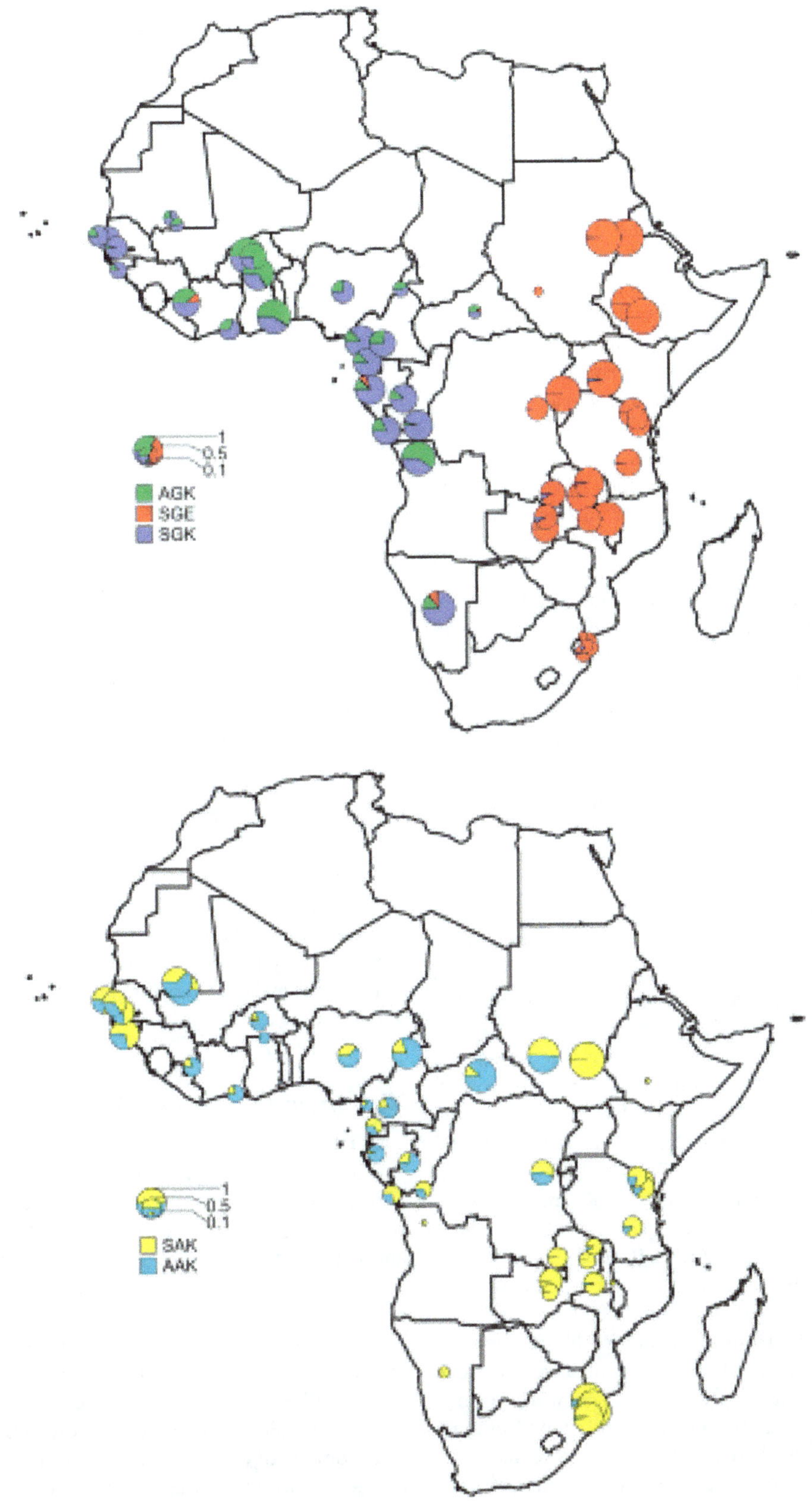

FIGURE 2 | The distribution of the major *pfdhps* alleles across sub-Saharan Africa. Resistant alleles; the upper map shows the relative proportions of the three major resistance alleles, SGK, AGK, and SGE. Wild-type alleles; the lower map shows the ratio of SAK and AAK alleles among wild-type *pfdhps* alleles (Pearce et al., 2009).

reported SP failure across East Africa, with Rwanda and Burundi exceeding the critical 25% value SP failure rates (Rapuoda et al., 2003); this could be due to a low uptake of SP by pregnant women due to weak health system and sub-optimal implementation policy, among other factors (Martin et al., 2020). The *pfdhps* A581G and *pfdhfr* I164L mutations, which confer SP resistance, have been found to be unevenly distributed across East Africa, suggesting a high level of SP resistance, as indicated by the prevalence of the K540E mutation, found across East Africa (Naidoo and Roper, 2011).

Zimbabwe reported high prevalence of *pfcrt* (K76T) to be 64%, 82%, and 92% in Chiredzi, Kariba, and Bindura, respectively. On the *pfdhfr* locus, the presence of triple mutations at codons N51I, C59R, and S108N was approximately 50% across the three locations, therefore indicative of widespread prevalence of molecular markers associated with CQ and PYR resistance in Zimbabwe (Schleicher et al., 2018). KwaZulu Natal in South Africa had reported SP resistance in 2000 and thus changed its malaria policy to the use of ACTs for malaria treatment (Knight et al., 2009).

In 2010, the quadruple mutation (A437G, N51I, C59R, and S108N) haplotypes were widespread throughout sub-Saharan Africa, particularly in Uganda, Mali, Kenya, and Malawi (Takechi et al., 2001; Osman et al., 2007), but the quintuple and sextuple mutants were found only in specific regions of Africa (Walker et al., 2017). The quintuple mutants, which plateaued in East and Southern Africa, were relatively rare in west Africa and parts of central Africa. Estimates of the prevalence of the *pfdhps*-A581G mutation suggest that the sextuple haplotype had become established in Rwanda, Burundi, D R Congo, southwestern Uganda, northwestern Tanzania, southeastern Kenyan, and northeastern Tanzanian borders.

Genotyping of *pfdhfr* responsible for PYR resistance showed no mutation in codons A16V, C59R, or I164L, while there was 84% mutation at codons N51I and S108N (Osman et al., 2007). Additionally, linkage exists between CQ mutation, *pfcrt* K76T, SDX mutation, *pfdhps* K540E, and PYR mutation *pfdhfr* (N51I and S108N), thus conferring parasite resistance against both CQ and SP. The C59R mutation observed in Mali, Kenya, and Malawi was, however, absent in Sudan in spite of 80% prevalence of *pfdhps* K540E. *Pfdhfr* N51I and S108N occurred in more than 80% (Osman et al., 2007). The A437G mutation at *pfdhps* and the triple mutation (N51I, C59R, and S108N) at *pfdhfr* associated with SP resistance is concurrent with those found even outside sub-Saharan Africa (Checchi et al., 2002). In six countries of Eastern and Southern Africa, more than 90% prevalence of *pfdhps*-K540E was implicated in SP resistance (Iriemenam et al., 2012). However, countries like Cameroon, Ghana, Zambia, Mozambique, Mali, and Zimbabwe had three doses of SP in their policy for all pregnant women, which seemed efficacious with resistant genotypes concurrently found in these countries (Mayor et al., 2008; Maiga et al., 2011; Kayentao et al., 2013). The quadruple mutation was uncommon compared with triple mutation, which confers a major resistance to SP in Africa (Peters et al., 2007). Conclusively, a systematic analysis conducted in African countries between 1996 and 2006 reported delayed clearance alluding to SP treatment failure (ter Kuile et al., 2015).

COMBATING CHLOROQUINE AND SULFADOXINE–PYRIMETHAMINE RESISTANCE

Several publications confirm the widespread resistance of CQ and SP, with substantial occurrence in Asian and African countries. The reasons for this hinged on various factors, which include, but is not limited to, the overuse of these antimalarial medications, underdosage of the medications in the treatment of active malaria infection, and high susceptibility of the parasite to adapt at the genetic metabolic levels rapidly (Hyde, 2007). General preventive as well as some of the specific measures have been considered as ways to combat further spread of antimalarial resistance.

Vector Control

Vector control makes use of ITNs/long-lasting insecticidal nets (LLINs) and IRS, which are the mainstay of malaria control. These two strategies have proven useful in the reduction of local malaria transmission by protecting susceptible individuals against infective mosquito bites, thereby leading to a reduction in the level of malaria intensity. When sleeping under the net, the net serves as a means of preventing mosquito contact or bite. Reducing the vector population through this means can indirectly serve as a measure to mitigate the spread of CQ- and SP-resistant *Plasmodium*. In fact, since 2007, the WHO has recommended universal coverage with ITN (Macintyre et al., 2011; World Health Organisation (WHO), 2011). IRS has also been reportedly effective in reducing the challenge of transmission. It serves as a means to terminating these vectors, thereby reducing the possible malaria morbidity and mortality (World Health Organisation (WHO), 2011). When vector control measures are well applied in combination, it is evident that the outcome of malaria transmission (CQ/SP resistant in this case) will be mitigated (World Health Organisation (WHO), 2010; Thu et al., 2017).

The Introduction of Artemisinin-Based Combination Therapies

An important strategy continues to be the use of effective antimalarials. However, this is threatened by the extensive resistance observed in the parasite toward the most affordable classes of drugs, thus highlighting the need for novel antimalarials (Winstanley et al., 2004) and ultimately a vaccine. The widespread resistance of the known frontline antimalarial drugs—CQ and SP—in April 2002 led to the introduction of ACTs as the first-line treatment for malaria by the WHO. Notably in the treatment of *P. falciparum*, it is recommended that two or more drugs must be combined. The combined drugs must have different modes of action. Since artemisinin-based compounds (dihydroartemisinin, artemether, and artesunate) are fast acting, they are usually combined with other classes of antimalarial with long half-life such as mefloquine, amodiaquine, lumefantrine, and piperaquine (Bell and Winstanley, 2005). The ACTs, which come in various combinations, is used to replace CQ and SP in order to prevent further increasing morbidity and mortality resulting from the observed resistance in the initial use of first-line medications (World Health Organisation (WHO), 2003; Dalrymple, 2009). The high efficacy and ability to interrupt the development of resistance supported the use of ACTs as the core of malaria treatment (Laxminarayan et al., 2006). The artemisinin component of ACTs has the ability to reduce parasitemia; thus, the progression from uncomplicated malaria to a severe form of the disease can be prevented by early treatment with ACTs, consequently reducing the amount of severe malaria cases and the rate of malaria mortality (Ndeffo Mbah et al., 2015). By June 2008, most malaria endemic nations have adopted the ACTs as its front-line antimalarial medication (World Health Organisation (WHO), 2008). Part of the measures put in place to avoid similar medication resistance as seen in CQ and SP is the disallowance of artemisinin monotherapy medications. This was part of the World Health Assembly resolution of 2007 (World Health Organisation (WHO), 2008).

Medication Adherence and Avoiding Self-Medication

Among humans, there are a variety of beliefs that can impact our behavior significantly. These beliefs are scarcely changed and can therefore affect adherence to antimalarials such as ACTs, thus highlighting the need for patients' beliefs to be considered when care is offered (Amponsah et al., 2015). Numerous interventions have been developed and employed in malaria endemic areas to promote adherence to medications. Clear guidelines to better adherence can be achieved through deeper understanding of the relative efficacy of each intervention (Fuangchan et al., 2014). The understanding of malaria treatment could be improved by community education, such as training of dispensers and promoting public awareness, thus improving adherence to antimalarials (Denis, 1998). To ensure malaria treatment approaches continue to be effective and improve the possibility of a positive outcome, medication adherence should be evaluated regularly, thereafter used as tools to encourage appropriate action, if necessary (Gerstl et al., 2015).

The CQ/SP resistance developed partly due to widespread presumptuous use of these medications without prior objective confirmation of the diagnosis. Due to the poverty and economic setting of many malaria endemic countries especially in sub-Saharan Africa, most people self-medicate and thereby inappropriately use CQ/SP (Idowu et al., 2006). To this end, the WHO essentially recommended and introduced affordable point-of-care rapid diagnostic tests for definitive malaria testing and diagnosing before the usage of an antimalarial even in under-resourced settings. This is expected to be accompanied by correct and complete usage of the antimalarial especially in this era of ACTs (White et al., 2009; Thu et al., 2017).

Combating the Counterfeit Medication Market

Generally, counterfeit medication presents a great challenge globally, thus contributing to the burden presented by the development of antimalarial drug resistance. Studies done in Eastern DR Congo showed that majority of the CQ has its active ingredient to be significantly underdosed while the SP was overdosed in terms of the active ingredients (Atemnkeng et al., 2007). A similar study in Nigeria corroborated the fact that the menace of counterfeit medication is huge, with 50% of CQ dispensed by street vendors underdosed of the active ingredients (Idowu et al., 2006). In light of this, the development of CQ and SP resistance is substantiated. However, going forward, this can be combatted by action at the policy level. Enacting the laws guiding counterfeit medications and strengthening of the institutions responsible will go a long way to reduce, if not totally remove, counterfeit medications in the society. This can mitigate the CQ/SP resistance in the long run (Yadav and Rawal, 2016). Another way to combat the problem of counterfeit medication is the provision of novel, effective, and affordable antimalarial drugs. This issue is addressed by the Medicines for Malaria Venture, whose aim consists of the discovery, development, and the facilitation of those antimalarials (Medicines for Malaria Venture [MMV], 2020). MMV is a non-profit Swiss foundation, officially introduced in 1999. It was one of the first public–private partnerships created to address the drug innovation gap of malaria (Bathurst and Hentschel, 2006). Developing medicines for children addresses the population most at risk of dying from malaria, thus serving as motivation for MMV to develop child-friendly formulations of current antimalarials and to develop next-generation medicines (Medicines for Malaria Venture [MMV], 2020). In 2009, Novartis and MMV developed an artemether–lumefantrine formulation, called *Coartem® Dispersible*, adapted to cater to the needs of children affected by *P. falciparum* malaria and was the first successfully co-developed product launched by the MMV, in which 400 million products were distributed (Premji, 2009; Medicines for Malaria Venture [MMV], 2020). MMV continues to develop and improve access to affordable medicines to lessen the global burden of malaria.

Reintroduction of Chloroquine in the Chloroquine-Sensitive Environment

Various studies have shown that with replacement of CQ/SP as the first line of treatment and subsequent replacement with ACTs, there was notable decrease in the prevalence of pfcrt K76T present in such communities. This was first demonstrated in Malawi in 2004, with the prevalence of pfcrt K76T reaching an undetectable level (Plowe, 2014).

Similar studies have validated this point in China and Zambia, with the outcome of both studies showing a resurgence of CQ sensitivity (Mwanza et al., 2016; Lu et al., 2017b). Considering the role of CQ/SP safety profile and affordability, this looks promising, and reintroduction of CQ/SP may be the way to go in the near future.

CONCLUSION

In sub-Saharan Africa, where the burden of malaria infection is great, one of the core challenges for malaria control is the emergence and spread of antimalarial drug resistance. Although other strategies are employed for malaria control such as ITNs and IRS, which are the foundation of the malaria control agenda, antimalarial drugs are essential to reduce transmission. However, because of their accessibility and affordability, CQ and SP—both first-line drugs in the past—were used excessively, which resulted in the establishment of resistance, which in turn hindered malaria control in sub-Saharan Africa. This prompted the introduction of ACTs, which decreased the pressure on CQ and SP in some regions of sub-Saharan Africa, thus encouraging their reintroduction in those regions. Ongoing antimalarial drug resistance should be closely monitored in sub-Saharan Africa to prevent the establishment and spread of resistance and to detect the return of sensitivity, which could result in the possible reintroduction of specific antimalarials.

AUTHOR CONTRIBUTIONS

AR: writing, editing, and collation. LM, OO, and OA: writing and editing. RM: supervision and editing. MA and MO: conceptualization, supervision, editing, and funding.

REFERENCES

Ahmed, A., Lumb, V., Das, M. K., Dev Wajihullah, V., and Sharma, Y. D. (2006). Prevalence of mutations associated with higher levels of sulfadoxine-pyrimethamine resistance in *plasmodium falciparum* isolates from car nicobar Island and Assam, India. *Antimicrob. Agents Chemother.* 50, 3934–3938. doi: 10.1128/aac.00732-06

Ajayi, N. A., and Ukwaja, K. N. (2013). Possible artemisinin-based combination therapy-resistant malaria in Nigeria: a report of three cases. *Rev. Soc. Bras. Med. Trop.* 46, 525–527. doi: 10.1590/0037-8682-0098-2013

Amponsah, A. O., Vosper, H., and Marfo, A. F. A. (2015). Patient related factors affecting adherence to antimalarial medication in an urban estate in ghana. *Malar. Res. Treat.* 2015, 452539–452539.

Atemnkeng, M. A., Chimanuka, B., and Plaizier-Vercammen, J. (2007). Quality evaluation of chloroquine, quinine, sulfadoxine–pyrimethamine and proguanil formulations sold on the market in East Congo DR. *J. Clin. Pharm. Ther.* 32, 123–132. doi: 10.1111/j.1365-2710.2007.00797.x

Awasthi, G., and Das, A. (2013). Genetics of chloroquine-resistant malaria: a haplotypic view. *Memor. Instit. Oswal. Cruz* 108, 947–961. doi: 10.1590/0074-0276130274

Baraka, V., Ishengoma, D. S., Fransis, F., Minja, D. T. R., Madebe, R. A., Ngatunga, D., et al. (2015). High-level *Plasmodium falciparum* sulfadoxine-pyrimethamine resistance with the concomitant occurrence of septuple haplotype in Tanzania. *Mal. J.* 14:439.

Basco, L. K., Tahar, R., and Ringwald, P. (1998). Molecular basis of in vivo resistance to sulfadoxine-pyrimethamine in African adult patients infected with *Plasmodium falciparum* malaria parasites. *Antimicr. Agents Chemother.* 42, 1811–1814. doi: 10.1128/aac.42.7.1811

Basco, L., Same-Ekobo, A., Ngane, V., Ndounga, M., Metoh, T., Ringwald, P., et al. (2002). Therapeutic efficacy of sulfadoxine-pyrimethamine, amodiaquine and the sulfadoxine-pyrimethamine-amodiaquine combination against uncomplicated *Plasmodium falciparum* malaria in young children in Cameroon. *Bull. World Health Organiz.* 80, 538–545.

Bathurst, I., and Hentschel, C. (2006). Medicines for malaria venture: sustaining antimalarial drug development. *Trends Parasitol.* 22, 301–307. doi: 10.1016/j.pt.2006.05.011

Bell, D., and Winstanley, P. (2005). Current issues in the treatment of uncomplicated malaria in Africa. *Br. Med. Bull.* 71, 29–43. doi: 10.1093/bmb/ldh031

Bertin, G., Briand, V., Bonaventure, D., Carrieu, A., Massougbodji, A., Cot, M., et al. (2011). Molecular markers of resistance to sulphadoxine-pyrimethamine during intermittent preventive treatment of pregnant women in Benin. *Mal. J.* 10:196. doi: 10.1186/1475-2875-10-196

Bin Dajem, S. M., and Al-Qahtani, A. (2010). Analysis of gene mutations involved in chloroquine resistance in *Plasmodium falciparum* parasites isolated from patients in the southwest of Saudi Arabia. *Ann. Saudi Med.* 30, 187–192. doi: 10.4103/0256-4947.62826

Birnbaum, J., Scharf, S., Schmidt, S., Jonscher, E., Hoeijmakers, W. A. M., Flemming, S., et al. (2020). A Kelch13-defined endocytosis pathway mediates artemisinin resistance in malaria parasites. *Science* 367:51. doi: 10.1126/science.aax4735

Bloland, P. B., Lackritz, E. M., Kazembe, P. N., Were, J. B., Steketee, R., and Campbell, C. C. (1993). Beyond chloroquine: implications of drug resistance for evaluating malaria therapy efficacy and treatment policy in Africa. *J. Infect. Dis.* 167, 932–937. doi: 10.1093/infdis/167.4.932

Bonnet, M., Roper, C., Félix, M., Coulibaly, L., Kankolongo, G. M., and Guthmann, J. P. (2007). Efficacy of antimalarial treatment in Guinea: in vivo study of two artemisinin combination therapies in Dabola and molecular markers of resistance to sulphadoxine-pyrimethamine in N'Zérékoré. *Malar. J.* 6:54.

Capan, M., Mombo-Ngoma, G., Makristathis, A., and Ramharter, M. (2010). Anti-bacterial activity of intermittent preventive treatment of malaria in pregnancy: comparative in vitro study of sulphadoxine-pyrimethamine, mefloquine, and azithromycin. *Mal J.* 9:303. doi: 10.1186/1475-2875-9-303

Chauvin, P., Menard, S., Iriart, X., Nsango, S. E., Tchioffo, M. T., Abate, L., et al. (2015). Prevalence of *Plasmodium falciparum* parasites resistant to sulfadoxine/pyrimethamine in pregnant women in Yaoundé, Cameroon: emergence of highly resistant *pfdhfr/pfdhps* alleles. *J. Antimicrob. Chemother.* 70, 2566–2571. doi: 10.1093/jac/dkv160

Checchi, F., Durand, R., Balkan, S., Vonhm, B. T., Kollie, J. Z., Biberson, P., et al. (2002). High *Plasmodium falciparum* resistance to chloroquine and sulfadoxine-pyrimethamine in Harper, Liberia: results in vivo and analysis of point mutations. *Transact. R. Soc. Trop. Med. Hygiene* 96, 664–669. doi: 10.1016/s0035-9203(02)90346-9

Chinappi, M., Via, A., Marcatili, P., and Tramontano, A. (2010). On the mechanism of chloroquine resistance in *Plasmodium falciparum*. *PLoS One* 5:e14064.

Chourasia, M. K., Raghavendra, K., Bhatt, R. M., Swain, D. K., Valecha, N., and Kleinschmidt, I. (2017). Burden of asymptomatic malaria among a tribal population in a forested village of central India: a hidden challenge for malaria control in India. *Public Health* 147, 92–97. doi: 10.1016/j.puhe.2017.02.010

Coban, C. (2020). The host targeting effect of chloroquine in malaria. *Curr. Opin. Immunol.* 66, 98–107. doi: 10.1016/j.coi.2020.07.005

Conrad, M. D., and Rosenthal, P. J. (2019). Antimalarial drug resistance in Africa: the calm before the storm? *Lancet Infect. Dis.* 19, e338–e351.

Conroy, A. L., Datta, D., and John, C. C. (2019). What causes severe malaria and its complications in children? Lessons learned over the past 15 years. *BMC Med.* 17:52.

Coulibaly, S. O., Kayentao, K., Taylor, S., Guirou, E. A., Khairallah, C., Guindo, N., et al. (2014). Parasite clearance following treatment with sulphadoxine-pyrimethamine for intermittent preventive treatment in Burkina-Faso and Mali: 42-day in vivo follow-up study. *Mal. J.* 13:41. doi: 10.1186/1475-2875-13-41

Cowman, A. F., Karcz, S., Galatis, D., and Culvenor, J. G. (1991). A P-glycoprotein homologue of *Plasmodium falciparum* is localized on the digestive vacuole. *J. Cell Biol.* 113, 1033–1042. doi: 10.1083/jcb.113.5.1033

Dagnogo, O., Ako, A. B., Ouattara, L., Dago, N. D., Coulibaly, D. N. g, Touré, A. O., et al. (2018). Towards a re-emergence of chloroquine sensitivity in Côte d'Ivoire? *Mal. J.* 17, 413–413.

D'Alessandro, U., and Buttiëns, H. (2001). History and importance of antimalarial drug resistance. *Trop Med. Int. Health* 6, 845–848. doi: 10.1046/j.1365-3156.2001.00819.x

Dalrymple, D. G. (2009). *Artemisia Annua, Artemisinin, ACTs and Malaria Control in Africa: The Interplay of Tradition, Science and Public Policy, Working Paper.* Geneva: Medicines for Malaria Venture.

De Kock, M., Tarning, J., Workman, L., Allen, E. N., Tekete, M. M., Djimde, A. A., et al. (2018). Population pharmacokinetic properties of sulfadoxine and pyrimethamine: a pooled analysis to inform optimal dosing in african children with uncomplicated Malaria. *Antimicr. Agents Chemother.* 62:e01370-17.

Denis, M. B. (1998). Improving compliance with quinine + tetracycline for treatment of malaria: evaluation of health education interventions in Cambodian villages. *Bull. World Health Organ.* 76(Suppl. 1), 43–49.

Desai, M., Gutman, J., Taylor, S. M., Wiegand, R. E., Khairallah, C., Kayentao, K., et al. (2015). Impact of sulfadoxine-pyrimethamine resistance on effectiveness of intermittent preventive therapy for malaria in pregnancy at clearing infections and preventing low birth weight. *Clin. Infect. Dis.* 62, 323–333. doi: 10.1093/cid/civ881

Dicko, A., Konare, M., Traore, D., Testa, J., Salamon, R., Doumbo, O., et al. (2012). The implementation of malaria intermittent preventive trialtreatment with sulphadoxine-pyrimethamine in infants reduced all-cause mortality in the district of Kolokani, Mali: results from a cluster randomized control. *Mal. J.* 11:73.

Dicko, A., Sagara, I., Djimdé, A. A., Touré, S. O., Traore, M., Dama, S., et al. (2010). Molecular markers of resistance to sulphadoxine-pyrimethamine one year after implementation of intermittent preventive treatment of malaria in infants in Mali. *Mal. J.* 9:9.

Dondorp, A. M., and Ringwald, P. (2013). Artemisinin resistance is a clear and present danger. *Trends Parasitol* 29, 359–360. doi: 10.1016/j.pt.2013.05.005

Dorsey, G., Kamya, M. R., Singh, A., and Rosenthal, P. J. (2001). Polymorphisms in the *Plasmodium falciparum pfcrt* and *pfmdr*-1 genes and clinical response to chloroquine in Kampala, Uganda. *J. Infect Dis.* 183, 1417–1420.

Durand, R., Gabbett, E., Di Piazza, J-P., Delabre, J-F., and Le Bras, J. (1999). Analysis of κ and ω repeats of the *cg2* gene and chloroquine susceptibility in isolates of *Plasmodium falciparum* from sub-Saharan Africa. *Mol. Biochem. Parasitol.* 101, 185–197. doi: 10.1016/s0166-6851(99)00073-0

Ebel, E. R., Reis, F., Petrov, D. A., and Beleza, S. (2020). Shifts in antimalarial drug policy since 2006 have rapidly selected *P. falciparum* resistance alleles in Angola. doi: 10.1101/2020.09.29.310706

Ecker, A., Lehane, A. M., Clain, J., and Fidock, D. A. (2012). *pfcrt* and its role in antimalarial drug resistance. *Trends Parasitol.* 28, 504–514. doi: 10.1016/j.pt.2012.08.002

Ehlgen, F., Pham, J. S., de Koning-Ward, T., Cowman, A. F., and Ralph, S. A. (2012). Investigation of the *Plasmodium falciparum* food vacuole through inducible expression of the chloroquine resistance transporter (PfCRT). *PLoS One* 7:e38781. doi: 10.1371/journal.pone.0038781

Enosse, S., Magnussen, P., Abacassamo, F., ómez-Olivé, X. G., Rønn, A. M., Thompson, R., et al. (2008). Rapid increase of *Plasmodium falciparum dhfr/dhps* resistant haplotypes, after the adoption of sulphadoxine-pyrimethamine as first line treatment in 2002, in southern Mozambique. *Mal. J.* 7:115.

Eriksen, J., Mwankusye, S., Mduma, S., Kitua, A., Swedberg, G., Tomson, G., et al. (2004). Patterns of resistance and DHFR/DHPS genotypes of *Plasmodium falciparum* in rural Tanzania prior to the adoption of sulfadoxine—pyrimethamine as first-line treatment. *Transact. R. Soc. Trop. Med. Hyg.* 98, 347–353. doi: 10.1016/j.trstmh.2003.10.010

Fairhurst, R. M., and Dondorp, A. M. (2016). Artemisinin-resistant *Plasmodium falciparum* malaria. *Microbiol. Spect.* 4:13. doi: 10.1128/microbiolspec.EI1110-0013-2016

Ferreira, P. E., Holmgren, G., Veiga, M. I., Uhlén, P., Kaneko, A., and Gil, J. P. (2011). Pfmdr1: Mechanisms of Transport Modulation by Functional Polymorphisms. *PLoS One* 6:e23875. doi: 10.1371/journal.pone.0023875

Fidock, D. A., Nomura, T., Talley, A. K., Cooper, R. A., Dzekunov, S. M., Ferdig, M. T., et al. (2000). Mutations in the *P. falciparum* digestive vacuole transmembrane protein PfCRT and evidence for their role in chloroquine resistance. *Mol. Cell* 6, 861–871. doi: 10.1016/s1097-2765(05)00077-8

Figueiredo, P., Benchimol, C., Lopes, D., Bernardino, L., do Rosário, V. E., Varandas, L., et al. (2008). Prevalence of *pfmdr1, pfcrt, pfdhfr* and *pfdhps* mutations associated with drug resistance, in Luanda, Angola. *Mal. J.* 7:236.

Flegg, J. A., Metcalf, C. J. E., Gharbi, M., Venkatesan, M., Shewchuk, T., Hopkins Sibley, C., et al. (2013). Trends in antimalarial drug use in Africa. *Am. J. Trop. Med. Hyg.* 89, 857–865.

Fortes, F., Dimbu, R., Figueiredo, P., Neto, Z., do Rosário, V. E., and Lopes, D. (2011). Evaluation of prevalence's of *pfdhfr* and *pfdhps* mutations in Angola. *Malaria J.* 10:22. doi: 10.1186/1475-2875-10-22

Frosch, A. E. P., Venkatesan, M., and Laufer, M. K. (2011). Patterns of chloroquine use and resistance in sub-Saharan Africa: a systematic review of household survey and molecular data. *Mal. J.* 10:116. doi: 10.1186/1475-2875-10-116

Fuangchan, A., Dhippayom, T., and Kongkaew, C. (2014). Intervention to promote patients' adherence to antimalarial medication: a systematic review. *Am. J. Trop. Med. Hyg.* 90, 11–19. doi: 10.4269/ajtmh.12-0598

Galatas, B., Nhamussua, L., Candrinho, B., Mabote, L., Cisteró, P., Gupta, H., et al. (2017). In-Vivo efficacy of chloroquine to clear asymptomatic infections in mozambican adults: a randomized, placebo-controlled trial with implications for elimination strategies. *Sci. Rep.* 7, 1356–1356.

Gatton, M. L., Martin, L. B., and Cheng, Q. (2004). Evolution of resistance to sulfadoxine-pyrimethamine in *Plasmodium falciparum*. *Antimicrob Agents Chemother.* 48, 2116–2123. doi: 10.1128/aac.48.6.2116-2123.2004

Gerstl, S., Namagana, A., Palacios, L., Mweshi, F., Aprile, S., and Lima, A. (2015). High adherence to malaria treatment: promising results of an adherence study in South Kivu, Democratic Republic of the Congo. *Mal. J.* 14:414.

Gesase, S., Gosling, R. D., Hashim, R., Ord, R., Naidoo, I., Madebe, R., et al. (2009). High resistance of *Plasmodium falciparum* to sulphadoxine/pyrimethamine in northern Tanzania and the emergence of dhps resistance mutation at Codon 581. *PLoS One* 4:e4569. doi: 10.1371/journal.pone.0004569

Grais, R. F. I., Laminou, M., Woi-Messe, L., Makarimi, R., Bouriema, S. H., Langendorf, C., et al. (2018). Molecular markers of resistance to amodiaquine plus sulfadoxine–pyrimethamine in an area with seasonal malaria chemoprevention in south central Niger. *Mal. J.* 17:98.

Greenwood, B. M., Bojang, K., Whitty, C. J., and Targett, G. A. (2005). Malaria. *Lancet* 365, 1487–1498.

Griffin, C. E., Hoke, J. M., Samarakoon, U., Duan, J., Mu, J., Ferdig, M. T., et al. (2012). Mutation in the *Plasmodium falciparum* CRT protein determines the stereospecific activity of antimalarial cinchona alkaloids. *Antimicrob Agents Chemother.* 56, 5356–5364. doi: 10.1128/aac.05667-11

Griffin, J. T., Cairns, M., Ghani, A. C., Roper, C., Schellenberg, D., Carneiro, I., et al. (2010). Protective efficacy of intermittent preventive treatment of malaria in infants (IPTi) using sulfadoxine-pyrimethamine and parasite resistance. *PLoS One* 5:e12618. doi: 10.1371/journal.pone.0012618

Grobusch, M. P., and Kremsner, P. G. (2005). Uncomplicated malaria. *Curr. Top. Microbiol. Immunol.* 295, 83–104.

Hailemeskel, E., Kassa, M., Taddesse, G., Mohammed, H., Woyessa, A., Tasew, G., et al. (2013). Prevalence of sulfadoxine-pyrimethamine resistance-associated mutations in *dhfr* and *dhps* genes of *Plasmodium falciparum* three years after SP withdrawal in Bahir Dar, Northwest Ethiopia. *Acta Trop.* 128, 636–641. doi: 10.1016/j.actatropica.2013.09.010

Hanboonkunupakarn, B., and White, N. J. (2016). The threat of antimalarial drug resistance. *Trop. Dis. Travel Med. Vacc.* 2:10.

Happi, C. T., Gbotosho, G. O., Folarin, O. A., Akinboye, D. O., Yusuf, B. O., Ebong, O. O., et al. (2005). Polymorphisms in *Plasmodium falciparum dhfr* and *dhps* genes and age related in vivo sulfadoxine–pyrimethamine resistance in malaria-infected patients from Nigeria. *Acta Trop.* 95, 183–193. doi: 10.1016/j.actatropica.2005.06.015

Harinasuta, T., Suntharasamai, P., and Viravan, C. (1965). Chloroquine-resistant *falciparum* malaria in Thailand. *Lancet* 2, 657–660. doi: 10.1016/s0140-6736(65)90395-8

Heinberg, A., and Kirkman, L. (2015). The molecular basis of antifolate resistance in *Plasmodium falciparum*: looking beyond point mutations. *Annal. N. Y. Acad. Sci.* 1342, 10–18. doi: 10.1111/nyas.12662

Homewood, C. A., Warhurst, D. C., Peters, W., and Baggaley, V. C. (1972). Lysosomes, pH and the Anti-malarial action of chloroquine. *Nature* 235, 50–52. doi: 10.1038/235050a0

Hyde, J. E. (2009). Exploring the folate pathway in *Plasmodium falciparum*. *Acta Trop.* 94, 191–206. doi: 10.1016/j.actatropica.2005.04.002

Hyde, J. E. (2007). Drug-resistant malaria - an insight. *FEBS J.* 274, 4688–4698. doi: 10.1111/j.1742-4658.2007.05999.x

Ibraheem, Z. O., Abd Majid, R., Noor, S. M., Sedik, H. M., and Basir, R. (2014). Role of different *pfcrt* and *pfmdr-1* mutations in conferring resistance to antimalaria drugs in *Plasmodium falciparum*. *Mal. Res. Treat.* 2014:950424.

Idowu, O. A., Apalara, S. B., and Lasisi, A. A. (2006). Assessment of quality of chloroquine tablets sold by drug vendors in Abeokuta, Nigeria. *Tanzan Health Res. Bull.* 8, 45–46.

Ikegbunam, M. N., Nkonganyi, C. N., Thomas, B. N., Esimone, C. O., Velavan, T. P., and Ojurongbe, O. (2019). Analysis of *Plasmodium falciparumpfcrt* and *pfmdr1* genes in parasite isolates from asymptomatic individuals in Southeast Nigeria 11 years after withdrawal of chloroquine. Malaria J. 18:343. doi: 10.1186/s12936-019-2977-6

Iriemenam, N. C., Shah, M., Gatei, W., van Eijk, A. M., Ayisi, J., Kariuki, S., et al. (2012). Temporal trends of sulphadoxine-pyrimethamine (SP) drug-resistance molecular markers in *Plasmodium falciparum* parasites from pregnant women in western Kenya. *Mal. J.* 11:134. doi: 10.1186/1475-2875-11-134

Jiang, T., Chen, J., Fu, H., Wu, K., Yao, Y., Eyi, J. U. M., et al. (2019). High prevalence of *pfdhfr-pfdhps* quadruple mutations associated with sulfadoxine-pyrimethamine resistance in *Plasmodium falciparum* isolates from Bioko Island, Equatorial Guinea. *Malaria J.* 18:101. doi: 10.1186/s12936-019-2734-x

Kajubi, R., Ochieng, T., Kakuru, A., Jagannathan, P., Nakalembe, M., Ruel, T., et al. (2019). Monthly sulfadoxine-pyrimethamine versus dihydroartemisinin-piperaquine for intermittent preventive treatment of malaria in pregnancy: a double-blind, randomised, controlled, superiority trial. *Lancet* 393, 1428–1439. doi: 10.1016/s0140-6736(18)32224-4

Kalanda, G. C., Hill, J., Verhoeff, F. H., and Brabin, B. J. (2006). Comparative efficacy of chloroquine and sulphadoxine–pyrimethamine in pregnant women and children: a meta-analysis. *Trop Med. Int. Health* 11, 569–577. doi: 10.1111/j.1365-3156.2006.01608.x

Kayentao, K., Garner, P., Maria van Eijk, A., Naidoo, I., Roper, C., Mulokozi, A., et al. (2013). Intermittent preventive therapy for malaria during pregnancy using 2 vs 3 or more doses of sulfadoxine-pyrimethamine and risk of low birth weight in africa: systematic review and meta-analysis. *JAMA* 309, 594–604. doi: 10.1001/jama.2012.216231

Knight, S. E., Anyachebelu, E. J., Geddes, R., and Maharaj, R. (2009). Impact of delayed introduction of sulfadoxine–pyrimethamine and arthemeter–lumefantrine on malaria epidemiology in KwaZulu-Natal, South Africa. *Trop Med. Int. Health* 14, 1086–1092. doi: 10.1111/j.1365-3156.2009.02333.x

Kublin, J. G., Cortese, J. F., Njunju, E. M., Mukadam, R. A., Wirima, J. J., Kazembe, P. N., et al. (2003). Reemergence of chloroquine-sensitive *Plasmodium falciparum* malaria after cessation of chloroquine use in Malawi. *J. Infect. Dis.* 187, 1870–1875. doi: 10.1086/375419

Kümpornsin, K., Modchang, C., Heinberg, A., Ekland, E. H., Jirawatcharadech, P., Chobson, P., et al. (2014). Origin of robustness in generating drug-resistant malaria parasites. *Mol. Biol. Evol.* 31, 1649–1660. doi: 10.1093/molbev/msu140

Lawrenson, A., Cooper, D., O'Neill, P., and Berry, N. (2018). Study of the antimalarial activity of 4-aminoquinoline compounds against chloroquine-sensitive and chloroquine-resistant parasite strains. *J. Mol. Model.* 24:237. doi: 10.1007/s00894-018-3755-z

Laxminarayan, R., Over, M., and Smith, D. L. (2006). Will a global subsidy of new antimalarials delay the emergence of resistance and save lives? *Health Aff. (Millwood)* 25, 325–336. doi: 10.1377/hlthaff.25.2.325

Lehane, A. M., and Kirk, K. (2008). Chloroquine resistance-conferring mutations in pfcrt give rise to a chloroquine-associated H+ leak from the malaria parasite's digestive vacuole. *Antimicrob Agents Chemothe.r* 52, 4374–4380. doi: 10.1128/aac.00666-08

Lehane, A. M., McDevitt, C. A., Kirk, K., and Fidock, D. A. (2012). Degrees of chloroquine resistance in *Plasmodium* - is the redox system involved? *Int. J. Parasitol. Drugs Drug Resist.* 2, 47–57. doi: 10.1016/j.ijpddr.2011.11.001

Loria, P., Miller, S., Foley, M., and Tilley, L. (1999). Inhibition of the peroxidative degradation of haem as the basis of action of chloroquine and other quinoline antimalarials. *Biochem. J.* 339(Pt 2), 363–370. doi: 10.1042/0264-6021:3390363

Lu, F., Culleton, R., Zhang, M., Ramaprasad, A., von Seidlein, L., Zhou, H., et al. (2017b). Emergence of indigenous artemisinin-resistant *Plasmodium falciparum* in Africa. *N. Engl. J. Med.* 376, 991–993.

Lu, F., Zhang, M., Culleton, R. L., Xu, S., Tang, J., Zhou, H., et al. (2017a). Return of chloroquine sensitivity to Africa? Surveillance of African *Plasmodium falciparum* chloroquine resistance through malaria imported to China. *Paras. Vect.* 10, 355.

Lusingu, J. P., and Von Seidlein, L. (2008). Challenges in malaria control in sub-Saharan Africa: the vaccine perspective. *Tanzan J. Health Res.* 10, 253–266.

Macintyre, K., Littrell, M., Keating, J., Hamainza, B., Miller, J., and Eisele, T. P. (2011). Determinants of hanging and use of ITNs in the context of near universal coverage in Zambia. *Health Policy Plann.* 27, 316–325. doi: 10.1093/heapol/czr042

Maharaj, R., Raman, J., Morris, N., Moonasar, D., Durrheim, D. N., Seocharan, I., et al. (2013). Epidemiology of malaria in South Africa: From control to elimination. *SAMJ South Afr. Med. J.* 103, 779–783. doi: 10.7196/samj.7441

Maiga, H., Djimde, A. A., Beavogui, A. H., Toure, O., Tekete, M., Sangare, C. P. O., et al. (2015). Efficacy of sulphadoxine-pyrimethamine + artesunate, sulphadoxine-pyrimethamine + amodiaquine, and sulphadoxine-pyrimethamine alone in uncomplicated *falciparum* malaria in Mali. *Mal. J.* 14:64. doi: 10.1186/s12936-015-0557-y

Maiga, O. M., Kayentao, K., Traoré, B. T., Djimde, A., Traoré, B., Diallo, M., et al. (2011). Superiority of 3 Over 2 doses of intermittent preventive treatment with sulfadoxine-pyrimethamine for the prevention of malaria during pregnancy in mali: a randomized controlled trial. *Clin. Infect. Dis.* 53, 215–223. doi: 10.1093/cid/cir374

Maitland, K. (2016). Severe malaria in african children – the need for continuing investment. *N. Engl. J. Med.* 375, 2416–2417. doi: 10.1056/nejmp1613528

Makono, R., and Sibanda, S. (1999). Review of the prevalence of malaria in Zimbabwe with specific reference to parasite drug resistance (1984-96). *Trans. R. Soc. Trop. Med. Hyg.* 93, 449–452. doi: 10.1016/s0035-9203(99)90331-0

Malisa, A. L., Pearce, R. J., Abdulla, S., Mshinda, H., Kachur, P. S., Bloland, P., et al. (2010). Drug coverage in treatment of malaria and the consequences for resistance evolution – evidence from the use of sulphadoxine/pyrimethamine. *Mal. J.* 9:190.

Marks, F., Evans, J., Meyer, C. G., Browne, E. N., Flessner, C., von Kalckreuth, V., et al. (2005). High prevalence of markers for sulfadoxine and pyrimethamine resistance in *Plasmodium falciparum* in the absence of drug pressure in the Ashanti region of Ghana. *Antimicrob Agents Chemother.* 49, 1101–1105. doi: 10.1128/aac.49.3.1101-1105.2005

Martin, M. K., Venantius, K. B., Patricia, N., Bernard, K., Keith, B., Allen, K., et al. (2020). Correlates of uptake of optimal doses of sulfadoxine-pyrimethamine for prevention of malaria during pregnancy in East-Central Uganda. *Mal. J.* 19:153.

Mayor, A., Serra-Casas, E., Sanz, S., Aponte, J. J., Macete, E., Mandomando, I., et al. (2008). Molecular Markers of resistance to sulfadoxine-pyrimethamine during intermittent preventive treatment for malaria in mozambican infants. *J. Infect. Dis.* 197, 1737–1742. doi: 10.1086/588144

Mbugi, E. V., Mutayoba, B. M., Malisa, A. L., Balthazary, S. T., Nyambo, T. B., and Mshinda, H. (2006). Drug resistance to sulphadoxine-pyrimethamine in *Plasmodium falciparum* malaria in Mlimba, Tanzania. *Mal. J.* 5:94.

Medicines for Malaria Venture (MMV) (2020). Available online at: www.mmv.org (accessed October 27, 2020).

Meshnick, S. R. (1998). Artemisinin antimalarials: mechanisms of action and resistance. *Med. Trop. (Mars)* 58(Suppl. 3), 13–17.

Mharakurwa, S., and Mugochi, T. (1994). Chloroquine-resistant *falciparum* malaria in an area of rising endemicity in Zimbabwe. *J. Trop. Med. Hyg.* 97, 39–45.

Mlambo, G., Sullivan, D., Mutambu, S. L., Soko, W., Mbedzi, J., Chivenga, J., et al. (2007). High prevalence of molecular markers for resistance to chloroquine and pyrimethamine in *Plasmodium falciparum* from Zimbabwe. *Parasitol. Res.* 101, 1147–1151. doi: 10.1007/s00436-007-0597-5

Mubyazi, G. M., and Gonzalez-Block, M. A. (2005). Research influence on antimalarial drug policy change in Tanzania: case study of replacing chloroquine with sulfadoxine-pyrimethamine as the first-line drug. *Mal. J.* 4, 51–51.

Mwanza, S., Joshi, S., Nambozi, M., Chileshe, J., Malunga, P., Kabuya, J-B., et al. (2016). The return of chloroquine-susceptible *Plasmodium falciparum* malaria in Zambia. *Malaria J.* 15, 584–584. doi: 10.1186/s12936-016-1637-3

Mwendera, C., de Jager, C., Longwe, H., Phiri, K., Hongoro, C., and Mutero, C. M. (2016). Malaria research and its influence on anti-malarial drug policy in Malawi: a case study. *Health Res. Policy Syst.* 14:41. doi: 10.1186/s12961-016-0108-1

Naidoo, I., and Roper, C. (2010). Following the path of most resistance: *dhps* K540E dispersal in African *Plasmodium falciparum*. *Trends Parasitol.* 26, 447–456. doi: 10.1016/j.pt.2010.05.001

Naidoo, I., and Roper, C. (2011). Drug resistance maps to guide intermittent preventive treatment of malaria in African infants. *Parasitology* 138, 1469–1479. doi: 10.1017/s0031182011000746

Najera, J. A., and Zaim, M. (2001). *Malaria Vector Control – Insecticides for Indoor Residual Spraying*. Geneva: World Health Organization Communicable Disease Control, Prevention and Eradication.

Ndeffo Mbah, M. L., Parikh, S., and Galvani, A. P. (2015). Comparing the impact of artemisinin-based combination therapies on malaria transmission in sub-Saharan Africa. *Am. J. Trop. Med. Hyg.* 92, 555–560. doi: 10.4269/ajtmh.14-0490

Ndiaye, M., Faye, B., Tine, R., Ndiaye, J. L., Lo, A., Abiola, A., et al. (2012). Assessment of the molecular marker of Plasmodium falciparum chloroquine resistance (Pfcrt) in Senegal after several years of chloroquine withdrawal. *Am. J. Trop. Med. Hyg.* 87, 640–645. doi: 10.4269/ajtmh.2012.11-0709

Njokah, M. J., Kang'ethe, J. N., Kinyua, J., Kariuki, D., and Kimani, F. T. (2016). In vitro selection of *Plasmodium falciparum pfcrt* and *pfmdr1* variants by artemisinin. *Malar. J.* 15:381.

Nuwaha, F. (2001). The challenge of chloroquine-resistant malaria in sub-Saharan Africa. *Health Policy Plann.* 16, 1–12. doi: 10.1093/heapol/16.1.1

Nzila, A. (2006). The past, present and future of antifolates in the treatment of *Plasmodium falciparum* infection. *J. Antimicrob. Chemother.* 57, 1043–1054. doi: 10.1093/jac/dkl104

Nzila, A. M., Mberu, E. K., Sulo, J., Dayo, H., Winstanley, P. A., Sibley, C. H., et al. (2000). Towards an understanding of the mechanism of pyrimethamine-sulfadoxine resistance in *Plasmodium falciparum*: genotyping of dihydrofolate reductase and dihydropteroate synthase of Kenyan parasites. *Antimicrob. Agents Chemother.* 44, 991–996. doi: 10.1128/aac.44.4.991-996.2000

Ogouyèmi-Hounto, A., Ndam, N. T., Kinde Gazard, D., d'Almeida, S., Koussihoude, L., Ollo, E., et al. (2013). Prevalence of the molecular marker of *Plasmodium falciparum* resistance to chloroquine and sulphadoxine/pyrimethamine in Benin seven years after the change of malaria treatment policy. *Mal. J.* 12:147.

Okumu, F. O., and Moore, S. J. (2011). Combining indoor residual spraying and insecticide-treated nets for malaria control in Africa: a review of possible outcomes and an outline of suggestions for the future. *Malar. J.* 10:208.

Oladipo, O. O., Wellington, O. A., and Sutherland, C. J. (2015). Persistence of chloroquine-resistant haplotypes of *Plasmodium falciparum* in children with uncomplicated Malaria in Lagos, Nigeria, four years after change of chloroquine as first-line antimalarial medicine. *Diagn. Pathol.* 10:41. doi: 10.1186/s13000-015-0276-2

Olapeju, B., Choiriyyah, I., Lynch, M., Acosta, A., Blaufuss, S., Filemyr, E., et al. (2018). Age and gender trends in insecticide-treated net use in sub-Saharan Africa: a multi-country analysis. *Mal. J.* 17:423.

Omar, S. A. I, Adagu, S., Gump, D. W., Ndaru, N. P., and Warhurst, D. C. (2001). *Plasmodium falciparum* in Kenya: high prevalence of drug-resistance-associated polymorphisms in hospital admissions with severe malaria in an epidemic area. *Annal. Trop. Med. Parasitol.* 95, 661–669. doi: 10.1080/00034980120103234

Osman, M. E., Mockenhaupt, F. P., Bienzle, U., Elbashir, M. I., and Giha, H. A. (2007). Field-based evidence for linkage of mutations associated with chloroquine (*pfcrt/pfmdr1*) and sulfadoxine-pyrimethamine (pfdhfr/pfdhps) resistance and for the fitness cost of multiple mutations in *P. falciparum*. *Infect. Genet. Evol.* 7, 52–59. doi: 10.1016/j.meegid.2006.03.008

Oyibo, W. A., and Agomo, C. O. (2011). Scaling up of intermittent preventive treatment of malaria in pregnancy using sulphadoxine-pyrimethamine: prospects and challenges. *Mat. Child Health J.* 15, 542–552. doi: 10.1007/s10995-010-0608-5

Parker, D., Carrara, V., Pukrittayakamee, S., McGready, R., and Nosten, F. (2015). Malaria ecology along the Thailand- Myanmar border. *Mal. J.* 14:921.

Pearce, R. J., Drakeley, C., Chandramohan, D., Mosha, F., and Roper, C. (2003). Molecular determination of point mutation haplotypes in the dihydrofolate reductase and dihydropteroate synthase of *Plasmodium falciparum* in three districts of northern Tanzania. *Antimicrob Agents Chemother.* 47, 1347–1354. doi: 10.1128/aac.47.4.1347-1354.2003

Pearce, R. J., Pota, H., Evehe, M. S., El-Hadj, B., Mombo-Ngoma, G., Malisa, A. L., et al. (2009). Multiple origins and regional dispersal of resistant dhps in African *Plasmodium falciparum* malaria. *PLoS Med.* 6:e1000055. doi: 10.1371/journal.pmed.1000055

Peters, P. J., Thigpen, M. C., Parise, M. E., and Newman, R. D. (2007). Safety and toxicity of sulfadoxine/pyrimethamine: implications for malaria prevention in pregnancy using intermittent preventive treatment. *Drug Saf.* 30, 481–501. doi: 10.2165/00002018-200730060-00003

Plowe, C. V. (2014). Resistance nailed. *Nature* 505, 30–31. doi: 10.1038/nature12845

Pluess, B., Tanser, F. C., Lengeler, C., and Sharp, B. L. (2010). Indoor residual spraying for preventing malaria. *Cochr. Database Syst. Rev.* 2010:CD006657.

Premji, Z. G. (2009). Coartem® : the journey to the clinic. *Mal. J.* 8:S3.

Pulcini, S., Staines, H. M., Lee, A. H., Shafik, S. H., Bouyer, G., Moore, C. M., et al. (2015). Mutations in the *Plasmodium falciparum* chloroquine resistance transporter, PfCRT, enlarge the parasite's food vacuole and alter drug sensitivities. *Sci. Rep.* 5:14552. doi: 10.1038/srep14552

Raman, J., Kagoro, F. M., Mabuza, A., Malatje, G., Reid, A., Frean, J., and Barnes, K. I. (2019). Absence of *kelch13* artemisinin resistance markers but strong selection for lumefantrine-tolerance molecular markers following 18 years of artemisinin-based combination therapy use in Mpumalanga Province, South Africa (2001–2018). *Malaria J.* 18:280. doi: 10.1186/s12936-019-2911-y

Raphemot, R., Posfai, D., and Derbyshire, E. R. (2016). Current therapies and future possibilities for drug development against liver-stage malaria. *J. Clin. Investigat.* 126, 2013–2020. doi: 10.1172/jci82981

Rapuoda, B., Ali, A., Bakyaita, N., Mutabingwa, T., Mwita, A., Rwagacondo, C., et al. (2003). The efficacy of antimalarial monotherapies, sulfadoxine-pyrimethamine and amodiaquine in East Africa: implication for sub-regional policy. The East African Network for Monitoring Antimalarial Treatment (EANMAT). *Trop. Med. Int. Health* 8, 860–867. doi: 10.1046/j.1360-2276.2003.01114.x

Recker, M., Bull, P. C., and Buckee, C. O. (2018). Recent advances in the molecular epidemiology of clinical malaria. *F1000Research* 7, F1000FacultyRev-1159.

Reiling, S. J., Krohne, G., Friedrich, O., Geary, T. G., and Rohrbach, P. (2018). Chloroquine exposure triggers distinct cellular responses in sensitive versus resistant Plasmodium falciparum parasites. *Sci. Rep.* 8:11137.

Roepe, P. D. (2011). PfCRT-mediated drug transport in malarial parasites. *Biochemistry* 50, 163–171. doi: 10.1021/bi101638n

Sandefur, C. I., Wooden, J. M. I, Quaye, K., Sirawaraporn, W., and Sibley, C. H. (2007). Pyrimethamine-resistant dihydrofolate reductase enzymes of *Plasmodium falciparum* are not enzymatically compromised in vitro. *Mol. Biochem. Parasitol.* 154, 1–5. doi: 10.1016/j.molbiopara.2007.03.009

Scates, S. S., Finn, T. P., Wisniewski, J., Dadi, D., Mandike, R., Khamis, M., et al. (2020). Costs of insecticide-treated bed net distribution systems in sub-Saharan Africa. *Mal. J.* 19, 105–105.

Schleicher, T. R., Yang, J., Freudzon, M., Rembisz, A., Craft, S., Hamilton, M., et al. (2018). A mosquito salivary gland protein partially inhibits *Plasmodium* sporozoite cell traversal and transmission. *Nat. Commun.* 9:2908.

Schönfeld, M., Barreto Miranda, I., Schunk, M., Maduhu, I., Maboko, L., Hoelscher, M., et al. (2007). Molecular surveillance of drug-resistance associated mutations of *Plasmodium falciparum* in south-west Tanzania. *Mal. J.* 6:2.

Shafik, S. H., Cobbold, S. A., Barkat, K., Richards, S. N., Lancaster, N. S., Llinás, M., et al. (2020). The natural function of the malaria parasite's chloroquine resistance transporter. *Nat. Commun.* 11:3922. doi: 10.1038/s41467-020-17781-6

Sharma, J., Khan, S., Dutta, P., and Mahanta, J. (2015). Molecular determination of antifolate resistance associated point mutations in *Plasmodium falciparum* dihydrofolate reductase (dhfr) and dihydropteroate synthetase (dhps) genes among the field samples in Arunachal Pradesh. *J. Vector Borne Dis.* 52, 116–121.

Shretta, R., Omumbo, J., Rapuoda, B., and Snow, R. W. (2000). Using evidence to change antimalarial drug policy in Kenya. *Trop. Med. Int. Health* 5, 755–764. doi: 10.1046/j.1365-3156.2000.00643.x

Siddiqui, F. A., Boonhok, R., Cabrera, M., Mbenda, H. G. N., Wang, M., Min, H., et al. (2020). Role of *Plasmodium falciparum* Kelch 13 protein mutations in *P. falciparum* populations from northeastern myanmar in mediating artemisinin resistance. *mBio* 11:e001134-19.

Slater, H. C., Griffin, J. T., Ghani, A. C., and Okell, L. C. (2016). Assessing the potential impact of artemisinin and partner drug resistance in sub-Saharan Africa. *Mal. J.* 15, 10–10.

Smith Gueye, C., Newby, G., Gosling, R. D., Whittaker, M. A., Chandramohan, D., Slutsker, L., et al. (2016). Strategies and approaches to vector control in nine malaria-eliminating countries: a cross-case study analysis. *Mal. J.* 15:2.

Sridaran, S., McClintock, S. K., Syphard, L. M., Herman, K. M., Barnwell, J. W., and Udhayakumar, V. (2010). Anti-folate drug resistance in Africa: meta-analysis of reported dihydrofolate reductase (*dhfr*) and dihydropteroate synthase (*dhps*) mutant genotype frequencies in African Plasmodium falciparum parasite populations. *Mal. J.* 9:247. doi: 10.1186/1475-2875-9-247

Steinhardt, L. C., Jean, Y. S., Impoinvil, D., Mace, K. E., Wiegand, R., Huber, C. S., et al. (2017). Effectiveness of insecticide-treated bednets in malaria prevention in Haiti: a case-control study. *Lancet Global Health* 5, e96–e103.

Tagbor, H., Bruce, J., Browne, E., Randal, A., Greenwood, B., and Chandramohan, D. (2006). Efficacy, safety, and tolerability of amodiaquine plus sulphadoxine-pyrimethamine used alone or in combination for malaria treatment in pregnancy: a randomised trial. *Lancet* 368, 1349–1356. doi: 10.1016/s0140-6736(06)69559-7

Takala-Harrison, S., and Laufer, M. K. (2015). Antimalarial drug resistance in Africa: key lessons for the future. *Annal. N. Y. Acad. Sci.* 1342, 62–67. doi: 10.1111/nyas.12766

Takechi, M., Matsuo, M., Ziba, C., Macheso, A., Butao, D. I, Zungu, L., et al. (2001). Therapeutic efficacy of sulphadoxine/pyrimethamine and susceptibility in vitro of P. falciparum isolates to sulphadoxine-pyremethamine and other antimalarial drugs in Malawian children. *Trop. Med. Int. Health* 6, 429–434. doi: 10.1046/j.1365-3156.2001.00735.x

Taylor, C., Florey, L., and Ye, Y. (2017). Equity trends in ownership of insecticide-treated nets in 19 sub-Saharan African countries. *Bull. World Health Organ.* 95, 322–332. doi: 10.2471/blt.16.172924

Tekete, M. M., Toure, S., Fredericks, A., Beavogui, A. H., Sangare, C. P. O., Evans, A., et al. (2011). Effects of amodiaquine and artesunate on sulphadoxine-pyrimethamine pharmacokinetic parameters in children under five in Mali. *Mal. J.* 10:275. doi: 10.1186/1475-2875-10-275

ter Kuile, F. O., van Eijk, A. M., and Filler, S. J. (2015). Effect of sulfadoxine-pyrimethamine resistance on the efficacy of intermittent preventive therapy for malaria control during pregnancy: a systematic review. *JAMA* 297, 2603–2616. doi: 10.1001/jama.297.23.2603

Terlouw, D. J., Nahlen, B. L., Courval, J. M., Kariuki, S. K., Rosenberg, O. S., Oloo, A. J., et al. (2003). Sulfadoxine-pyrimethamine in treatment of malaria in Western Kenya: increasing resistance and underdosing. *Antimicrob Agents Chemother.* 47, 2929–2932. doi: 10.1128/aac.47.9.2929-2932.2003

Thomsen, T. T., Madsen, L. B., Hansson, H. H., Tomás, E. V., Charlwood, D. I, Bygbjerg, C., et al. (2013). Rapid selection of *Plasmodium falciparum* chloroquine resistance transporter gene and multidrug resistance gene-1 haplotypes associated with past chloroquine and present artemether-lumefantrine use in Inhambane District, southern Mozambique. *Am. J. Trop. Med. Hyg.* 88, 536–541. doi: 10.4269/ajtmh.12-0525

Thu, A. M., Phyo, A. P., Landier, J., Parker, D. M., and Nosten, F. H. (2017). Combating multidrug-resistant *Plasmodium falciparum* malaria. *FEBS J.* 284, 2569–2578.

Tizifa, T. A., Kabaghe, A. N., McCann, R. S., van den Berg, H., Van Vugt, M., and Phiri, K. S. (2018). Prevention efforts for Malaria. *Curr. Trop. Med. Rep.* 5, 41–50.

Trape, J. F. (2001). The public health impact of chloroquine resistance in Africa. *Am. J. Trop. Med. Hyg.* 64, 12–17. doi: 10.4269/ajtmh.2001.64.12

Trape, J. F., Pison, G., Preziosi, M. P., Enel, C., Desgrées du Loû, A., Delaunay, V., et al. (1998). Impact of chloroquine resistance on malaria mortality. *C R Acad. Sci. III* 321, 689–697.

Ukpe, I. S., Moonasar, D., Raman, J., Barnes, K. I., Baker, L., and Blumberg, L. (2013). Case management of malaria: Treatment and chemoprophylaxis. *S. Afr. Med. J.* 103(10 Pt 2), 793–798. doi: 10.7196/samj.7443

Veiga, M. I., Dhingra, S. K., Henrich, P. P., Straimer, J., Gnädig, N., Uhlemann, A-C., et al. (2016). Globally prevalent *pfmdr1* mutations modulate *Plasmodium falciparum* susceptibility to artemisinin-based combination therapies. *Nat. Commun.* 7:11553. doi: 10.1038/ncomms11553

Viana, G. M. R., Machado, R. L. D., Calvosa, V. S. P., and Póvoa, M. M. (2006). Mutations in the *pfmdr1, cg2,* and *pfcrt* genes in *Plasmodium falciparum* samples from endemic malaria areas in Rondonia and Pará State, Brazilian Amazon Region. *Cad Saude Publica* 22, 2703–2711. doi: 10.1590/s0102-311x2006001200019

von Seidlein, L., and Dondorp, A. (2015). Fighting fire with fire: mass antimalarial drug administrations in an era of antimalarial resistance. *Exp. Rev. Anti. Infect. Ther.* 13, 715–730. doi: 10.1586/14787210.2015.1031744

Walker, P. G. T., Floyd, J., ter Kuile, F., and Cairns, M. (2017). Estimated impact on birth weight of scaling up intermittent preventive treatment of malaria in pregnancy given sulphadoxine-pyrimethamine resistance in Africa: a mathematical model. *PLoS Med.* 14:e1002243. doi: 10.1371/journal.pmed.1002243

Wernsdorfer, W. H. (1994). Epidemiology of drug resistance in malaria. *Acta Tropica* 56, 143–156. doi: 10.1016/0001-706x(94)90060-4

White, N. J., Pongtavornpinyo, W., Maude, R. J., Saralamba, S., Aguas, R., Stepniewska, K., et al. (2009). Hyperparasitaemia and low dosing are an important source of anti-malarial drug resistance. *Mal. J.* 8:253.

Wicht, K. J., Mok, S., and Fidock, D. A. (2020). Molecular Mechanisms of drug resistance in *Plasmodium falciparum* malaria. *Annu. Rev. Microbiol.* 74, 431–454. doi: 10.1146/annurev-micro-020518-115546

Winstanley, P., Ward, S., Snow, R., and Breckenridge, A. (2004). Therapy of falciparum malaria in sub-saharan Africa: from molecule to policy. *Clin. Microbiol. Rev.* 17, 612–637. doi: 10.1128/cmr.17.3.612-637.2004

World Health Organisation (WHO) (2008). *World Malaria Report 2007.* Geneva: World Health Organization.

World Health Organisation (WHO) (2003). *World Malaria Report 2002.* Geneva: World Health Organization.

World Health Organisation (WHO) (2010). *WHO Technical Report Series 957.* Geneva: World Health Organization.

World Health Organisation (WHO) (2011). *World Malaria Report 2010.* Geneva: World Health Organization.

World Health Organisation (WHO) (2017). *World Malaria Report 2016.* Geneva: World Health Organization.

World Health Organisation (WHO) (2019). *World Malaria Report 2018.* Geneva: World Health Organization.

World Health Organisation (WHO) (2020). *World Malaria Report 2018.* Geneva: World Health Organization.

Xia, Z.-G., Wang, R.-B., Wang, D.-Q., Feng, J., Zheng, Q., Deng, C.-S., et al. (2014). China-Africa cooperation initiatives in malaria control and elimination. *Adv. Parasitol.* 86, 319–337. doi: 10.1016/b978-0-12-800869-0.00012-3

Xie, S. C., Ralph, S. A., and Tilley, L. (2020). K13, the cytostome, and artemisinin resistance. *Trends Parasitol.* 36, 533–544. doi: 10.1016/j.pt.2020.03.006

Yadav, S., and Rawal, G. (2016). The menace due to fake antimalarial drugs. *Int. J. Pharmaceut. Chem. Anal.* 3, 53–55. doi: 10.5958/2394-2797.2016.00007.1

Yeka, A., Gasasira, A., Mpimbaza, A., Achan, J., Nankabirwa, J., Nsobya, S., et al. (2012). Malaria in Uganda: challenges to control on the long road to elimination: I. Epidemiology and current control efforts. *Acta Trop.* 121, 184–195. doi: 10.1016/j.actatropica.2011.03.004

Young, M. D., and Moore, D. V. (1961). Chloroquine resistance in *Plasmodium falciparum. Am. J. Trop. Med. Hyg.* 10, 317–320.

Zareen, S., Ur Rehman, H., Gul, N., Ur Rehman, M., Bibi, S., Bakht, A., et al. (2016). Malaria is still a life-threatening disease review. *J. Entomol. Zool. Stud. JEZS* 105, 105–112.

Zhao, L., Pi, L., Qin, Y., Lu, Y., Zeng, W., Xiang, Z., et al. (2020). Widespread resistance mutations to sulfadoxine-pyrimethamine in malaria parasites imported to China from Central and Western Africa. *Int. J. Parasitol. Drugs Drug Resist.* 12, 1–6. doi: 10.1016/j.ijpddr.2019.11.002

21

Impact of Highland Topography Changes on Exposure to Malaria Vectors and Immunity in Western Kenya

Christine Ludwin Wanjala[1,2] *and Eliningaya J. Kweka*[3,4*]

[1] *Centre for Global Health Research, Kenya Medical Research Institute, Kisumu, Kenya,* [2] *Department of Medical Laboratory Sciences, Masinde Muliro University of Science and Technology, Kakamega, Kenya,* [3] *Mosquito Section, Division of Livestock and Human Diseases Vector Control, Tropical Pesticides Research Institute, Arusha, Tanzania,* [4] *Department of Medical Parasitology and Entomology, Catholic University of Health and Allied Sciences, Mwanza, Tanzania*

Edited by:
Efstratios Vogiannis, Evangeliki Model School of Smyrna – Athens, Greece

Reviewed by:
Gulnihal Ozbay, Delaware State University, USA
Konstantina Svoli, Evangeliki Model School of Smyrna – Athens, Greece

***Correspondence:**
Eliningaya J. Kweka
kwekae@tpri.or.tz

Background: It is almost an axiom that in the African highlands (above 1,500 m) transmission of *Plasmodium falciparum* is limited primarily by low ambient temperature and that small changes in temperature could result in temporary favorable conditions for unstable transmission within populations that have acquired little functional immunity. The pattern of malaria transmission in the highland plateau ecosystems is less distinct due to the flat topography and diffuse hydrology resulting from numerous streams. The non-homogeneous distribution of larval breeding habitats in east African highlands obviously affects *Anopheles* spatial distribution which, consequently, leads to heterogeneous human exposure to malaria. Another delicate parameter in the fragile transmission risk of malaria in the highlands is the rapid loss of primary forest due to subsistence agriculture. The implication of this change in land cover on malaria transmission is that deforestation can lead to changes in microclimate of both adult and larval habitats hence increase larvae survival, population density, and gametocytes development in adult mosquitoes. Deforestation has been documented to enhancing vectorial capacity of *Anopheles gambiae* by nearly 100% compared to forested areas.

Method: The study was conducted in five different ecosystems in the western Kenya highlands, two U-shaped valleys (Iguhu, Emutete), two V-shaped valleys (Marani, Fort Ternan), and one plateau (Shikondi) for 16 months among 6- to 15-year-old children. Exposure to malaria was tested using circumsporozoite protein (CSP) and merozoite surface protein immunochromatographic antibody tests. Malaria parasite was examined using different tools, which include microscopy based on blood smears, rapid diagnostic test based on HRP 2 proteins, and serology based on human immune response to parasite and vector antigens have been also examined in the highlands in comparison with different topographical systems of western Kenya.

Results: The results suggested that changes in the topography had implication on transmission in highlands of western Kenya and appropriate diagnosis, treatment, and control tool

Abbreviations: CSP, circumsporozoite protein; IgG, immuno globulin G; MSP, merozoite surface protein antibodies.

needed to be considered accordingly. Both plateau and U-shaped valley found to have higher parasite density than V-shaped valley. People in V-valley were less immune than in plateau and U-valley residents.

Conclusion: Topography diversity in western Kenya highlands has a significant impact on exposure rates of human to malaria vectors and parasite. The residents of V-shaped valleys are at risk of having explosive malaria outbreaks during hyper-transmission periods due to low exposure to malaria parasite; hence, they have low immune response to malaria, while the U-shaped valleys have stable malaria transmission, therefore, the human population has developed immunity to malaria due to continuous exposure to malaria.

Keywords: topography, V-valley, U-valley, immunity, exposure, rapid diagnostic kit, highland

INTRODUCTION

Malaria is a major human health threat that occurs globally in tropical and sub-tropical regions. Though malaria has been declining from 1.5 million mortality cases to 438,000 cases in 2014 (1), efforts has to be made to investigate the underlying causes of these hundreds of death cases. The mounting threat is evidence witnessed by increased numbers of malaria outbreaks in the Kenyan highlands (elevation >1,500 m), where malaria was previously rare (2, 3). Malaria outbreaks occurred sporadically in the highlands of western Kenya from the 1920s to the 1950s (4, 5). Since 1988, however, malaria epidemics have occurred with heightened frequency throughout the Kenyan highlands, causing serious mortality and morbidity (2, 3). Malaria in the Western Kenya Highland is characterized by unstable and high-transmission variability (6, 7), which results into epidemics during periods of suitable climatic conditions. Depending on drainage characteristics of the highland vector ecosystems, different transmission intensities results into heterogeneous exposure and development of immunity (6, 8–10). The sensitivity of a site to malaria epidemics is dependent on the level of immunity of the human population. In the last two decades, malaria epidemics have increased in frequency and intensity in the East Africa highlands in populations that have little or no exposure to plasmodial infections (3, 11–13). Research indicates that the mechanisms leading to epidemic malaria in the highlands are complex and are probably due to the concerted effects of factors, such as topography, hydrology, climate variability, land-use/land-cover change, and drug resistance (6, 8–10, 14). Effective disease control calls for a clear understanding of the interaction between these epidemiologic factors (9).

In this study, the highlands topography was classified into three ecosystems these being the flat bottomed valleys (U-shaped), the narrow bottomed valley (V shaped), and the plateau. A longitudinal cohort study was carried out with a primary focus on a spatial-temporal qualitative assessment of exposure to infections using immunological markers in the different ecosystems. Parasitological surveys were carried out to provide baseline data on the effects of ecosystem characteristics on malaria prevalence. Malaria epidemics in western Kenya highlands are driven by climate variability. However, environmental terrain characteristics can modify the level of malaria transmission and the rate of development of immunity (10). Immunity to severe malaria generally requires only a few infections at any level of endemicity (15–17). However, the long interval between infections and the spatial variability of transmission in areas of unstable endemicity fail to provide frequent enough challenge to sustain much disease-modulating immunity. Recent studies suggested that residents of highland areas generally lack immunity to *Plasmodium falciparum* and are particularly vulnerable to malaria infection (18–20). The proportion of asymptomatic individuals is usually lower in highlands than in high-transmission areas where there is small among-season variation in *P. falciparum* prevalence and parasite densities (21); thus, a small increase in the abundance of vectors may lead to a significant malaria outbreak in the highlands. At high altitudes in the highlands and on hilltops, where malaria transmission intensity is low, human populations have poorly developed immunity to malaria because exposures are infrequent, and persons are vulnerable to severe clinical illness and complications from *Plasmodium* infection (22). High risk for severe malaria is seen in persons living in areas with low-to-moderate transmission intensities (23). In such areas, the proportion of asymptomatic persons is usually lower than in high-transmission areas, where *P. falciparum* prevalence and parasite density varies little between seasons (24). As a consequence of low immunity in the human population of the highlands, malaria epidemics have caused significant human mortality (6). Compared to the malaria situation between the 1920s and 1950s, the current pattern of malaria epidemics in the highlands is characterized by increased frequencies (23), expanded geographic areas (8, 25), and increased case-fatality rates (3). The reemergence of epidemic malaria is likely due to local malaria transmission in the highlands (2, 7, 26, 27). In the late 1980s and early 1990s, a series of malaria epidemics were reported in the western highlands of Kenya and other communities at high altitude in Africa (28–30). Whereas substantial progress has been made on epidemiology and ecology of malaria in highlands, little is known on what proportion of human population exposed to malaria has mounted an immune response. This study was designed to identify how major environmental terrain characteristics that control the breeding of malaria vectors in the western Kenya highlands can influence exposure to transmission and the development of an immune response.

MATERIALS AND METHODS

Study Sites

Study sites where characterized into three topographical types.

"U"-Shaped Valleys

Iguhu in Kakamega

Iguhu village (00°17′ N, 34°74′ E and elevation 1,450–1,580 m above sea level) is located in Kakamega district, western Kenya, with population ≈11,000 (**Figure 1**). This area experiences two rainy seasons and averages 2,000 mm rainfall per year. The long rainy season usually occurs between April and May, with an average monthly rainfall 150–260 mm, while the short rainy season usually occurs between September and October, with an average monthly rainfall 165 mm. Malaria prevalence peaks usually lag 1–2 months after the rain. The mean annual daily temperature is 20.8°C. The area has experienced extensive deforestation and swamp reclamation in recent years as a result of rapid human population growth and the demand for settlement and agricultural land; therefore, only patches of forest remain. Malaria vectors in the area are *Anopheles gambiae* sensu stricto and *Anopheles funestus* (31–33). Maize is the principal subsistence crop with vegetables grown on small irrigated plots in valley bottoms. The Yala River bisects the area; most mosquito larval habitats are found on riverbanks in the bottom of the valley and on the banks of streams during both dry and rainy seasons (34).

Emutete in Emuhaya

Emutete village (00°22′ N, 34°64′ E and elevation 1,463–1,603 m above the sea level) is located in Emuhaya district (**Figure 1**). This area is hilly characterized by steep-sided valleys with flat bottoms and plateaus where most homes are built. Small streams run along the valley bottoms and papyrus swamps are common. The valleys are approximately 2.4 km^2 in area and at least 1 km apart. This area is densely populated, with malaria prevalence of 39.6% (35). This area experiences two rainy seasons and averages 2,500 mm rainfall per year. Malaria prevalence peaks usually lag 1–2 months after the rain. The mean annual daily temperature is 20.5°C.

"V"-Shaped Valleys

Marani in Kisii

Marani (00°02′ N, 34°48′ E and elevation 1,520–1,700 m above the sea level) is located on the highland plateau adjacent to the Lake Victoria Basin and 17 km north of Kisii (**Figure 1**). This area is in a steep valley where the Marani River flows through a shallow gorge on the western side, and river banks are forested with *Eucalyptus* trees. Malaria epidemics have occurred frequently in this area in the last 15 years.

Fort Tenan in Kericho

Fort Ternan (00°12′ S, 35°21′ E and elevation 1,500–1,600 m above the sea level) is found in Kericho District (**Figure 1**). Malaria prevalence in this area is unstable varying annually between 10 and 60%, due to this instability, epidemics are common with a high morbidity and mortality rates. Depending on the temperature during a specific year, transmission risk in this area is either seasonal or sporadic (2). This area consists of a variety of land covers ranging from shore regions to hilly areas and from

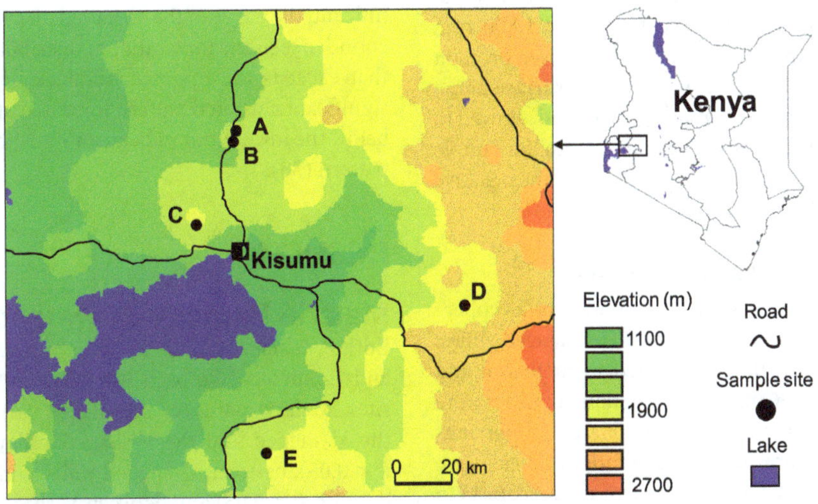

A. Shikondi
B. Iguhu
C. Emutete
D. Fort Ternan
E. Marani

FIGURE 1 | A map showing the location of the study sites.

rainy forests to tea plantations. Agricultural activities in these area are dominated by cash crops, e.g., sugarcane, tea, and coffee.

Plateau

Shikondi in Kakamega

Shikondi (00°19′ N, 34°76′ E, elevation 1,533–1,576 m above the sea level) is a plateau found in Kakamega district, Western Kenya (**Figure 1**). This area experiences two rainy seasons and averages 2,000 mm rainfall per year. The long rainy season usually occurs between April and May, with an average monthly rainfall 150–260 mm, while the short rainy season usually occurs between September and October, with an average monthly rainfall 165 mm. Malaria prevalence peaks usually lag 1–2 months after the rain. The mean annual daily temperature is 20.8°C.

Laboratory Analysis

Immunoassay for Exposure to Malaria

Exposure to malaria parasites is indicated by the presence of circumsporozoite proteins (CSPs) antibodies and the merozoite surface protein (MSP) antibodies in the serum. These antibodies persist even if the individual is cured of the parasite. Malaria P.f./P.v. 3 line test device consist of a sample window containing an absorbent pad where the serum/plasma are to be added. It contains a membrane strip, which is pre-coated with recombinant malaria P.f. capture antigens (MSP, CSP) on the test band P.f. region and with recombinant malaria P.v. capture antigens (MSP, CSP) on the test band P.v. region. The recombinant malaria P.v./P.f. antigen (MSP, CSP)-colloidal gold conjugate and serum sample moves along the membrane chromatographically to the test region (P.f., P.v.) and forms a visible line as antibody–antigen gold particle complex forms with high degree of sensitivity and specificity. Blood samples were collected by a standard finger prick and put in capillary tubes, then centrifuged at 1,800 rpm for 5 min to obtain the serum. After the test, kit had been brought to room temperature, the device was put on a flat surface and a drop of serum was added in to the sample window and allowed to soak in, then two drops of the diluent was added into the sample window. The positive results were read in 10 min and the negative results in 20 min.

Microscopic Analysis of Malaria Parasites

Standard finger-prick method was used for blood samples collection and thick and thin smears prepared on well labeled slides. After smears were air dried, they were fixed in methanol and stained with 4% Giemsa for 30 min (36). The stained smears were then examined using the magnification of 1,000× oil immersions to identify and count the parasite species. Random checks were carried out on the slide counts by independent microscopists to ensure quality control. Parasite density was scored against leukocytes (8,000 cells/μl of blood) positive slide; otherwise, the whole slide was carefully scanned before being declared negative (37).

Weather Data

Meteorological data collected were mean monthly rainfall, maximum, and minimum temperature for each study site. Data were obtained from the Kenya Department of Meteorology.

Data Analysis

Malaria parasites site-specific prevalence rates were determined by expressing positive blood smears as a percentage of all the examined blood smears. Geometric mean parasite density was calculated for each site considering only true positive slides. The paired t-test was used to determine differences of the prevalence of antibody and malaria parasites infections among the sites at 0.05 significance level. K function was used to determine if spatial distribution of infections in the sites was significantly clustered or it was random. In this method, the distance interval is specified, and then the GIS calculates the average number of infections within the distance of each infection. Increasing distances at a specified interval shows at what distance the concentration of infections is the greatest. If the average number of infections found at a distance is greater than that for a random distribution throughout the study area, then the distribution is considered clustered. The GIS finds the distance from each point to every other point, and then, for each point, counts up the number of surrounding points within the given distance. I is a weight and is either 1 if the neighboring point is within the distance of the target point or 0 if it is not. To see if there is a pattern, the observed K values at each distance is compared to the expected values for a random distribution. This is done by plotting the values on the chart, with the K values on the y-axis against the distance on the x-axis. The K value gets very large as the distance increases to reduce the height of the y-axis and make the chart easier to read, log transformed values are plotted instead of the raw K values. $L(d)$ is a variation of the K values. At any distance, if the line for the observed L values is above that of the expected values, the distribution is more clustered than expected for random distribution. If it is below the line for the expected values, the distribution is more dispersed. To determine if the pattern is statistically significant, the curve of the observed distribution is compared to the confidence limits for a random distribution. An observed L value that exceeds the upper confidence limit indicated statistically significant clustered pattern for that distance, while one that falls below the lower limit indicates a statistically significant dispersed pattern (38).

RESULTS

Malaria Parasite Prevalence

Both *P. falciparum* and *Plasmodium malariae* was found in Iguhu and Emutete while only *P. falciparum* was found in the other sites. Malaria parasites prevalence varied significantly between the U-shaped and the V-shaped valleys (t = 12.036, df = 12, $P < 0.05$), between U-shaped valley and the plateau ($t = -11.65$, df = 12, $P < 0.05$) and between V-shaped valleys and the plateau ($t = -2.76$, df = 12, $P < 0.05$). There was no significant difference in the parasite prevalence within the U-shaped valleys (t = 1.27, df = 12, $P > 0.05$), and within the V-shaped valleys ($t = -4.44$, df = 12, $P > 0.05$). The mean parasite prevalence in the U-shaped valleys was 22.12%, in the V-shaped valleys was 2.76% and at the plateau was 4.42% over the study period. There was 5.0-fold greater parasite prevalence in the U-shaped compared to the V-shaped valleys.

Parasite Density

Population living in U-shaped valleys had higher parasite density compared to the V-shaped valleys but varied at the plateau. Geometric means varied significantly between the V-shaped valleys and the plateau ($t = -2.72$, df = 12, $P < 0.05$) and between the V-shaped valleys and the U-shaped valleys ($t = -7.03$, df = 12, $P < 0.05$). There was no significant difference in the geometric means within the V-shaped valleys ($t = -2.1$, df = 12, $P > 0.05$), within the U-shaped valleys ($t = -1.73$, df = 12, $P > 0.05$) and between the U-shaped valley and the plateau ($t = 1.38$, df = 12, $P > 0.05$).

Gametocyte Prevalence

The U-shaped valleys had higher *P. falciparum* gametocytes prevalence compared to the V-shaped valleys and at the plateau. Gametocytes prevalence varied significantly between the V-shaped valleys and the U-shaped valleys ($t = 6.60$, df = 12, $P < 0.05$), between V-shaped valleys and the plateau ($t = 3.13$, df = 12, $P < 0.05$) and between U-shaped valleys and the plateau ($t = 3.34$, df = 12, $P < 0.05$). There was no significant difference in the gametocytes prevalence within the V-shaped valleys ($t = 0.30$, df = 12, $P > 0.05$), within the U-shaped valleys ($t = -0.20$, df = 12, $P > 0.05$). No gametocytes found in Marani during the period of the study (**Figure 2**).

Antibodies Prevalence

The U-shaped and V-shaped valleys had significant variations on antibodies prevalence varied between them ($t = 6.23$, df = 12, $P < 0.05$) and between the U-shaped valleys and the plateau ($t = 6.18$, df = 12, $P < 0.05$). There was no significant difference in the antibodies prevalence within U-shaped valleys ($t = -0.66$, df = 12, $P > 0.05$), within V-shaped valleys ($t = 0.68$, df = 12, $P > 0.05$) and between V-shaped valleys and the plateau ($t = -0.99$, df = 12, $P > 0.05$). The mean antibody prevalence in the U-shaped valley was 24.19%, in the V-shaped valley was 10.13% and at the plateau was 12.23% over the period of the study. There was 2.0-fold greater antibody prevalence in the U-shaped compared to the V-shaped valleys.

Spatial Distribution of Malaria Infections

The global weighted K function, $L(d)$, was used to examine the spatial distribution of malaria infection by household over an interpoint distance of 100–1,400 m for all the sites. **Figure 3** shows measures of the observed $L(d)$ and the 95% CI plotted for various values of interpoint distance for the Surveys in Emutete and Iguhu, respectively. The spatial distribution of infections is considered evenly dispersed if the observed K function values are below the lower limit of the 95% CI, clustered if above the upper limit, or random if within the 95% CI. The weighted K function indicated that the malaria infection distribution pattern was significantly different than expected under complete spatial randomness in the U-shaped valley (**Figure 4**) but was random in the V-shaped valley (**Figure 3**) and the plateau (**Figure 5**). Spatial clustering occurred at the swamps in the U-shaped valleys (**Figure 4**), it was less clustered at the plateau at low altitude but random in the V-shaped valley (**Figure 3**). The majority of

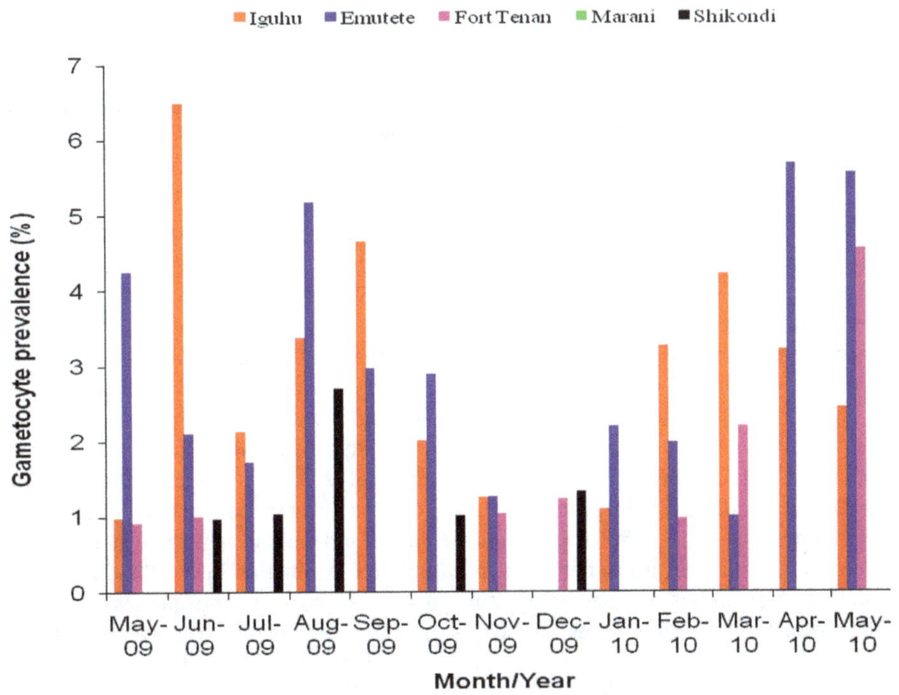

FIGURE 2 | Gametocytes prevalence rates in the five sites, no gametocytes were observed at Marani, Kisii during the period of study.

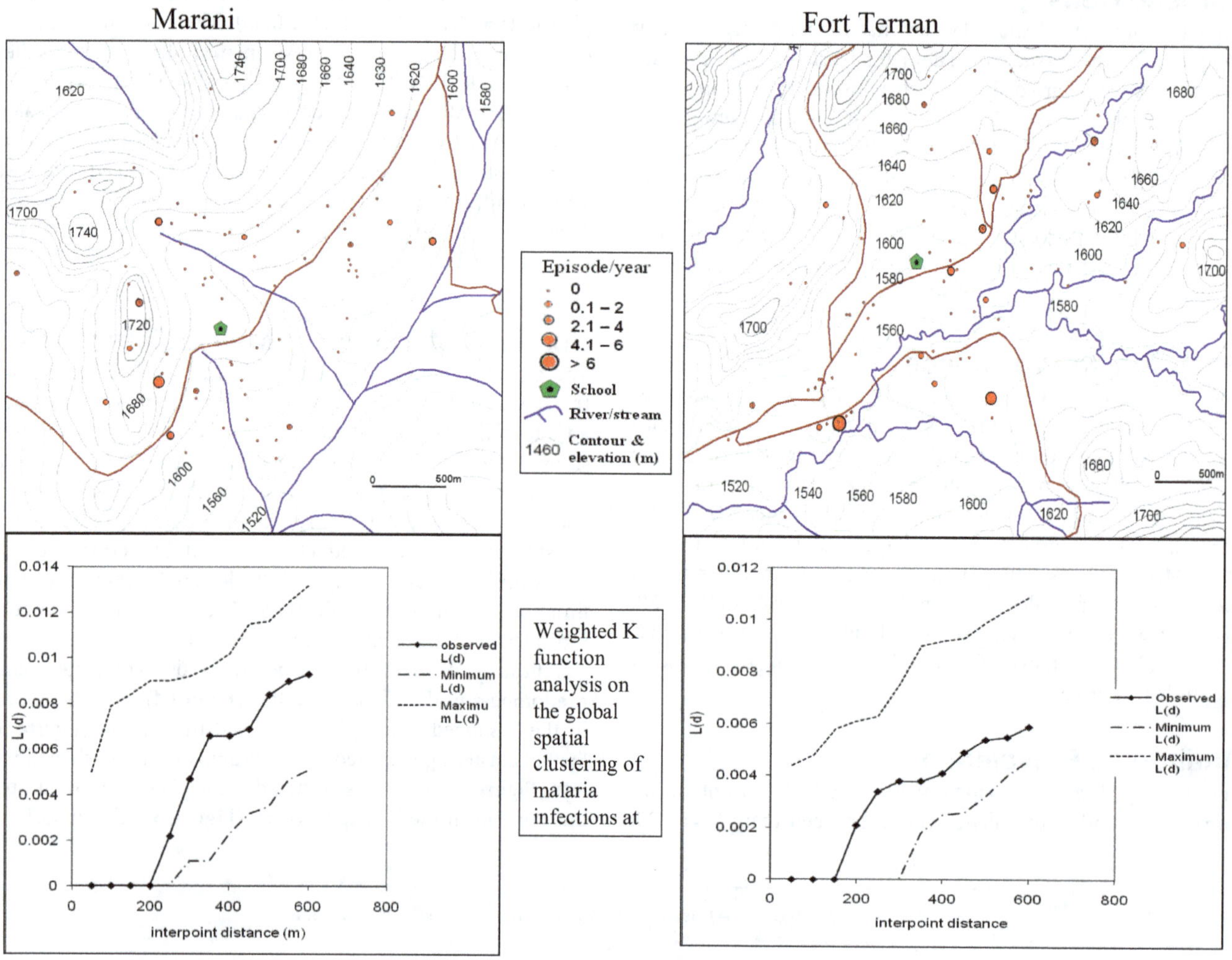

FIGURE 3 | Showing spatial distribution of malaria infections and cluster analysis in the "V"-shaped valleys of Marani and Fort Ternan (Weighted *K* function analysis shows that there was no significant clustering of malaria infections in Marani and Fort Ternan).

children with parasite positive blood smears in the U-shaped valleys were found infected 4–6 occasions during 12 months, while those in the V-shaped valleys and the plateau had 1–2 infections per year. Thus, the children in the U-shaped valleys were infected for a longer period (**Figures 3** and **4**).

DISCUSSION

This study has revealed that the western Kenya highland topography is a complex ecosystem comprising of hills, plateaus, valleys, rivers, streams, and swamps. This ecosystem has profound effects on the level of malaria transmission. It has been shown that malaria transmission in the highlands is heterogeneous with the highest incidence being found at valley bottoms followed by hillsides and hilltops (9, 10, 14, 39). In this study, we found that the prevalence of malaria infections was fivefold higher in children living in the U-shaped valleys than in the children living in the V-shaped valleys and the prevalence of malaria infections at the plateau was similar to that of the V-shaped valleys. Similar findings have been reported in different topography in highlands (10, 16, 40, 41). The prevalence of malaria parasites antibodies was twofold higher in the children living in the U-shaped valleys than in the children living in the V-shaped valleys. Similar findings have been shown in western Kenya highlands with serological markers, where the residents at the valley bottom are more exposed to mosquitoes infectious bites than those living in uphill's (42, 43). The gametocytes prevalence was also high in the children living in the U-shaped valleys compared to the V-shaped valleys and the plateau with no gametocytes observed at Kisii. The children population in U-valleys previously were found to have higher exposure to mosquitoes that subsequently have caused them to be in higher risk of *P. falciparum* gametocytes carriage (10, 16, 42, 43). Parasite densities were high in the children living in the U-shaped valley compared to the V-shaped valleys and varied greatly at the plateau. Similar findings were present previously with the human population in broad valleys having more

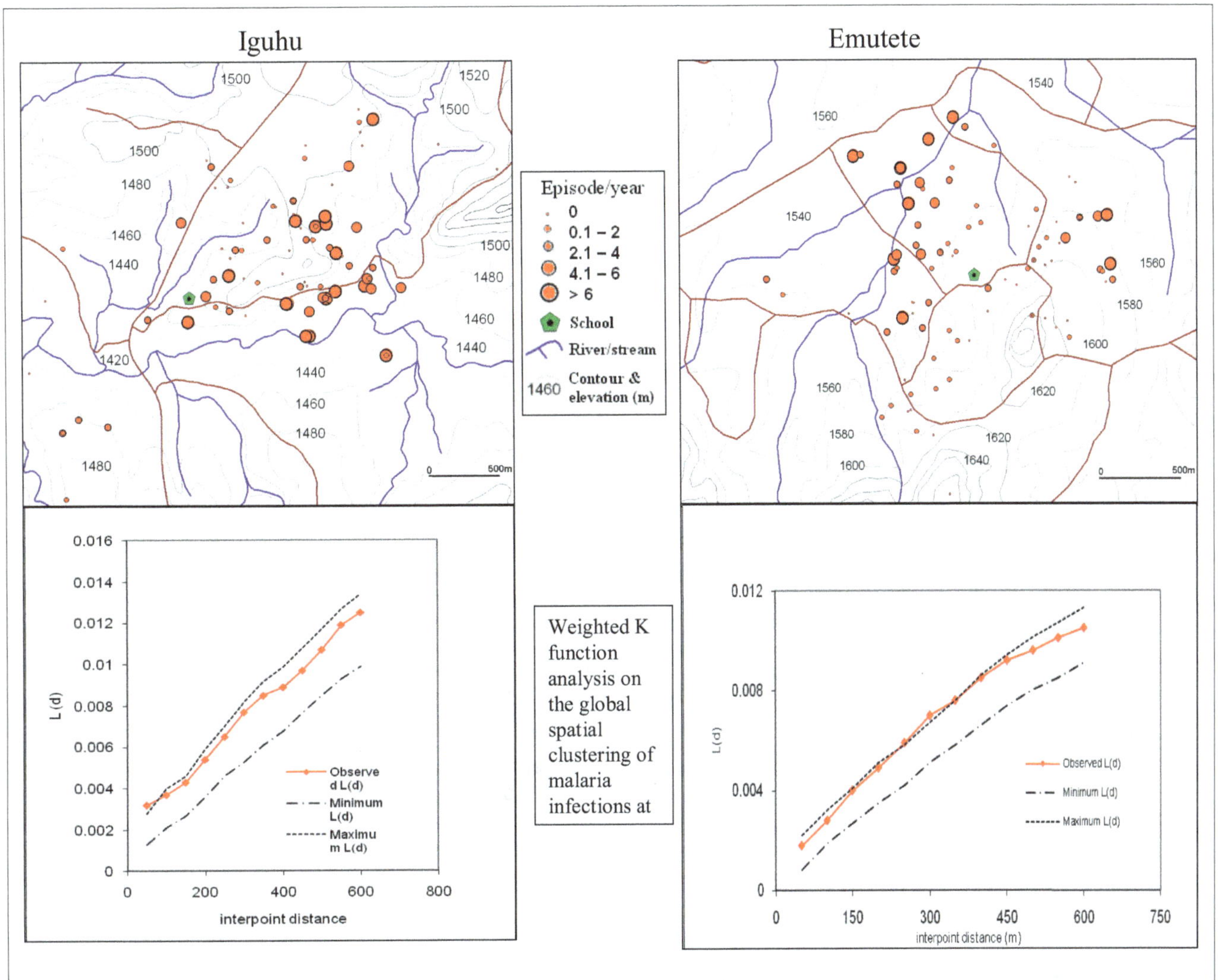

FIGURE 4 | Showing spatial distribution of malaria cases and cluster analysis in the "U" shaped valleys of Iguhu and Emutete. The infections were clustered around low altitude areas and also around swamps (Weighted *K* function shows significant clustering of malaria infections in Emutete and Iguhu).

exposure to mosquitoes and higher infection rates (9, 10, 44, 45). We also found out that there was clustering of infections at the swamps in the U-shaped valleys but the infections were randomly distributed in the V-shaped valley and the plateau. Topographic features of the highlands restrict the spatial distribution of vector breeding habitats; this, ultimately, affects malaria transmission, exposure of the human population to malaria infection, and development of immunity of human populations to malaria (9, 43, 45).

In the highlands, most severe malaria cases during an epidemic come from uphill human populations that have not been regularly exposed to malaria infection (7, 10, 44, 46–48). Studies of malaria in highland areas have generally concentrated on malaria parasites densities and vector densities in malaria stable areas within the highlands. Literature searches did not reveal studies that have assessed the immune profile of the population in the highlands and whether topography especially the shape of the valleys in the highlands and plateaus are consistently associated with malaria risk. Our study addresses this gap in knowledge and demonstrates that topography in this case the shape of the valley and plateaus affects exposure of the human population to malaria and immune response to malaria. These findings suggest that within the highlands some areas have stable malaria transmission and the human population in these areas has developed immunity to malaria; in low and unstable malaria transmission areas, the human population lack immunity to malaria and are likely to suffer severe clinical malaria and subsequently malaria epidemics.

High malaria parasites prevalence in the U-shaped valleys compared to the V-shaped valleys indicates that malaria transmission in the U-shaped valley is more stable. Our findings are similar to later studies which indicated that children in the malaria stable transmission areas have asymptomatic parasitemia and that children under this condition are able to suppress high parasitemia and presumably avoid severe disease (9, 45). The twofold higher mean antibodies prevalence than the

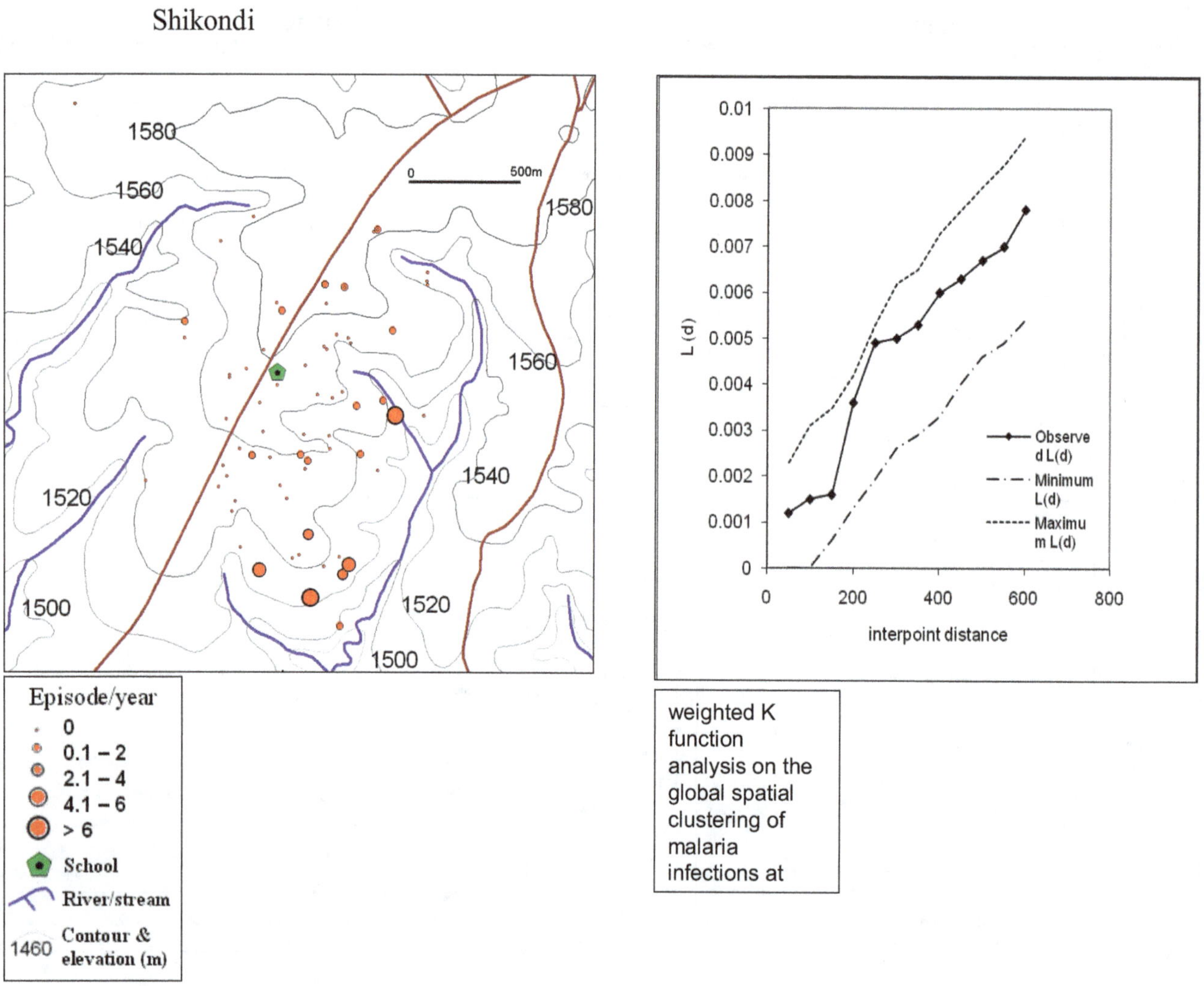

FIGURE 5 | Showing spatial distribution of malaria cases and cluster analysis from the Shikondi plateau. The infections were randomly distributed with a few clusters around the low altitude (Weighted *K* function analysis indicates that there was no significant clustering of malaria infections at the plateau).

mean parasites prevalence in the V-shaped valleys may suggest that malaria in the V-shaped valley is symptomatic, most cases are treated and more antibodies are detected since the parasites are cleared by the drugs. Other studies have shown a log-linear relationship between exposure and child prevalence predicted by mathematical models assuming exposure-dependent immunity (49). The log-linear relationship between transmission intensity and prevalence of both infections and enlarged spleens, thus, support the existence of exposure-dependent acquired immunity (50). Our results also indicate that children in the U-shaped valley were able to maintain the same level of parasite densities throughout the study, but children in the V-shaped valley took long to achieve the same levels of parasite densities as those in the U-shaped valleys, this suggests that children in stable malaria transmission areas are able to control the numbers of parasites in the blood during a period of increased exposure to infected mosquitoes in the main transmission season (10, 42, 43). Apart from *P. falciparum*, *P. malariae* was observed in the U-shaped valleys but only *P. falciparum* was observed in the V-shaped valleys and the plateau, this suggest that residents of malaria stable transmission areas often have mixed infections but only *Plasmodium* species is found in unstable malaria transmission areas (51).

There was also great variation of the parasites densities at the plateau that is indicated by the magnitude of the error bars, this can be explained by the flat topography and the more diffuse hydrology resulting from numerous streams at the plateau. Other studies have shown that malaria transmission at the plateau ranges from low on the hilltops to high to a level as high as that at the valley bottoms (10, 42, 44). According to the Ministry of Health in Burundi, malaria in the high plateau is hypo- to meso-endemic and prone to epidemics (52). Our results have shown clearly that malaria prevalence in the highland is greatly affected by the terrain characteristics of the highland, the dynamics of malaria infections were significantly different among the two valley systems and the plateau indicating that malaria transmission in the highlands is heterogeneous due to its complex topographical features. The shape of the valley affects the availability of mosquito breeding habitats, thus affecting malaria transmission. U-shaped valleys have poor drainage and this causes accumulation of water during rainy seasons creating excellent breeding habitats for malaria vectors; by contrast, there is no accumulation of water in the V-shaped valleys due to good drainage.

The high gametocytes prevalence rates in the U-shaped valleys compared to the V-shaped valleys indicate that the reservoir of malaria infections in the U-shaped valleys is higher than in the V-shaped valleys and the plateau. While the population living in the U-shaped valley maintains a large reservoir of infectious gametocytes, the people living in the V-shaped valley comprise a high proportion of susceptible individuals. Under permissive climatic conditions, the infectious vector population could increase, leading to higher rates of malaria prevalence. In our study, the mean gametocyte density varied significantly between the V-shaped and the U-shaped valleys, and between each of the two valley systems and the plateau. The low prevalence of gametocytes in the V-shaped valleys with no gametocytes observed in Kisii indicates that there is a weak transmission system in the V-shaped valley (15, 16).

High antibody prevalence in the U-shaped valley compared to the V-shaped valleys and at the plateau indicates that children in the U-shaped valley are regularly exposed to malaria parasites due to stable malaria transmission in these areas and, therefore, they have developed immunity to malaria parasites. Majority of residents in the U-shaped valleys suffer 2–6 episodes of malaria per year or are continuously infected for 6 months where as in the V-shaped valley and the plateau majority of the residents suffer 1–2 malaria episodes per year or are continuously infected for 2 months (42, 43). This shows that individual in the U-shaped valleys have developed immunity to malaria due to continuous exposure to malaria parasites. Similar studies have shown that the majority of breeding habitats in the hilly highlands are confined to the valley bottoms because the hillside gradients provide efficient drainage, this areas are, therefore, characterized by well-established transmission, with the majority of children 6–13 years old maintaining asymptomatic parasitemia (9, 10, 40). Previous studies using human sera from individuals in malaria endemic populations have found evidence of association between total IgG levels MSP2 with a reduced subsequent risk of clinical malaria (3, 19, 42–44). Other studies have shown that in regions where malaria is hyperendemic, adults develop potent but non-sterile immunity against malaria in which individuals chronically harbor low-grade parasitemia and only occasionally suffer from mild clinical malaria (53). Soe and others also showed that there is an association between antigen-specific antibody responses and protection against clinical malaria in Southeast Asia (53). Segeja and colleagues in Tanzania showed that individuals with higher levels of IgG are partially protected from malaria infections (54). The findings of our study indicate that the high prevalence of antibodies in the U-shaped valleys is responsible for asymptomatic malaria in these areas. In spite of high prevalence of malaria in the U-shaped valleys, individuals in the U-shaped valley have developed immunity to clinical malaria, individuals in the V-shaped valleys, on the other hand, have low prevalence of malaria but they also lack immunity to malaria and, therefore, they are more prone to malaria epidemics during hyper-transmission periods. Spatial analysis of the malaria antibodies and infections indicated that there was a significant positive clustering around swamps and marshes in the U-shaped valleys of western Kenya highlands.

CONCLUSION

The findings of this study indicate that the topography characteristics of the highland valleys systems affect the exposure of the human population to malaria parasites and the immune response to malaria. The residents of V-shaped valleys are at risk of having explosive malaria outbreaks during hyper-transmission periods due to low exposure to malaria parasite; hence, they have low immune response to malaria, while the U-shaped valleys have stable malaria transmission; therefore, the human population has developed immunity to malaria due to continuous exposure to malaria. The spatial distribution maps have found clustering of malaria infections around the swamps and at low altitude in the U-shaped valleys and random distribution of malaria in the V-shaped valleys, implementation of malaria control treats the highlands as a homogeneous entity and does not take into consideration the high heterogeneity of transmission and incidence. Thus, the distribution of interventions does not take in care the different transmission intensities and disease incidence, topography maps can be reliably used to identify the affected areas and the scarce resources focused to these areas to control malaria.

AUTHOR CONTRIBUTIONS

CW conceived and designed the study, did data collection, and analysis. EK drafted the manuscript. Both revised and agreed upon submission.

ACKNOWLEDGMENTS

Authors acknowledge the field Assistants who did data collection, namely, David Cheryot, Nicolas Juma, Jared Rioba, Lucy Atieli, Judith Otete, Eliud Simiyu, and Edna ototo, for their technical assistance. Most but important, acknowledging the International Development Research Centre, Canada (IDRC) and DFID (UK) for funding this project (Project ID: 104707-001) through the Climate Change Adaptation in Africa (CCAA) program. The funder had no role in data collection, data analysis, or influence on the outcome of the study. This manuscript has been published with the permission of the Director, Kenya Medical Research Institute, Kisumu.

REFERENCES

1. WHO. *Factsheet on the World Malaria Report 2015*. Geneva: World Health Organisation (2015).
2. Malakooti MA, Biomndo K, Shanks GD. Reemergence of epidemic malaria in the highlands of western Kenya. *Emerg Infect Dis* (1998) 4(4):671–6. doi:10.3201/eid0404.980422
3. Shanks GD, Biomndo K, Hay SI, Snow RW. Changing patterns of clinical malaria since 1965 among a tea estate population located in the Kenyan highlands. *Trans R Soc Trop Med Hyg* (2000) 94(3):253–5. doi:10.1016/S0035-9203(00)90310-9
4. Garnham P. The incidence of malaria at high altitudes. *J Natl Malar Soc* (1948) 7(4):275–84.
5. Roberts J. The control of epidemic malaria in the highlands of western Kenya. Part II. The campaign. *J Trop Med Hyg* (1964) 67(8):191–9.
6. Hay SI, Cox J, Rogers DJ, Randolph SE, Stern DI, Shanks GD, et al. Climate change and the resurgence of malaria in the East African highlands. *Nature* (2002) 415(6874):905–9. doi:10.1038/415905a
7. Zhou G, Minakawa N, Githeko AK, Yan G. Association between climate variability and malaria epidemics in the East African highlands. *Proc Natl Acad Sci U S A* (2004) 101(8):2375–80. doi:10.1073/pnas.0308714100
8. Githeko AK, Lindsay SW, Confalonieri UE, Patz JA. Climate change and vector-borne diseases: a regional analysis. *Bull World Health Organ* (2000) 78(9):1136–47.
9. Githeko AK, Ayisi JM, Odada PK, Atieli FK, Ndenga BA, Githure JI, et al. Topography and malaria transmission heterogeneity in western Kenya highlands: prospects for focal vector control. *Malar J* (2006) 5(1):1–9. doi:10.1186/1475-2875-5-107
10. Atieli HE, Zhou G, Lee M-C, Kweka EJ, Afrane Y, Mwanzo I, et al. Topography as a modifier of breeding habitats and concurrent vulnerability to malaria risk in the western Kenya highlands. *Parasit Vectors* (2011) 4(1):1–12. doi:10.1186/1756-3305-4-241
11. Rono J, Färnert A, Murungi L, Ojal J, Kamuyu G, Guleid F, et al. Multiple clinical episodes of *Plasmodium falciparum* malaria in a low transmission intensity setting: exposure versus immunity. *BMC Med* (2015) 13(1):1–11. doi:10.1186/s12916-015-0354-z
12. Stevenson JC, Stresman GH, Baidjoe A, Okoth A, Oriango R, Owaga C, et al. Use of different transmission metrics to describe malaria epidemiology in the highlands of western Kenya. *Malar J* (2015) 14(1):1–13. doi:10.1186/s12936-015-0944-4
13. Kangoye DT, Mensah VA, Murungi LM, Nkumama I, Nebie I, Marsh K, et al. Dynamics and role of antibodies to *Plasmodium falciparum* merozoite antigens in children living in two settings with differing malaria transmission intensity. *Vaccine* (2016) 34(1):160–6. doi:10.1016/j.vaccine.2015.10.058
14. Himeidan YE-S, Kweka E. Malaria in east African highlands during the past 30 years: impact of environmental changes. *Front Physiol* (2012) 3:315. doi:10.3389/fphys.2012.00315
15. Githeko AK, Ototo EN, Guiyun Y. Progress towards understanding the ecology and epidemiology of malaria in the western Kenya highlands: opportunities and challenges for control under climate change risk. *Acta Trop* (2012) 121(1):19–25. doi:10.1016/j.actatropica.2011.10.002
16. Wanjala CL, Waitumbi J, Zhou G, Githeko AK. Identification of malaria transmission and epidemic hotspots in the western Kenya highlands: its application to malaria epidemic prediction. *Parasit Vectors* (2011) 4(1):1–13. doi:10.1186/1756-3305-4-81
17. Mouchet J, Laventure S, Blanchy S, Fioramonti R, Rakotonjanabelo A, Rabarison P, et al. The reconquest of the Madagascar highlands by malaria. *Bulletin de la Societe de pathologie exotique (1990)* (1996) 90(3):162–8.
18. Frosch AEP, John CC. Immunomodulation in *Plasmodium falciparum* malaria: experiments in nature and their conflicting implications for potential therapeutic agents. *Expert Rev Anti Infect Ther* (2012) 10(11):1343–56. doi:10.1586/eri.12.118
19. Rolfes MA, McCarra M, Magak NG, Ernst KC, Dent AE, Lindblade KA, et al. Development of clinical immunity to malaria in highland areas of low and unstable transmission. *Am J Trop Med Hyg* (2012) 87(5):806–12. doi:10.4269/ajtmh.2012.11-0530
20. John CC, Ouma JH, Sumba PO, Hollingdale MR, Kazura JW, King CL. Lymphocyte proliferation and antibody responses to *Plasmodium falciparum* liver-stage antigen-1 in a highland area of Kenya with seasonal variation in malaria transmission. *Am J Trop Med Hyg* (2002) 66(4):372–8.
21. Smith H, Crandall I, Prudhomme J, Sherman I. Optimization and inhibition of the adherent ability of *Plasmodium falciparum*-infected erythrocytes. *Memórias do Instituto Oswaldo Cruz* (1992) 87:303–12. doi:10.1590/S0074-02761992000700052
22. Snow R, Craig M, Newton C, Steketee R. *The Public Health Burden of Plasmodium falciparum Malaria in Africa: Deriving the Numbers. The Disease Control Priorities Project (DCPP) Working Paper Number 11, 2003.* Washington, DC (2008).
23. Snow RW, Omumbo JA, Lowe B, Molyneux CS, Obiero J-O, Palmer A, et al. Relation between severe malaria morbidity in children and level of *Plasmodium falciparum* transmission in Africa. *Lancet* (1997) 349(9066):1650–4. doi:10.1016/S0140-6736(97)02038-2
24. Smith T, Charlwood JD, Kihonda J, Mwankusye S, Billingsley P, Meuwissen J, et al. Absence of seasonal variation in malaria parasitaemia in an area of intense seasonal transmission. *Acta Trop* (1993) 54(1):55–72. doi:10.1016/0001-706X(93)90068-M
25. Githeko AK, Ndegwa W. Predicting malaria epidemics in the Kenyan highlands using climate data: a tool for decision makers. *Glob Change Hum Health* (2001) 2(1):54–63. doi:10.1023/A:1011943131643
26. Omumbo JA, Lyon B, Waweru SM, Connor SJ, Thomson MC. Raised temperatures over the Kericho tea estates: revisiting the climate in the East African highlands malaria debate. *Malar J* (2011) 10(1):1–16. doi:10.1186/1475-2875-10-12
27. Alonso D, Bouma MJ, Pascual M. Epidemic malaria and warmer temperatures in recent decades in an East African highland. *Proc Biol Sci* (2011) 278(1712):1661–9. doi:10.1098/rspb.2010.2020
28. Lindblade KA, Walker ED, Onapa AW, Katungu J, Wilson ML. Land use change alters malaria transmission parameters by modifying temperature in a highland area of Uganda. *Trop Med Int Health* (2000) 5(4):263–74. doi:10.1046/j.1365-3156.2000.00551.x
29. Lindblade KA, Walker ED, Wilson ML. Early warning of malaria epidemics in African highlands using *Anopheles* (Diptera: Culicidae) indoor resting density. *J Med Entomol* (2000) 37(5):664–74. doi:10.1603/0022-2585-37.5.664
30. Lindblade KA, Walker ED, Onapa AW, Katungu J, Wilson ML. Highland malaria in Uganda: prospective analysis of an epidemic associated with El Niño. *Trans R Soc Trop Med Hyg* (1999) 93(5):480–7. doi:10.1016/S0035-9203(99)90344-9
31. Kweka EJ, Zhou G, Munga S, Lee M-C, Atieli HE, Nyindo M, et al. Anopheline larval habitats seasonality and species distribution: a prerequisite for effective targeted larval habitats control programmes. *PLoS One* (2012) 7(12):e52084. doi:10.1371/journal.pone.0052084
32. Kweka EJ, Kamau L, Munga S, Lee M-C, Githeko AK, Yan G. A first report of *Anopheles funestus* sibling species in western Kenya highlands. *Acta Trop* (2013) 128(1):158–61. doi:10.1016/j.actatropica.2013.06.006
33. Kweka EJ, Zhou G, Lee M-C, Gilbreath TM, Mosha F, Munga S, et al. Evaluation of two methods of estimating larval habitat productivity in western Kenya highlands. *Parasit Vectors* (2011) 4(1):1–9. doi:10.1186/1756-3305-4-110
34. Minakawa N, Sonye G, Mogi M, Yan G. Habitat characteristics of *Anopheles gambiae* s.s. larvae in a Kenyan highland. *Med Vet Entomol* (2004) 18(3):301–5. doi:10.1111/j.0269-283X.2004.00503.x
35. Fillinger U, Ndenga B, Githeko A, Lindsay SW. Integrated malaria vector control with microbial larvicides and insecticide-treated nets in western Kenya: a controlled trial. *Bull World Health Organ* (2009) 87:655–65. doi:10.2471/BLT.08.055632
36. Iqbal J, Hira P, Al-Ali F, Khalid N, Sher A. Modified Giemsa staining for rapid diagnosis of malaria infection. *Med Princ Pract* (2003) 12(3):156–9. doi:10.1159/000070751
37. Slutsker L, Taylor TE, Wirima JJ, Steketee RW. In-hospital morbidity and mortality due to malaria-associated severe anaemia in two areas of Malawi with different patterns of malaria infection. *Trans R Soc Trop Med Hyg* (1994) 88(5):548–51. doi:10.1016/0035-9203(94)90157-0

38. Mitchell C, Adebajo A, Hay E, Carr A. Shoulder pain: diagnosis and management in primary care. *BMJ* (2005) 331(7525):1124–8. doi:10.1136/bmj.331.7525.1124
39. Himeidan YE, Zhou G, Yakob L, Afrane Y, Munga S, Atieli H, et al. Habitat stability and occurrences of malaria vector larvae in western Kenya highlands. *Malar J* (2009) 8(1):1–6. doi:10.1186/1475-2875-8-234
40. Githeko AK, Ogallo L, Lemnge M, Okia M, Ototo EN. Development and validation of climate and ecosystem-based early malaria epidemic prediction models in East Africa. *Malar J* (2014) 13(1):1–11. doi:10.1186/1475-2875-13-329
41. Ototo EN, Githeko AK, Wanjala CL, Scott TW. Surveillance of vector populations and malaria transmission during the 2009/10 El Niño event in the western Kenya highlands: opportunities for early detection of malaria hyper-transmission. *Parasit Vectors* (2011) 4(1):1–9. doi:10.1186/1756-3305-4-144
42. Badu K, Afrane YA, Larbi J, Stewart VA, Waitumbi J, Angov E, et al. Marked variation in MSP-119 antibody responses to malaria in western Kenyan highlands. *BMC Infect Dis* (2012) 12(1):1–9. doi:10.1186/1471-2334-12-50
43. Badu K, Siangla J, Larbi J, Lawson BW, Afrane Y, Ong'echa J, et al. Variation in exposure to *Anopheles gambiae* salivary gland peptide (gSG6-P1) across different malaria transmission settings in the western Kenya highlands. *Malar J* (2012) 11(1):1–9. doi:10.1186/1475-2875-11-318
44. Afrane YA, Zhou G, Githeko AK, Yan G. Clinical malaria case definition and malaria attributable fraction in the highlands of western Kenya. *Malar J* (2014) 13(1):1–7. doi:10.1186/1475-2875-13-405
45. Zhou G, Munga S, Minakawa N, Githeko AK, Yan G. Spatial relationship between adult malaria vector abundance and environmental factors in western Kenya highlands. *Am J Trop Med Hyg* (2007) 77(1):29–35.
46. Stern DI, Gething PW, Kabaria CW, Temperley WH, Noor AM, Okiro EA, et al. Temperature and malaria trends in highland East Africa. *PLoS One* (2011) 6(9):e24524. doi:10.1371/journal.pone.0024524
47. Baum E, Badu K, Molina DM, Liang X, Felgner PL, Yan G. Protein microarray analysis of antibody responses to *Plasmodium falciparum* in Western Kenyan highland sites with differing transmission levels. *PLoS One* (2013) 8(12):e82246. doi:10.1371/journal.pone.0082246
48. Tchuinkam T, Nyih-Kong B, Fopa F, Simard F, Antonio-Nkondjio C, Awono-Ambene H-P, et al. Distribution of *Plasmodium falciparum* gametocytes and malaria-attributable fraction of fever episodes along an altitudinal transect in Western Cameroon. *Malar J* (2015) 14(1):1–15. doi:10.1186/s12936-015-0594-6
49. Gupta S, Snow RW, Donnelly CA, Marsh K, Newbold C. Immunity to non-cerebral severe malaria is acquired after one or two infections. *Nat Med* (1999) 5(3):340–3. doi:10.1038/6560
50. Bødker R, Msangeni HA, Kisinza W, Lindsay SW. Relationship between the intensity of exposure to malaria parasites and infection in the Usambara Mountains, Tanzania. *Am J Trop Med Hyg* (2006) 74(5):716–23.
51. Bousema JT, Drakeley CJ, Mens PF, Arens T, Houben R, Omar SA, et al. Increased *Plasmodium falciparum* gametocyte production in mixed infections with *P. malariae*. *Am J Trop Med Hyg* (2008) 78(3):442–8.
52. Protopopoff N, Van Bortel W, Marcotty T, Van Herp M, Maes P, Baza D, et al. Spatial targeted vector control is able to reduce malaria prevalence in the highlands of Burundi. *Am J Trop Med Hyg* (2008) 79(1):12–8.
53. Soe S, Theisen M, Roussilhon C, Aye K-S, Druilhe P. Association between protection against clinical malaria and antibodies to merozoite surface antigens in an area of hyperendemicity in Myanmar: complementarity between responses to merozoite surface protein 3 and the 220-kilodalton glutamate-rich protein. *Infect Immun* (2004) 72(1):247–52. doi:10.1128/iai.72.1.247-252.2004
54. Segeja MD, Mmbando BP, Seth MD, Lusingu JP, Lemnge MM. Acquisition of antibodies to merozoite surface protein 3 among residents of Korogwe, north eastern Tanzania. *BMC Infect Dis* (2010) 10(1):1–7. doi:10.1186/1471-2334-10-55

Permissions

All chapters in this book were first published in CTM, by InTech Open; hereby published with permission under the Creative Commons Attribution License or equivalent. Every chapter published in this book has been scrutinized by our experts. Their significance has been extensively debated. The topics covered herein carry significant findings which will fuel the growth of the discipline. They may even be implemented as practical applications or may be referred to as a beginning point for another development.

The contributors of this book come from diverse backgrounds, making this book a truly international effort. This book will bring forth new frontiers with its revolutionizing research information and detailed analysis of the nascent developments around the world.

We would like to thank all the contributing authors for lending their expertise to make the book truly unique. They have played a crucial role in the development of this book. Without their invaluable contributions this book wouldn't have been possible. They have made vital efforts to compile up to date information on the varied aspects of this subject to make this book a valuable addition to the collection of many professionals and students.

This book was conceptualized with the vision of imparting up-to-date information and advanced data in this field. To ensure the same, a matchless editorial board was set up. Every individual on the board went through rigorous rounds of assessment to prove their worth. After which they invested a large part of their time researching and compiling the most relevant data for our readers.

The editorial board has been involved in producing this book since its inception. They have spent rigorous hours researching and exploring the diverse topics which have resulted in the successful publishing of this book. They have passed on their knowledge of decades through this book. To expedite this challenging task, the publisher supported the team at every step. A small team of assistant editors was also appointed to further simplify the editing procedure and attain best results for the readers.

Apart from the editorial board, the designing team has also invested a significant amount of their time in understanding the subject and creating the most relevant covers. They scrutinized every image to scout for the most suitable representation of the subject and create an appropriate cover for the book.

The publishing team has been an ardent support to the editorial, designing and production team. Their endless efforts to recruit the best for this project, has resulted in the accomplishment of this book. They are a veteran in the field of academics and their pool of knowledge is as vast as their experience in printing. Their expertise and guidance has proved useful at every step. Their uncompromising quality standards have made this book an exceptional effort. Their encouragement from time to time has been an inspiration for everyone.

The publisher and the editorial board hope that this book will prove to be a valuable piece of knowledge for researchers, students, practitioners and scholars across the globe.

List of Contributors

Elizabeth H. Aitken, Agersew Alemu and Stephen J. Rogerson
Department of Medicine at Royal Melbourne Hospital, Peter Doherty Institute, University of Melbourne, Melbourne, VIC, Australia

Ann Ly and Diana S. Hansen
The Walter and Eliza Hall Institute of Medical Research, Parkville, VIC, Australia
Department of Medical Biology, The University of Melbourne, Parkville, VIC, Australia

Totino, Cláudio T. Daniel-Ribeiro and Maria de Fátima Ferreira-da-Cruz
Laboratory of Malaria Research, Instituto Oswaldo Cruz, Fundação Oswaldo Cruz, Rio de Janeiro, Brazil

Regina Joice Cordy
Department of Biology, Wake Forest University, Winston-Salem, NC, United States,
Department of Microbiology and Immunology, Wake Forest School of Medicine, Winston-Salem, NC, United States

Kai Matuschewski
Parasitology Unit, Max Planck Institute for Infection Biology, Berlin, Germany
Institute of Chemistry and Biochemistry, Free University, Berlin, Germany

Josefine Dunst and Faustin Kamena
Parasitology Unit, Max Planck Institute for Infection Biology, Berlin, Germany
Institute of Chemistry and Biochemistry, Free University, Berlin, Germany
Molecular Parasitology, Institute of Biology, Humboldt University, Berlin, Germany

Ib C. Bygbjerg and Karin L. Schiøler
Department of Public Health, University of Copenhagen, Copenhagen, Denmark

Lone Simonsen
Department of Science and Environment, Roskilde University, Roskilde, Denmark

Xi Zen Yap
Burnet Institute, Melbourne, VIC, Australia
Department of Medicine, Dentistry, and Health Sciences, The University of Melbourne, Parkville, VIC, Australia

Rachel J. Lundie and Meredith O'Keeffe
Burnet Institute, Melbourne, VIC, Australia

Department of Biochemistry and Molecular Biology, Biomedicine Discovery Institute, Monash University, Clayton, VIC, Australia

James G. Beeson and G. Beeson
Burnet Institute, Melbourne, VIC, Australia
Department of Medicine, Dentistry, and Health Sciences, The University of Melbourne, Parkville, VIC, Australia
Department of Microbiology and Central Clinical school, Monash University, VIC, Australia

Isabel K. Fletcher
Centre on Climate Change and Planetary Health, London School of Hygiene & Tropical Medicine, London, United Kingdom
Centre for Mathematical Modelling of Infectious Diseases, London School of Hygiene & Tropical Medicine, London, United Kingdom

Anna M. Stewart-Ibarra
Inter-American Institute for Global Change Research, Montevideo, Uruguay

Rachel Sippy
Institute for Global Health and Translational Science, SUNY Upstate Medical University, Syracuse, NY, United States

Gabriel Carrasco-Escobar
Health Innovation Laboratory, Institute of Tropical Medicine "Alexander von Humboldt", Universidad Peruana Cayetano Heredia, Lima, Peru
Division of Infectious Diseases and Global Public Health, Department of Medicine, University of California, San Diego, San Diego, CA, United States

Mercy Silva
Hospital Teofilo Davila, Ministerio de Salud Pública, Quito, Ecuador

Efrain Beltran-Ayala
Facultad de Medicina, Universidad Tecnica de Machala, Machala, Ecuador

Tania Ordoñez
Distrito de Salud 07D02 del Ministerio de Salud Pública, Quito, Ecuador

Jefferson Adrian
Departamento de Ciencias de la Computación y Electrónica, Universidad Técnica Particular de Loja, Loja, Ecuador

Fabián E. Sáenz
Centro de Investigación para la Salud en América Latina, Facultad de Ciencias Exactas y Naturales, Pontificia Universidad Católica del Ecuador, Quito, Ecuador

Chris Drakeley
Department of Infection Biology, Faculty of Infectious and Tropical Diseases, London School of Hygiene & Tropical Medicine, London, United Kingdom

Kate E. Jones
Centre for Biodiversity and Environment Research, Department of Genetics, Evolution and Environment, University College London, London, United Kingdom

Rachel Lowe
Centre on Climate Change and Planetary Health, London School of Hygiene & Tropical Medicine, London, United Kingdom
Centre for Mathematical Modelling of Infectious Diseases, London School of Hygiene & Tropical Medicine, London, United Kingdom,
Barcelona Institute for Global Health (ISGlobal), Barcelona, Spain

Giulia Siciliano and Pietro Alano
Dipartimento di Malattie Infettive, Parassitarie ed Immunomediate, Istituto Superiore di Sanità, Rome, Italy

Mingqiang Li, Fei Tuo, Ruixiang Tan, Qi Wang, Qin Xu, Jianping Song, Wenfeng Guo and Changsheng Deng
Artemisinin Research Center, Guangzhou University of Chinese Medicine, Guangzhou, China

Hongying Zhang, Shaoqin Zheng and Hong Yan
Science and Technology Park, Guangzhou University of Chinese Medicine, Guangzhou, China

Xinbing Yu and Fangli Lu
Department of Parasitology, Zhongshan School of Medicine, Sun Yat-Sen University, Guangzhou, China

Zhibing Wu
The First Affiliated Hospital of Guangzhou University of Chinese Medicine, Guangzhou, China

Jun Huang
Sino-French Hoffmann Institute, Guangzhou Medical University, Guangzhou, China

Herodes Sacramento Rampao and Carlos Alberto Bandeira D'almeida
Centro Nacional de Endemias, Ministry of Health, São Tomé, São Tomé and Príncipe

Danilo Buonsenso
Department of Woman and Child Health and Public Health, Fondazione Policlinico Universitario A. Gemelli IRCCS, Rome, Italy
Dipartimento di Scienze Biotecnologiche di Base, Cliniche Intensivologiche e Perioperatorie, Università Cattolica del Sacro Cuore, Rome, Italy
Center for Global Health Research and Studies, Università Cattolica del Sacro Cuore, Rome, Italy

Francesco Iodice
Institute of Neurology, Fondazione Policlinico Universitario A. Gemelli IRCCS, Rome, Italy

Bianca Cinicola
Department of Pediatrics, Sapienza University of Rome, Policliclinico Umberto I, Rome, Italy

Francesca Raffaelli
Dipartimento Scienze di Laboratorio e Infettivologiche, Fondazione Policlinico Universitario Agostino Gemelli IRCCS, Rome, Italy

Solia Sowa
Konta Wallah Community Health Center, Port Loko, Sierra Leone

Walter Ricciardi
Department of Woman and Child Health and Public Health, Fondazione Policlinico Universitario A. Gemelli IRCCS, Rome, Italy
Sezione di Igiene, Istituto di Sanità Pubblica, Università Cattolica del Sacro Cuore, Rome, Italy

Lea-Christina Kaminski, Mathias Riehn, Annemieke Abel, Christiane Steeg and Thomas Jacobs
Protozoa Immunology, Bernhard Nocht Institute for Tropical Medicine, Hamburg, Germany

Denis Dekugmen Yar, Francis Aminkiah and Ellis Owusu Dabo
Kumasi Centre for Collaborative Research in Tropical Medicine, Kumasi, Ghana

Maria Sophia Mackroth
Protozoa Immunology, Bernhard Nocht Institute for Tropical Medicine, Hamburg, Germany
Divisions of Tropical Medicine and Infectious Diseases, I. Medical Department, University Medical Centre Hamburg, Germany

Otchere Addai-Mensah
Department of Medical Laboratory Technology, Faculty of Allied Health Sciences, Kwame Nkrumah University of Science and Technology, Kumasi, Ghana

Kevin Wamae
KEMRI-Wellcome Trust Research Programme, CGMRC, Kilifi, Kenya

Kelvin M. Kimenyi
KEMRI-Wellcome Trust Research Programme, CGMRC, Kilifi, Kenya
Centre for Biotechnology and Bioinformatics, University of Nairobi, Nairobi, Kenya

Lynette Isabella Ochola-Oyier
KEMRI-Wellcome Trust Research Programme, CGMRC, Kilifi, Kenya
Pwani University Bioscience Research Centre, Pwani University, Kilifi, Kenya

Rhea J. Longley, Adrian V. S. Hill and Alexandra J. Spencer
The Jenner Institute, Nuffield Department of Medicine, University of Oxford, Oxford, UK

Tatiana Almeida Pádua and Mariana Conceição Souza
Laboratory of Applied Pharmacology, Institute of Drug Technology (Farmanguinhos), Oswaldo Cruz Foundation, Rio de Janeiro, Brazil

Suzana Zakovic and Elena A. Levashina
Vector Biology, Max-Planck Institute for Infection Biology, Berlin, Germany

Sarat Kumar Dalai, Naveen Yadav, Manoj Patidar and Hardik Patel
Institute of Science, Nirma University, Ahmedabad, India

Agam Prasad Singh
Infectious Diseases Laboratory, National Institute of Immunology, New Delhi, India

Tejram Sahu, Lynn Lambert, Jessica Herrod, Solomon Conteh, Sachy Orr-Gonzalez, Dariyen Carter and Patrick E. Duffy
Laboratory of Malaria Immunology and Vaccinology, National Institute of Allergy and Infectious Diseases, National Institutes of Health, Rockville, MD, USA

Ute Frevert
Division of Medical Parasitology, Department of Microbiology, New York University School of Medicine, New York, NY, USA

Urszula Krzych
Division of Malaria Vaccine Development, Department of Cellular Immunology, Walter Reed Army Institute of Research, Silver Spring, MD, USA

Luiza Carvalho Mourão, Gustavo Pereira Cardoso-Oliveira and Érika Martins Braga
Departamento de Parasitologia, Instituto de Ciências Biológicas, Universidade Federal de Minas Gerais, Belo Horizonte, Brazil

Alexandra T. Roux, Leah Maharaj, Olukunle Oyegoke, Oluwasegun P. Akoniyon, Matthew Adekunle Adeleke and Moses Okpeku
Discipline of Genetics, School of Life Sciences, University of KwaZulu-Natal, Westville, South Africa

Rajendra Maharaj
Office of Malaria Research, South African Medical Research Council, Cape Town, South Africa

Christine Ludwin Wanjala
Centre for Global Health Research, Kenya Medical Research Institute, Kisumu, Kenya
Department of Medical Laboratory Sciences, Masinde Muliro University of Science and Technology, Kakamega, Kenya

Eliningaya J. Kweka
Mosquito Section, Division of Livestock and Human Diseases Vector Control, Tropical Pesticides Research Institute, Arusha, Tanzania
Department of Medical Parasitology and Entomology, Catholic University of Health and Allied Sciences, Mwanza, Tanzania

Index

www.ingramcontent.com/pod-product-compliance
Lightning Source LLC
LaVergne TN
LVHW060533210926
848485LV00005B/1188
* 9 7 8 1 6 3 9 8 7 3 4 8 7 *